PLASTIC SURGERY

Indications, Operations, and Outcomes

Bruce M. Achauer, MD, FACS
Professor of Surgery,
Division of Plastic Surgery,
University of California Irvine,
California College of Medicine,
Orange, California

Elof Eriksson, MD, PhD, FACS
Joseph E. Murray Professor of Plastic and Reconstructive Surgery,
Harvard Medical School;
Chief, Division of Plastic Surgery,
Brigham and Women's Hospital,
Chief, Division of Plastic Surgery,
Children's Hospital,
Boston, Massachusetts

Bahman Guyuron, MD, FACS
Clinical Professor of Plastic Surgery,
Case Western Reserve University,
Cleveland, Ohio;
Medical Director,
Zeeba Medical Campus,
Lyndhurst, Ohio

John J. Coleman III, MD, FACS
Professor of Surgery;
Chief of Plastic Surgery;
Staff Physician,
Indiana University Medical Center;
Director, Pediatric Burn Unit;
Staff Physician,
Riley Children's Hospital;
Staff Physician,
Wishard Memorial Hospital,
Indianapolis, Indiana

Robert C. Russell, MD, FRACS, FACS
Clinical Professor of Surgery,
Division of Plastic Surgery,
Southern Illinois University School of Medicine;
Springfield, Illinois

Craig A. Vander Kolk, MD, FACS
Associate Professor of Plastic Surgery;
Director, Cleft and Craniofacial Center,
Johns Hopkins University School of Medicine,
Baltimore, Maryland

PLASTIC SURGERY

Indications, Operations, and Outcomes

Volume Three

Head and Neck Surgery

· EDITOR
John J. Coleman III, MD, FACS
Professor of Surgery;
Chief of Plastic Surgery;
Staff Physician,
Indiana University Medical Center;
Director, Pediatric Burn Unit;
Staff Physician,
Riley Children's Hospital;
Staff Physician,
Wishard Memorial Hospital,
Indianapolis, Indiana

OUTCOMES EDITOR
Edwin G. Wilkins, MD, MS
Associate Professor of Plastic Surgery,
University of Michigan Health Systems,
Ann Arbor, Michigan

MANAGING EDITOR
Victoria M. VanderKam, RN, BS, CPSN
Clinical Nurse, Division of Plastic Surgery,
University of California Irvine Medical Center,
Orange, California

ILLUSTRATIONS BY
Min Li, MD
Indiana University School of Medicine,
Department of Surgery, Section of Plastic Surgery,
Indianapolis, Indiana

with 6279 illustrations, including 963 in color, and 18 color plates

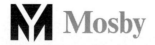

A Harcourt Health Sciences Company

St. Louis   London   Philadelphia   Sydney   Toronto

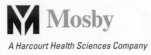

A Harcourt Health Sciences Company

Acquisitions Editor: Richard Zorab
Developmental Editor: Dolores Meloni
Project Manager: Carol Sullivan Weis
Senior Production Editor: David Stein
Designers: Dave Zielinski/Mark Oberkrom

Mosby, Inc.
A Harcourt Health Sciences Company
11830 Westline Industrial Drive
St. Louis, Missouri 63146

Printed in the United States of America

Volume 3 ISBN 0-8151-1023-5
Set ISBN 0-8151-0984-9

00 01 02 03 04 GW/MVY 9 8 7 6 5 4 3 2 1

Contributors

BRUCE M. ACHAUER, MD, FACS
Professor of Surgery,
Division of Plastic Surgery,
University of California Irvine,
California College of Medicine,
Orange, California

GREGORY J. ADAMSON, MD
Clinical Instructor of Orthopedics,
University of Illinois College of Medicine at Peoria;
Staff, St. Francis Medical Center,
Peoria, Illinois

GHADA Y. AFIFI, MD
Clinical Assistant Professor,
Division of Plastic Surgery,
Department of Surgery,
Loma Linda University Medical Center and Children's
Hospital;
Attending Surgeon, Plastic Surgery,
Jerry L. Pettis Memorial Veterans Affairs Medical Center,
Loma Linda, California;
Private Practice,
Newport Beach, California

RICHARD D. ANDERSON, MD
Plastic Surgery Staff,
Scottsdale Healthcare Hospitals;
Private Practice,
Scottsdale, Arizona

JAMES P. ANTHONY, MD
Associate Professor of Surgery,
Division of Plastic Surgery,
University of California–San Francisco,
San Francisco, California

HÉCTOR ARÁMBULA, MD
Professor of Plastic Surgery,
Postgraduate Division of Medicine,
Universidad Nacional Autonoma de Mexico;
Chairman, Plastic Surgery Service,
Hospital de Traumatologia Magdalena de las Salinas,
Instituto Mexicano del Seguro Social, IMSS,
Mexico City, Mexico

LOUIS C. ARGENTA, MD
Julius A. Howell Professor and Chairman,
Department of Plastic Surgery,
Wake Forest University School of Medicine;
Professor and Chairman,
Department of Plastic and Reconstructive Surgery,
North Carolina Baptist Hospital,
Winston-Salem, North Carolina

DUFFIELD ASHMEAD IV, MD
Assistant Clinical Professor of Plastic Surgery and
Orthopedics,
University of Connecticut School of Medicine,
Farmington, Connecticut;
Director, Division of Hand Surgery,
Connecticut Children's Medical Center,
Hartford, Connecticut

CHRISTOPHER J. ASSAD, BS, MD, FRCSC
Plastic and Reconstructive Surgeon;
Associate Staff,
Halton Health Care Services Corporation,
Milton District Hospital,
Milton, Ontario, Canada

THOMAS J. BAKER, MD
Professor of Plastic Surgery–Voluntary,
University of Miami School of Medicine;
Senior Attending Physician,
Mercy Hospital,
Miami, Florida

TRACY M. BAKER, MD
Instructor in Plastic Surgery,
University of Miami School of Medicine,
Miami, Florida

JUAN P. BARRET, MD
Professor, Rijksuniversiteit Groningen;
Plastic and Reconstructive Surgeon,
University Hospital Groningen,
Groningen, The Netherlands

MUNISH K. BATRA, MD
Assistant Clinical Instructor–Voluntary,
Division of Plastic Surgery,
University of California–San Diego Medical Center,
San Diego, California;
Private Practice,
Del Mar, California

BRUCE S. BAUER, MD, FACS
Associate Professor of Surgery,
Northwestern University Medical School;
Head, Division of Plastic Surgery,
The Children's Memorial Hospital,
Chicago, Illinois

STEPHEN P. BEALS, MD, FACS, FAAP,
Assistant Professor of Plastic Surgery,
Mayo Medical School;
Adjunct Professor,
Department of Speech and Hearing Science,
Arizona State University;
Craniofacial Consultant,
Barrow Neurological Institute
Phoenix, Arizona

MICHAEL S. BEDNAR, MD
Associate Professor,
Department of Orthopedic Surgery and Rehabilitation,
Stritch School of Medicine,
Loyola University–Chicago,
Maywood, Illinois

RAMIN A. BEHMAND, MD
Chief Resident,
Division of Plastic and Reconstructive Surgery,
University of Michigan Hospitals,
Ann Arbor, Michigan

RUSSELL W. BESSETTE, DDS, MD
Clinical Professor of Plastic Surgery,
State University of New York–Buffalo,
School of Medicine;
Executive Director of Research,
Sisters Hospital,
Buffalo, New York

MARINA D. BIZZARRI-SCHMID, MD
Instructor in Anesthesia,
Harvard Medical School;
Anesthesiologist,
Brigham and Women's Hospital,
Boston, Massachusetts

GREG BORSCHEL, MD
Plastic Surgery Resident,
University of Michigan Hospitals,
Ann Arbor, Michigan

MARK T. BOSCHERT, MS, MD
Attending Physician,
St. Joseph Health Center;
Private Practice,
St. Charles, Missouri,
Attending Physician,
Barnes-St. Peters Hospital,
St. Peters, Missouri

JOHN BOSTWICK, MD, FACS
Professor and Chairman of Plastic Surgery,
Emory University School of Medicine;
Chief of Plastic Surgery,
Emory University Hospital,
Atlanta, Georgia

J. BRIAN BOYD, MB, ChB, MD, FRCSC, FACS
Professor of Surgery,
The Ohio State University College of Medicine,
Columbus, Ohio;
Chairman of Plastic Surgery,
Cleveland Clinic–Florida,
Fort Lauderdale, Florida

WILLIAM R. BOYDSTON, MD, PhD
Pediatric Neurosurgeon,
Children's Healthcare of Atlanta,
Scottish Rite Children's Hospital,
Atlanta, Georgia

KARL H. BREUING, MD
Instructor in Surgery,
Harvard Medical School;
Attending Physician, Plastic Surgery,
Brigham and Women's Hospital;
Attending Physician, Plastic Surgery,
Children's Hospital;
Attending Physician, Plastic Surgery,
Faulkner Hospital;
Attending Physician, Plastic Surgery,
Dana Farber Cancer Institute,
Boston, Massachusetts

FORST E. BROWN, MD
Emeritus Professor of Plastic Surgery,
Dartmouth Medical School,
Hanover, New Hampshire;
Consultant,
Veterans Administration Hospital,
White River Junction, Vermont

RICHARD E. BROWN, MD, FACS
Clinical Associate Professor;
Hand Fellowship Director,
Division of Plastic Surgery,
Southern Illinois University School of Medicine,
Springfield, Illinois

MARIE-CLAIRE BUCKLEY, MD
Plastic Surgery Fellow,
University of Minnesota Medical School,
Division of Plastic and Reconstructive Surgery,
Minneapolis, Minnesota

GREGORY M. BUNCKE, MD, FACS
Clinical Assistant Professor of Surgery,
University of California–San Francisco,
San Francisco, California;
Clinical Assistant Professor of Surgery,
Stanford University,
Stanford, California;
Co-Director, Division of Microsurgery,
California Pacific Medical Center,
San Francisco, California

HARRY J. BUNCKE, MD
Clinical Professor of Surgery,
University of California–San Francisco,
San Francisco, California;
Associate Clinical Professor of Surgery,
Stanford Medical School,
Stanford, California;
Director, Microsurgical Transplantation–Replantation
    Service,
California Pacific Medical Center–Davies,
San Francisco, California

RUDOLF BUNTIC, MD
Clinical Instructor,
Division of Plastic Surgery,
Stanford University,
Stanford, California;
Attending Microsurgeon,
California Pacific Medical Center,
San Francisco, California

ELISA A. BURGESS, MD
Resident in Plastic Surgery,
Oregon Health Sciences University,
Portland, Oregon

FERNANDO D. BURSTEIN, MD
Clinical Associate Professor,
Plastic and Reconstructive Surgery,
Emory University School of Medicine;
Chief, Plastic and Reconstructive Surgery;
Co-Director, Center for Craniofacial Disorders,
Scottish Rite Children's Medical Center,
Atlanta, Georgia

GRANT W. CARLSON, MD
Professor of Surgery,
Emory University School of Medicine;
Chief of Surgical Services,
Crawford Long Hospital;
Chief of Surgical Oncology,
Emory Clinic,
Atlanta, Georgia

JAMES CARRAWAY, MD, AB
Professor of Plastic Surgery;
Chairman, Division of Plastic Surgery,
Eastern Virginia Medical School,
Norfolk, Virginia

STANLEY A. CASTOR, MD
Plastic Surgery Staff Physician,
The Watson Clinic,
Lakeland, Florida

BERNARD CHANG, MD
Director, Plastic and Reconstructive Surgery,
Mercy Medical Center,
Baltimore, Maryland

YU-RAY CHEN, MD
Professor, Department of Plastic Surgery,
Chang Gung University Medical School
Tao-Yuan, Taiwan;
Superintendent and Attending Surgeon,
Department of Plastic Surgery,
Chang Gung Memorial Hospital,
Taipei, Taiwan

ANDREAS CHIMONIDES, BS, MD
Staff Physician,
Butler Memorial Hospital,
Butler, Pennsylvania;
Staff Physician,
St. Francis Medical Center;
Staff Physician,
University of Pennsylvania Medical Center–St. Margaret's
  Hospital,
Pittsburgh, Pennsylvania

MARK A. CODNER, MD
Clinical Assistant Professor,
Emory University School of Medicine;
Private Practice,
Atlanta, Georgia

I. KELMAN COHEN, MD
Professor of Surgery;
Director, Wound Healing Center,
Medical College of Virginia,
Virginia Commonwealth University,
Richmond, Virginia

MYLES J. COHEN, MD
Clinical Assistant Professor of Surgery,
University of Southern California School of Medicine;
Attending Physician,
Cedars Sinai Medical Center,
Los Angeles, California

STEVEN R. COHEN, MD
Associate Clinical Professor,
Division of Plastic and Reconstructive Surgery,
University of California Medical Center–San Diego;
Chief, Craniofacial Surgery,
Children's Hospital of San Diego,
San Diego, California

VICTOR COHEN, MD
Resident Physician,
McGill University Health Center,
McGill University School of Medicine,
Montreal, Quebec, Canada

JOHN J. COLEMAN III, MD, FACS
Professor of Surgery;
Chief of Plastic Surgery;
Staff Physician,
Indiana University Medical Center;
Director, Pediatric Burn Unit;
Staff Physician,
Riley Children's Hospital;
Staff Physician,
Wishard Memorial Hospital,
Indianapolis, Indiana

LAWRENCE B. COLEN, MD
Associate Professor of Plastic and Reconstructive Surgery,
Eastern Virginia Medical School,
Norfolk, Virginia

E. DALE COLLINS, MD, MS
Assistant Professor of Surgery,
Dartmouth Medical School,
Hanover, New Hampshire;
Medical Director, Comprehensive Breast Program,
Dartmouth-Hitchcock Medical Center,
Lebanon, New Hampshire

MATTHEW J. CONCANNON, MD, FACS
Assistant Professor;
Director of Hand and Microsurgery,
University of Missouri,
Columbia, Missouri

BRUCE F. CONNELL, MD
Clinical Professor of Surgery,
University of California Irvine,
California College of Medicine,
Orange, California

AISLING CONRAN, MD
Assistant Professor, Clinical Anesthesia,
University of Chicago,
Chicago, Illinois

PAUL C. COTTERILL, BS, MD, ABHRS,
Honorary Lecturer,
Sunnybrook Hospital,
Department of Dermatology,
University of Toronto,
Toronto, Ontario, Canada

KIMBALL MAURICE CROFTS, MD
Staff Physician,
Utah Valley Regional Medical Center,
Provo, Utah;
Staff Physician,
Timpanogos Regional Hospital,
Orem, Utah;
Staff Physician,
Mt. View Hospital,
Payson, Utah;
Staff Physician,
Sevier Valley Hospital,
Richfield, Utah

LISA R. DAVID, MD
Assistant Professor,
Department of Plastic and Reconstructive Surgery,
Wake Forest University School of Medicine;
Attending Physician,
North Carolina Baptist Hospital,
Winston-Salem, North Carolina

WILLIAM M. DAVIDSON, AB, DMD, PhD
Professor and Chairman,
Department of Orthodontics,
University of Maryland Dental School;
Associate Staff, Dentistry,
Johns Hopkins Hospital,
Baltimore, Maryland

MARK A. DEITCH, MD
Assistant Professor of Surgery,
Division of Orthopedic Surgery,
University of Maryland School of Medicine,
Baltimore, Maryland

MARK D. DeLACURE, MD, FACS
Chief, Division of Head and Neck Surgery and Oncology;
Associate Professor of Otolaryngology–Head and Neck
    Surgery,
Department of Otolaryngology;
Associate Professor of Reconstructive Plastic Surgery,
Institute of Reconstructive Plastic Surgery,
Department of Surgery,
New York University School of Medicine,
New York, New York

VALERIE BURKE DeLEON, MA,
Department of Cell Biology and Anatomy,
Johns Hopkins University School of Medicine,
Baltimore, Maryland

JOHN Di SAIA, MD
Assistant Clinical Professor,
Division of Plastic Surgery,
University of California Irvine,
California College of Medicine,
Orange, California

RICHARD V. DOWDEN, MD
Clinical Assistant Professor,
Case Western Reserve University,
Cleveland, Ohio

CRAIG R. DUFRESNE, MD, FACS
Clinical Professor of Plastic Surgery,
Georgetown University,
Washington, DC;
Plastic Surgery Section Chief;
Co-Director, Center for Facial Rehabilitation,
Fairfax Hospital,
Inova Hospital System,
Fairfax, Virginia

FELMONT F. EAVES III, MD, FACS
Assistant Clinical Professor,
University of North Carolina,
Chapel Hill, North Carolina;
Attending Physician,
Charlotte Plastic Surgery Center;
Attending Physician,
Carolinas Medical Center;
Attending Physician,
Presbyterian Hospital;
Attending Physician,
Mercy Hospital,
Charlotte, North Carolina

PHILIP EDELMAN, MD
Associate Professor of Medicine;
Director, Toxicology and Clinical Services,
Division of Occupational and Environmental Medicine,
George Washington University School of Medicine,
Washington, DC

ERIC T. EMERSON, MD
Private Practice,
Gastonia, North Carolina

TODD B. ENGEN, MD
Clinical Faculty,
University of Utah School of Medicine,
Salt Lake City, Utah;
Clinical Director,
Excel Cosmetic Surgery Center,
Orem, Utah

BARRY L. EPPLEY, MD, DMD
Assistant Professor of Plastic Surgery,
Indiana University School of Medicine,
Indianapolis, Indiana

ELOF ERIKSSON, MD, PhD, FACS
Joseph E. Murray Professor of Plastic and Reconstructive
    Surgery,
Harvard Medical School;
Chief, Division of Plastic Surgery,
Brigham and Women's Hospital;
Chief, Division of Plastic Surgery,
Children's Hospital,
Boston, Massachusetts

GREGORY R.D. EVANS, MD, FACS
Professor of Surgery;
Chair, Division of Plastic Surgery,
University of California Irvine,
California College of Medicine
Orange, California

JEFFREY A. FEARON, MD, FACS, FAAP
Director, The Craniofacial Center,
North Texas Hospital for Children at Medical City Dallas,
Dallas, Texas

LYNNE M. FEEHAN, MS, PT
Senior Hand Therapist,
Hand Program,
Workers' Compensation Board of British Columbia,
Richmond, British Columbia, Canada

RANDALL S. FEINGOLD, MD, FACS
Assistant Clinical Professor, Plastic and Reconstructive
    Surgery,
Albert Einstein College of Medicine,
Bronx, New York;
Attending Surgeon,
Long Island Jewish Medical Center,
New Hyde Park, New York;
Chief, Division of Plastic Surgery,
North Shore University Hospital at Forest Hills,
Forest Hills, New York

ROBERT D. FOSTER, MD
Assistant Professor in Residence,
Division of Plastic and Reconstructive Surgery,
University of California–San Francisco,
San Francisco, California

FRANK J. FRASSICA, MD
Professor of Orthopedic Surgery and Oncology,
Johns Hopkins University School of Medicine,
Baltimore, Maryland

ALAN E. FREELAND, MD
Professor, Department of Orthopedic Surgery;
Director, Hand Surgery Service,
The University of Mississippi Medical Center,
Jackson, Mississippi

MENNEN T. GALLAS, MD
Junior Faculty Associate,
University of Texas M.D. Anderson Cancer Center,
Houston, Texas

BING SIANG GAN, MD, PhD, FRCSC
Assistant Professor,
Departments of Surgery and Pharmacology-Toxicology,
University of Western Ontario;
Staff Surgeon,
Hand and Upper Limb Centre;
Staff Surgeon,
St. Joseph's Health Centre,
London, Ontario, Canada

WARREN L. GARNER, MD
Associate Professor of Surgery,
University of Southern California;
Associate Professor of Plastic Surgery;
Director, LAC & USC Burn Center,
Los Angeles, California

DAVID G. GENECOV, MD
Attending Surgeon,
International Craniofacial Institute,
Dallas, Texas

GEORGE K. GITTES, MD
Associate Professor,
Department of Surgery,
University of Missouri–Kansas City;
Holder and Ashcraft Chair of Pediatric Surgical Research,
Children's Mercy Hospital,
Kansas City, Missouri

JEFFREY A. GOLDSTEIN, MD
Associate Professor of Surgery,
Case Western Reserve University;
Medical Director, Craniofacial Center;
Chief of Plastic and Reconstructive Surgery,
Rainbow Babies and Children's Hospital,
Cleveland, Ohio

HECTOR GONZALEZ-MIRAMONTES, MD
Private Practice,
Guadalajara, Mexico

LAWRENCE J. GOTTLIEB, MD
Professor of Clinical Surgery,
University of Chicago,
Pritzker School of Medicine,
Chicago, Illinois

MARK S. GRANICK, MD
Professor of Surgery;
Chief of Plastic Surgery,
MCP-Hahnemann University,
Philadelphia, Pennsylvania

FREDERICK M. GRAZER, MD, FACS
Associate Clinical Professor,
Division of Plastic Surgery,
University of California Irvine,
California College of Medicine;
Staff Physician,
University of California Irvine Medical Center,
Orange, California;
Clinical Professor of Surgery,
The Pennsylvania State University Milton S. Hershey
    Medical Center College of Medicine,
Hershey, Pennsylvania;
Staff Physician,
Hoag Memorial Hospital Presbyterian,
Newport Beach, California

JON M. GRAZER, MD, MPH
Staff Physician,
Hoag Memorial Hospital Presbyterian,
Newport Beach, California;
Staff Physician,
Western Medical Center,
Santa Ana, California

JUDITH M. GURLEY, MD
Assistant Professor of Surgery,
Division of Plastic and Reconstructive Surgery,
Washington University School of Medicine;
Attending Physician,
St. Louis Children's Hospital;
Attending Physician,
Shriner's Hospital for Children,
St. Louis, Missouri

BAHMAN GUYURON, MD, FACS
Clinical Professor of Plastic Surgery,
Case Western Reserve University,
Cleveland, Ohio;
Medical Director,
Zeeba Medical Campus,
Lyndhurst, Ohio

HONGSHIK HAN, MD
Plastic Surgery Resident,
Division of Plastic Surgery,
Northwestern University Medical School,
Chicago, Illinois

ROBERT A. HARDESTY, MD
Professor,
Loma Linda University School of Medicine;
Medical Staff President;
Chief of Plastic Surgery,
Loma Linda University Medical Center,
Loma Linda, California

MAUREEN HARDY, PT, MS, CHT
Clinical Assistant Professor,
University of Mississippi Medical Center;
Director, Hand Management Center,
St. Dominic Hospital,
Jackson, Mississippi

ALAN SCOTT HARMATZ, BS, MD
Assistant Professor of Surgery,
University of Vermont College of Medicine,
Burlington, Vermont;
Attending Physician,
Maine Medical Center,
Portland, Maine

STEPHEN U. HARRIS, MD
Staff Physician,
Nassau County Medical Center,
East Meadow, New York;
Staff Physician,
North Shore Hospital,
Manhasset, New York;
Staff Physician,
Winthrop University Hospital,
Mineola, New York;
Plastic Surgeon,
Long Island Plastic Surgical Group,
Garden City, New York

ROBERT J. HAVLIK, MD
Associate Professor of Surgery,
Indiana University School of Medicine,
Indianapolis, Indiana

DETLEV HEBEBRAND, MD, PhD
Attending Physician,
Hand and Burn Center,
Bergmannsheil Clinic,
Ruhr University,
Bochum, Germany

MARC H. HEDRICK, MD
Assistant Professor of Surgery and Pediatrics,
Division of Plastic and Reconstructive Surgery,
University of California–Los Angeles School of Medicine,
Los Angeles, California

DOMINIC F. HEFFEL, MD
Resident, General Surgery,
University of California–Los Angeles Center for Health
    Sciences,
Los Angeles, California

CHRIS S. HELMSTEDTER, MD
Director of Orthopedic Oncology–Southern California,
Kaiser Permanente,
Baldwin Park, California;
Assistant Clinical Professor, Orthopedics and Surgery,
University of Southern California School of Medicine,
Los Angeles, California

VINCENT R. HENTZ, MD
Professor of Functional Restoration (Hand Surgery),
Stanford University School of Medicine,
Stanford, California

JEFFREY HOLLINGER, DDS, PhD
Professor, Biology and Biomedical Health Engineering;
Director, Center for Bone Tissue Engineering,
Carnegie Mellon University,
Pittsburgh, Pennsylvania

HEINZ-HERBERT HOMANN, MD
Attending Physician,
Hand and Burn Center,
Bergmannsheil Clinic,
Ruhr University,
Bochum, Germany

CHARLES E. HORTON, MD, FACS, FRCSC
Professor of Plastic Surgery,
Eastern Virginia Medical School,
Norfolk, Virginia;
Clinical Professor of Surgery,
Medical College of Virginia,
Richmond, Virginia

CHARLES E. HORTON, Jr., MD
Assistant Professor of Urology,
Eastern Virginia Medical School;
Chief, Department of Urology,
Children's Hospital of the King's Daughters,
Norfolk, Virginia

ERIC H. HUBLI, MD, FACS, FAAP
Craniomaxillofacial Surgeon,
International Craniofacial Institute,
Dallas, Texas

ROGER J. HUDGINS, MD
Assistant Professor,
Morehouse University School of Medicine;
Chief of Pediatric Neurosurgery,
Children's Healthcare of Atlanta,
Scottish Rite Children's Hospital,
Atlanta, Georgia

LAWRENCE N. HURST, MD, FRCSC
Professor and Chairman,
Division of Plastic Surgery,
The University of Western Ontario;
Chief, Division of Plastic Surgery
London Health Sciences Centre, University Campus,
London, Ontario, Canada

ETHYLIN WANG JABS, MD
Dr. Frank V. Sutland Professor of Pediatric Genetics;
Professor of Pediatrics, Medicine, and Plastic Surgery,
John Hopkins University School of Medicine,
Baltimore, Maryland

MOULTON K. JOHNSON, MD
Associate Professor of Orthopedic Surgery,
University of California–Los Angeles,
Los Angeles, California

GLYN JONES, MD, FRCS, FCS
Associate Professor of Plastic Surgery;
Chief of Plastic Surgery,
Crawford Long Hospital,
Emory Clinic,
Atlanta, Georgia

NEIL F. JONES, MD
Professor, Division of Plastic and Reconstructive Surgery,
Department of Orthopedic Surgery,
University of California–Los Angeles;
Chief of Hand Surgery,
University of California–Los Angeles Medical Center,
Los Angeles, California

JESSE B. JUPITER, MD
Professor of Orthopedic Surgery,
Harvard Medical School;
Head, Orthopedic Hand Service,
Massachusetts General Hospital,
Boston, Massachusetts

M.J. JURKIEWICZ, MD, DDS
Professor of Surgery, Emeritus,
Emory University School of Medicine,
Atlanta, Georgia

MADELYN D. KAHANA, MD
Associate Professor of Anesthesiology and Pediatrics,
The University of Chicago Hospital,
Chicago, Illinois

CHIA CHI KAO, MD
Fellow, Department of Reconstructive and Plastic Surgery,
University of Southern California,
Los Angeles, California

AJAYA KASHYAP, MD
Assistant Professor,
University of Massachusetts Medical Center,
Worcester, Massachusetts;
Attending Plastic Surgeon,
Metrowest Medical Center,
Framingham, Massachusetts

JULIA A. KATARINCIC, MD
Consultant, Department of Orthopedic Surgery,
Mayo Clinic,
Rochester, Minnesota

DANIEL J. KELLEY, MD
Assistant Professor;
Director, Head and Neck Oncology/Skull Base Surgery,
Department of Otolaryngology and Bronchoesophagology,
Temple University School of Medicine,
Philadelphia, Pennsylvania

KEVIN J. KELLY, DDS, MD
Associate Professor,
Department of Plastic Surgery,
Vanderbilt University School of Medicine;
Director, Craniofacial Surgery,
Department of Plastic Surgery,
Vanderbilt Medical Center,
Nashville, Tennessee

PRASAD G. KILARU, MD
Clinical Assistant Professor of Surgery,
University of Southern California–Los Angeles,
Los Angeles, California;
Staff Physician,
City of Hope National Medical Center,
Duarte, California

GABRIEL M. KIND, MD
Assistant Clinical Professor,
Department of Surgery,
Division of Plastic and Reconstructive Surgery,
University of California–San Francisco;
Assistant Director of Research;
Assistant Fellowship Director,
The Buncke Clinic,
San Francisco, California

BRIAN M. KINNEY, MD, FACS, MSME
Clinical Assistant Professor of Plastic Surgery,
University of Southern California–Los Angeles;
Former Chief,
Century City Hospital,
Los Angeles, California

ELIZABETH M. KIRALY, MD
Fellow, Hand and Microvascular Surgery,
University of Nevada School of Medicine,
Department of Surgery,
Division of Plastic Surgery,
Las Vegas, Nevada

JOHN O. KUCAN, MD
Professor of Surgery,
Institute of Plastic Surgery,
Southern Illinois University School of Medicine,
Springfield, Illinois

M. ABRAHAM KURIAKOSE, MD, DDS, FACS
Assistant Professor of Otolaryngology,
Division of Head and Neck Surgery,
Department of Otolaryngology,
New York University School of Medicine;
Attending Surgeon,
New York University Medical Center,
New York, New York

AMY L. LADD, MD
Associate Professor,
Division of Hand and Upper Extremity,
Department of Functional Restoration,
Stanford University;
Chief, Hand and Upper Extremity Clinic,
Lucile Salter Packard Children's Hospital,
Stanford, California

PATRICK W. LAPPERT, MD
Assistant Professor of Surgery,
Uniformed Services University of the Health Sciences,
Bethesda, Maryland;
Chief, Department of Plastic Surgery,
Naval Medical Center,
Portsmouth, Virginia

DON LaROSSA, MD
Professor of Plastic Surgery,
The University of Pennsylvania School of Medicine;
Staff Physician,
Hospital of The University of Pennsylvania;
Senior Surgeon,
Children's Hospital of Philadelphia,
Philadelphia, Pennsylvania

DAVID L. LARSON, MD
Professor and Chair of Plastic and Reconstructive Surgery,
Medical College of Wisconsin,
Milwaukee, Wisconsin

DONALD R. LAUB, Jr., MS, MD
Assistant Professor,
Departments of Surgery and Orthopedics,
University of Vermont;
Attending Plastic and Hand Surgeon,
Fletcher Allen Health Care,
Burlington, Vermont

MICHAEL LAW, MD
Fellow, Microsurgery,
University of Southern California–Los Angeles,
Division of Plastic Surgery,
Los Angeles, California

W. THOMAS LAWRENCE, MPH, MD
Professor and Chief,
Section of Plastic Surgery,
University of Kansas Medical Center,
Kansas City, Kansas

W.P. ANDREW LEE, MD, FACS
Assistant Professor of Surgery,
Harvard Medical School;
Chief of Hand Service,
Department of Surgery,
Massachusetts General Hospital,
Boston, Massachusetts

SALVATORE LETTIERI, MD
Senior Associate Consultant,
Mayo Clinic,
Division of Plastic and Reconstructive Surgery,
Rochester, Minnesota

JAN S. LEWIN, PhD
Assistant Professor and Director,
Speech Pathology and Audiology Section,
University of Texas M.D. Anderson Cancer Center,
Houston, Texas

TERRY R. LIGHT, MD
Dr. William M. Scholl Professor;
Chairman, Department of Orthopedic Surgery and
    Rehabilitation,
Stritch School of Medicine,
Loyola University–Chicago,
Maywood, Illinois

SEAN LILLE, MD
Research Professor,
Department of Chemistry and Biochemistry,
Arizona State University,
Tempe, Arizona;
Research Scientist,
Mayo Clinic–Scottsdale,
Scottsdale, Arizona;
Private Practice,
Phoenix, Arizona

TED LOCKWOOD, MD
Associate Clinical Professor,
University of Kansas Medical School;
Assistant Clinical Professor,
University of Missouri–Kansas City Medical School,
Kansas City, Missouri

MICHAEL T. LONGAKER, MD, FACS
John Marquis Converse Professor of Plastic Surgery Research;
Director of Surgical Research,
New York University School of Medicine;
Attending Plastic Surgeon,
New York University Medical Center,
New York, New York

H. PETER LORENZ, MD
Assistant Professor of Plastic Surgery,
University of California–Los Angeles School of Medicine,
Los Angeles, California

GEORGE L. LUCAS, MD
Professor and Chairman,
Orthopedic Surgery;
Program Director,
University of Kansas Wichita;
Orthopedic Surgeon,
Via Christi Hospital;
Orthopedic Surgeon,
Wesley Medical Center,
Wichita, Kansas

PETER J. LUND, BS, MD
Orthopedic/Hand Surgery,
Methodist Volunteer General Hospital,
Martin, Tennessee

STEVEN D. MACHT, MD, DDS
Clinical Professor of Plastic Surgery,
George Washington University,
Washington, DC

JOHN S. MANCOLL, MD
Private Practice,
Fort Wayne, Indiana

GREGORY A. MANTOOTH, MD
Chief Resident,
Division of Plastic and Reconstructive Surgery,
Indiana University,
Indianapolis, Indiana

BENJAMIN M. MASER, MD
Community Physician,
Department of Functional Restoration,
Stanford University,
Stanford, California

BRUCE A. MAST, MD
Assistant Professor,
Department of Surgery,
Division of Plastic and Reconstructive Surgery,
University of Florida;
Chief, Section of Plastic Surgery,
Malcolm Randall Gainesville Veterans Administration
    Medical Center,
Gainesville, Florida

ALAN MATARASSO, MD
Clinical Associate Professor of Plastic Surgery,
Albert Einstein College of Medicine;
Surgeon,
Manhattan Eye, Ear, Throat Hospital,
New York, New York

G. PATRICK MAXWELL, MD
Assistant Professor of Plastic Surgery,
Vanderbilt University;
Director, Institute for Aesthetic Surgery,
Baptist Hospital,
Nashville, Tennessee

MICHAEL H. MAYER, MD
Physician and Surgeon,
Plastic and Reconstructive Surgery,
Portland, Oregon

TRACY E. McCALL, MD
Chief Plastic Surgery Resident,
State University of New York,
Health Science Center at Brooklyn,
Brooklyn, New York

ROBERT L. McCAULEY, MD
Chief, Plastic and Reconstructive Surgery,
Shriners Burns Hospital Galveston;
Professor of Surgery and Pediatrics,
University of Texas Medical Branch,
Galveston, Texas

LAWRENCE R. MENENDEZ, MD
Associate Professor, Clinical Orthopedics;
Associate Professor, Department of Surgery,
Division of Tumor and Endocrine,
University of Southern California;
Chief of Orthopedics,
Kenneth Norris Jr. Cancer Hospital,
Los Angeles, California

FREDERICK J. MENICK, MD
Private Practice,
Tucson, Arizona

WYNDELL H. MERRITT, MD, FACS
Clinical Assistant Professor of Surgery,
Medical College of Virginia,
Richmond, Virginia

BRYAN J. MICHELOW, MBBCh, FRCS
Clinical Assistant Professor,
Case Western Reserve University,
Cleveland, Ohio

SCOTT R. MILLER, MD
Clinical Instructor of Plastic Surgery,
University of California–San Diego,
San Diego, California;
Attending Surgeon,
Scripps Memorial Hospital,
La Jolla, California

TIMOTHY A. MILLER, MD
Professor,
University of California–Los Angeles;
Chief, Plastic Surgery,
Wadsworth Veterans Administration Medical Center,
Los Angeles, California

FERNANDO MOLINA, MD
Professor, Plastic, Aesthetic, and Reconstructive Surgery;
Head, Division of Plastic and Reconstructive Surgery,
Hospital General Dr. Manual Gea Gonzalez,
Mexico City, Mexico

ROBERT E. MONTROY, MD
Associate Clinical Professor,
Division of Plastic Surgery,
University of California Irvine,
California College of Medicine,
Orange, California;
Chief, Plastic Surgery Section;
Assistant Chief, Spinal Cord Injury/Disease Health Care
    Group,
Department of Veterans Affairs Medical Center,
Long Beach, California

THOMAS S. MOORE, MD
Clinical Professor of Plastic Surgery,
Indiana University School of Medicine;
Chairman, Department of Plastic Surgery,
St. Vincent Hospital,
Indianapolis, Indiana

FARAMARZ MOVAGHARNIA, DO
Plastic Surgeon;
Staff Physician,
Emory Northlake Regional Medical Center,
Atlanta, Georgia

ARIAN MOWLAVI, MD
Plastic Surgery Resident,
Southern Illinois University School of Medicine,
Springfield, Illinois

JOSEPH E. MURRAY, MD
Emeritus Professor of Surgery,
Harvard Medical School,
Boston, Massachusetts

THOMAS A. MUSTOE, MD
Professor and Chief, Division of Plastic Surgery,
Northwestern University Medical School,
Chicago, Illinois

ARSHAD R. MUZAFFAR, MD
Chief Resident,
Department of Plastic Surgery,
University of Texas Southwestern Medical Center,
Parkland Memorial Hospital,
Dallas, Texas

NASH H. NAAM, MD, FACS
Clinical Professor,
Department of Plastic and Reconstructive Surgery,
Southern Illinois University School of Medicine,
Springfield, Illinois;
Director, Southern Illinois Hand Center,
Effingham, Illinois

SATORU NAGATA, MD, PhD
Visiting Professor,
Division of Plastic Surgery,
University of California Irvine,
California College of Medicine,
Orange, California;
Department Director,
Reconstructive Plastic Surgery,
Chiba Tokushukai Hospital,
Narashinodai, Funabashi, Chiba, Japan

DANIEL J. NAGLE, MD
Associate Clinical Professor of Orthopedic Surgery,
Northwestern University Medical School;
Attending Hand and Microsurgeon,
Northwestern Memorial Hospital,
Chicago, Illinois

FOAD NAHAI, MD, FACS
Private Practice,
Atlanta, Georgia

DAVID T. NETSCHER, MD, FACS
Associate Professor,
Division of Plastic Surgery,
Baylor College of Medicine;
Chief, Plastic Surgery,
Veterans Affairs Medical Center,
Houston, Texas

MICHAEL W. NEUMEISTER, MD
Assistant Professor;
Plastic Surgery Program Director;
Chief, Microsurgery and Research,
Southern Illinois University School of Medicine;
Director, Hyperbaric Oxygen Unit,
Co-Director, Regional Burn Unit,
Memorial Medical Center,
Springfield, Illinois

RONALD E. PALMER, MD
Clinical Assistant Professor,
University of Illinois College of Medicine at Peoria,
Peoria, Illinois

FRANK A. PAPAY, MS, MD, FACS, FAAP
Assistant Clinical Professor,
The Ohio State University College of Medicine,
Columbus, Ohio;
Staff Surgeon;
Head, Section of Craniofacial and Pediatric Plastic Surgery,
The Cleveland Clinic Foundation,
Department of Plastic and Reconstructive Surgery,
Cleveland, Ohio

ROBERT W. PARSONS, MD
Professor Emeritus in Plastic Surgery and Pediatrics,
University of Chicago,
Pritzker School of Medicine,
Chicago, Illinois

WILLIAM C. PEDERSON, MD, FACS
Clinical Associate Professor,
Department of Surgery and Orthopedic Surgery,
University of Texas Health Science Center–San Antonio,
San Antonio, Texas

LINDA G. PHILLIPS, MD
Professor of Plastic Surgery;
Chief, Division of Plastic Surgery,
University of Texas Medical Branch,
Galveston, Texas

GEORGE J. PICHA, MD, PhD, FACS
Clinical Assistant Professor,
Division of Plastic Surgery,
Case Western Reserve University,
Cleveland, Ohio;
Private Practice,
Lyndhurst, Ohio

JEFFREY C. POSNICK, DMD, MD, FRCSC, FACS
Clinical Professor, Plastic Surgery, Pediatrics, Oral and
    Maxillofacial Surgery, and Otolaryngology/Head and Neck
    Surgery,
Georgetown University,
Washington, DC;
Director, Posnick Center for Facial Plastic Surgery,
Chevy Chase, Maryland

JASON N. POZNER, MD
Private Practice,
Boca Raton, Florida

STEFAN PREUSS, MD
Fellow, Plastic and Reconstructive Surgery,
Harvard Medical School;
Staff Physician,
Brigham and Women's Hospital;
Staff Physician,
Children's Hospital,
Boston, Massachusetts

JULIAN J. PRIBAZ, MD
Associate Professor of Surgery;
Program Director,
Harvard Plastic Surgery Residency Training Program,
Harvard Medical School;
Associate Surgeon,
Brigham and Women's Hospital;
Associate Surgeon,
Children's Hospital,
Boston, Massachusetts

C. LIN PUCKETT, MD, FACS
Professor and Head, Division of Plastic Surgery,
University of Missouri,
Columbia, Missouri

OSCAR M. RAMIREZ, MD
Clinical Assistant Professor,
Johns Hopkins University School of Medicine;
Clinical Assistant Professor,
University of Maryland,
Baltimore, Maryland;
Director,
Esthétique International,
Plastic Surgical Center,
Timonium, Maryland

GERALD V. RAYMOND, MD
Assistant Professor,
John Hopkins University School of Medicine;
Neurologist,
Kennedy Krieger Institute,
Baltimore, Maryland

RILEY REES, MD
Professor of Plastic and Reconstructive Surgery,
University of Michigan Medical Center;
Chief, Plastic Surgeon Section,
Veterans Administration Medical Center,
Ann Arbor, Michigan,
Associate,
Chelsea Community Hospital,
Chelsea, Michigan

DANIEL REICHNER, MD
Plastic Surgery Resident,
University of California Irvine,
California College of Medicine,
Orange, California

JOAN RICHTSMEIER, MA, PhD
Professor, Department of Cell Biology and Anatomy,
Department of Plastic Surgery,
Johns Hopkins University School of Medicine,
Baltimore, Maryland

DAVID RING, MD
Fellow, Orthopedic Hand Service,
Massachusetts General Hospital,
Boston, Massachusetts

THOMAS L. ROBERTS III, MD
Associate Clinical Professor of Surgery,
Medical University of South Carolina at Spartanburg,
Spartanburg, South Carolina

ROD J. ROHRICH, MD, FACS
Professor and Chairman,
Department of Plastic Surgery,
University of Texas Medical Center at Dallas,
Dallas, Texas

LORNE E. ROTSTEIN, MD, FRCSC, FACS
Associate Professor,
Department of Surgery,
University of Toronto;
Staff Surgeon,
Princess Margaret Hospital,
The Toronto General Hospital University Health Network,
Toronto, Ontario, Canada

J. PETER RUBIN, MD
Fellow in Plastic Surgery,
Harvard Medical School,
Boston, Massachusetts

ROBERT C. RUSSELL, MD, FRACS, FACS
Clinical Professor of Surgery,
Division of Plastic Surgery,
Southern Illinois University School of Medicine,
Springfield, Illinois

A. MICHAEL SADOVE, MD
Professor of Surgery (Plastics),
Indiana University School of Medicine;
Chief, Plastic Surgery,
James Whitcomb Riley Hospital for Children,
Indianapolis, Indiana

KENNETH E. SALYER, MD
Adjunct Professor, Department of Orthodontics,
Baylor College of Dentistry,
Baylor University,
Dallas, Texas;
Clinical Professor, Department of Surgery,
Division of Plastic and Reconstructive Surgery,
University of Texas Health Science Center at San Antonio,
San Antonio, Texas;
Founding Director,
International Craniofacial Institute,
Cleft Lip and Palate Treatment Center,
Dallas, Texas

NICOLAS SASTRE, MD
Professor of Plastic Surgery,
Postgraduate Division of Medical Faculty,
Universidad Nacional Autonoma de Mexico;
Chairman, Plastic Surgery Department,
Hospital General de Mexico,
Mexico City, Mexico

STEPHEN A. SCHENDEL, MD, DDS
Professor and Head, Division of Plastic and Reconstructive
   Surgery;
Chairman, Department of Functional Restoration,
Stanford University,
Stanford, California

STEPHEN B. SCHNALL, MD
Associate Professor of Clinical Orthopedics,
University of Southern California School of Medicine,
Los Angeles, California

ALAN E. SEYFER, MD
Chief, Plastic Surgery,
Professor of Surgery, Anatomy, and Cell Developmental
   Biology,
Oregon Health Sciences University;
Chief, Plastic Surgery,
Doernbecher Childrens Hospital;
Staff Surgeon,
Shriners' Hospital for Crippled Children;
Portland Veterans Administration Medical Center,
Portland, Oregon

JATIN P. SHAH, MD, FACS, FRCS, FDSRCS
Professor of Surgery,
Weill Medical College,
Cornell University;
E.W. Strong Chair in Head and Neck Oncology;
Chief, Head and Neck Service,
Memorial Sloan-Kettering Cancer Center,
New York, New York

ARTHUR SHEKTMAN, MD
Attending Surgeon,
Newton-Wellesley Hospital,
Newton, Massachusetts;
Attending Surgeon,
St. Elizabeth's Medical Center,
Boston, Massachusetts

RANDY SHERMAN, MD
Professor and Chief,
Division of Plastic and Reconstructive Surgery,
University of Southern California–Los Angeles;
Chief, Plastic Surgery,
University of Southern California University Hospital;
Chief, Plastic Surgery,
Los Angeles County Hospital,
Los Angeles, California

PETER P. SIKO, MD
Research Manager,
The Buncke Clinic,
San Francisco, California

CARL E. SILVER, MD
Professor of Surgery,
Albert Einstein College of Medicine;
Chief, Head and Neck Surgery,
Montefiore Medical Center,
Bronx, New York

JEFFREY D. SMITH, MD
Clinical Fellow in Surgery,
Harvard Medical School;
Chief Resident, Plastic Surgery,
Brigham and Women's Hospital;
Chief Resident, Plastic Surgery,
Children's Hospital,
Boston, Massachusetts

NICOLE ZOOK SOMMER, MD
Plastic Surgery Resident,
Southern Illinois University School of Medicine,
Springfield, Illinois

RAJIV SOOD, MD
Associate Professor of Plastic Surgery,
Indiana University Medical Center;
Chief, Plastic Surgery Section,
Wishard Memorial Hospital,
Indianapolis, Indiana

CAROL L. SORENSEN, PsyD
Adjunct Professor of Psychology,
Concordia University,
Irvine, California

PANAYOTIS N. SOUCACOS, MD, FACS
Professor and Chairman,
Department of Orthopedics,
University of Ioannina School of Medicine,
Ioannina, Greece

MYRON SPECTOR, BS, MS, PhD
Professor of Orthopedic Surgery (Biomaterials),
Harvard Medical School;
Director of Orthopedic Research,
Department of Orthopedic Surgery,
Brigham and Women's Hospital,
Boston, Massachusetts

MELVIN SPIRA, MD, DDS
Professor of Surgery,
Division of Plastic Surgery,
Baylor College of Medicine,
Houston, Texas

HANS U. STEINAU, MD
Professor, Department of Plastic Surgery,
Director, Clinic for Plastic Surgery,
Hand and Burn Center,
Bergmannsheil Clinic,
Ruhr University,
Bochum, Germany

PETER J. STERN, MD
Professor and Chairman,
Department of Orthopedic Surgery,
University of Cincinnati College of Medicine,
Cincinnati, Ohio

BERISH STRAUCH, MD
Professor and Chairman,
Department of Plastic Surgery,
Albert Einstein College of Medicine,
Montefiore Medical Center,
Bronx, New York

JAMES M. STUZIN, MD
Clinical Assistant Professor of Plastic Surgery–Voluntary,
University of Miami School of Medicine;
Senior Attending Physician,
Mercy Hospital,
Miami, Florida

MARK R. SULTAN, MD
Associate Clinical Professor of Surgery,
Columbia University;
Chief, Division of Plastic Surgery,
Beth Israel Medical Center,
New York, New York

WILLIAM M. SWARTZ, MD, FACS
Clinical Associate Professor,
Department of Surgery,
University of Pittsburgh,
Pittsburgh, Pennsylvania

JULIA K. TERZIS, MD, PhD, FRCSC
Professor, Department of Surgery,
Division of Plastic and Reconstructive Surgery;
Director, Microsurgery Program,
Eastern Virginia Medical School,
Microsurgical Research Center,
Norfolk, Virginia

VIVIAN TING, MD
Resident in General Surgery,
University of Rochester Medical Center,
Strong Memorial Hospital,
Rochester, New York

BRYANT A. TOTH, MD, FACS
Assistant Clinical Professor of Surgery,
Department of Surgery,
University of California–San Francisco;
Attending Surgeon,
California Pacific Medical Center,
San Francisco, California;
Chief, Division of Plastic Surgery,
Children's Hospital of Northern California,
Oakland, California

LAWRENCE C. TSEN, MD
Assistant Professor of Anesthesia,
Harvard Medical School;
Attending Anesthesiologist,
Department of Anesthesiology,
Perioperative and Pain Medicine,
Brigham and Women's Hospital,
Boston, Massachusetts

MARTIN G. UNGER, MD, FRCSC, ABCS, ABHRS
Clinical Teacher and Lecturer,
University of Toronto;
Chief of Plastic Surgery,
One Medical Place Hospital,
Toronto, Ontario, Canada

ALLEN L. VAN BEEK, BS, MD
Clinical Associate Professor,
University of Minnesota,
Department of Surgery,
Minneapolis, Minnesota

VICTORIA M. VANDERKAM, RN, BS, CPSN
Clinical Nurse, Division of Plastic Surgery,
University of California Irvine Medical Center,
Orange, California

CRAIG A. VANDER KOLK, MD, FACS
Associate Professor of Plastic Surgery,
Director, Cleft and Craniofacial Center,
Johns Hopkins University School of Medicine,
Baltimore, Maryland

NICHOLAS VEDDER, MD
Associate Professor,
University of Washington,
Seattle, Washington

MARIOS D. VEKRIS, MD
Orthopedic Attending Surgeon,
Ioannina University Hospital,
Ioannina Medical School,
Ioannina, Greece

PETER M. VOGT, MD, PhD
Associate Professor;
Attending Physician,
Hand and Burn Center,
Bergmannsheil Clinic,
Ruhr University,
Bochum, Germany

JEFFREY D. WAGNER, MD
Associate Professor of Surgery,
Department of Surgery,
Division of Plastic and Reconstructive Surgery,
Indiana University School of Medicine,
Indianapolis, Indiana

ROBERT L. WALTON, MD, FACS
Professor of Surgery,
University of Chicago School of Medicine;
Chief, Section of Plastic Surgery,
University of Chicago Hospitals,
Chicago, Illinois

BERNADETTE WANG, MD
Fellow, Hand and Microsurgery,
Curtis National Hand Center,
Union Memorial Hospital,
Baltimore, Maryland

H. KIRK WATSON, MD
Director, Connecticut Combined Hand Surgery Fellowship;
Assistant Clinical Professor of Orthopedics, Rehabilitation,
    and Plastic Surgery,
Yale University School of Medicine,
New Haven, Connecticut;
Clinical Professor, Department of Orthopedics,
University of Connecticut School of Medicine,
Farmington, Connecticut;
Senior Staff,
Hartford Hospital;
Connecticut Children's Medical Center,
Hartford, Connecticut

M. SHARON WEBB, MD, PhD, JD
Attorney-at-Law,
Boston, Massachusetts

DENTON D. WEISS, LCDR, MC, USNR
Department of Plastic Surgery,
Naval Medical Center Portsmouth,
Portsmouth, Virginia

KATHLEEN J. WELCH, MD, MPH
Instructor in Anesthesia,
Harvard Medical School;
Director of Plastic Surgical Anesthesia,
Brigham and Women's Hospital,
Boston, Massachusetts

DEBORAH J. WHITE, MD
Staff Physician,
Scottsdale Healthcare,
Scottsdale, Arizona

GORDON H. WILKES, BS, MD, FRCSC
Clinical Professor of Surgery,
University of Alberta;
Chief of Surgery,
Misericordia Hospital,
Edmonton, Alberta, Canada

J. KERWIN WILLIAMS, MD
Clinical Associate Professor,
Division of Plastic Surgery,
Emory University School of Medicine;
Attending Physician,
Pediatric and Craniofacial Associates,
Atlanta Plastic Surgery,
Atlanta, Georgia

TODD WILLIAMS, MD
Chief Plastic Surgery Fellow,
Southern Illinois University School of Medicine,
Institute for Plastic and Reconstructive Surgery,
Springfield, Illinois

PETER D. WITT, MD, FACS
Associate Professor of Plastic Surgery;
Director, Pediatric Plastic Surgery,
Sutherland Institute,
University of Kansas School of Medicine,
Kansas City, Kansas

JOHN F. WOLFAARDT, BDS, MDent, PhD
Professor,
Faculty of Medicine and Dentistry,
University of Alberta;
Director, Craniofacial Osseointegration and Maxillofacial
    Prosthetic Rehabilitation Unit,
Misericordia Hospital,
Edmonton, Alberta, Canada

WILLIAM A. ZAMBONI, MD
Professor and Chief,
Division of Plastic Surgery,
University of Nevada School of Medicine,
Las Vegas, Nevada

JAMES E. ZINS, MD
Chairman, Department of Plastic Surgery,
The Cleveland Clinic Foundation,
Cleveland, Ohio

ELVIN G. ZOOK, MD
Professor of Plastic Surgery,
Southern Illinois University School of Medicine;
Chairman, Department of Plastic Surgery,
Memorial Medical Center,
Springfield, Illinois

RONALD M. ZUKER, MD, FRCSC,
FACS, FAAP
Professor of Surgery,
University of Toronto;
Head, Division of Plastic Surgery,
The Hospital for Sick Children,
Toronto, Ontario, Canada

*To Janice, my most accurate critic, my best helper
with love and thanks*

General Preface

This large project is dedicated to our colleagues who have contributed individual chapters to this textbook. Those who write chapters for books know that they are the unsung heroes of the medical publishing business. The chapter authors are recognized experts in their fields who have given their time in an effort to communicate their knowledge to the rest of the world. This unselfish work involves a long time commitment and a multistaged process. We would not have plastic surgery textbooks if it were not for the many people who give so freely of their time and expertise. We thank each of our chapter authors; this project is by you and for you, and we hope that you are proud of the finished product.

Plastic Surgery: Indications, Operations, and Outcomes was envisioned as a comprehensive overview of the entire discipline of plastic surgery. The concept was to create a practical book that would be useful for plastic surgeons in practice and for those in training. Each clinical chapter follows a standard format as closely as possible; the chapters first describe the indications for surgery, then discuss the operation of choice, including procedural details, and finally present outcomes information when available.

A project such as this has a history of its own. Bruce Achauer started the process in 1992 by talking to publishers and potential coeditors. He has provided leadership throughout the project. Working together, Achauer, Elof Eriksson, and Bahman Guyuron determined the title, focus, outline, and editors. In the fall of 1995, Achauer, Eriksson, and Guyuron signed a contract with Mosby, agreeing that they would edit the textbook. Jack Coleman, Bob Russell, and Craig Vander Kolk agreed to serve as volume editors.

Early on it was decided that the authors would focus on outcomes as much as possible, although we knew full well that there was little information on outcomes in plastic surgery. The goal was to increase awareness of this need and guide readers to begin thinking toward measuring outcomes. Ed Wilkins accepted the challenge of serving as outcomes editor.

The actual writing of the text began in 1996. The entire process of writing and editing took several years and involved a long-term commitment. The publishing business, like many others, has undergone tremendous change, including consolidation and the creation of larger firms from several companies. There was also an inevitable change of personnel during the process. Although Mosby started the project, Harcourt Health Sciences completed it. Throughout the years, our editorial staff has been extremely helpful.

Many individuals have been involved with this project. We extend our gratitude to the following people: John DeCarville and Bob Hurley, who captured our vision from the start and fully embraced it; Richard Zorab, Senior Editor, and Dolores Meloni, Senior Developmental Editor, of Harcourt Health Sciences, who saw the project through to its fruition; our tireless production staff of Carol Weis, Project Manager, and Florence Achenbach, Rick Dudley, Karen Rehwinkel, Christine Schwepker, and David Stein, Production Editors; and finally, Victoria VanderKam, who was willing to do anything necessary to see this project through.

It has been a fabulous experience, and we are grateful for the opportunity to participate. We thank everybody (authors, illustrators, and editors) for their commitment, hard work, and friendship and for creating this excellent textbook for plastic surgery.

BRUCE M. ACHAUER
ELOF ERIKSSON
BAHMAN GUYURON
JOHN J. COLEMAN
ROBERT C. RUSSELL
CRAIG A. VANDER KOLK

Preface to the Third Volume

The head and face are the most dramatically defining human characteristics. Unlike most animals, we humans use the tools of facial expression and verbal interaction frequently and effectively in our dealings with our environment. Within the anatomical confines of the head and neck lie the organs responsible for reason and complex thought, the assessment of spatial relationships (with vision, hearing, and to a much lesser degree olfaction), the initiation of respiration and speech, and the preparation and passage of nutrients into the alimentary tract. The delicate functional synergy of this area and its external structure allow us to face the world and our fellow human beings, to interact with them, and to survive alone or in the company of others. It is not surprising, then, to consider the devastation visited upon the individual who suffers from a significant structural or functional disorder of the head and neck. This person's ability to survive is impaired, and his or her acceptance by society is greatly diminished. Facial deformity and dysfunction create social isolation and bar afflicted individuals from normal life, curtailing their participation in the pleasures of social interaction and, because appearance is often the initiating aspect of sexual activity, limiting their ability to contribute their genotype to the human gene pool.

Attempts to alleviate the suffering caused by deformity of the head and neck, both congenital and acquired, account for a large part of the past and present activities of plastic surgery and plastic surgeons. In the last 20 years, remarkable progress made in plastic surgery has had an immediate benefit for these patients. The elucidation, development, and refinement of the musculocutaneous concept and the interest in the vascular anatomy of the tissues that it has engendered have populated a once sparse and limited armamentarium with numerous versatile techniques that can be used to correct deformity and dysfunction in the head and neck. When this powerful concept is combined with the technique of microvascular transfer, the number of weapons increases. Moreover, careful selection and execution of these methods minimize associated donor site or adjacent local deformity and dysfunction.

Advances in reconstructive plastic surgery have been particularly dramatic in the treatment of those with malignancy in the head and neck area. These patients, like all others seeking the help of physicians, have a hierarchy of priorities that should be reflected in the particular treatment chosen to correct their problem. Foremost in the treatment of patients with head and neck malignancy, as in those with any illness, is their survival. Extirpative surgery or radiotherapy usually addresses this priority.

Except for the development of craniofacial surgery, little has changed in this aspect of treatment in the last 50 years. The next priorities are function and appearance, usually in that order. Clearly the advances of the recent years in reconstructive plastic surgery have dramatically improved the surgeon's ability to preserve or restore reasonably normal function and to recreate a socially acceptable appearance. The next priority is efficiency, or the ability to deliver the therapy in a time period relevant to the natural history of the disease or deformity. It is perfectly reasonable to address the deformity of cleft lip and palate with multiple, staged procedures over a period of 10 to 15 years. To offer such a plan to the patient with $T_4N_1M_0$ carcinoma of the floor of the mouth who is undergoing composite resection would be ridiculous and futile. Single-stage reconstruction with microvascular surgery in musculocutaneous flaps has made an enormous difference in allowing patients with serious head and neck deformity or disease a rapid, efficient return to society. The rapid evolution of these techniques over the past 20 years has changed the approach to head and neck cancer, allowing a more aggressive yet safer attack on the specific problem. Encouraged by the success in reconstructive malignancy, surgeons have extended these methods to other less deadly problems. Although in the past free tissue transfer was reserved for only the most desperate of conditions, it is now considered a useful tool in almost any situation requiring tissue replacement or augmentation.

Having witnessed most of this evolution during my career, I frequently wonder at the persistence and patience of those surgeons who endeavored to treat such problems before the late 1970s and at the faith and courage of the patients subjected to these treatments.

Advances in head and neck surgery have come from several specialties. Since the inception of the specialty, the plastic surgeon has taken skills and concepts from the broad arena of surgical technique and knowledge and applied them to the problems arising in this anatomical area. Innovation, as well as testing, verification, and modification of therapies, has been the purview of plastic surgery. This volume attempts to provide comprehensive analysis of those head and neck problems not addressed in the aesthetic and craniofacial volumes and proposes presently accepted therapies. Notably, all chapters, except for those on the larynx and gastric transposition, were written by plastic surgeons who are actively engaged in the practice of surgery and the attempt to alleviate the suffering of and improve the quality of life for those patients affected with disorders of the head and neck. Future research, technique development, and therapy assessment will remain the privileges and responsibilities of plastic surgery.

My thanks to Mrs. Donna Heifner for her rapid and efficient preparation of the manuscripts and revisions and to my collaborator, friend, and fellow plastic surgeon, Min Li, for his expert creation of the illustrations and his continued good-natured willingness to modify them at my frequent request.

JOHN J. COLEMAN III

Outcomes Preface

At the dawn of a new millennium, we are witnessing the most dramatic overhaul of the American health care system in more than a century. Health care reform is well underway, driven by economic and political forces within both the public and private sectors. The watchwords of this not-so-quiet revolution, terms such as *efficiency, cost-effectiveness,* and *value,* reflect the new demand by payers that health care interventions deliver measurable benefit at reasonable costs. Contrary to long-standing traditions in the United States, exactly what constitutes a "reasonable" cost is determined not by those who provide health care but rather by those who foot the bill. The growing emphasis on cost-effectiveness, or "value" for every dollar spent, is forcing providers to fundamentally rethink traditional patterns of care. In this brave new world, medical decisions are made only after the perceived benefits have been weighed against the risks *and* costs of treatment.

Recent reforms also reflect changes in the traditional standards by which we have assessed the effectiveness of care. Treatment options are no longer being judged simply in terms of morbidity and mortality. Instead, interventions are evaluated by studying their impacts on long-term functioning, well-being, and quality of life. This new emphasis on measurement of outcomes from the "patient's viewpoint" is of particular interest to plastic surgeons. Unlike cardiac or transplant surgeries, aesthetic and reconstructive procedures usually do not produce life-saving results. Instead, plastic surgeons endeavor to bestow more subtle benefits on their clientele, improving their body image, psychosocial well-being, and physical functioning. Lest plastic surgeons downplay the significance of their work, it is important to note that health services researchers and payers now evaluate the value of health care interventions in terms of quality-adjusted life years (QALYs) contributed. Interventions that substantially improve quality of life may be viewed as comparable (or superior) to treatment options that increase longevity.

Clearly, assessment of patient-centered outcomes is of critical importance not only to plastic surgeons but to all health care providers. Outcomes data are playing increasingly important roles in determining which treatment modalities are supported by payers and managed care providers. Research assessing the results and costs of care also may determine where and by whom that care is delivered. Outcomes studies also provide key information to patients and providers to assist in medical decision-making. In managing health care delivery systems, outcomes data (such as patient satisfaction) identify potential targets for quality improvement efforts and provide meaningful yardsticks with which to assess progress.

Given the growing importance of assessing and reporting patient-centered results of care, the chapter authors of this textbook have included "Outcomes" sections where appropriate. Available data on a diverse array of outcomes parameters are referenced. However, as the reader will note, considerable gaps still exist in our knowledge of surgical outcomes, particularly in the areas of quality of life and cost analyses. While we attempt to summarize existing outcomes data in each chapter, we also have endeavored to highlight some areas in which more research is needed. For many aesthetic and reconstructive problems and procedures, the quantity of unanswered research questions dwarfs our current body of knowledge. It is the hope of the volume authors and editors that some of the issues raised in these chapters will stimulate new outcomes studies to answer these questions.

EDWIN G. WILKINS

Contents

VOLUME TWO CRANIOMAXILLOFACIAL, CLEFT, AND PEDIATRIC SURGERY
Craig A. Vander Kolk, Editor

PART III   MAXILLOFACIAL SURGERY

PART IV   PEDIATRIC PLASTIC SURGERY

VOLUME THREE   HEAD AND NECK SURGERY
John J. Coleman III, Editor

VOLUME FOUR   HAND SURGERY
Robert C. Russell, Editor

Oncologic and Reconstructive Principles

Grant W. Carlson

INDICATIONS

EPIDEMIOLOGY

The majority of head and neck cancers are squamous cell carcinomas (SCC) of the upper aerodigestive tract. Most of the remaining tumors are adenocarcinomas of the salivary glands, melanomas, and soft tissue sarcomas. Usually a disease of men in their fifth or sixth decade, cancer of the head and neck represents about 4% of all malignant tumors in the United States. The male to female ratio is 4:1 but this is decreasing because of an increase in female tobacco use. In 1992, 42,800 new cases of SCC were diagnosed in the United States, resulting in 11,600 deaths.[7] The disease is endemic in other parts of the world such as India and Southeast Asia, where cancer of the oral cavity represents about 35% of all malignant tumors. Again, the vast majority of cases are related to tobacco use. The risk of developing a head and neck SCC is proportional to the overall amount of tobacco smoked.[39] Ethanol consumption potentiates tobacco-related carcinogenesis and is also an independent risk factor. A nondrinker who smokes has a fivefold increased risk of developing a head and neck cancer, whereas an ethanol drinker who smokes has a fifteenfold increase.[41] Smokeless tobacco has become increasingly popular among young people, resulting in a rise in oral cavity cancers in this age group. Advanced head and neck cancer has also been reported in habitual marijuana users.

Occupational risk factors including nickel refining, woodworking, and exposure to textile fibers may predispose to cancers of the nasal cavity and paranasal sinuses.[9,15,21,30] There appears to be an inverse relationship between the consumption of fruits and vegetables and the incidence of head and neck cancer, with recent evidence suggesting that dietary carotenoids may have a protective effect in patients at high risk.[24]

Viruses probably play a role in head and neck carcinogenesis. DNA of the human papillomavirus has been detected in laryngeal SCC.[44] Infection with Epstein-Barr virus is associated with nasopharyngeal carcinoma with DNA from the virus isolated from all histologic types. There is some genetic predisposition for head and neck cancer because of the sporadic occurrences in young adults and nonusers of tobacco and ethanol.[25]

BIOLOGY

The carcinogens tobacco and ethanol affect the entire mucosal surface of the upper aerodigestive tract, lungs, and esophagus. This is termed *field carcinogenesis,* and accounts for the ~5% to 7% incidence of synchronous cancers seen in the head and neck.[37] Metachronous cancers will develop in 30% to 40% of patients if they continue to smoke, but the risk decreases to 6% in those who quit.[29] Randomized trials of isotretinoin, a synthetic retinoid, taken orally to prevent the development of second malignancies after treatment of various head and neck cancers have shown a reduction in new cancers but at the high cost of drug toxicity.[20]

Premalignant lesions can be observed during careful intraoral examination of high risk patients. Leukoplakia, defined as a white, keratotic area that cannot be scraped off, is frequently seen in patients with head and neck cancer. Histologic examination of leukoplakia reveals 11% to 15% incidence of dysplasia. About 3% to 5% of leukoplakia will eventually degenerate into carcinoma.[43] Epithelial changes of premalignancy are more common in leukoplakia found in the floor of the mouth or tongue than at other oral cavity sites, portending the higher frequency of malignancy in those areas. Erythroplasia, reddened areas of oral mucosa, is associated with in situ or invasive cancer in 54% to 64% of lesions.[26]

There is mounting evidence for a genetic basis to the multistep process of head and neck carcinogenesis.[13] Chromosome analysis has revealed nonrandom deletions and rearrangements. This has been manifested in molecular changes such as the overexpression of the receptor for epidermal growth factor. Amplification on int-2 and bcl-1 oncogenes has been found in some SCC cell lines. Frequent deletions of chromosome 18q have suggested that tumor suppressor genes may be affected.

DIAGNOSIS AND STAGING

The signs and symptoms of cancer of the upper aerodigestive tract vary with the location of the primary site and the stage of the cancer. Approximately one third of patients will present

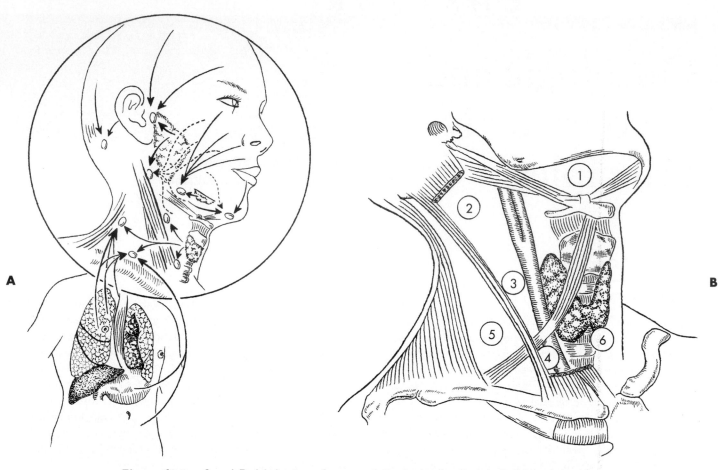

Figure 68-1. **A** and **B,** Likely sites of metastasis in the head and neck. *1,* Submental nodes; *2,* jugulodigastric nodes; *3,* midjugular nodes; *4,* juguloomohyoid nodes; *5,* posterior triangle nodes; *6,* Delphian node.

with early stage disease and have vague symptoms and minimal physical findings. These patients usually present to the general internist or dentist, who must have a high index of suspicion when patients with a history of tobacco and ethanol use complain of problems in the head and neck region.

Cancer of the nasopharynx may present with nasal obstruction, epistaxis, or serous otitis media from obstruction of the eustachian tube. Advanced lesions present with cranial neuropathies and posterior cervical lymphadenopathy. Early oral cavity cancers may present with pain, ulcers that fail to heal, or a change in fit of dentures. Cancers of the oropharynx, hypopharynx, or supraglottic larynx rarely produce early symptoms and are usually diagnosed in the late stages. Persistent unilateral sore throat may be a manifestation of an oropharyngeal cancer. Otalgia may result from referred pain pathways from cranial nerves V, IX, and X, and as an isolated finding in patients of this risk group should initiate a complete examination of the upper aerodigestive tract. Dysphagia and odynophagia may signal hypopharyngeal or supraglottic laryngeal cancer and hoarseness.

A mass in the neck is the initial presenting symptom in 25% of patients with oral or oropharyngeal SCC and in 50% of patients with nasopharyngeal SCC. Chronology, patient's age, and mass location are important diagnostic factors. Inflammatory lesions generally have a brief duration and are common in

the pediatric and teenage population. A solitary mass in the neck of an adult that has been present for over 6 weeks should be presumed to be cancer until proven otherwise. The vast majority of adult solitary non-thyroidal neck masses are metastatic cancers originating from a primary above the clavicles. The location of the mass may suggest the locations of the primary cancer (Figure 68-1) (Table 68-1).

Physical examination can identify greater than 90% of cancers of the upper aerodigestive tract that have metastasized to the neck. Examination requires inspection of all visible mucosal surfaces. Palpation is useful for lesions of the floor of mouth, tongue, and tonsils. Indirect laryngoscopy can usually be performed without topical anesthesia to visualize the larynx and hypopharynx. The base of tongue, tonsillar fossa, nasopharynx and pyriform sinuses are the most common areas for occult SCC. Flexible nasopharyngoscopy can be performed without sedation and is useful in patients in whom indirect laryngoscopy is not possible or is equivocal. The extent of tumor can usually be assessed by direct visualization, but in certain cases vital dye staining with toluidine blue may help delineate the extent of malignancy and identify premalignant changes.

Radiologic examination by computed tomography (CT) or magnetic resonance imaging (MRI) is useful to assess the extent of local or regional spread of tumor, particularly in infiltrative

Table 68-1.
Levels of Cervical Lymph Nodes

LOCATION	PRIMARY SITE
Level 1 (submandibular, submental)	Anterior tongue, floor of mouth, anterior alveolar ridge
Level 2 (jugulodigastric, upper jugular)	Oropharynx, nasopharynx
Level 3 (midjugular)	Hypopharynx, larynx, lateral tongue
Level 4 (low jugular)	Usually subclavicular: breast, lung, kidney, GI tract
Level 5 (posterior triangle, spinal accessory)	Scalp, nasopharynx, parotid

cancers where the depth of invasion is difficult to evaluate and in difficult to examine areas such as the parapharyngeal space, larynx, pyriform sinus, and nasopharynx. Bony invasion or tumor proximity to bone is better evaluated by CT scan, whereas soft tissue and nerve infiltration or differentiation of tumor from surrounding inflammation is better appreciated on MRI. The CT scan is also useful in diagnosis of subclinical lymphatic metastases to the neck. Changes suggestive of malignancy are diameter greater than 1.5 cm and spherical shape; in three studies comparing CT scans to physical examination, CT scans demonstrated superiority of 82% vs. 75%, 93% vs. 70%, and 90% vs. 82% evidence of central necrosis.[38] Plain x-rays including panorex and soft tissue films may be helpful for oral cavity lesions to evaluate possible mandibular involvement or calculus disease of the salivary glands. Shaha compared the diagnostic effectiveness of clinical evaluation, panorex films, and CT scans in 60 patients with carcinoma of the floor of the mouth. He found that clinical evaluation was superior to all other modalities.[36]

Examination under anesthesia is helpful to fully evaluate the primary cancer and to obtain biopsies. Triple endoscopy (direct laryngoscopy, bronchoscopy, and esophagoscopy) to evaluate for synchronous malignancies is not cost-effective and is not performed unless warranted by clinical suspicion.[5]

Although diagnosis can sometimes be made by scraping accessible lesions for cytology, most lesions of the oral cavity are amenable to incisional biopsy under local anesthesia. Excisional biopsy is warranted only for small lesions. Fine-needle aspiration is simple and cost-effective for masses in the head and neck, especially lymph nodes. It has a 96% to 100% accuracy but a negative aspirate does not rule out cancer.[35]

Staging is critical for planning the appropriate treatment for prognosis and for stratification in clinical trials. The American

Joint Committee of Cancer TNM staging system is prevalent in the United States based on clinical and diagnostic tests at the time of initial presentation of the cancer. The T stands for tumor size and extent and has specific parameters within the upper aerodigestive tract. The N defines nodal involvement and the M metastatic spread (Figure 68-2) (Table 68-2). Unlike other cancer sites, head and neck cancer may be Stage IV without distant metastases. Pretreatment screening includes a chest x-ray, liver function tests, and an alkaline phosphatase assay. If abnormalities are found, CT scan and bone specific to the abnormality will more clearly delineate the extent of disease.

NATURAL HISTORY AND STANDARD THERAPY

The majority of head and neck cancer patients present with locally and regionally advanced disease. Standard therapy usually combines surgery and radiation therapy. This combination has been shown to improve local and regional control over each modality used alone, but this has not resulted in an increase in survival. Chemotherapy is only accepted as a standard for recurrent or metastatic disease. Induction chemotherapy and radiation therapy have been used for organ preservation in cancer of the larynx.[16]

Stage I and Stage II diseases respond to single-modality therapy, either surgery or radiation, with a control rate of 60% to 90%. The choice of treatment depends on potential morbidity as well as the risk of developing a second malignancy, since radiation can only be administered once. Oral cavity and oral pharyngeal cancers are usually treated with surgery, excision with a margin of 2 cm of normal tissue around the tumor. Because achievement of an adequate surgical margin around laryngeal or most hypopharyngeal lesions would require laryngectomy with the concomitant loss of speech, Stage I and Stage II cancers in this area are usually treated with definitive radiotherapy or surgery reserved for failure and salvage.

Stage III and Stage IV diseases generally require multimodality treatment including extensive surgery followed by radiation. Disease control ranges from 30% to 60%, and many patients die with locally or regionally persistent or recurrent disease. Those unable to tolerate extensive surgery or those with unresectable disease are treated with palliative radiation therapy.

Although SCC demonstrates a high response rate to cytotoxic chemotherapy, with single agent responses to methotrexate, cisplatin, 5-FU, and bleomycin ranging from 24% to 40% and combination therapies ranging from 60% to 100% partial response and 5% to 50% complete response, no randomized trial of chemotherapy to date has demonstrated a survival advantage over conventional treatment with surgery and radiotherapy. Despite this poor performance, the concept of neoadjuvant chemotherapy for organ preservation has become prevalent for hypopharyngeal and laryngeal malignancy. If patients treated with cisplatin and 5-FU followed by radiation therapy demonstrate a complete response, they are followed. Surgery is reserved for those not responding or for those who recur after radiotherapy. Although there is a small survival

Data Form for Cancer Staging

Patient identification
Name _____
Address _____
Hospital or clinic number _____
Age _____ Sex _____ Race _____

Institutional identification
Hospital or clinic _____
Address _____

Oncology Record

Anatomic site of cancer _____

Chronology of classification*   [ ] Clinical-diagnostic (cTNM)
                                 [ ] Surgical-evaluative (sTNM)

Date of classification _____

Histologic type† _____ Grade (G) _____

[ ] Postsurgical resection–pathologic (pTNM)
[ ] Retreatment (rTNM)   [ ] Autopsy (aTNM)

Definitions for All Time Periods

Primary Tumor (T)
[ ] TX   Minimum requirements to assess the primary tumor cannot be met.
[ ] T0   No evidence of primary tumor
[ ] Tis   Carcinoma *in situ*
[ ] T1   Greatest diameter of primary tumor 2 cm or less
[ ] T2   Greatest diameter of primary tumor more than 2 cm but not more than 4 cm
[ ] T3   Greatest diameter of primary tumor more than 4 cm
[ ] T4   Massive tumor more than 4 cm in diameter with deep invasion to involve antrum, pterygoid muscles, base of tongue, skin of neck

Lymph Nodes (N)
Same definitions to be used if postsurgical treatment–pathologic staging is used:

[ ] NX   Minimum requirements to assess the regional nodes cannot be met.
[ ] N0   No clinically positive node
[ ] N1   Single clinically positive homolateral node 3 cm or less in diameter
[ ] N2   Single clinically positive homolateral node more than 3 but not more than 6 cm in diameter or multiple clinically positive homolateral nodes, none more than 6 cm in diameter
  [ ] N2a   Single clinically positive homolateral node more than 3 cm but not more than 6 cm in diameter
  [ ] N2b   Multiple clinically positive homolateral nodes, none more than 6 cm in diameter
[ ] N3   Massive homolateral node(s), bilateral nodes, or contralateral node(s)
  [ ] N3a   Clinically positive homolateral node(s), one more than 6 cm in diameter
  [ ] N3b   Bilateral clinically positive nodes (in this situation, each side of the neck should be staged separately; *i.e.*, N3b: right, N2a; left, N1)
  [ ] N3c   Contralateral clinically positive node(s) only

Distant Metastasis (M)
[ ] MX   Minimum requirements to assess the presence of distant metastasis
[ ] M0   No (known) distant metastasis
[ ] M1   Distant metastasis present
      Specify _____

* Use a separate form each time a case is staged.
† See next page for additional information.

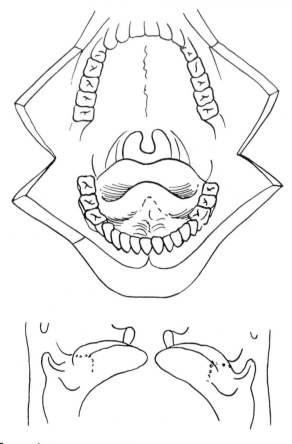

Tumor size: _____ cm

Location of Tumor

[ ] Lips: Upper
        Lower
[ ] Buccal mucosa
[ ] Floor of mouth
[ ] Oral tongue
[ ] Hard palate
[ ] Gingivae: Upper
          Lower
          Retromolar trigone

Examination by _____ M.D.
Date _____

Figure 68-2. American Joint Committee on Cancer staging form of carcinoma of the oral cavity. Accurate recording and transmission of stage is crucial to subsequent therapy. (From the American Joint Committee on Cancer.) *Continued*

Characteristics of Tumor

[ ] Exophytic
[ ] Superficial
[ ] Moderately infiltrating
[ ] Deeply infiltrating
[ ] Ulcerated
[ ] Extends to or overlies bone
[ ] Gross erosion of bone
[ ] Radiographic destruction of bone

Involvement of Neighboring Regions

[ ] Tonsillar pillar or soft palate
[ ] Nasal cavity or antrum
[ ] Nasopharynx
[ ] Pterygoid muscles
[ ] Soft tissues or skin of neck

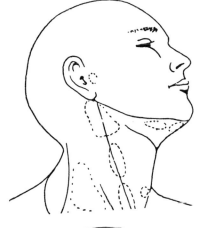

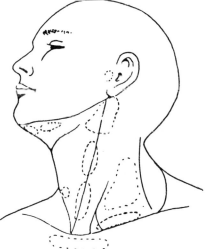

Indicate on diagram primary tumor and regional nodes involved.

Stage Grouping

[ ] Stage I   T1, N0, M0
[ ] Stage II   T2, N0, M0
[ ] Stage III   T3, N0, M0
                 T1, T2, T3; N1, M0
[ ] Stage IV   T4, N0, N1; M0
                 Any T, N2, N3; M0
                 Any T, any N, M1

Staging Procedures

A variety of procedures and special studies may be employed in the process of staging a given tumor. Both the clinical usefulness and cost efficiency must be considered. The following suggestions are made for staging a cancer of the oral cavity.

Essential for staging

1. Complete physical examination of the head and neck including indirect laryngoscopy and nasopharyngoscopy
2. Biopsy of primary tumor
3. Chest roentgenogram
4. Panorex films or other x-ray films for tumors overlying the jaws
5. Roentgenograms of paranasal sinuses for tumors overlying the palate

May be useful for staging or patient management

1. Multichemistry screen
2. Staining of surface mucosa with toluidine blue
3. Performance status (Karnofsky or ECOG scale)

May be useful for future staging systems or research studies

1. Panendoscopy (direct laryngoscopy, bronchoscopy, esophagoscopy)
2. Studies of immune competence

Histologic Type of Cancer

Predominant cancer is squamous cell carcinoma.

Histologic Grade

[ ] G1   Well differentiated
[ ] G2   Moderately well differentiated
[ ] G3–G4 Poorly to very poorly differentiated

Postsurgical Resection–Pathologic Residual Tumor (R)

This does not enter into staging but may be a factor in deciding further treatment.

[ ] R0   No residual tumor
[ ] R1   Microscopic residual tumor
[ ] R2   Macroscopic residual tumor
           Specify_____

Performance Status of Host (H)

Several systems for recording a patient's activity and symptoms are in use and are more or less equivalent, as follows:

AJCC	Performance	ECOG Scale	Karnofsky Scale (%)
[ ] H0	Normal activity	0	90-100
[ ] H1	Symptomatic but ambulatory; cares for self	1	70-80
[ ] H2	Ambulatory more than 50% of time; occasionally needs assistance	2	50-60
[ ] H3	Ambulatory 50% or less of time; nursing care needed	3	30-40
[ ] H4	Bedridden; may need hospitalization	4	10-20

Figure 68-2, cont'd.   For legend see opposite page.

Table 68-2.
Classification of Head and Neck Cancers

PRIMARY TUMOR (T)	DESCRIPTION
GENERAL, FOR ALL SITES	
TX	No available information of primary tumor
T0	No evidence of primary tumor
TIS	Carcinoma in situ
ORAL CAVITY, OROPHARYNX	
T1	Greatest diameter of primary tumor ≤ 2 cm
T2	>2 cm or = 4 cm
T3	>4 cm
T4	Massive tumor, with deep invasion into maxilla, mandible, pterygoids, soft tissue of neck
HYPOPHARYNX	
T1	Tumor confined to region of origin
T2	Extension into adjacent region or site, without fixation of hemilarynx
T3	Extension into adjacent region or site, with fixation of hemilarynx
T4	Massive tumor, invading bone or soft tissue of neck
LARYNX, GLOTTIC	
T1	Confined to true vocal cords; normal mobility
T2	Supraglottic or subglottic extension; normal or impaired mobility
T3	Confined to larynx proper; cord fixation
T4	Cartilage destruction and/or extension out of larynx
SUPRAGLOTTIC	
T1	Confined to site of origin; normal mobility
T2	Extension to glottis or adjacent supraglottic site; normal/impaired mobility
T3	Confined to larynx proper; cord fixation and/or extension hypopharynx or preepiglottic space
T4	Massive tumor; cartilage destruction and/or extension out of larynx
NODAL METASTASIS (N)	
NX	Nodes cannot be assessed
N0	No clinically positive nodes
N1	Single, clinically positive, ipsilateral node ≤ 3 cm
N2A	Single, clinically positive, ipsilateral node >3 cm or = 6 cm
N2B	Multiple, clinically positive, ipsilateral nodes; all ≤ 6 cm
N3A	Clinically positive, ipsilateral node(s); one >6 cm
N3B	Bilateral, clinically positive nodes (each side subclassified)
N3C	Contralateral, clinically positive nodes(s), only
DISTANT METASTASIS (M)	
MX	Not assessed
M0	No distant metastases identified
M1	Distant metastases present
STAGE GROUPINGS	
Stage I	$T_1N_0M_0$
Stage II	$T_2N_0M_0$
Stage III	$T_3N_0M_0$, T_1, T_2, or $T_3N_1M_0$
Stage IV	T_4N_0 or N_1M_0
	Any T N_2 or N_3M_0
	Any T, any N, M_1

Table 68-3.
Response Rates to Chemotherapy Regimens for Primary Head and Neck Cancer

AGENT	NO. OF PATIENTS	COMPLETE RESPONSE (%)	PARTIAL RESPONSE (%)
Cisplatin, 5-FU	117	49	49
Cisplatin, 5-FU	103	35	49
Methotrexate, vincristine	158	19	51
Methotrexate, leukourin	82	6	34

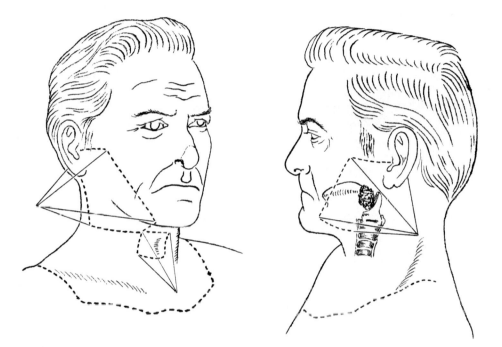

Figure 68-3. Radiation fields and doses for treatment by external beam (teletherapy) radiotherapy of a $T_2N_1M_0$ squamous cell carcinoma of the tongue.

disadvantage in this group, more natural speech is preserved in most cases (Table 68-3).

When radiotherapy is selected as the definitive or potentially curative treatment modality, tumoricidal doses in the range of 6000 to 7000 cGy must be used for the primary site. Depending on the site and the risk of subclinical nodal metastases, one or both necks must also be treated with 5000 to 5500 cGy. When radiotherapy is used as an adjuvant therapy to surgery, the primary site and surrounding tissues are usually treated with 5000 to 5500 cGy and the neck or necks with 4500-5500 cGy (Figure 68-3). These doses and fields may result in early edema and inflammation in the oral cavity and neck followed by fibrosis and a gradually progressive local tissue ischemia. A number of series have demonstrated increased complications in surgery performed in previously unradiated patients. Interstitial radiotherapy or brachytherapy is sometimes useful in oral cavity SCC, since large doses of radiation can be delivered to a localized area, with rapid falloff of dose and less effect on adjacent tissues. This, however, is usually combined with external field radiation (teletherapy) in primary disease.

Nasopharynx

Nasopharyngeal carcinoma is rare in the United States but common in parts of China and Southeast Asia. The majority of patients present with nodal metastases in the posterior neck. A histologic variant, lymphoepithelioma has a better prognosis than SCC. These tumors are highly radiosensitive, especially lymphoepithelioma, and radiation is the treatment of choice. Neck dissections are performed for persistent nodal disease.

Oral Cavity

The oral cavity is the most common site of head and neck cancer. It is bordered by the lip vermilion, the junction of the hard/soft palate, anterior tonsillar pillar, and the circumvallate papillae (Figure 68-4). It includes the lip, floor of mouth, anterior tongue to the circumvallate papillae, buccal mucosa, alveolar ridge, retromolar trigone, and hard palate. Treatment choice depends on stage, the anticipated functional result, patient performance status, and the need for treatment of the neck, but usually involves surgical resection.

Alveolar Ridge

Carcinoma of the alveolar ridge is less directly related to tobacco and ethanol than other oral cavity cancers. It is sometimes related to poor oral hygiene and ill-fitting dentures. Direct mandibular invasion through the periosteum is common in patients with teeth, spread through the occlusal ridge and dental orifice; subsequent perineural invasion is common in edentulous patients (Figure 68-5).

Floor of Mouth

The floor of mouth is the area between the tongue and the inner surface of the mandible. Tumors may involve Wharton's duct, resulting in submandibular gland enlargement mimicking metastatic spread. Small cancers can be treated with transoral excision or radiation therapy via an intraoral cone or brachytherapy. If the tumor abuts but does not seem to invade the mandible, a rim mandibulectomy may be performed. Advanced lesions may require a partial mandibulectomy. Large tumors are treated with surgery followed by radiation. There is a high incidence of clinical and subclinical neck metastasis, so treatment of the neck is important with lesions greater than T1 (2 cm).

Anterior Tongue

Carcinoma of the anterior or mobile tongue usually occurs as a chronic nonhealing ulcer along the lateral aspect. Second only to the lip as site for malignancy, the tongue contains a rich lymphatic supply so that greater than one third of patients have lymph node involvement at the time of diagnosis of the primary cancer. Small lesions may be treated with surgery or radiation with equivalent survival. Larger lesions require surgery includ-

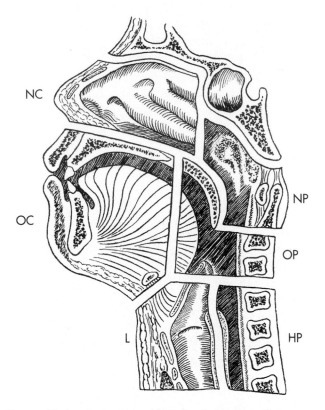

Figure 68-4. Anatomic and functional divisions of the upper aerodigestive tract. *L,* Larynx; *OC,* oral cavity; *NC,* nasal cavity; *NP,* nasopharynx; *OP,* oropharynx; *HP,* hypopharynx.

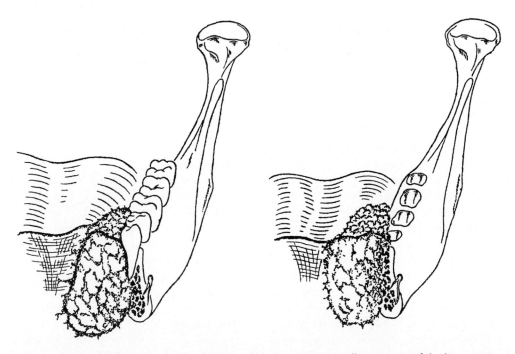

Figure 68-5. Method of invasion of the mandible by squamous cell carcinoma of the lip, tongue, or floor of mouth in patients with and without dentition.

ing neck dissection and flap reconstruction, with adjuvant radiation administered if perineural lymphatic invasion is found and in cases with nodal metastases (Figure 68-6).

Lip

The lip is the most common site of cancer in the oral cavity. Although lower lip SCC largely occurs in men with a history of smoking and prolonged sun exposure, basal cell carcinoma predominates in the upper lip (Figure 68-7). Primary lesions are usually treated by surgical excision and primary closure after repair of the orbicularis muscle. Up to one third of the lower lip can be resected and closed primarily. Larger lesions may require a staged lip switch, which transfers upper lip tissue pedicled on the labial artery by the Abbe technique. This procedure preserves the oral commissure and can close defects up to two thirds of the width of the lower lip. The Karapandzic technique (i.e., rotation-advancement of the remaining skin, orbicularis muscle, and mucosa, with the motor and sensory innervation intact) is useful to preserve oral continuity in moderately large lip lesions but carries with it the problem of microstomia.[22] Total lower lip reconstruction can be accomplished with fan flaps, gate flaps, or a radial forearm free flap using a tongue flap to restore the vermilion.[19,28,32] In selected lesions of the oral commissure, radiation therapy may be used to reduce morbidity, except in very large or histologically aggressive lesions. Lymph node metastases are uncommon and elective node dissection is not indicated. Aggressive SCC of the lower lip has a predilection for perineural invasion along the mental nerve, and involvement of the mandible may come via the mental foramen as well as by direct extension.

Buccal Mucosa

Cancer of the buccal mucosa is relatively uncommon in the United States, accounting for only 5% of oral cavity cancers. It is common in areas where chewing tobacco and betel nut is practiced such as India, Venezuela, and Southeast Asia. In the United States, most buccal cancers tend to be well differentiated, slow growing, and, despite their large size, less likely than tumors of other oral sites to have subclinical metastases to the neck. Verrucous carcinoma, a common form of buccal cancer, exhibits an exophytic, frondlike growth pattern; is a well-differentiated SCC; and rarely spreads to lymph nodes.

Surgical resection may create a full-thickness defect of mucosa, muscle, and skin. Reconstruction of these defects requires restoration of internal lining as well as external skin coverage. Fasciocutaneous free flaps such as the scapula or radial forearm are useful in these cases. Although skin grafts are useful to restore mucosal surfaces, they frequently result in fibrosis, tethering the tongue and jaw.

Oropharynx

The oropharynx is bounded by junction of the hard and soft palate anteriorly, extending to the level of the hyoid bone (see

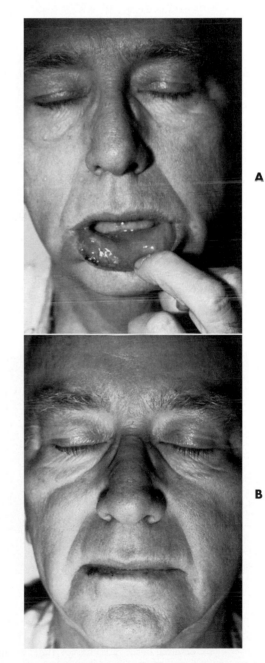

Figure 68-7. **A** and **B,** Squamous cell carcinoma of the lip.

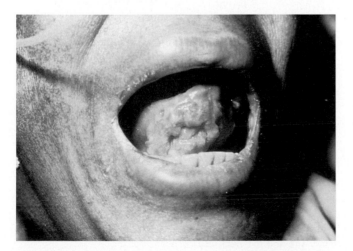

Figure 68-6. Squamous cell carcinoma of the anterior (immobile) tongue. Note raised margins and ulcerated center.

Figure 68-4) and includes soft palate, uvula, tonsil, pharyngeal wall, and the base of tongue. Carcinoma of the oropharynx is frequently poorly differentiated, having a greater propensity for nodal metastases and worse survival than oral cavity cancer.

Soft Palate

The soft palate is the only site in the oropharynx where cancer is consistently diagnosed at an early stage. Radiation therapy gives excellent local control. Surgery is usually reserved for very small and very large tumors because of the morbidity associated with loss of the soft palate.

Base of Tongue

The tongue base is posterior to the circumvallate papillae, extending to the vallecula. Cancer of the base of tongue is often occult and presents with nodal spread in 75% of cases. Surgical therapy is difficult and morbid because of the functional importance of this area adjacent to the larynx and because of its inaccessibility. A mandibulotomy or lateral pharyngotomy is often required for exposure, and fistula formation, inability to swallow, and aspiration frequently result. The 5-year survival

is ~50% for stage I and 10% to 20% for stage IV disease. Early exophytic lesions may be treated with radiation, either teletherapy or combined brachytherapy and teletherapy. Advanced, deeply invasive tumors are treated with surgery followed by radiation (Figure 68-8).

Tonsil

Cancer in the tonsil can be exophytic or deeply invasive. Anterior tonsillar pillar lesions tend to have a better prognosis and are grouped with retromolar trigone cancers of the oral cavity. Tonsillar fossa tumors are the more common and all tonsillar cancers appear to be more radiosensitive than other primary sites. Radiation is used with curative intent in the majority of T_1-T_3 cases, but combined therapy is indicated for large tumors or those that abut or invade the mandible or pterygoid muscles.

Hypopharynx

The area from the level of the hyoid bone to the lower border of the cricoid cartilage is composed of two distinct areas: the larynx and hypopharynx (see Figure 68-4). The pyriform sinus

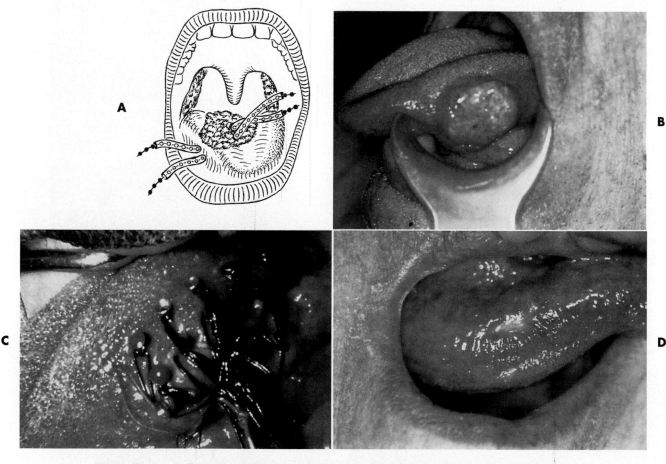

Figure 68-8. **A,** Brachytherapy or interstitial therapy of squamous cell carcinoma of the tongue. Catheters are placed through the tumor in an array to provide a high dose of radiation to the local area with a low dose to the adjacent areas. The radiation source is loaded into the catheters and removed after several days, at which time the catheters are removed. This is usually supplemented by external beam radiotherapy (teletherapy) to the primary site and the neck. **B,** Exophytic tongue lesion. **C,** Brachytherapy catheters in place. **D,** Postradiotherapy appearance.

is the site of the majority of the cancers seen in the hypopharynx. Lesions remain occult until they achieve large size, often invading the larynx and metastasizing to the cervical lymph nodes. Nodal spread occurs in over 66% of cases and is often bilateral, requiring a laryngopharyngectomy and bilateral neck dissections followed by radiation therapy. The rare T_1-T_2 lesions may be treated with a partial laryngopharyngectomy or radiation alone.

Larynx

The larynx is the most frequent site of SCC of the head and neck outside of the oral cavity. It has three anatomic areas with unique clinical features. The supraglottic larynx is composed of the epiglottis, aryepiglottic fold, and false vocal cords. Cancers in this area are frequently nonsymptomatic, causing hoarseness and dysphagia only when they reach large size or involve the epiglottis. Unlike the tumors of the intrinsic larynx, they metastasize to lymph nodes at an early stage and may involve jugular, submental, and submandibular nodes. Early stage disease can be treated effectively with a supraglottic laryngectomy or radiation therapy. More extensive disease involving the intrinsic larynx or base of tongue requires total laryngectomy and radiotherapy with neck dissection and possible reconstruction.

The glottis comprises the true vocal cords. The area has a paucity of lymphatics, and patients tend to present early with hoarseness or cough without neck metastases. Early glottic cancer can be treated effectively with radiation to the primary site alone. T_2 and T_3 lesions (cord fixation) can be treated with induction chemotherapy and radiation, preserving the larynx in over 60% of cases.[16]

The subglottic larynx below the true vocal cords is an infrequent site of laryngeal cancer. These cancers are difficult to diagnose and usually present in a late stage. Treatment is surgery followed by radiation. The prognosis in primary subglottic cancer is generally poor because of submucosal spread into the trachea and late diagnosis.

Paranasal Sinuses

Cancer of the paranasal sinuses is rare; it occurs most commonly in the maxillary sinus, with the ethmoid sinus being the second most frequent site. Most are epidermoid carcinomas, but 10% are of minor salivary gland origin, and 10% are lymphomas, sarcomas, or melanomas. T_1 and T_2 lesions of the maxillary sinus can be treated with surgery or radiation. More advanced lesions may invade the infratemporal fossa, the pterygoid muscles, or the orbit and nasal cavity, and require surgery and adjuvant radiotherapy. Lesions that invade or encroach on the skull base can be extirpated by a combined intracranial-extracranial approach.

MANAGEMENT OF THE NECK

Detailed knowledge of the cervical lymphatics is necessary to diagnose and treat cancer of the head and neck.[10] One third of the lymph nodes in the body are concentrated in the head and neck region. At the junction of the head and neck are groups of nodes named for their location: occipital, retroauricular, parotid, submandibular, submental, and retropharyngeal nodes. These nodes are frequently involved with metastatic skin cancer like melanoma. The second echelon nodes course along the internal jugular vein and spinal accessory nerve.

Standardization of description of the location of lymph node groups has been an important advance in studying the natural history of head and neck cancer and is useful in prognosis and treatment planning (see Figure 68-1).

Level I	Submental group: nodal tissue between the anterior belly of the digastric muscles and above the hyoid bone. Submandibular group: nodal tissue in the triangular area bounded by the anterior and posterior bellies of the digastric muscle and the inferior border of the mandible.
Level II	Upper jugular or jugulodigastric group: nodal tissue around upper portion internal jugular vein and the upper spinal accessory nerve. It extends from the skull base to the bifurcation of the carotid artery or the hyoid bone, the posterior limit is the posterior border of the sternocleidomastoid muscle, and the anterior border is the lateral border of the sternohyoid muscle.
Level III	Middle jugular group: nodal tissue around the middle third of the internal jugular vein from the inferior border of Level II to the omohyoid muscle. The anterior and posterior borders are the same as those for Level II.
Level IV	Lower jugular group: nodal tissue around the inferior third of the internal jugular vein from the inferior border of level III to the clavicle. The anterior and posterior borders are the same as those for Levels II and III.
Level V	Posterior triangle group: nodal tissue around the lower portion of the spinal accessory nerve and along the transverse cervical vessels. It is bounded by the triangle formed by the clavicle, posterior border of the sternocleidomastoid muscle, and anterior border of the trapezius muscle.
Level VI	Anterior compartment group: lymph nodes surrounding the midline visceral structures of the neck extending from the level of the hyoid bone superiorly to the suprasternal notch inferiorly. The lateral border is the medial border of the carotid sheath. Included are the parathyroidal and paratracheal lymph nodes and those along the recurrent laryngeal nerves.

The lymph nodes in the posterior triangle course along the spinal accessory nerve. The upper nodes in this group are in the anterior neck where there is a coalescence of nodes from both the upper jugular and spinal accessory group. These nodes are the drainage of the nose and upper extent of the aerodigestive tract. The spinal accessory nodes are infrequently involved in metastases from the oral cavity but preservation may be impossible because of proximity to the anterior jugular chain. Small nodes course along the transverse cervical vessels communicating with both the spinal accessory and jugular chains. They receive drainage from the skin of the lateral neck and chest. The nodes in this group are more frequently involved by metastatic carcinoma from below the clavicle (breast, lung, kidney, stomach, or lower gastrointestinal [GI] tract) than from the neck itself (e.g., Virchow's node).

The lymphatics of the anterior triangle course along the internal jugular vein. They are embedded in the fascia of the carotid sheath, and the majority lie on the anterolateral aspect of the vein. In the upper neck are found the jugulodigastric nodes, which are below the posterior belly of the digastric muscle behind the angle of the mandible. This important surgical area is a frequent site of cervical metastases, since it is the way station not only for drainage from Level I nodes in the neck, but also for the preauricular parotid and other facial nodes. Because of the common occurrence of extracapsular spread of lymph node metastases in this area, the spinal accessory nerve must be sacrificed to adequately remove nodes in this area. The jugular nodes are found where the omohyoid muscle crosses the carotid sheath. These drain the middle part of the aerodigestive tract, larynx, hypopharynx, and thyroid. The inferior nodes are below the omohyoid and drain the thyroid, esophagus, and trachea.

The risk of cervical node involvement is related to tumor stage/thickness, degree of vascular/neural invasion, and tumor angiogenesis.[45] The management of the neck is not site specific. The goals are to accurately stage the disease and decrease the likelihood of regional recurrence. Metastatic involvement of the cervical lymphatics reduces survival by 20% to 50% for all sites and is the single best prognostic factor in head and neck cancer. The most common manifestation of recurrence is regional relapse, so adequate treatment of the neck is mandatory.

The traditional primary role of lymph node dissection in head and neck cancer is to achieve locoregional control. Radical neck dissection, the removal of the envelope of tissue that contains the cervical lymph nodes, was first described by Crile in 1906.[14] The procedure removes all the lymph node–bearing tissue from the midline of the neck to the anterior border of the trapezius muscle and from the horizontal ramus of the mandible to the clavicle (levels I-V). The classic operation, popularized by Martin in the 1940s, includes the removal of the sternocleidomastoid muscle, internal jugular vein, and spinal accessory nerve. The upper portion of the nerve exits the jugular foramen in close proximity to the internal jugular vein. Dissection of the nerve in this area of the neck violates the anterior fascial compartment. The nerve then passes through the fascial envelope of the posterior triangle to innervate the trapezius muscle. Martin stressed that the nerve must be sacrificed to adequately extirpate the cervical lymphatics in the jugulodigastric area and posterior triangle. Metastases to the posterior triangle are extremely rare unless Level I-IV nodes are involved.

Sacrifice of the spinal accessory nerve is very debilitating. Nahum et al described the shoulder syndrome of pain and droop with scapular displacement in 1961.[31] Trapezius muscle paralysis limits abduction and support of the shoulder. Several studies have demonstrated successful grafting of the resected nerve with a portion of greater auricular nerve. Modifications of the radical neck dissection have been developed to preserve the spinal accessory nerve in early stage neck disease where Level V metastases are infrequent.

The recurrence rate for tumor in the neck following radical neck dissection has been reported from 10% to 70%. Failure of locoregional following radical neck dissection has been related to failure at the tumor primary site. Strong demonstrated 71% recurrence in the neck if multiple levels of nodes were involved at initial staging.[40] In this series there was 25% primary site failure as well.

Schneider et al found neck recurrences of 11% for N1 disease and 19% for N2 disease with the primary tumor controlled.[33] DeSanto reported recurrence rates in dissected necks at 2 years as: N0 7.5%, N1 20.2%, and N2 37.4%.[17] These results suggest that the efficacy of radical neck dissection decreases as the amount of disease in the neck increases and that there is a higher failure rate for advanced stage disease.

A number of modifications of radical neck dissection have been proposed to preserve one or more of the nonlymphatic structures ordinarily sacrificed in a radical neck dissection. Modified neck dissection has also been termed *functional neck dissection*. Bocca and Pignataro suggested removal of Levels I-V with preservation of the spinal accessory nerve, sternocleidomastoid muscle, and internal jugular vein.[6] The theoretic advantages of modified neck dissection are:
- Preservation of neck and shoulder girdle function.
- Better cosmetic contour of the neck.
- Protection of the internal carotid artery.
- Ability to perform simultaneous bilateral procedures safely.
- Use as an elective operation in clinical N0 necks.

Preservation of the spinal accessory nerve is an attempt to reduce the shoulder morbidity seen with a radical neck dissection. It is usually followed by a temporary, reversible phase of dysfunction resulting from traction or devascularization of the nerve. Preservation of the sternocleidomastoid muscle may improve the cosmetic contour of the neck and protect the carotid artery.

Bilateral cervical lymph node metastases are not an infrequent occurrence. Bilateral radical neck dissections are usually performed as staged procedures several weeks apart. Loss of both internal jugular veins may alter cerebral and facial circulation, although Crile believed that the vertebral venous system would provide adequate collateral circulation.[14] The perceived risks of bilateral jugular vein loss include death, brain damage, blindness, and permanent facial distortion. Ballantyne and Jackson reported a series of 179 synchronous bilateral radical neck dissections with a mortality rate of 3.4% comparable to unilateral neck dissection.[4] Elevation of the head, judicious fluid administration, and leaving one vein are cited as mechanisms to avoid complications.

As single-center experience with SCC of the upper aerodigestive tract has increased, pathologic analysis of prophylactic or elective neck dissection has suggested the actual risk of lymph node metastases to specific neck levels from any given primary site in the upper aerodigestive tract. This knowledge has given rise to the concept of *selective* neck dissection or removal only of those lymph nodes that are statistically likely to be involved. Thus, for a T_2N_0 anterior floor of mouth SCC, the *selective* neck dissection would remove levels I, II, and III only, since the likelihood of metastases to levels IV and V is extremely

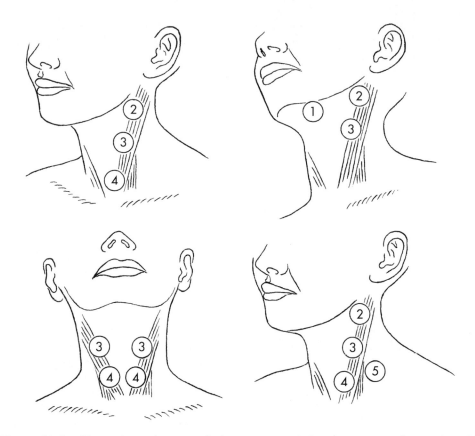

Figure 68-9. The various selective neck dissections are designed to remove the at-risk nodal stations for a given primary site when the neck is N_0 (no clinically palpable lymph nodes), while preserving the nonaffected structures. *1*, Submental nodes; *2*, jugulodigastric nodes; *3*, midjugular nodes; *4*, juguloomohyoid nodes; *5*, posterior triangle nodes.

small. Similarly, for a T_2N_0 lateral pyriform sinus SCC, the selective neck dissection would remove levels II, III, and IV, since subclinical metastasis would be rare in levels I and V (Figure 68-9). The presence of clinically apparent lymph node metastases or a previous dissection of some part of the neck makes the selective neck dissection concept less reliable.

Although less predictive in the head and neck than in the trunk and extremities, sentinel lymph node mapping by either vital dye staining or lymphoscintigraphy will undoubtedly increase our knowledge of lymph node metastatic patterns and probably influence future therapy.

CHEMOTHERAPY

The treatment of SCC of the head and neck metastatic to distinct sites is largely palliative. Radiation therapy to bony metastases can be important for pain relief and stabilization. Because of the shared risk factors of smoking, esophageal and lung cancers are common in patients presenting with or having been treated for SCC of the head and neck. A solitary lung mass in a patient with SCC of the head and neck is statistically more likely to be a primary lung cancer than a metastasis and should be fully evaluated.

OPERATIONS

SURGICAL APPROACH TO THE ORAL CAVITY AND OROPHARYNX

Since cure of SCC of the head and neck depends to a great degree on the adequacy of excision, good surgical exposure is of paramount importance. Small tumors of the anterior floor of mouth and tongue may be approached through the mouth. When the perioral exposure is limited, a midline lip splitting procedure is necessary. This minimizes injury to the lip musculature, vessels, and nerves. The vertical incision is halted at the deepest part of the chin cleft (Figure 68-10). It then follows a circular curve around the chin prominence to reach the midline below it. The incision can be continued to expose the submandibular area if a neck dissection is performed. The half circle is concave to the side of the neck dissection to prevent skin necrosis and facilitate a mandibulotomy. Whenever possible to preserve sensation to the lip, the mandible should be divided between the mental foramen and the insertion of the anterior belly of the digastric muscle to increase exposure. Although numerous patterns have been suggested, a straight bony cut is easiest and least traumatic to the dentition and can be easily reapproximated with a mandibular plate. This approach divides only the lingual mucosa and the mylohyoid muscle to allow the "mandibular swing" (Figure 68-11). The insertions of the

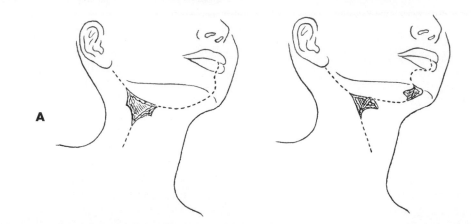

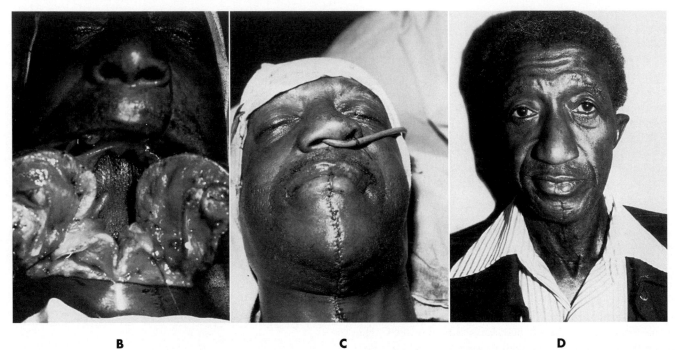

Figure 68-10. **A** to **D,** Midline lip splitting incision extended for exposure of upper neck.

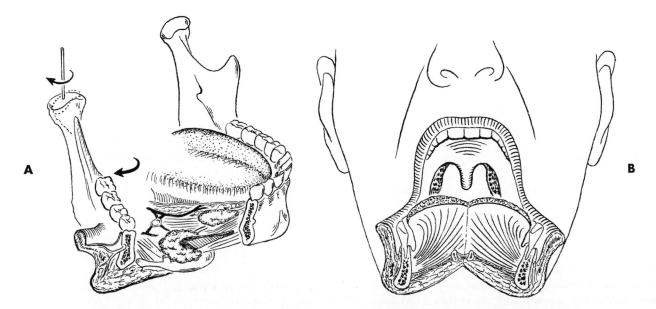

Figure 68-11. **A,** Mandibular swing procedure. Paramedian incisions preserve muscle attachments to the mandible. **B,** The midline Trotter approach provides excellent exposure of the base of tongue and posterior phalanges.

genioglossus, geniohyoid, and anterior digastric muscles are preserved, which may improve the blood supply to the mandible. The approach to superior lesions described by Trotter involves midline lip mandible and tongue split and has minimal interference with function.

SURGICAL MARGINS

Tumor recurrences are likely if surgical margins are positive, within 5 mm, or contain premalignant changes. The impact of positive margins is considerable. Vikram found a 73% recurrence rate when margins were positive for tumor compared with 39% when the margins were negative.[42] Multiple frozen sections from the excised specimen or from the remaining tissue are important to ensure tumor-free margins. In addition to conventional hematoxylin and eosin staining of oral tissues for margin analysis and tumor characterization, a number of more sensitive tests have been recently developed.

Mutations in p53 suppressor gene are found in 45% of invasive head and neck SCC. Polymerase chain reaction can sequence primary tumor DNA and make a probe specific to that tumor. Using this technique, surgical margins that are histologically negative may be found to contain cancer cells.[8] This may have clinical utility in the future.

RADICAL NECK DISSECTION

Sequence of Dissection
The classic description of radical neck dissection begins with the division of the sternocleidomastoid muscle and the internal jugular vein at the base of the neck. The operation then proceeds in the cephalad direction. This is technically easy but involves sacrifice of the spinal accessory nerve without assessment of the upper neck. This approach also increases venous engorgement of the upper end of the internal jugular vein and its tributaries, making ligation more difficult and increasing bleeding. It also fails to take advantage of the fact that the major vessels of the neck have no posterior branches except the occipital artery arising under the posterior belly of the digastric muscle. The resectability of the nodal metastases cannot be assessed until the neck dissection is almost completed.

Beginning in the submandibular triangle and proceeding laterally and inferiorly has several advantages. The majority of nodal metastases are in the upper neck and this allows early assessment of operability. This sequence allows assessment of the spinal accessory nerve's relationship to nodal metastases for possible nerve preservation. This operation is an attack on the tumor and not on the neck.

Surgical Exposure and Incisions
A superiorly based subplatysmal apron flap that extends from the mastoid tip to the mandibular symphysis provides good surgical exposure and adequate soft tissue coverage of the major vessels. A vertical extension along the anterior border of the trapezius muscle can provide additional exposure to the

posterior triangle (Figure 68-12). The incision can be incorporated into a lip splitting incision.

The skin flap is elevated over the inferior edge of the mandible and fixed with sutures. The greater auricular nerve and the external jugular vein are preserved for possible nerve grafting or recipient vessels for microvascular transfer.

Many different incisions for neck dissection have been advocated. The most useful incision will have a number of characteristics: ease of exposure of the underlying structures, adequate blood supply to the skin flaps, minimal effect on the vascularity of the facial skin, coverage of the carotid should wound dehiscence occur, convenience of extension for intraoral exposure, and acceptable early and late appearance. The McFee incision with two parallel transverse incisions, one in the upper neck from the hyoid to the border of the trapezius and the other just above the clavicle from the medial border of the sternocleidomastoid muscle to the border of the trapezius, encompasses all of the advantages.

Submental and Submandibular Dissection: Level I
This dissection begins with identification of the marginal mandibular nerve. It usually has multiple branches, which run

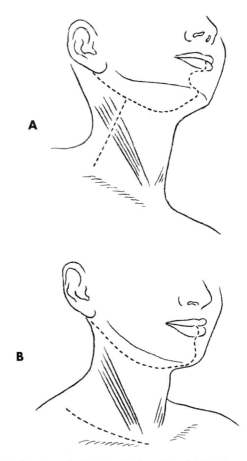

Figure 68-12. **A,** Superiorly based apron flap provides good exposure to the neck. An oblique extension can improve exposure to the posterior triangle. **B,** The parallel McFee incisions minimize exposure of the carotid artery in the event of a wound separation.

in areolar tissue between the platysma and the fascia surrounding the submandibular gland. The facial vessels are identified crossing the inferior border of the mandible at the anterior border of the masseter muscle. The nerve branches course superficial and variably cephalad or caudal to these vessels at the mandibles. The vessels are ligated below the nerve and retracted superiorly to get the marginal nerve branches out of the operative field.

The submental dissection begins by incising the deep cervical fascia off the contralateral anterior digastric muscle and along the inferior border of the mandible. The dissection begins by grasping the fascia and carefully dissecting it off the mylohyoid muscle, which forms the floor of the submental triangle. The dissection is continued laterally to the ipsilateral digastric muscle where the submental vessels branching from the facial vessels are encountered. These are ligated and divided and the submandibular dissection begun.

The digastric muscles provide a safe plane in which to operate. The submandibular gland is retracted laterally to expose the ipsilateral mylohyoid muscle (Figure 68-13, A). The free posterior margin of the mylohyoid is key to the submandibular dissection. It is retracted medially to reveal the deep portion of the submandibular gland lying on the hyoglossus muscle. The lingual nerve is located cephalad beneath the mandible and is attached to the gland by the submandibular ganglion. It must be carefully ligated to avoid troublesome bleeding. Wharton's duct is deep to the lingual nerve and is ligated carefully to avoid nerve injury. The hypoglossal nerve is located inferiorly below the digastric muscle (see Figure 68-8). It is accompanied by a plexus of veins. The fascia and gland are mobilized laterally. The facial artery is again ligated as it courses from deep to the digastric muscle around the posterior surface of the gland.

Upper Neck Dissection: Level II

The posterior belly of the digastric muscle is key to the dissection in this area. It is superficial to the vessels of the carotid sheath and hypoglossal nerve. The tail of the parotid gland is carefully divided to expose the retromandibular vein, which is ligated and divided. The insertion of the sternocleidomastoid muscle is divided with the electrocautery and retracted inferiorly to expose the posterior digastric muscle (Figure 68-13, B). The occipital artery runs parallel and deep to the muscle, which is retracted with a vein retractor to expose the internal jugular vein and splenius capitis muscle. Cranial nerve XII crosses over the bifurcation of the carotid vessels at a variable distance above the bifurcation. The ansa cervicalis, which provides motor innervation to the strap muscles, branches from the hypoglossal nerve and is divided. The vagus nerve can be identified between the internal jugular vein and the carotid artery. Exposure and manipulation of the carotid bifurcation may result in bradycardia and hypotension. Injection of 1% lidocaine into the adventitia of the carotid at the bifurcation

will alleviate this problem. The spinal accessory nerve is identified exiting the jugular foramen superficial to the internal jugular vein. In up to 30% of cases, it travels deep to the vein. If there is bulky nodal disease around the nerve or clinical evidence of extracapsular tumor spread, it is probably unsafe to attempt nerve preservation. If a short segment of nerve is adherent to tumor, it may be resected and a greater auricular nerve graft interposed using 9-0 nylon interrupted epineural sutures. The internal jugular vein is divided after placing two clamps proximal and one distal. The proximal stump is suture ligated followed by a second tie placed behind the second clamp. The contents of the submandibular triangle and upper neck dissection are now reflected inferiorly (Figure 68-14, A).

Posterior Neck Dissection

The posterior neck is dissected in continuity with the midneck dissection. The sternocleidomastoid muscle, nodal contents, and internal jugular vein have been reflected inferiorly and anteriorly baring the splenius capitis muscle, which forms the floor (Figure 68-14, B). The prevertebral fascia is identified and removed with the specimen, thus transecting the cervical plexus branches of C2-4 as they emerge from the fascia. At this point care must be taken not to pull the phrenic nerve up into the dissection. Dissection continues along the anterior border of the trapezius muscle, exposing the levator scapulae muscle until the omohyoid muscle is identified. The spinal accessory nerve emerges from under the sternocleidomastoid muscle at the midpoint of the muscle. This posterior plane is relatively avascular.

Lower Neck Dissection

The omohyoid muscle is key to the inferior neck dissection. It is superficial to the carotid sheath and is used as a guide to divide the sternocleidomastoid muscle. The brachial plexus and the phrenic nerve are behind and on top of the anterior scalene muscle respectively and are carefully preserved. The subclavian vein or artery may extend up into the neck and may be encountered behind the clavicle and in front of the scalene muscle. The thoracic duct is located behind the junction of the internal jugular vein and subclavian vein, so careful ligation of the fatty areola tissue in this area is important to avoid chyle fistula.

The sternal and clavicular heads of the sternocleidomastoid muscle are divided, exposing the omohyoid muscle, which is also divided. The proximal portion of the internal jugular vein is ligated in a similar manner to that previously described. The supraclavicular fat surrounding the omohyoid muscle contains the transverse cervical vessels. The vein is more superficial than the artery and courses parallel to the omohyoid muscle, which may be superficial or deep to it. The vein enters the internal or external jugular vein laterally. These vessels are excellent recipient vessels for free tissue transfer in the head and neck. Care is taken to avoid pulling the fatty tissue from behind the clavicle or damaging the apex of the pleura. The entire specimen is removed en bloc.

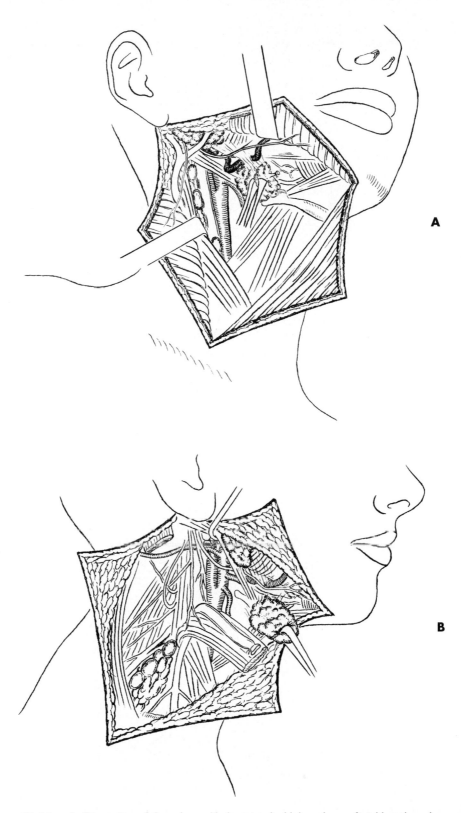

Figure 68-13. **A,** Dissection of the submandibular triangle. Unless the prefacial lymph nodes are involved by the cancer, the marginal mandibular nerve is preserved. The submandibular fascia is continuous with the parotid fascia by the pars interglandularis, which envelopes the contents superficial to the posterior belly of the digastric. **B,** Division of the attachments to the splenius capitis allows dissection along the posterior belly of the digastric, which exposes the jugular vein, accessory nerve, and occipital artery.

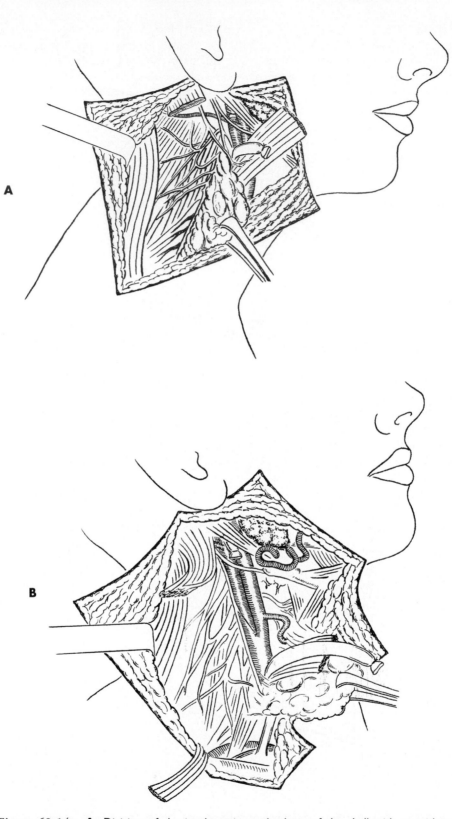

Figure 68-14. A, Division of the jugular vein at the base of the skull with or without the accessory nerve decreases the venous hypertension in the dissection. The attachments to the trapezius are divided, and the dissection is carried down into the posterior triangle, taking care not to place excess traction on the cervical plexus branches, thus injuring the phrenic nerve. **B,** Division of the posterior triangle fat and lymphatics and the omohyoid muscle reveals the jugular vein in the lower neck. Careful attention to ligation at the base of the jugular will minimize chyle leak. Division of the inferior jugular vein and freeing the fascial attachments to the strap muscles allow en bloc removal of the neck contents.

MODIFIED NECK DISSECTION

Various modifications of classical neck dissection have been advocated for elective or prophylactic neck dissection or when the extent of metabolic disease is minimal.

Surgical Approach

The cervical lymphatics are removed by careful dissection of the investing and prevertebral layers of the deep cervical fascia (see Figure 68-16). The sternocleidomastoid muscle, internal jugular vein, and spinal accessory nerve are dissected free of the fascia. The entire dissection is performed through an anterior approach by retracting the sternocleidomastoid muscle laterally. The posterior triangle is dissected from underneath the muscle with preservation of the cervical plexus. The exposure and submandibular dissection are identical for that described for the radical neck dissection.

Fascial Dissection

The investing layer of the deep cervical fascia is incised along the anterior border of the sternocleidomastoid muscle. When possible, the greater auricular nerve is preserved by carefully dissecting it out of the parotid tail. The investing fascia is grasped and retracted medially. The sternocleidomastoid muscle is retracted laterally and the small perforating vessels entering the muscle from the fascia are cauterized. The fascial dissection is carried to the posterior edge of the sternocleidomastoid muscle where the investing fascia joins the prevertebral fascia. This fascia is reflected medially off the deep cervical muscles (splenius capitis, levator scapulae, and scalene muscles), preserving the cervical plexus and phrenic nerve branches (see Figure 68-13).

Posterior Neck Dissection

The spinal accessory nerve exits behind the sternocleidomastoid muscle at approximately its midpoint (Erb's point). The greater auricular nerve courses obliquely over the sternocleidomastoid muscle at this point. Working from underneath the sternocleidomastoid muscle, the contents of the posterior triangle are reflected medially. The posterior margin of dissection is several centimeters from the edge of the trapezius muscle. The inferior limit of the dissection is the transverse cervical artery and the omohyoid muscle. This is usually several centimeters above the clavicle.

Central Neck Dissection

Normally, the jugular vein is lateral but traction of the investing fascia pulls it medial to the carotid artery. Thus the carotid artery is encountered first with dissection of the central neck. Sharp scalpel dissection directly against the vessel releases the fascia and adventitia. The vagus nerve is identified between the vessels, and the hypoglossal nerve is seen crossing the carotid artery at approximately its bifurcation. The fascial and nodal contents are then reflected over the internal jugular vein. The facial vein is ligated proximally to release the contents of the submandibular triangle.

Upper Neck Dissection

The dissection of the upper neck is the most important and difficult portion of a modified neck dissection. Clinical judgment is necessary to determine whether the spinal accessory nerve can be preserved while adequately removing the cervical lymphatics. The upper third of the nerve must be identified prior to its entrance into the sternocleidomastoid muscle (Figure 68-15). The tail of the parotid is divided with the electrocautery and the posterior facial vein divided to expose the posterior belly of the digastric muscle. The spinal accessory nerve is identified exiting the jugular foramen underneath the digastric muscle. The nerve is carefully dissected out of the surrounding tissue until it enters the sternocleidomastoid muscle. It is retracted medially with a vein retractor and the sternocleidomastoid muscle retracted laterally to expose the upper spinal accessory nodal tissue lateral to the nerve. The fascia overlying the splenius capitis muscle is incised, grasped, and reflected under the nerve and over the internal jugular vein and carotid artery to join the contents of the central neck dissection (Figure 68-16).

HEAD AND NECK RECONSTRUCTION

Reconstruction after extirpation of head and neck cancer continues to be a surgical challenge. The majority of patients are debilitated and present with locally advanced disease. Poor long-term survival and the need for adjuvant radiotherapy demand that in most cases the reconstruction should be immediate and single stage, should allow a rapid restoration of function, and should have a low morbidity.

Edgerton introduced the concept of immediate reconstruction after resection of head and neck cancer in 1951.[18] Unfortunately at that time there were limited options for reconstruction and most efforts were multistaged, with each stage at high risk of failure. McGregor introduced the axial patterned forehead flap in 1963 based on the superficial temporal vessels; this advanced the concept of primary reconstruction, bringing it closer to single stage.[27] Bakamjian, in 1965, introduced the deltopectoral flap based on the axial extension of branches of the internal mammary artery entering the skin of the chest wall through the second, third, and fourth intercostal spaces. This would become the reconstructive workhorse for over a decade.[3]

In the 1970s the concept of the musculocutaneous flap was elucidated, greatly improving the ability to transfer in a single stage a large amount of well-vascularized skin and muscle into the head and neck. The pectoralis major musculocutaneous flap was promulgated by Ariyan in 1979.[2] Based on the thoracoacromial vessels, it is a reliable, bulky flap near the extirpative operative field with a favorable rotation arc (see Figure 68-18). Careful reconstructive planning allows the use of both the deltopectoral and the pectoralis major flap in the same patient (Figure 68-17, A). It continues to be used successfully in many sites in the head and neck including the oral cavity, oropharynx, and hypopharynx.

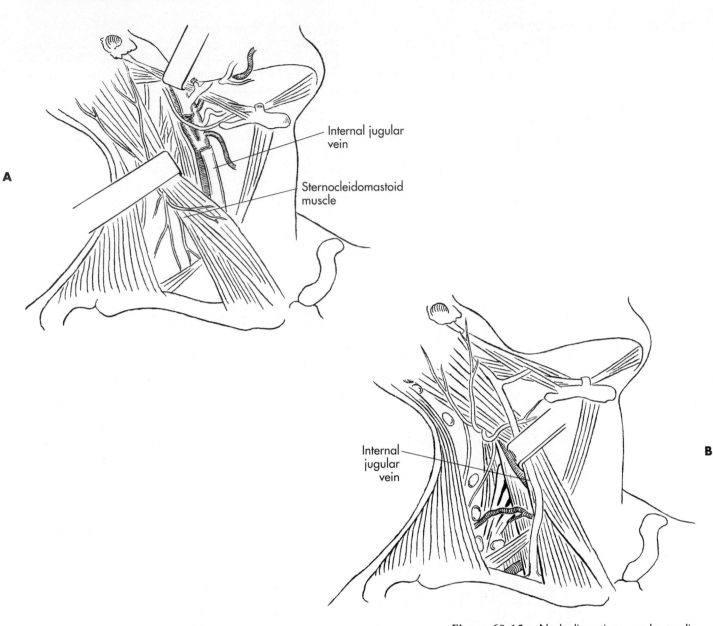

A

Internal jugular vein

Sternocleidomastoid muscle

Internal jugular vein

B

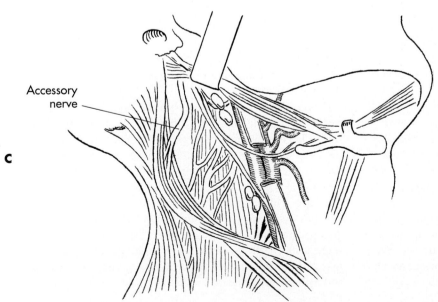

Accessory nerve

C

Figure 68-15. Neck dissections can be modified to preserve the sternocleidomastoid muscle **(A)**, the jugular vein **(B)**, and the accessory nerve **(C).** *Continued*

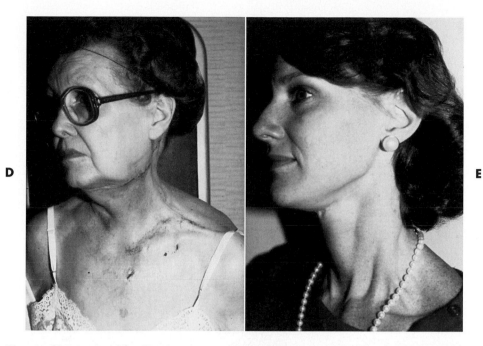

Figure 68-15, cont'd. D, Appearance after standard radical neck dissection removing sternocleidomastoid muscle, jugular vein, and accessory nerve. **E,** Appearance of the modified neck dissection preserving sternocleidomastoid muscle and accessory nerve but taking the jugular vein.

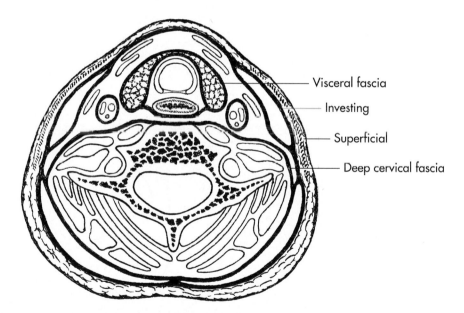

— Visceral fascia

— Investing

— Superficial

— Deep cervical fascia

Figure 68-16. The fascial layers of the neck: *Superficial* (platysma and superficial musculoaponeurotic system); *investing* (surrounds sternocleidomastoid and lymph nodes, also referred to as superficial layer of the deep cervical fascia); *deep cervical fascia* (surrounds trapezius, scalenes, etc.); and *visceral fascia* (surrounds thyroid and trachea).

Microvascular free tissue transfer has supplanted the pectoralis major flap for the majority of head and neck reconstruction. It is a great advance in the treatment of head and neck cancer because it provides restoration of form and function not possible using conventional flaps; unique, specialized tissue with an independent blood supply can be used; and there is freedom from rotation arcs. Disadvantages include the demands for microsurgical expertise and equip-ment, prolonged operative times, and a 3% to 7% risk of flap failure.

Preoperative Evaluation

Major head and neck reconstruction requires coordination between the ablative and reconstructive surgeon. A preopera-tive assessment of the anticipated defect includes size, mu-cosal lining, bone, and soft tissue coverage. The patient's

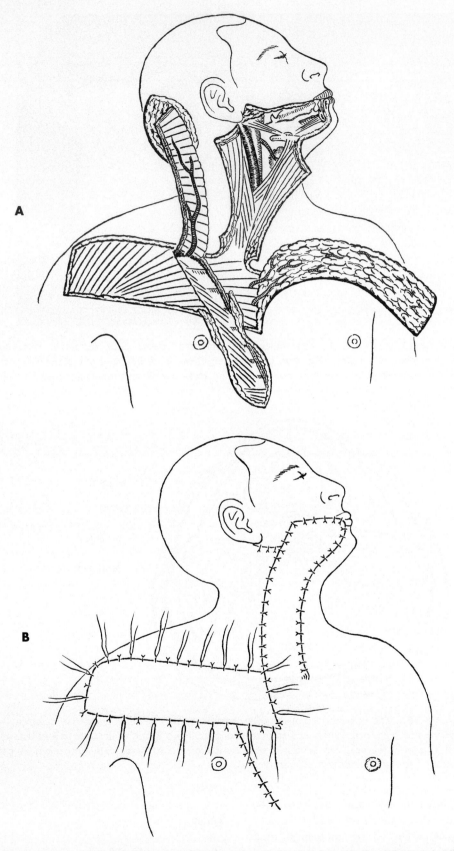

Figure 68-17. **A** and **B,** The pectoralis major flap can be designed with the deltopectoral flap to provide good coverage in the head and neck both for oral lining and muscle cover of the carotid artery.

overall medical condition and performance status must be considered prior to planning a potentially long and complicated reconstruction.

Oral Cavity Reconstruction

Reconstruction in the oral cavity must preserve tongue mobility for speech and swallowing. Small defects can be closed with skin grafts or local mucosal or skin nasolabial flaps. Tongue flaps are occasionally useful but must be designed so as not to interfere with residual tongue mobility. Defects larger than several centimeters require flap closure to prevent tongue tethering. The radial forearm free flap has become the flap of choice for intraoral reconstruction. It is a thin, pliable fasciocutaneous flap based on the radial artery and accompanying veins. The remote donor site is advantageous for a two-team operative approach, reducing procedure time. It can be used as a sensate flap by suturing the lingual nerve to the lateral antebrachial cutaneous nerve. Other skin flaps useful in oral reconstruction are the scapula flap, lateral arm flap, lateral thigh flap, and the various groin flaps.

There is no satisfactory method to reconstruct the tongue. Reconstructive priorities include airway protection, swallowing, and articulation. Although creation of an adequate conduit between lips and esophagus is the primary goal, some surgeons believe the donor tissue should be bulky enough to fill the oral cavity and allow a seal to form against the palate. This may seal and assist in the propulsion of food and articulation. A pectoralis major musculocutaneous flap or a rectus abdominis free flap can be used to restore tongue bulk when a total glossectomy or base of tongue resection is performed. A functional advantage of one method over the other has never been documented. Laryngeal suspension in a cephalad and anterior vector is one of the most important parts of the reconstruction and will allow decannulation in the majority of patients when the larynx is preserved. The majority of patients maintain intelligible speech and swallow without aspiration.

Mandibular Reconstruction

The method of reconstruction depends on the defect size, location, and soft tissue involvement. Loss of the lateral mandible may be well tolerated without reconstruction, but unopposed masticatory muscle pull can occasionally result in pain and dysphagia. Defects involving anterior arches alone or in combination with other sites demand reconstruction because of loss of support for the tongue and larynx. Alloplastic reconstruction plates can restore the mandibular contour but will not permit dental restoration and have a high extrusion rate at all sites but especially in the anterior dental arch. Autogenous bone grafts tolerate radiation poorly and have a limited role in the primary or secondary reconstruction of head and neck cancer patients.

Vascularized free bone flaps, such as the fibula, iliac crest, radius, and scapula, have become the method of choice. They promote primary bone healing, resist radiotherapy, and allow dental restoration with osseointegrated implants. The fibula free flap can provide a segment of sturdy bone and overlying skin 25-cm or longer depending on body habit. It is based on

numerous segmental perforators from the peroneal artery. The remote donor site is advantageous, and loss of the fibula is well tolerated both aesthetically and functionally.

Hypopharyngeal Reconstruction

The pectoralis major musculocutaneous flap is useful to repair partial pharyngectomy defects and fistulas that develop after laryngectomy. Its bulk makes it a poor choice for total reconstruction of the hypopharynx and cervical esophagus. Free jejunal transfer has become the method of choice for circumferential reconstruction. A segment of proximal jejunum is isolated on its mesentery and bowel continuity reestablished. The segment is transferred to the neck and sutured to the base of tongue and cervical esophagus in an isoperistaltic manner. Microvascular anastomoses are then performed to vessels in the neck. A tubed radial forearm free flap can be used in instances where a laparotomy is not possible, and this method is particularly good when a patch closure is appropriate or the neck has been previously dissected and vascular anastomosis must be carried out in the lower neck or supraclavicular area. The potential for lower donor site morbidity and improved prosthetic voice restoration are advantages in this technique.[1] When an esophagectomy is required, a gastric transposition based on the right gastric and epiploic arteries can reestablish enteric continuity.

OUTCOMES

NATURAL HISTORY OF SQUAMOUS CELL CARCINOMA OF THE HEAD AND NECK

Stage I disease has a greater than 80% cure rate when treated with radiation therapy or surgery. Stage II disease has a greater than 60% cure rate when treated with either modality. In these patients, other diseases and the development of second primary cancers pose a greater threat to survival than recurrences of the primary head and neck cancer.

Cervical lymph node metastases reduce survival by approximately 50%. Extracapsular nodal disease is a particularly bad prognostic sign. Fewer than 30% of patients with locally advanced disease (Stage III/IV) are cured. The outcome is slightly better for patients with Stage III laryngeal cancer. The majority of patients die with locally or regionally persistent or recurrent disease as well as disseminated disease.

COMPLICATIONS

Infection

Neck dissection alone is clean, uncontaminated surgery and requires no antibiotic prophylaxis; however, the majority of head and neck surgery is contaminated, and prophylactic antibiotics are necessary for at least 24 hours after surgery to cover indigenous aerobic and anaerobic organisms, especially gram-positive bacteria.

The risk of infection is greater in patients who have advanced disease, who have concurrent systemic illnesses like diabetes, and who have received preoperative radiotherapy. Despite prophylactic antibiotic therapy, wound infection is a major source of morbidity after contaminated head and neck surgery. Wound infection has also been associated with a higher tumor recurrence rate.

Neck Dissection

Conley cited an operative mortality of 1% and a wound complication rate of 5% to 10% for cervical lymphadenectomy.[12] Closed suction drainage has decreased the incidence of seromas and hematomas.

A chylous fistula may result from division of the main or accessory thoracic duct. It results in massive plasma loss and hypoalbuminemia. The initial treatment is adequate drainage and pressure dressings. Dietary restriction of fats may be beneficial. Earlier reoperation is indicated for patients with greater than 60 cc/24-hours drainage. An infusion of intralipid causes the chyle to become milky and may help identify the disrupted lymphatics at the time of surgery. Tetracycline sclerotherapy of the area surrounding the leak has been shown to be helpful in select cases.

Oropharyngocutaneous Fistula

Early postoperative fistula formation is a consequence of mucosal suture line disruption secondary to technical error such as suturing inadequate mucosa under tension. Conley reported a 10% to 30% incidence after composite resection and a 22% to 50% incidence after laryngectomy.[12] Fistula or suture line leakage can result in infection or abscess formation in the neck, which may thrombose the blood supply to the reconstruction, resulting in flap failure. Definitive therapy depends on the fistula location and on whether prior irradiation had been administered. A small fistula in a nonirradiated patient will almost always close spontaneously with local wound care and adequate nutrition. Prompt surgery is indicated for any fistula that contaminates the carotid artery in an irradiated neck to prevent *carotid artery blowout,* which is associated with a mortality approaching 50%. Treatment requires resection of the involved vessel, arterial repair if possible, and muscle flap coverage usually with a pectoralis major muscle flap (Figure 68-18).

Radiotherapy

Complications include xerostomia, delayed wound healing, fibrosis, trismus, and soft tissue necrosis. *Osteoradionecrosis of the mandible* is an infrequent but serious consequence of radiotherapy to the oral cavity. Symptoms including pain, trismus, and fistula formation usually become apparent only after the bone has become septic. Conservative management includes oral hygiene, antibiotics, minor debridement, and hyperbaric oxygen. Surgery is indicated for intractable pain, persistent bone exposure, fistula, and pathologic fracture. Surgical treatment includes aggressive debridement and flap coverage.

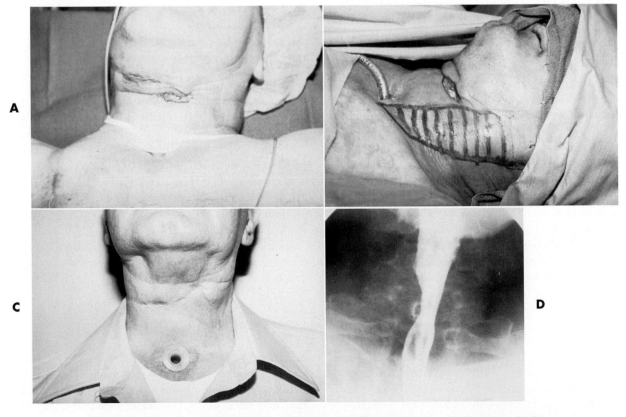

Figure 68-18. **A** to **D,** Closure of a small pharyngocutaneous fistula with the sternocleidomastoid musculocutaneous flap in a patient who underwent salvage laryngectomy after radiation failure.

Pedicled Versus Free Flap Reconstruction

There are little data in the literature comparing the results of pedicled vs. free flaps in head and neck reconstruction. Carlson et al examined various methods used to reconstruct the hypopharynx and cervical esophagus.[11] Free jejunal transfer resulted in shorter hospitalization, more rapid restoration of oral intake, and a lower incidence of flap necrosis than pedicled musculocutaneous flaps. The M.D. Anderson Cancer Center published results comparing pectoralis major musculocutaneous flaps with radial forearm and rectus abdominis free flaps.[23,24] Free flap reconstruction was found to have lower complication rates, better aesthetic outcomes, less donor site morbidity, and shorter hospital stay, and provided superior cost-effectiveness in head and neck reconstruction compared with pedicled flaps.

Because many patients who develop head and neck cancers present with advanced stage disease and the overall cure rate is only 30% to 50% in these patients, it is crucial that the therapeutic interventions that are chosen are most efficient in restoring optimal function and as normal an appearance as possible. Derangement of the main vegetative functions of the human organism, respiration and alimentation (and their corollary functions, speech and swallowing), is a common consequence of therapy. The advent of microvascular surgery and the elucidation of vascular anatomy encouraged by the musculocutaneous concept have greatly enhanced the principle of single-stage radical resection and reconstruction. Thus, although 89% of failures of therapy with advanced head and neck cancer will occur within 2 years, many of these patients can experience comfortable, functional lives without the need for multistaged operative reconstructions.

REFERENCES

1. Anthony JP, Singer MI, Mathes SJ: Pharyngoesophageal reconstruction using the tubed radial forearm flap, *Clin Plast Surg* 21:137-147, 1994.

2. Ariyan S: The pectoralis major myocutaneous flap: a versatile flap for reconstruction in the head and neck, *Plast Reconstr Surg* 63:73, 1979.

3. Bakamjian VY: A two-stage method for pharyngoesophageal reconstruction with a primary pectoral skin flap, *Plast Reconstr Surg* 36:173, 1965.

4. Ballantyne AJ, Jackson GL: Synchronous bilateral neck dissection, *Am J Surg* 144:452-455, 1982.

5. Benninger MS, Enrique RR, Nichols RD: Symptom-directed selective endoscopy and cost containment for evaluation of head and neck cancer, *Head Neck* 15:532-536, 1993.

6. Bocca E, Pignataro O: A conservation technique in radical neck dissection, *Ann Otol Rhinol Laryngol* 76:975-979, 1967.

7. Boring CC, Squires TS, Tong T: Cancer statistics, 1992, *CA Cancer J Clin* 42:19-38, 1992.

8. Brennan JA: Molecular assessment of histopathological staging in squamous-cell carcinoma of the head and neck, *N Engl J Med* 332:1995, 1995.

9. Brown LM, Mason TJ, Pickle LW: Occupational risk factors for laryngeal cancer on the Texas Gulf Coast, *Cancer Res* 48:1960-1964, 1988.

10. Carlson GW: Surgical anatomy of the neck, *Surg Clin North Am* 73:837-852, 1993.

11. Carlson GW, Schusterman MA, Guillamondegui OM: Total reconstruction of the hypopharynx and cervical esophagus: a 20-year experience, *Ann Plast Surg* 29:408-412, 1992.

12. Conley JJ: Oropharyngocutaneous fistula. In Conley JJ, editor: *Complications of head and neck surgery,* Philadelphia, 1979, WB Saunders, p 92-98.

13. Cowan JM, et al: Cytogenic evidence of the multistep origin of head and neck squamous cell carcinomas, *J Natl Cancer Inst* 84:793-797, 1992.

14. Crile G: Excision of cancer of the head and neck: with special reference to the plan of dissection based upon 132 operations, *J Am Med Assoc* 47:1780-1785, 1906.

15. Decker J, Goldstein JC: Risk factors in head and neck cancer, *N Engl J Med* 306:1151-1155, 1982.

16. Department of Veterans Affairs Laryngeal Cancer Study Group: Induction chemotherapy plus radiation compared with surgery plus radiation in patients with advanced laryngeal cancer, *N Engl J Med* 324:1685-1690, 1991.

17. DeSanto LW: Neck dissection: is it worthwhile? *Laryngoscope* 92:502, 1982.

18. Edgerton MT: Replacement of lining to oral cavity following surgery, *Cancer* 4:110, 1951.

19. Fujimori R: "Gate flap" for the total reconstruction of the lower lip, *Br J Plast Surg* 33:340, 1980.

20. Hong WK, et al: Prevention of second primary tumors with isotretinoin in squamous-cell carcinoma of the head and neck, *N Engl J Med* 323;795-801, 1990.

21. Jacobs CD: Etiologic considerations for head and neck squamous cancers. In Jacobs CD, Editor: *Carcinomas of the head and neck: evaluation and management,* Boston, 1990, Kluwer Academic, p 265-282.

22. Karapandzic M: Reconstruction of lip defects by local arterial flaps, *Br J Plast Surg* 27:93, 1974.

23. Kroll SS, Reece GP, Miller MJ, et al: Comparison of the rectus abdominis free flap with the pectoralis major myocutaneous flap for reconstructions in the head and neck, *Am J Surg* 164:615-618, 1992.

24. Lippman SM, et al: Comparison of low-dose isotretinoin with beta carotene to prevent oral carcinogenesis, *N Engl J Med* 328:15-20, 1993.

25. Lund VJ, Howard DJ: Head and neck cancer in the young: a prognostic evaluation of head and neck masses, *Am J Surg* 159:482-485, 1990.

26. Mashberg A, Feldman LJ: Clinical criteria for identifying early oral and oropharyngeal carcinoma: erythroplasia revisited, *Am J Surg* 156:273, 1988.

27. McGregor IA: Temporal flap in intraoral cancer: its use in repairing the post-excisional defect, *Br J Surg* 16:318, 1963.

28. McGregor IA: Reconstruction of the lower lip, *Br J Plast Surg* 36:40, 1983.

29. Moore C: Cigarette smoking and cancer of the mouth, pharynx, and larynx, *JAMA* 218:553, 1971.

30. Muscat JE, Wynder EL: Tobacco, alcohol, asbestos, and occupational risk factors for laryngeal cancer, *Cancer* 69:2244-2251, 1992.

31. Nahum AM, Mullaly W, Marmor L: A syndrome resulting from radical neck dissection, *Arch Otol* 74:82-86, 1961.

32. Sadove RC, Luce EA, McGrath PC: Reconstruction of the lower lip and chin with the composite radial forearm-palmaris longus free flap, *Plast Reconstr Surg* 88:209, 1991.

33. Schneider JJ: Control by irradiation alone of nonfixed clinically positive lymph nodes from squamous cell carcinoma of the oral cavity, oropharynx, supraglottic larynx, and hypopharynx, *Am J Roentgenol* 123:42, 1975.

34. Schusterman MA, Kroll SS, Weber RS, et al: Intraoral soft tissue reconstruction after cancer ablation: a comparison of the pectoralis major flap and the radial forearm flap, *Am J Surg* 162:397-399, 1991.

35. Schwartz R, Chan NH, MacFarlane JK: Fine needle aspiration cytology in the evaluation of head and neck masses, *Am J Surg* 159:482-485, 1990.

36. Shaha AR: Preoperative evaluation of the mandible in patients with carcinoma of the floor of mouth, *Head Neck* 13:398-402, 1991.

37. Slaughter DP, Southwick HW, Smejkal W: Field cancerization in oral stratified squamous epithelium, *Cancer* 6:963, 1953.

38. Som PM: Detection of metastasis in cervical lymph nodes: CT and MR criteria and differential diagnosis, *AJR* 158:961-969, 1992.

39. Spitz MR, Fueger JJ, Goepfert H: Squamous cell carcinoma of the aerodigestive tract: a case comparison analysis, *Cancer* 61:203, 1988.

40. Strong EW: Preoperative radiation and radical neck dissection, *Surg Clin North Am* 49:271-276, 1969.

41. Thompson LW: Head and neck cancer: early detection, *Semin Surg Oncol* 5:168, 1989.

42. Vikram B: Failure at the primary site following multimodality treatment in advanced head and neck cancer, *Head Neck Surg* 6:720, 1984.

43. Waldron CA, Shafer WG: Leukoplakia revisited: a clinicopathologic study of 3256 oral leukoplakias, *Cancer* 36:1386, 1975.

44. Watts SL, Brewer EE, Fry TL: Human papillomavirus DNA types in squamous cell carcinomas of the head and neck, *Oral Surg Oral Med Oral Pathol* 71:701-707, 1991.

45. Williams JK, et al: Tumor angiogenesis as a prognostic factor in oral cavity tumors, *Am J Surg* 168:373-380, 1994.

Dental and Maxillofacial Considerations

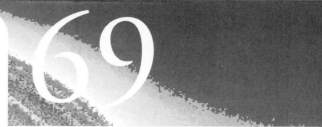

Barry L. Eppley

INTRODUCTION

The oral cavity and its surrounding maxillofacial skeletal encasement not only are situated at the central point of the head and neck but also offer the main portal of entry into this region. They constitute a remarkable articulating skeletal structure (mandible) that unites with a fixed well-aerated set of paired bones (maxilla) that serves to separate the mouth from the nose. At the interface of these maxillofacial skeletal structures is the dentition, a set of 28 to 32 harder-than-bone units, whose interdigitation is responsible for mastication and deglutition but is also a reflection of facial skeletal balance and temporomandibular joint function.

Understanding occlusal and facial skeletal anatomy and physiology is paramount to a satisfactory facial reconstruction. It is no longer adequate to accept an orofacial reconstruction where a mass of tissue, albeit well vascularized, fills in the deficit. The large number of reconstructive procedures and flaps now available makes it possible to specifically "tailor" most orofacial reconstructions. Despite this tremendous diversity of contemporary plastic surgery procedures, a proper functioning and anatomically correct reconstruction may not be achieved if basic dental and maxillofacial principles are not applied.

INDICATIONS

Diagnostic and therapeutic endeavors of the head and neck require an appreciation and understanding of those structures that constitute the oral cavity and render its function, the teeth, the jaws, and the soft tissue that envelops them.

DENTAL ANATOMY

An individual tooth has three subunits: the *crown* (exposed portion of the tooth assuming a healthy periodontium), the *neck* (submerged portion beneath the periodontium that extends down to the alveolus), and the *root* (portion contained within the bone).[1] Each portion of a tooth is composed of different specialized hard tissue that serves a specific function. The crown is covered with enamel, which can tolerate the forces required for chewing and grinding. Cementum, a much softer substance than enamel, surrounds the outer portion of the neck and root of the tooth, providing connective tissue attachment to the adjacent periodontium and alveolar bone.[4] Any force or trauma that fractures or separates the roots of teeth makes them unsalvageable. Separation of the crown or neck from the root, however, may still allow prosthetic restoration (Figure 69-1).

The development and eruption of teeth occur through primary (deciduous) and secondary (permanent) dentition phases.[5] At birth, the tooth-bearing processes of both the maxilla and mandible contain the partially formed crowns of the 20 deciduous teeth. In the first 2 years, all of the deciduous teeth erupt into the oral cavity, initiated by the central incisors (with the lower central incisors typically preceding the upper central incisors) and followed by the first molars, the cuspids, and the second molars (Figure 69-2). The most common nomenclature to identify these deciduous teeth by quadrant is:

(maxillary right)	e d c b a / a b c d e	(maxillary left)
(mandibular right)	e d c b a / a b c d e	(mandibular left)

Where:

a = Primary central incisor
b = Primary lateral incisor
c = Primary cuspid (canine)
d = Primary first molar
e = Primary second molar

They may also be described in successive alphabetical fashion (a to t) starting at the right maxillary second molar (a), extending around the arch to the left maxillary second molar (j), dropping down to the mandibular left second molar (k),

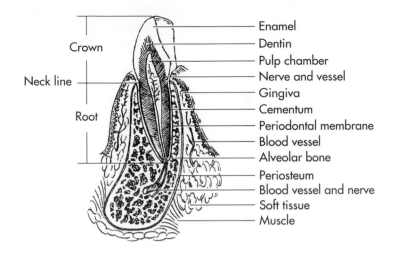

Figure 69-1. Dental anatomy and local relationships to the bony and soft tissue components of the mandible.

Crown
Neck line
Root

Enamel
Dentin
Pulp chamber
Nerve and vessel
Gingiva
Cementum
Periodontal membrane
Blood vessel
Alveolar bone
Periosteum
Blood vessel and nerve
Soft tissue
Muscle

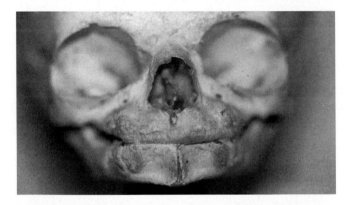

Figure 69-2. Fetal maxillomandibular skeleton. The entire maxilla and mandible are filled with developing primary teeth surrounded by thin overlying bone.

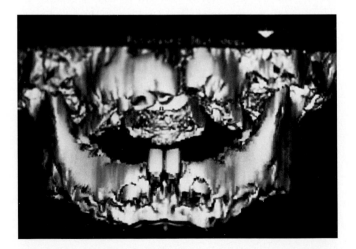

Figure 69-3. Three-dimensional CT scan of 6-month-old infant with fully erupted mandibular primary central incisors. The symphysis and body of the mandible can be seen to be filled with developing teeth.

and going around the mandibular arch to the right maxillary second molar (t) (Figure 69-3).

$$\frac{a\ b\ c\ d\ e\ /\ f\ g\ h\ i\ j}{t\ s\ r\ q\ p\ /\ o\ n\ m\ l\ k}$$

Between the ages of 3 and 6 years, no other teeth usually erupt into the oral cavity. The developing permanent teeth within the jaws continue to grow, and the alveolar processes—which develop as supporting structures for the teeth—contribute to the increased vertical dimension of the jaws and the lower portion of the face. The transverse growth of the jaws is usually evident by the spacing that occurs between the deciduous incisor teeth. It is important to appreciate that during this age period the entire midfacial and lower facial skeleton, from the infraorbital rims to the inferior border of the mandible, is completely filled with erupted primary teeth and unerupted and developing permanent teeth (Figure 69-4).

By the age of 6, the first permanent molar teeth erupt, beginning a 6-year transitional period in which the primary dentition will exfoliate and be replaced by the permanent dentition. Each of the primary teeth will be replaced by a permanent tooth of the same type except the primary molars, which will be replaced by permanent bicuspid teeth, and the permanent first, second, and third molars, which develop posterior to the second primary molar and thus have no antecedent teeth. Therefore the permanent dentition has 12 more teeth (a total of 32) than the primary dentition. The order of permanent tooth eruption is typically central and lateral incisors (6, 7, and 8 years of age), cuspids (9 and 10 years of age), bicuspids (10, 11, and 12 years of age), and first and second molars (12 and 13 years of age). The third molars (often referred to as wisdom teeth) do not erupt until the cessation of jaw growth between 17 to 21 years of age (Figure 69-5). As with the primary dentition, the permanent dentition is usually

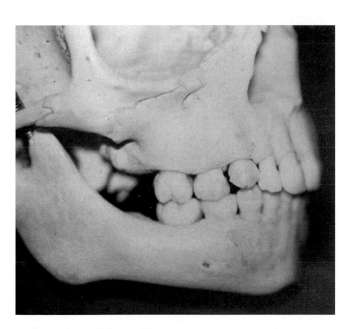

Figure 69-4. Pediatric (3-year-old) facial skeleton with fully erupted primary dentition. The surrounding maxilla and mandible are now filled with the developing permanent teeth from the infraorbital foramen to the inferior border of the mandible.

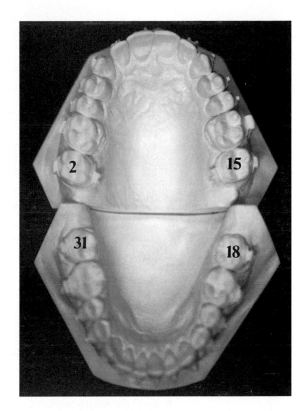

Figure 69-5. Plaster casts of permanent teeth including their numbering. Note that the third molars (numbers 1, 16, 17, and 32) have been removed in this patient.

described by quadrants, although with numbers rather than letters:

$$\frac{8\ 7\ 6\ 5\ 4\ 3\ 2\ 1\ /\ 1\ 2\ 3\ 4\ 5\ 6\ 7\ 8}{8\ 7\ 6\ 5\ 4\ 3\ 2\ 1\ /\ 1\ 2\ 3\ 4\ 5\ 6\ 7\ 8}$$

Where:

1 = Permanent central incisor
2 = Permanent lateral incisor
3 = Permanent cuspid (canine)
4 = Permanent first premolar
5 = Permanent second premolar
6 = Permanent first molar
7 = Permanent second molar
8 = Permanent third molar

It can also be described in successive numerical fashion, from 1 to 32:

$$\frac{1\ \ 2\ \ 3\ \ 4\ \ 5\ \ 6\ \ 7\ \ 8\ /\ 9\ \ 10\ \ 11\ \ 12\ \ 13\ \ 14\ \ 15\ \ 16}{32\ \ 31\ \ 30\ \ 29\ \ 28\ \ 27\ \ 26\ \ 25\ /\ 24\ \ 23\ \ 22\ \ 21\ \ 20\ \ 19\ \ 18\ \ 17}$$

Radiographic evaluation of the teeth includes small films whose intent is to assess either the root structure for abscess or cyst pathology *(periapical films),* the crown or neck for dental

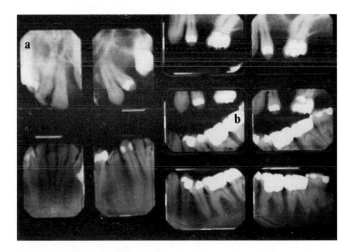

Figure 69-6. Dental radiograph films. Their improved resolution over conventional medical films allows interdental decay and alveolar bone loss to be seen. *a,* Periapical films; *b,* bitewing films.

disease or alveolar bone loss *(bitewing films),* or problems with the supporting maxillary/palatal or mandibular bone structure *(occlusal films).* These smaller films (Figure 69-6) should be differentiated from larger films such as the orthopantomogram, cephalometric films, or anteroposterior (AP) and lateral skull films, which include cranial and facial skeletal structures and whose resolution is inadequate for evaluation of the dentition (Table 69-1).

Table 69-1.
Dental and Maxillofacial Radiography

DIAGNOSTIC FILM TYPE	OPTIMAL USE
Periapical films	Vertical tooth structures, dental caries, root problems
Bitewing films	Molar tooth (nonroot) structures, interdental caries
Occlusal films	Anterior maxillary/mandibular structures, periapical bone pathology
Panorex (pantomograph)	Maxilla and mandible, assess number and location of teeth, mandibular ramus and TMJs
Cephalograms	Lateral and frontal craniofacial structures, preoperative/postoperative assessment for orthognathic and craniofacial surgery
Computed tomography	Bony maxillofacial anatomy
Magnetic resonance imaging	Soft tissue maxillofacial anatomy

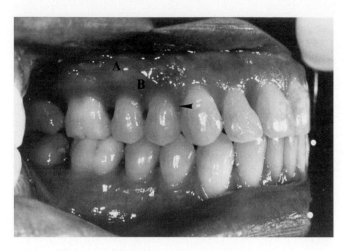

Figure 69-7. Periodontal tissues surrounding the teeth. *A,* Mucosa; *B,* attached gingiva; *arrow,* gingival papillae.

ORAL ANATOMY

The oral cavity extends from the lips to the anterior pillar of the fauces and consists of the *vestibule* (mucosal lining between the lips and cheeks and the teeth and alveoli, which creates a small antechamber) and the *mouth proper* (space enclosed by the teeth and alveolus, which creates a larger inner chamber).[4] The mucosal lining of the vestibule, palate, and floor of the mouth should be differentiated from the tissue that surrounds the teeth. The gums, or *periodontium,* are a specialized dense fibrous tissue covered with mucous membrane that attach to the cervical margin of the roots of the teeth and the alveolus of the jaws. They are unique in that they provide specialized connective tissue fibers that can attach to the cervical portion of the tooth, providing a bond between hard and soft tissue. Long-term survival of teeth necessitates this periodontal attachment (Figure 69-7). Other mucosal tissue or skin grafts will not attach to teeth and ultimately will result in the teeth being lost due to infection and alveolar bone resorption.

The vestibule plays an important but often underappreciated role in oral function. When the mouth is closed only a potential space exists between the outer and inner surfaces of the vestibule as they are in contact with the teeth and gums.

When the lips are distended by air, food, or fluids, a space is established between these otherwise closely adapted structures. Moreover, an open communication exists between the vestibule and the larger portion of the space of the mouth behind the last molar teeth, providing an avenue for fluid passage or tube placement in the event of restricted oral opening or maxillomandibular fixation. When the vestibule is lost from either resection, reconstruction, or scar contracture, control of food and fluid boluses is impaired because of decreased oral capacity and compliance, and the amount of vertical oral opening may be decreased. In the edentulous patient, the size or depth of the vestibule plays a critical role in the ability to adequately wear a dental prosthesis (denture). Without adequate vestibular depth, the flange of the denture is short and the mucosal surface area in contact with the denture is decreased. This results in inadequate suction force so that the denture remains mobile rather than stabilized on the remaining alveolar ridge or basal bone. Mastication is thus difficult and mucosal ulcerations may develop with an ill-fitting and mobile dental prosthesis. Vestibuloplasty, which creates or extends vestibular depth, is frequently necessary in the edentulous adult to expose and line an adequate bony-bearing ridge for prosthesis retention.

MAXILLOFACIAL ANATOMY

The jaws or maxillomandibular complex is a study of contrasting skeletal structures. The maxilla is primarily composed of the alveolar processes that support the teeth. Its paired members are united across the hard palate and attach to the upper facial skeleton by thick cortical buttresses underneath the nose and zygomas. Much of the maxilla is aerated by the sinuses and nasal passages, creating a thin unicortical bony structure for its walls. Intraoral exposure of the maxilla is quite easy through a high vestibular incision. There are very few structures that can be injured on the face of the maxilla. Identification of the infraorbital nerve superiorly and an appreciation of the level of the roots of the maxillary teeth

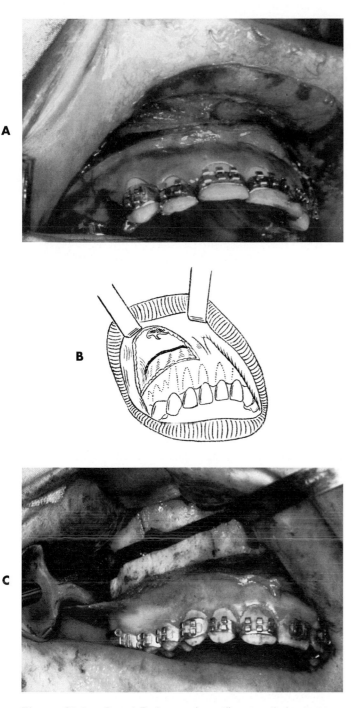

Figure 69-8. **A** and **B,** Intraoral maxillary vestibular incision. Note that the incision should be placed above the junction of the gingiva and attached mucosa to have adequate tissue for closure. **C,** Once the anterior surface of the maxilla is exposed, a 2-to 3-cm zone of bone is available that avoids the roots of the maxillary teeth inferiorly and the infraorbital nerve superiorly. This permits procedures, such as this Le Fort I osteotomy, to be safely done through this area.

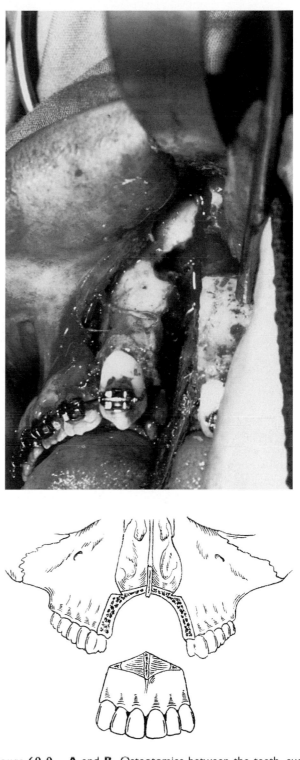

Figure 69-9. **A** and **B,** Osteotomies between the teeth, such as this premaxillary osteotomy between the canine and premolar, are possible because of the conical nature of the tooth roots.

inferiorly provide a 2-to 3-cm width of bone that can be safely cut and manipulated (Figure 69-8). The best method to avoid injuring the maxillary teeth is to identify the canine, since this tooth has the longest root and its most apical portion is easily identified just lateral and inferior to the pyriform aperture. Ostectomies, osteotomies, or device placement can be safely

done above this level. The conical shape of the incisors and canine roots allows osteotomy between these teeth in order to perform hemimaxillectomies or segmentalized Le Fort osteotomies (Figure 69-9). The diverging and multiple roots of the premolars and molars, however, make this procedure much more difficult and likely to damage teeth in the distal arch.

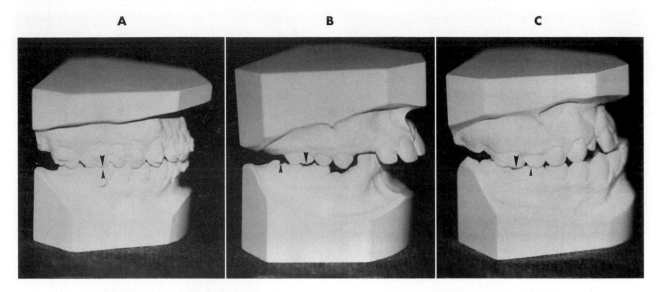

Figure 69-10. Angle's classification of occlusion. Note the relationship of the mesiobuccal cusp of the maxillary first molar *(larger arrow)* to the buccal groove of the mandibular first molar. **A,** Class I. **B,** Class II. **C,** Class III.

In sharp contrast, the mandible is a thick bicortical structure that exceeds all other bones of the facial skeleton in size and strength. It is L-shaped, with a horizontal portion (body and symphysis) containing the alveolar processes and teeth and two vertical portions (rami) on which the muscles of mastication attach. The pair of condyles at the cephalad extremities of the rami ride against the articular disks, which are interposed between them and the glenoid fossa of the temporal bone, and permit the mandibles range of motion. The mandible illustrates quite well the evolutionary concept of the relation between anatomic form and function. The angle, coronoid process, symphysis, and condylar neck provide the sites of muscular attachment responsible for movement and mastication. The alveolar supporting processes of the teeth and the condyle provide a means of articulation with other craniofacial bones. Functionally, the mandible is often considered a lever mechanism, with its paired L-shaped parabolic bones moving on the condyles as fulcrums. This simplistic explanation of mandibular function is most likely not biomechanically correct.

An anatomically correct skeletal relationship between the maxilla and mandible is important for proper oral opening (temporomandibular joint function) and masticatory efficiency. The maxillomandibular skeletal relationship is well described by the occlusal classification system of Angle (Figure 69-10). The occlusion of the teeth is a reflection of the anatomic positioning of the two jaws that contain them.[2,9] In the dentate individual, this occlusal typing provides a diagnostic means to choose between surgical (skeletal repositioning) and nonsurgical (occlusal equilibration, orthodontia) therapies. In the edentulous patient, however, the intricate interdigitation of the teeth is lost. With tooth loss, the supporting trabeculated alveolar bone is resorbed. In the mandible, alveolar bone loss occurs down to the level of the basal bone, and the translocation of the mental foramen to

the top of the remaining ridge is not uncommon. Although vertical bone height is lost, the horizontal dimensions of the body and symphysis of the mandible remain. In contrast, the maxilla loses both horizontal and vertical dimensions with alveolar resorption, and often only a very thin layer of bone exists between the maxillary sinuses and the remaining ridge. As a result of this differential alveolar bone resorption pattern, mandibular "overclosure" occurs with the appearance of a pseudoprominent chin (Figure 69-11). The width of the maxillary arch may now fit inside the mandibular arch width and contributes to reconstructive prosthetic instability.[3]

The temporomandibular joint (TMJ) deserves special consideration because it is an important but often misunderstood component of maxillomandibular anatomy and function. Contrary to many lower animal species, human oral opening is not performed by two moving jaws but by moving the mandible alone. This is made possible by the unique features of the TMJ that distinguish it from the other joints of the body.[6] The TMJ forms the bilateral movable attachments of the mandible with the skull. Because it has the dual properties of both hinged (ginglymoid) and gliding (arthrodial) attachment, it is termed a *ginglymoarthrodial joint.* Superior and inferior joint compartments are separated by an interposed meniscus. The articular surfaces of the inferiorly positioned mandibular condyle and the superiorly positioned glenoid fossa of the temporal bone are lined by dense fibrocartilage, unlike the hyaline cartilage found in most other joints. The meniscus is attached anteriorly to the articular eminence and superior head of the lateral pterygoid muscle and posteriorly to the glenoid fossa and squamotympanic suture. These internal joint structures are enclosed by a capsule of dense collagen tissue on the medial, lateral, and posterior walls of the joint (Figure 69-12). Internal joint function is a complex interplay of movement between the condyle and meniscus, which at certain points is completely diametric. Initial opening

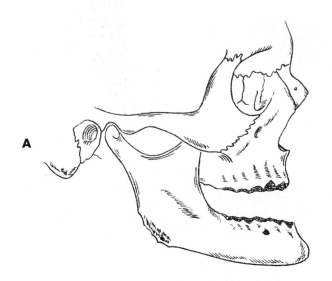

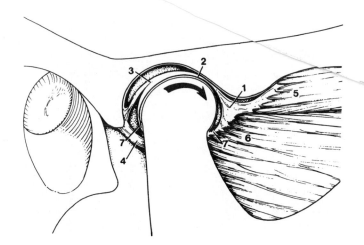

Figure 69-12. Diagrammatic sagittal temporomandibular joint anatomy. *1*, Anterior meniscus, which is attached to the pterygoid muscles; *2*, thinner midportion of the meniscus, which is prone to tears and perforations; *3*, thicker posterior meniscus, which is attached to the posterior portion of the glenoid fossa; *4*, posterior portion of capsular ligaments; *5* and *6*, medial and lateral pterygoid muscles; *7*, synovial lining.

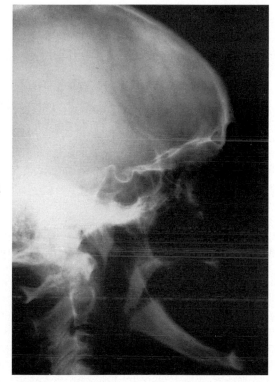

Figure 69-11. **A** and **B**, Lateral cephalogram in a long-standing edentulous patient demonstrating the severe alveolar resorption of the maxilla and mandible.

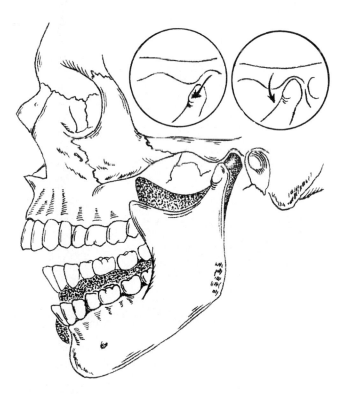

Figure 69-13. The initial 10-15 mm of jaw opening is provided by rotational motion of the condyle while the next 30-35 mm is provided by anterior translational movement.

is primarily a hinged movement with an anterior clockwise rotation of the condyle and a static positioning of the meniscus. This accounts for 10 to 15 mm of vertical interincisal opening. As opening increases, the condyle along with the meniscus begins to move anterior and inferior along the posterior slope of the articular eminence. This movement represents condylar translation (in contrast to hinged condylar rotation) and accounts for the ability to increase interincisal opening to a normal range of 35 to 50 mm. What is most interesting about condylar translation is the carrying forward of the meniscus with the condyle during initial movement

down the eminence but the necessity of the meniscus to then slide posteriorly over the condylar head as translation continues. Eventually, the condyle will reach the inferior peak of the eminence or even move anterior to the eminence to achieve maximal interincisal opening (Figure 69-13). If the meniscal

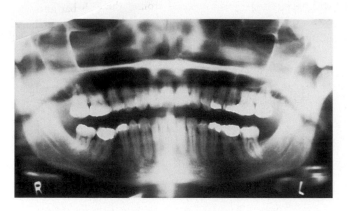

Figure 69-14. Orthopantographic film (i.e., panorex).

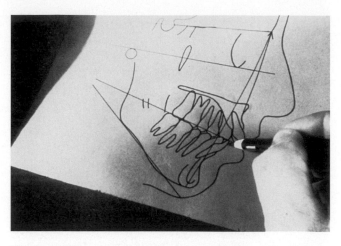

Figure 69-16. Tracing of cephalometric film for orthodontic or orthognathic treatment planning.

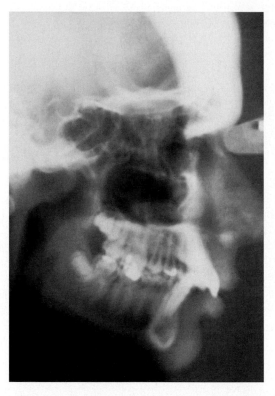

Figure 69-15. Lateral cephalometric film, which provides a clear view of both skeletal and soft tissue profiles.

movement should become impeded (due to stretching, tearing, or scarring of the meniscus from traumatic injury or chronic dysfunction), condylar translation is impeded and oral opening becomes limited to hinged movement only. Surgery may then be necessary to either repair the meniscus or increase superior joint space by reduction of the height of the eminence.

There are a variety of techniques available for radiographic assessment of the maxillofacial complex, including pantographic, cephalometric, computed tomography (CT), or magnetic resonance imaging (MRI). Pantographic radiography remains a common screening film in both dental and hospital settings. A form of tomography with an arc movement of the film and radiation source around the patient, this lays out the mandible in much the same way that a map is a two-dimensional representation of a spherical globe (Figure 69-14). Both TMJs can be simultaneously evaluated and measurements can be made of the mandible. Due to the arc movement in the taking of the film, however, anatomy is distorted at both the central and most lateral portions of the film, and it is more useful as a preliminary film in mandibular trauma screening for fractures. To evaluate the maxillary sinus or nasal airway, the Water's view is better. A cephalometric radiograph is a lateral film taken at a fixed distance from the patient. The patient is positioned with the lips in repose, in centric occlusion, and with the teeth slightly touching so that the soft tissue profile as well as the teeth and jaws can be seen (Figure 69-15). This permits analysis of the patient's hard and soft tissue profiles. This type of film can be distinguished from a lateral skull film by the presence of circular radiolucencies in the auditory canals (positioning ear rods) and the presence of a soft tissue profile on the film. By alignment of bilateral skeletal structures on the cephalometric film, detailed measurements and mathematical analyses of facial skeletal relationships can be performed (Figure 69-16).[10]

The diagnostic value of CT and MRI is well known for head and neck pathology. Three-dimensional CT reconstructions are particularly helpful in evaluation of maxillomandibular skeletal morphology and relationships. The use of MRI in TMJ dysfunction enables an unparalleled understanding of meniscocondylar interaction in static and translatory excursions (Figure 69-17).

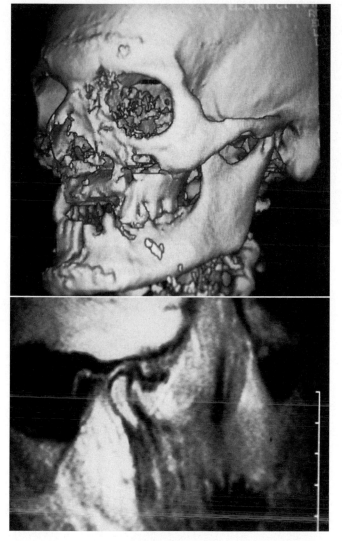

Figure 69-17. Radiographic technologies for detailed maxillofacial assessment. **A,** Three-dimensional CT scan after reconstruction from a facial gunshot injury. **B,** MRI of temporomandibular joint.

OPERATIONS

MAXILLOMANDIBULAR FIXATION

The retention or the restoration of a patient's pretherapy occlusal relationship (provided that it is acceptable and functional) is important prior to surgical manipulation or resection of the mid-facial or lower facial skeleton. This immobilization in proper occlusion has been termed placing the patient in *intermaxillary fixation* (IMF) but is probably more accurately termed *maxillomandibular fixation* (MMF). Many methods have been described to achieve MMF, but they essentially involve either the use of wires alone, wires and metal bars, or acrylic splints and wires.[7] The use of prefabricated flexible stainless steel bars (Erich arch bars) is probably the most frequent method undertaken. This bar is

easily contoured to the dental arch and is ligated to the teeth with stainless steel wires passed around the arch bar and the necks of the teeth. Cleats on the arch bar provide purchase points for interarch wire loops or elastic bands that complete the MMF (Figure 69-18). This method provides very accurate and stable occlusal fixation but is tedious to apply and is not particularly comfortable for the patient, even with local anesthesia. The use of interarch wires placed around the necks of one tooth in each arch and then cross-arch ligated (Ivy loops) is much quicker and easier but is less stable, is prone to loosening, and precludes the option of using rubber bands. As an intraoperative method of occlusal registration when postoperative maintenance of the fixation is not necessary, however, it is quite satisfactory. In the edentulous patient with no tooth roots to anchor wires, alveolar arch acrylic splints (sometimes referred to as Gunning's splints) are useful. These splints are either wired or screwed to the underlying bone, and the jaws are fixed in MMF by cross arch wires attached to the metal arch bars prefabricated into the splints. Although this method is effective, it requires preoperative arch impressions and fabrication of the splints, which may not always be possible. The simple intraoperative placement of a plate with screw attachment to the maxillary and mandibular arches is rapid and stable, and provides adequate access around the plates for postoperative feeding and oral hygiene (Figure 69-19).

TOOTH REPLANTATION

Avulsed intact teeth may be successfully replanted in a high percentage of cases. The avulsed tooth is replaced in the alveolus or kept in a moist wrap until replantation. If the extraoral time is short (less than 2 hours), reattachment of the tooth to the alveolar socket is common, although root resorption or ankylosis may still occur years later.

Surgical replantation requires cleaning but not sterilizing the tooth; irrigating but not curetting the recipient alveolar socket; replacement and stabilization of the replanted tooth, checking its position by radiographs and occlusion; and closure of any gingival lacerations. Stabilization of the replanted tooth can be done by interdental (Essig) wiring, arch bars, or acid-etch bonding of wire or acrylic splints (the preferred method). The stabilization time depends on the condition of the surrounding alveolar bone. If the alveolus is not fractured, the splinting method may be removed in 2 weeks. If extensive alveolar damage is present, 4 to 6 weeks of stabilization are required.

VESTIBULOPLASTY

Vestibuloplasty is useful when no sulcus depth is available for prosthetic retention and support due to either severe alveolar ridge resorption (years after tooth loss), muscle or mucosal attachments that occur on or near the crest of the alveolar

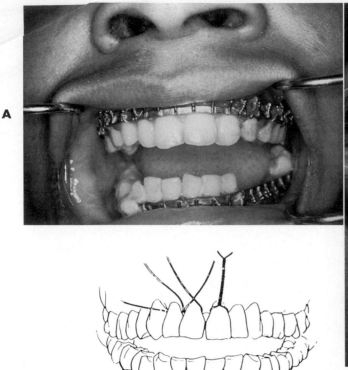

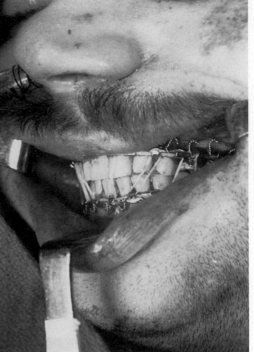

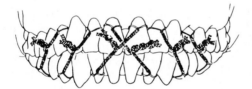

Figure 69-18. Methods of maxillomandibular fixation (MMF). **A,** Cleated arch bars with interdental wires. **B,** Elastic bands used to complete MMF. **C,** Interdental wires cross-arch ligated to achieve MMF.

Figure 69-19. One plate on each side of the mandibular and maxillary arch fixed by screws provides stable fixation.

ridge, or extensive scarring that exists between the buccal mucosa and the alveolar ridge. It is very important to determine the amount of remaining maxillary or mandibular bone before proceeding with soft tissue procedures. When adequate alveolar height remains (>10-to 15-mm vertical bone height), a soft tissue vestibuloplasty procedure alone can work well. With greater resorption and loss of vertical bone height, alveolar augmentation with alloplastic (e.g., hydroxyapatite) materials may be necessary prior to soft tissue surgery. With the emergence, reliability, and stability of endosseous implants and transmandibular implants over the past 15 years, however, many patients now opt for a fixed prosthesis rather than a removable denture. Therefore one-or two-stage alveolar ridge reconstructions (vestibuloplasty with or without prior ridge augmentation) have become far less common.

Although numerous methods of vestibuloplasty have been described, the development of mucosal flaps from a crestal incision, inferior repositioning of attached muscles,

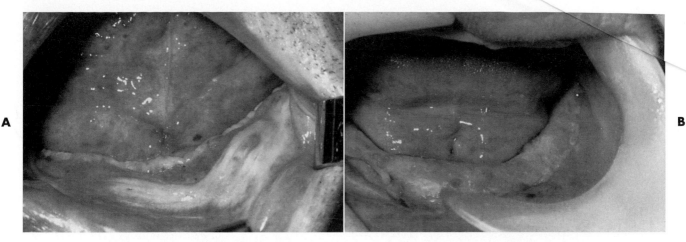

Figure 69-20. Mandibular vestibuloplasty with split-thickness skin graft. **A,** Atrophic alveolus with loss of vestibule. **B,** Postoperative result with vestibular lengthening and skin graft coverage.

and coverage with a non-meshed split-thickness skin via a fixed intraoral splint produce a consistent and stable result (Figure 69-20).

ENDOSSEOUS DENTAL IMPLANTS

Endosseous dental implants are described elsewhere in Volume 3.

MAXILLARY AND MANDIBULAR RECONSTRUCTION

Maxillary and mandibular reconstruction is described in Chapters 78 and 85.

MAXILLOFACIAL OSTEOTOMIES

Maxillofacial osteotomies are described elsewhere in Volume 3.

RIGID FIXATION

The dental implication for using metallic rigid fixation in maxillomandibular reconstruction is the avoidance of placing screws directly into the underlying root structures. This is easily understood and avoided in the mandible by staying below the level of the mental foramen (Figure 69-21). As the neurovascular supply enters the tooth root from below, this inferior area represents a very safe zone for bicortical screw placement. In the maxilla, however, there is no well-defined neurovascular canal. Therefore inserting screws above the horizontal level of the canine root (longest tooth) ensures against dental injury.

Monocortical screws can be used at almost any level of the maxilla or mandible. However, smaller screws (1.0 to 1.5 mm) with short insertion lengths (3 to 4 mm) can be used on the

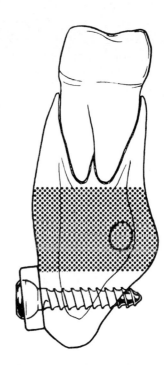

Figure 69-21. Placement of bicortical screws at the inferior border of the mandible protects tooth roots and the neurovascular bundle.

thicker outer cortex of the mandible, even directly over tooth roots. In the maxilla, the cortex over the buccal tooth roots is very thin to nonexistent, and any screw insertion should be avoided.

TEMPOROMANDIBULAR JOINT SURGERY

Surgical manipulation of the TMJ may be conceived as either intracapsular or extracapsular procedures. Intracapsular procedures are used when meniscocondylar dysfunction is present or when degeneration of the cartilage lining of the glenoid fossa or condyle has occurred.[8] Historically, this was done as an

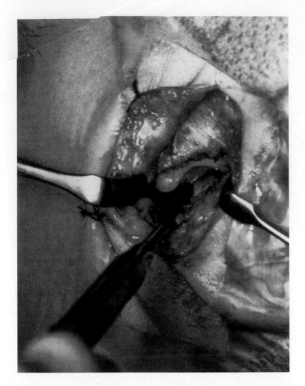

Figure 69-22. Exposure of the temporomandibular joint through a preauricular incision. The glenoid fossa, articular eminence, superior joint space, and meniscus are visualized.

open procedure through a preauricular incision (Figure 69-22). More recently, arthroscopic techniques have replaced the open approach as both a diagnostic and therapeutic procedure with apparently equivalent results. Extracapsular procedures are still indicated either to replace a resected or congenitally missing condyle or to release a fibrous or bony ankylosis of the joint. A basic concept in reconstruction of the TMJ is that autogenous materials such as rib and cartilage are almost always superior when dealing with condyle, meniscus, or fossa (Figure 69-23). The last 15 years have painfully demonstrated the complications of prosthetic TMJ reconstruction. The historic use of metal condyles and fossa implants, as well as alloplastic meniscal replacements, has clearly shown that contemporary biomaterials and engineering have yet to produce a long-term satisfactory TMJ replacement.

OUTCOMES

DENTAL REPLACEMENT

During the last 15 years, the high success rate, even in irradiated tissues, of endosseous tooth implants has markedly improved dental reconstruction. This method provides a more secure means of attaching tooth replacements than the traditional removable dentures or even transmandibular (e.g., staple) type implants. Consistent success rates as high as 90% to 95% retention of the devices after 5 to 10 years have been

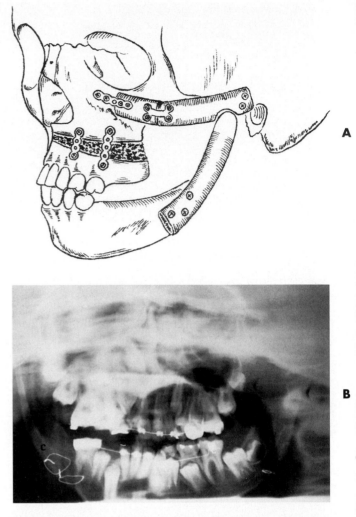

Figure 69-23. A and **B,** Costochondral graft reconstruction (c) of ramus and condyle in a hemifacial microsomia patient. Note large number of unerupted mandibular and maxillary teeth.

reported. This has understandably created great enthusiasm for their use, particularly after head and neck cancer reconstruction. However, certain practical concepts about endosseous dental implants are easily overlooked by those not familiar with them. An important issue is cost. Expenses could easily total $1,000 to $1,500 per tooth replaced, including the surgeon's placement fee, the cost of the devices, and the expenses incurred by the prosthodontist for the dental reconstruction attached to the implants. Endosseous implant reconstruction in an oral cancer reconstruction patient (e.g., hemimandibulectomy with free fibular osteocutaneous reconstruction)[11] could easily cost $5,000 to $7,500 as a conservative estimate. Since medical or dental insurance only rarely covers such expenses, this would place a considerable, and often impractical, burden on many patients. In addition, the long-term success of endosseous implants is highly dependent on the patient's level of oral hygiene and periodontal care. If the patient has a history of poor hygiene and has surrounding dentition with advanced periodontal disease, it is unlikely that the effort and cost of the implants can be justified. Therefore, although endosseous implants offer an ideal method of dental replacement, they are not a practical technology for every patient.

MAXILLOMANDIBULAR FIXATION

The use of MMF serves as an effective and inexpensive method of maintaining or effecting optimal occlusal interdigitation. Orthognathic surgery, facial fracture repair, or maxillomandibular resection should not be done without first establishing an intraoperative method of ensuring occlusal placement and a postoperative method of occlusal adjustment. For a few dollars worth of metal bars and wires and less than an hour of operative time, a functional occlusion can be obtained and immobility of the maxillomandibular skeleton ensured. Few complications are associated with its use short of minor dental discomfort and periodontal soft tissue injury while in place. After removal, however, periodontal regeneration can occur, provided the patient's level of hygiene is adequate. Failure to achieve dental occlusion can, however, cause extensive morbidity in the postoperative period including pain locally and in the TMJ, dental erosion, soft tissue injury, and TMJ arthritis or degeneration.

REFERENCES

1. Abrams J, ed: *Kraus' dental anatomy and occlusion,* ed 2, St Louis, 1992, Mosby.

2. Ash MM Jr: Philosophy of occlusion: past and present, *Dent Clin North Am* 39:233-255, 1995.

3. Bays RA, Maron B: The pathophysiology and anatomy of edentulous bone loss, In Fonseca RJ, Davis WH, editors: *Reconstructive preprosthetic oral and maxillofacial surgery,* ed 2, Philadelphia, 1995, WB Saunders, pp 19-40.

4. Brand RW, Isselhard DE: Oral cavity. In Brand RW, Isselhard DE, editors: *Anatomy of orofacial structures,* ed 4, St Louis, 1990, Mosby, pp 3-13.

5. Brand RW, Isselhard DE: Eruption and shedding of teeth. In Brand RW, Isselhard DE, editors: *Anatomy of orofacial structures,* ed 4, St Louis, 1990, Mosby, pp 84-89.

6. Brand RW, Isselhard DE: Temporomandibular joint. In Brand RW, Isselhard DE, editors: *Anatomy of orofacial structures,* ed 4, St Louis, 1990, Mosby, pp 152-157.

7. Brown T, Abbott JR, Daenke LL: Dental injuries. In David DJ, Simpson DA, editors: *Craniomaxillofacial trauma,* New York, 1996, Churchill Livingstone, pp 333-366.

8. Dautrey J, Pepersack W: Functional surgery of the TMJ, *Clin Plast Surg* 91:591-601, 1982.

9. dos Santos J Jr, ed: *Occlusion: principles and concepts,* ed 2, St Louis, 1996, Ishiyaku EuroAmerica.

10. Jacobsen A, editor: *Radiographic cephalometry, from basics to videoimaging,* Chicago, 1995, Quintessence Publishing.

11. Roumanas ED, Markowitz BL, Lorant JA, et al: Reconstructed mandibular defects: fibula free flaps and osseointegrated implants, *Plast Reconstr Surg* 99:356-365, 1997.

Radiation Treatment of Head and Neck Cancer

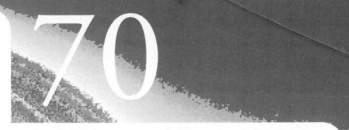

Faramarz Movagharnia
Mark S. Granick

INDICATIONS

Squamous cell carcinoma (SCC) is the most common malignant neoplasm of the head and neck (H&N). In its earliest stages, SCC may be asymptomatic or may present with only minor nonspecific symptoms, which may delay diagnosis.[7] Surgical resection is the treatment of choice for most H&N tumors, but radiotherapy is an alternative primary or adjuvant therapy. Radiation therapy (XRT) as a primary modality may effectively eradicate local disease and early-stage lesions. The combination of surgery and therapeutic irradiation (preoperative, postoperative, or intraoperative) is most helpful in advanced disease, where either surgery or radiotherapy alone is inadequate. Tumors at high risk for local recurrence and lymphatic metastasis may benefit from a combination of surgery and irradiation.

Combined surgery and XRT does not offer a dramatic increase in survival rate, since most of these patients have poor survival prospects at the time of initial therapy.[18] Radiotherapy as a surgical adjunct seems to be equally effective at tumor control, whether it is administered preoperatively or postoperatively. The purported rationale for preoperative XRT is to eradicate subclinical disease beyond the planned margin of surgical resection. It is also believed to diminish tumor implantation by decreasing the number of viable cells within the operative field, to decrease the potential for distant metastasis, and to convert an unresectable neoplasm into an operable lesion.[14] Preoperative XRT should allow for an ablation of reduced dimensions.

On the other hand, preoperative XRT interferes with the normal healing process. It damages all of the tissues, including the normal tissues surrounding the tumor, and can make distinguishing between tumor and normal tissues difficult.[5]

The indications for postoperative irradiation include positive or close surgical margins, large (T3 or T4) primary tumors, multiple positive nodes, nodes with extracapsular involvement (or size greater than 3 cm), and tumor invasion of vascular, lymphatic, and perineural tissue or adjacent structures. Proponents of postoperative radiation therapy claim that it does not adversely affect the surgery, since the wounds have healed. Consequently, higher doses can be given.[1,10,16] A potential disadvantage of postoperative radiotherapy is that cancer cell repopulation can occur if radiation therapy is delayed as a result of surgical complications.

Intraoperative radiotherapy is available and has some demonstrated benefit for patients who have extensive late-stage tumors.[6]

OPERATIONS

Irradiation of living tissue leads to the absorption of energy and excitation of tissue electrons. When the electrons are sufficiently energized, they can be ejected from an atom; this is referred to as the process of ionization. The end point of this reaction is that a large amount of energy is released and can cause significant damage to the cell. The nuclear DNA is the portion of the cell most sensitive to ionizing radiation.[2] Destruction of the nuclear DNA leads to cellular degeneration or progressive cell destruction after several divisions. Malignant neoplasms contain rapidly growing abnormal cellular populations that can be specifically inhibited by XRT. However, DNA is damaged by radiation in both normal and malignant cells. The therapeutic usefulness of XRT depends on both the sensitivity of the tumor to radiation and the consequent destruction of the tumor, as well as on the ability to minimize the effect on normal tissues. This can be controlled to an extent by careful treatment planning.

Ionizing radiation occurs as either electromagnetic waves or particulate forms.[8] Electromagnetic radiation pertains to electrical or magnetic energy that can occur in emissions of various wave lengths. The shorter wave lengths include x-rays and gamma rays. At the long end of the wave length spectrum are microwaves and radio waves, which are not used in therapeutic XRT treatment. Electromagnetic radiation also can occur in discrete energy packets referred to as photons. X-rays and gamma rays are delivered as high-energy photons of short wave length and are capable of causing an ionizing reaction in cellular tissue. Gamma rays are created for use in XRT from the unstable nuclei of radioactive substances such as cobalt, radium, or other isotopes. X-rays are produced in a device that accelerates electrons to very high energy and then aims them at a target that emits x-rays. Particulate irradiation consists of small energized particles such as electrons, neutrons, protons, alpha particles, pi-mesons, and others. These are generally high-energy particles that can cause ionization and destruction of tissues that they enter. Irradiation in any of its forms can directly destroy a cell by interfering with the DNA content. Another form of cellular destruction can occur as a result of the release of free radicals, highly reactive chemical ions that are created by the energy imparted by radiation.

Radiation therapy is generally delivered in one of two manners.[8] In the first technique, radioactive emissions can be generated by machines and aimed as an external beam at a patient's tumor. The other technique is brachytherapy, which involves implantation of radioactive sources directly into a patient's tumor. Tissue penetration by radiation is directly proportional to the energy level. The higher the energy, the deeper the tissue penetration. The gray (Gy) and centigray (cGy) are the units of measurement for radiation. One cGy is equivalent to one rad, the previously used measure. Treatment planning is a highly technical process. The proper fields and tumor sites must be precisely delineated. Dosage curves are then created by mathematical formulas characteristic of the tissue, the energy source, and the site of disease to minimize delivery of radiation to normal tissue and to achieve maximum dose at the tumor site.

Cells that are actively dividing are the most sensitive to radiation treatment. It was recognized early that if all of the radiation dose was given in one treatment, cells that were not in a phase of active cell division would be less sensitive and would be likely to survive. By breaking the treatments into multiple fractions (fractionating) more cells will theoretically rotate through the active stage of cell division and ultimately be destroyed during those radiosensitive phases. Furthermore, breaking the treatment dosage into multiple small fractions heightens the opportunity to maximize tumor cell damage and minimize normal tissue damage, taking advantage of the difference in responsiveness between normal and malignant tissues, the difference in the activity of the cell cycles in normal versus malignant tissues, and the increased efficiency of cell repair in normal tissues.

External beam irradiation is the most common form of XRT. Linear accelerators produce beams of electrons. Electrons are directly ionizing on the impacted tissues and, consequently, are rapidly absorbed and used for treatment of superficial lesions.

Photons are short pulses of high energy produced approximately 1 meter from the patient. The dose within the tissue is determined by both the distance from the source of the target tissues and the attenuation of radiation with the tissue. Photons are absorbed in tissues depending on their energy level. The photon beam will pass through superficial tissues without absorption and consequently without damage to these tissues. Megavoltage treatments therefore are skin sparing.

In actual practice, low-energy photons (approximately 150 KeV) can be used for treatment of superficial lesions; they are absorbed at levels close to the patient's skin surface. At orthovoltage levels (300 KeV) cobalt sources are used and the superficial tissues are relatively spared, while the deeper tissues are affected. However, with the currently used megavoltage treatment (1.2 MeV), or even with high megavoltage (4 to 18 MeV), photons are produced by linear accelerators as opposed to a source of radioactive material. These high-energy photons are absorbed at much deeper levels and are well suited for treatment of deep-seated tumors with excellent skin sparing.[4,13]

Brachytherapy is a form of implantation of radioactive material. Radium needles and seeds were used originally but are now obsolete. Currently, the radioactive sources usually consist of iridium 192, which is implanted in wires. This minimizes exposure to the staff and is much easier to insert. These implants are placed directly into the tumor by passing hollow plastic tubes (after loading catheters) using steel needles directly through the lesion. When employed for treatment of primary tumors, this is usually done in the operating room by both surgeon and radiotherapist. For base of tongue tumors or other bulky oral or pharyngeal lesions, prophylactic tracheostomy may be necessary to avoid upper airway obstruction from posttherapy swelling. Where used as an adjuvant to surgery, the radiotherapist usually places the catheters before the skin flaps are closed. The tubes are then loaded with radioactive seeds in the patient's room. After the calculated optimal dose of radiation has been delivered to the tissues, the implant and the after-loading catheters are removed.[8,13] Brachytherapy has been particularly successful in the treatment of tongue and mouth lesions because of the accessibility of these organs to the placement of needles and tubes through tumor masses.

Treatment planning is critical to a successful outcome. To determine optimal dosage, a planning session is required in which direct measurements of radiation dosages in tissue-equivalent phantoms are made and modified to the clinical situation. Radiation energy is absorbed by tissues in a predictable and calculable fashion. A computerized treatment-planning apparatus generates isodose curves or lines of equivalent radiation around the area of the tumor. A composite isodose plan is a distribution of the individual beams of radiation energy and how they impact and increase total dosage patterns within the tissues. The beams may be modified by using wedges or compensators, which absorb some of the energy, or by angling the fields and redirecting the beams. Patients are tattooed with Indian ink so that the fields are standardized from one treatment to the next. A mold of the patient's head or body part is commonly used to maintain patient position in each treatment session. Treatment planning includes localization of the tumor, estimating the volume of the lesion to be treated, localizing the target tissues with reference to the normal anatomy, producing the isodose plan and prescribing a tumoricidal dose to treat the lesion, simulating the planned fields on computerized equipment, and verifying the fields on the linear accelerator. Finally, the treatment must be delivered in a satisfactory pattern of

Table 70-1.
Tolerance Doses of Tissues Based on a Large Volume of Treatment

TISSUE	$TD_{5/5}$ cGy	$TD_{50/5}$ cGy	COMPLICATION
Skin	5500	7000	Necrosis/ulcer
Larynx	5000	7000	Edema, chondronecrosis
Esophagus	5500	6800	Stricture, perforation
Jejunum	4000	5500	Stricture, perforation
Spinal cord	4700	7000	Myelitis, necrosis
Parotid	3200	4000	Xerostomia
Brain	4500	6000	Necrosis

Adapted from Burman C, Kutcher GJ, Emami B, et al: Fitting of normal tissue tolerance data to an analytic function, *Int J Radiat Oncol Biol Phys* 21:123, 1991.

appropriate fractions and doses. Since the effect of the radiation is cumulative, the total dosage is the important final factor.

The typical management of a patient with head and neck cancer consists of primary treatment with megavoltage radiations, such as those produced by 4-to 6-MeV linear accelerators.[17] The most common technique is to use opposing upper lateral ports for the first 45 Gy. The portals are reduced to protect the spinal cord, and additional therapy is used to carry the total dose to 65 to 70 Gy. An attempt is made to spare the parotid glands in order to reduce xerostomia. Other treatment plans allow inclusion of the lymph nodes of the neck along with the primary site. During treatment, a patient's head is usually stabilized with a plastic cutout in order to prevent any variation from treatment session to treatment session. The tongue is also immobilized by placing a cork and tongue blade or a special bite block within the mouth.

After treatment with ionizing radiation, cells can be damaged in a number of ways. When a cell is irreversibly damaged, cellular death will occur; however, with sublethal damage, the cell can be repaired over a period of time. Repair requires not only time, but adequate nutrition and oxygen. At lower dosages, some cells can receive potentially lethal damage, which can be modified by altering the cellular environment. Certain rapidly dividing tissues (e.g., intestinal mucosa, skin, bone marrow) cannot survive radiation at this level; however, other less actively dividing cells can do well. Consequently, there are a number of different parameters necessary for the treatment of tumors in order to maximize the ionizing damage to tumor and minimize the damage to normal tissues. The total dosage is critical. Without sufficient dosage tumors are more likely to recur. In the head-neck region, the total dose of 50 to 70 Gy is appropriate for cure.[17] Each tumor histology has a certain range of total dose that is likely to achieve cure in a high percentage of cases, and this total dose varies dramatically from 2500 cGy in some hematopoietic tumors to 7500 cGy in some nerve and cartilage malignancies. This total

Table 70-2.
Tumor Lethal Doses

TISSUE	TUMOR LETHAL DOSE cGy
Seminoma	3500
Hodgkin's disease	4500
Basal cell carcinoma	4500
No nodal metastasis	5000
T_1 Larynx	6000-6500
T_2 Oral cavity	7000-7500
T_3 Oral cavity	8000+
Sarcoma	8000+

dose is signified as TD_5, TD_{50}, and TD_{90}, or the total dose that will eradicate 5%, 50%, and 90% of tumors, respectively. Just as tumors demonstrate a range of response, so do normal tissues, except that the relevant parameter with normal tissues is the toxicity, or inversely, the ability of the tissue to recover from a given dose of radiotherapy. There is comparable sensitivity of malignant and benign tissues, so hematopoietic gut mucosa and other rapidly dividing cells are highly sensitive, whereas nerve, bone, and muscles are much less sensitive. The measurement of sensitivity of normal tissues to the toxic effects of radiotherapy is LD_5, LD_{50}, and LD_{90} of the given tissue, or that dose that would be lethal to 5%, 50%, and 90% of tissues (Tables 70-1 and 70-2).

Dose fraction size is also quite important. Most doses are fractionated to about 200 cGy per treatment. The total volume of tissue treated is critical. Microscopic tumors obviously will do better, since the tumor load is less. Larger tumors tend to be ischemic in their central portions, and the cells are relatively protected in that environment. A final factor is the elapsed time during irradiation. There is an opportunity for cellular recovery to occur during delays in treatment.

OUTCOMES

Patients with head and neck SCC with small T1 or T2 lesions do well with primary radiation therapy or with surgery and have comparable cure rates, which range between 75% and 90% disease-free survival for 2 to 3 years. The 2-to 3-year period after initial treatment is adequate for following of patients with head and neck SCC, since the vast majority of these lesions will recur within 2 years if the recurrence is due to treatment failure.[17]

Patients with advanced T3 or T4 lesions tend to do poorly regardless of whether radiation therapy is used as a primary treatment or as a postoperative adjuvant. The survival rate is between 20% and 60% and decreases by 50% if a patient has positive cervical nodes.

That outcome of XRT of most concern to surgeons consists of the therapy's complications and long-term effects. The frequency and severity of sequelae of XRT is correlated to the specific sites of the treated tissues, the dose of radiation, how it is fractionated, how it is applied, what kind of radiation is used, and intercurrent diseases and medications. Complications occur not only as an acute effect of XRT but also as a different, more insidious long-term set of problems.

The acute problems consist of erythema and tenderness and possibly sloughing of mucosa in the oral cavity, hypopharynx, and cervical esophagus. These problems are exacerbated by continued smoking and alcohol abuse. Mucositis depends on the sensitivity of the particular patient, along with the dosage and fractionation pattern of the radiation that is given, being greater with higher doses and more rapid fractionation. It generally subsides with local therapy and occasionally requires a brief pause in the treatment program. Loss of taste is common if the tongue or salivary glands are within the radiation field. This may further impair the patient's ability to maintain his or her nutrition and may last for months after the treatment is complete.

Xerostomia is common if the minor and the major salivary glands are encompassed within the radiation field and a total dose of greater than 4000 cGy is administered. A dryness of the mucosa develops that is permanent and progressive. It can be treated with topical hydrating agents, but generally leads to loss of appetite, difficulty manipulating food particles in the mouth, and a continuous uncomfortable sensation for the patient, as well as increased risk of dental caries because of loss of the antibacterial effects of saliva.

Acute radiation dermatitis is characterized by erythema and an exudative skin slough. Hair loss occurs acutely and may grow back with a different density, color, and texture. The skin changes are analogous to mucositis and generally resolve in the acute phase with local care.

The long-term effects of radiation therapy are more severe. Although the treatment course is usually physically exhausting, short-term effects are usually self-limited and resolve after termination of therapy. The long-term effects of radiation are, however, progressive and worsen over time. The mucous membranes become dry and uncomfortable; the skin commonly exhibits some atrophy, discoloration, and hardening (Figure 70-1); and the ability of the skin to heal is markedly diminished, so that any surgical approach to irradiated tissue is at higher risk of postoperative healing problems.

The teeth present a particular problem in radiotherapy of the head and neck, since most cancers require inclusion of the dentition within the field. Good oral hygiene and fluoride gel used along with other fluoride carriers during radiation therapy are important to prevent a loss of teeth. Prior to radiation therapy, oral hygiene and dental status need to be optimized. Extractions, fluoride treatments, restorations, and periodontal treatments should be completed prior to the onset of radiation therapy, and all wounds should be fully healed. Artificial saliva must be provided for patients with xerostomia, and good oral hygiene and surveillance are a lifelong necessity after treatment. Secondary dental caries and destruction of the periodontal tissues are frequent occurrences. Periodontitis secondary to radiation therapy can lead to infection of the underlying mandible, with consequent osteoradionecrosis, a devastating disorder that may require more aggressive treatment than the initial tumor. Although the true incidence of this problem is unknown, the reported range of complications is from less than 1% to as high as 30%.[15] Predisposing factors for development of osteoradionecrosis are abuse of tobacco and alcohol, poor oral hygiene, and a total dose of radiation greater than 70 Gy. Once a patient has developed radionecrosis the

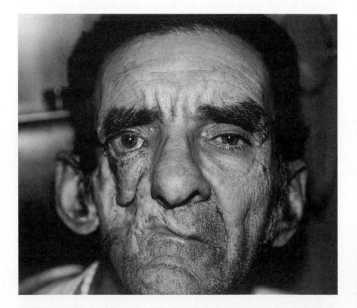

Figure 70-1.   Extreme case of chronic radiation injury to soft tissues in a patient primarily irradiated (>70 Gy) for maxillary SCC. Note the skin atrophy, contractures, and edema.

treatment options are hyperbaric oxygen treatment and, in some cases, resection of the affected tissues and replacement with well-vascularized tissue.[3,9,15] Forty-one percent of the patients with osteoradionecrosis of the mandible required hemimandibulectomy to manage this problem (Figure 70-2). When significant osteoradionecrosis presents, early resection of affected areas and replacement with a fibula or other osteocutaneous flap will avoid lengthy courses of minor debridements and hyperbaric oxygen treatment.

L'hermittes syndrome is a neuroma-like syndrome in the upper extremities brought on by neck flexion. Due to radiation of the cervical spinal cord, it is a chronic, progressive, and painful disorder manifesting with intermittent severe paresthesias. Other late effects of radiation therapy are hypothyroidism, pituitary insufficiency, lymphatic obstruction, growth retardation, hearing loss, stricture of mucosal-lined cavities and conduits, muscle fibrosis, and trismus. Carcinogenesis is a known risk, particularly in patients with an expected long life span. Patients exposed to low-dose XRT in the head and neck are at increased risk for the late development of thyroid tumors and salivary gland tumors. Patients who have had radiation exposure to the skin are at high risk for developing skin cancer within the zone of radiation or along its borders. Therapeutic irradiation also increases the risk of soft tissue sarcoma developing in the peripheral field at a later date, the median time being 15 years.

Larson et al[11,12] have developed a grading system for the extent of morbidity associated with late radiation changes. The grading system progresses from 0, indicating no long-term effects, to IV, indicating life-threatening effects. In a series of 569 patients, 128 patients were evaluated for grade IV radiation effects. Spontaneous ulceration of the mucous membranes, soft tissue radionecrosis, and osteoradionecrosis were the sequelae that these patients suffered.

Another complication of irradiation, particularly problematic in the head and neck, is the development of spontaneous fistulization between the oral cavity and the skin.[3] When orocutaneous fistula (Figure 70-3) presents in an

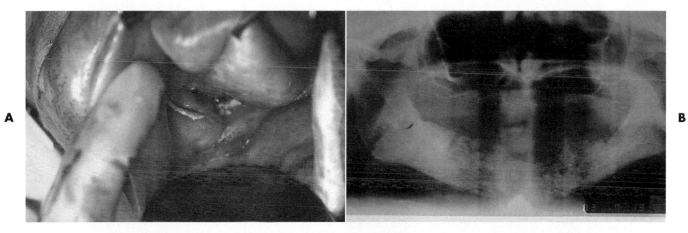

Figure 70-2. **A,** Intraoral view of radionecrotic mandible extruding through oral mucosa. **B,** Panorex demonstrating extensive osteonecrosis necessitating wide mandibulectomy and free flap reconstruction.

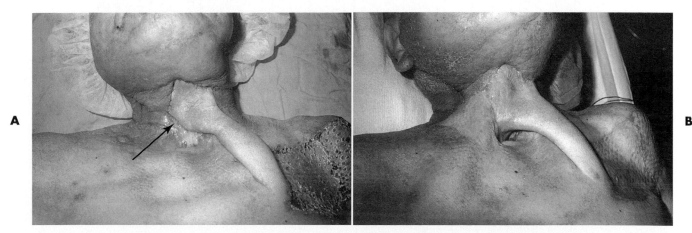

Figure 70-3. **A,** This patient developed a pharyngocutaneous fistula *(arrow)* after being treated by laryngectomy and postoperative XRT for SCC. The tubed deltopectoral flap, placed by the referring service, failed to obliterate the fistula. **B,** Fistula healed after reconstruction with a pectoralis major muscle flap.

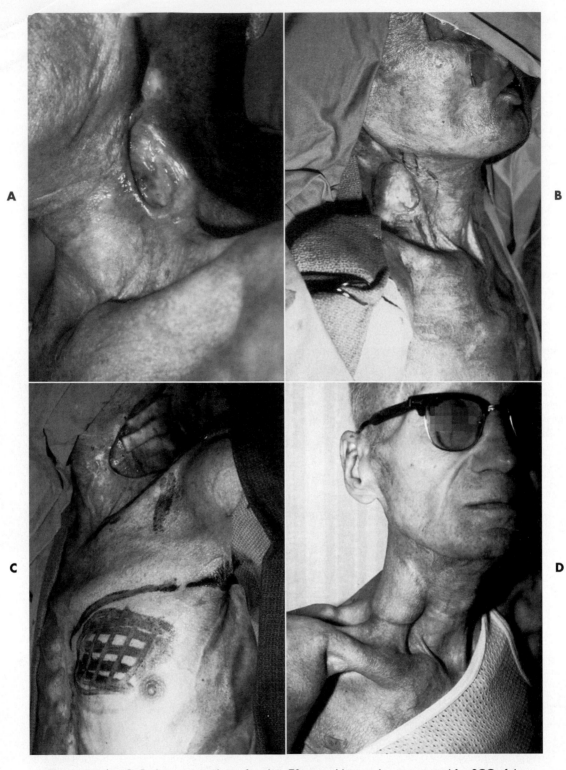

Figure 70-4. **A,** Radionecrotic ulcer of neck in 70-year-old man who was treated for SCC of the tonsil 12 years earlier by neck dissection and adjuvant radiotherapy. This ulcer developed acutely after an episode of hypotension caused by upper gastrointestinal bleeding. **B,** Outline of proposed resection of radionecrotic skin. **C,** The carotid artery was not invaded by infection but was exposed by the infection. Design of pectoralis major musculocutaneous flap preserving the blood supply to the deltopectoral flap as a salvage mechanism. **D,** Postoperative result.

irradiated neck, there is the risk of infection around the great vessels. Ionizing radiation has a predictable effect on the vasorum of the carotid artery, resulting in intimal fibrosis and relative ischemia of the vessel wall. Exposure of such an irradiated vessel without the normal blood supply, and thus the normal ability to create granulation tissue and heal, will result in desiccation, invasive infection of the vessel wall, and either catastrophic hemorrhage into the neck or oral cavity, or septic thrombosis with possible subsequent septic emboli to the brain. Exposure of the radiated carotid is a surgical emergency, and immediate coverage with well-vascularized tissue such as a pectoralis muscle flap should be performed. Closure of any accompanying fistula should be performed at the same time. If the carotid is invasively infected, it should be resected to proximal and distal unaffected tissue and either ligated or bypassed, depending on the status of the cerebral circulation (Figure 70-4).

Radiation necrosis in the head and neck may manifest as osteoradionecrosis, spontaneous fistula, carotid necrosis, skin flap necrosis, brain necrosis, or disorders of any other tissue within the field of therapy. Since radiotherapy is particularly effective in the treatment of laryngeal SCC, expansion of medications for therapy has resulted in trials of combined chemotherapy and radiotherapy in the attempt to preserve the organ of speech. Chondronecrosis of the larynx may occur in these trials because of the sensitizing effect of cisplatinum on normal tissues, although it also occurs without adjuvant chemotherapy as well. Although early disease may respond to local therapy with or without hyperbaric oxygen, most clinically significant cases will require laryngectomy and reconstruction with well-vascularized tissue, by either a thoracic musculocutaneous flap or a microvascular free autograft, to restore alimentary continuity, since surrounding affected tissues must be resected as well. Because the entire field of radiated tissue is affected to some degree, careful clinical assessment of tissue viability at the margin of resection of diseased tissue is important. Resection of questionably vascularized tissue, as well as obviously necrotic tissue, and replacement with well-vascularized tissue are key to resolution of the problem.

REFERENCES

1. Amdur RJ, Parsons JT, Mendenhall WM, et al: Postoperative irradiation for squamous cell carcinoma of the head and neck: analysis of treatment results and complications, *Int J Radiat Oncol Biol Phys* 16:25-36, 1989.

2. Bernstein EF, Sullivan FJ, Mitchell JB, et al: Biology of chronic radiation effect on tissues and wound healing, *Clin Plast Surg* 20(3):435-453, 1993.

3. Coleman JJ III: Management of radiation-induced soft-tissue injury to the head and neck, *Clin Plast Surg* 20:517-530, 1993.

4. Dearnaley OP: Principles of radiotherapy. In Hurwich A, editor: *Oncology: a multidisciplinary textbook,* New York, 1995, Chapman & Hall Medical, pp 119-136.

5. DeSanto LW, Beahrs OH, Holt JJ, et al: Neck dissection and combined therapy. Study of the effectiveness, *Arch Otolaryngol* 111(6):366-370, 1985.

6. Freeman SB, Hamaker RC, Rate WR, et al: Management of advanced cervical metastasis using intraoperative radiotherapy, *Laryngoscope* 105:575-578, 1995.

7. Guggenheimer J, Verbin RS, Johnston JT, et al: Factors delaying the diagnosis of oral and oropharyngeal carcinomas, *Cancer* 64:932-935, 1989.

8. Illidge TM, Hamilton CR: Principles of clinical radiation oncology. In Love RR, editor: *Manual of clinical oncology,* ed 6, Berlin, 1994, Springer-Verlage, pp 176-185.

9. Kindwall EP: Hyperbaric oxygen's effect on radiation necrosis, *Clin Plast Surg* 20:473-484, 1993.

10. Kramer S, Gelber RD, Snow JB, et al: Combined radiation therapy and surgery in the management of advanced head and neck cancer· final report of study 73-03 of the radiation therapy oncology group, *Head Neck Surg* 10:19-30, 1987.

11. Larson DL: Long term effects of radiation therapy in the head and neck, *Clin Plast Surg* 20:485-490, 1993.

12. Larson DL, Lindberg RL, Lanc E, et al: Major complications of radiotherapy in cancer of the oral cavity and oropharynx, *Am J Surg* 146:532-535, 1983.

13. Murnro A, Walsh-Waring G: Head and neck. In Sekora K, Halman KE, editors: *Treatment of cancer,* ed 2, London, 1990, Chapman & Hall Medical, pp 264-269.

14. O'Brien JC: *Head and neck 1: tumors: selected readings in plastic surgery.* Vol. 8, No. 9, 1995; 1-44.

15. Sanger JR, Matloub HS, Yousif NJ, et al: Management of osteoradionecrosis of the mandible, *Clin Plast Surg* 20:517-530, 1993.

16. Vikram B, Strong EW, Shah J, et al: Elective postoperative radiation therapy in stage III and IV epidermoid carcinoma of the head and neck, *Am J Surg* 140:580-584, 1980.

17. Wang CC: Oral cavity. In Perez CA, Brady LW, editors: *Principles and practices of radiation oncology,* ed 2, Philadelphia, 1992, JB Lippincott, pp 672-678.

18. Wasserman TH, Kligerman MM: Chemical modifiers of radiation. In Perez CA, Brady LW, editors: *Principles and practices of radiation oncology,* ed 2, Philadelphia, 1992, JB Lippincott, pp 455-456.

CHAPTER

Functional Outcome Considerations in Upper Aerodigestive Tract Reconstruction

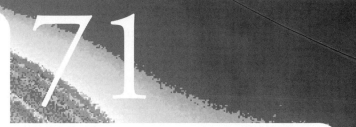

Mennen T. Gallas
Jan S. Lewin
Gregory R.D. Evans

INDICATIONS

The goal of this chapter is to outline those aspects in head and neck reconstruction that lead to significant alterations in functional outcome, specifically regarding speech and swallowing, and to identify measures important in assessing these functional parameters following various reconstructive options. Because the field is diverse, and individual tumor sites in the oral cavity alter the criteria for speech and swallowing restoration and evaluation, it would be impossible to generalize reconstructive evaluations and outcomes in head and neck defects. Consequently, three representative operations and reconstructions have been selected to exemplify the influence of resection and reconstruction on the evaluation and rehabilitation of these functional processes: mandibulectomy, glossectomy, and total laryngopharyngectomy. The chapter is formatted into three sections. First a historical review and overall rehabilitative goal is presented. Second, the three representative surgeries are discussed as they relate to speech and swallowing regarding defect site and size, reconstructive considerations, and outcome assessment. Lastly, the impact of functional outcome on quality of life is discussed.

HISTORICAL PERSPECTIVE

Reconstructive head and neck surgery has undergone revolutionary changes over the past 20 years. Once considered routine, the prolonged reconstruction of large defects involving multiple stages has been supplanted by evolving methods of single-stage reconstruction, from primary closure to utilization of regional or distant tissue. Further influenced by developments in radiology, anesthesia, and microsurgery, reconstruction of the upper aerodigestive tract has introduced new concepts to the surgical management of the head and neck patient. Traditionally, surgical goals in the head and neck were directed toward the alleviation of pain with improved survival. These goals were initially attempted by reconstruction focusing on wound closure through the advancement of local tissue and the use of skin grafts. A compromise in form and function with these early techniques was acceptable, with the objectives of providing safe wound healing and improving patient comfort for tumor removal. With the development of newer techniques including the use of axial pattern flaps and pedicled myocutaneous flaps, the level of care and possibilities of improvement increased, shifting the reconstructive focus toward the restoration of better form with enhanced function. These methods allowed faster recovery and more aggressive surgical extirpation, leading to an improved quality of life. No longer was the cure considered worse than the disease. The standard of care had extended beyond previously limited expectations for repair and closure to surgical approaches and therapeutic endpoints, with even greater expectations for functional and aesthetic outcomes. Thus the trend has shifted from extending the duration of life to improving the quality of life. There is a need to better define the extent of operative intervention and predictably measure its overall effect on patient rehabilitation as a result of these changes.

The present generation of reconstructive technology incorporating the use of microsurgery for tissue transfer has allowed surgeons to be more aggressive, with less morbidity and mortality, resulting in improved outcomes.[62] Despite these developments, however, overall survival has changed little. The importance of form and function in the setting of limited life expectancy becomes clearly evident.

GENERAL RECONSTRUCTIVE CONSIDERATIONS

The head and neck subserves a multitude of functions central to survival. Aside from providing the basic functions of chewing, swallowing, and speaking, the upper aerodigestive tract facilitates the specialized senses including taste, touch, and smell. The obvious visibility of the head and neck renders patients vulnerable to public scrutiny and draws undesirable attention to any disfigurement and functional alterations. Consequently, surgery involving this region produces not only a physical deformity with its attendant functional deficits, but also alters the patient's perception of reality, as well as the patient's ability to interact with his or her surroundings. Inevitably, the head and neck patient is influenced by an altered self-image and experiences a compromised ability to cope.[8,16,26] The extent to which this affects a particular patient is directly related to surgical outcome.

Central to the theme of providing optimal care is the ability to match patient expectation with outcome. The primary goal of surgical therapy is to adequately resect all of the cancer; however, reconstruction is critical to ultimate patient success. Reconstructive concerns should neither compromise nor supplant surgical ablation; nevertheless, they are critical to the overall surgical plan.

Modern reconstructive methodology, including flap selection, should have these optimal characteristics: reliability, expediency, adequate functional results, and acceptable cosmesis. Reliability is perhaps the most important factor in any type of oncologic reconstruction. Patients usually have advanced disease, indicating either a limited survival or the need for adjuvant therapy. A failed reconstruction that prolongs hospitalization and delays adjuvant therapy does not improve the quality of life. Furthermore, prolonged reconstruction and recovery not only delay optimal therapy but also waste quality "family" time and increase cost. A reliable reconstructive technique reduces temporal demands.

Expediency must also be considered, especially in today's managed care market. The cost-to-utility ratio will necessarily influence the management plan of these complicated patients. Modern reconstruction is effectively performed with microsurgery through a single-stage technique.[29] Cost utilization is maximized, and hospitalization time is minimized.[34,35] Finally, in addition to reliability and expediency, reconstruction must provide for basic function and acceptable cosmesis.

GENERAL SPEECH AND SWALLOWING CONSIDERATIONS

The site of the tumor and the method of reconstruction, among other factors, will significantly impact the patient's ability to speak and swallow postoperatively. The literature demonstrates differing success rates associated with specific types of reconstructive procedures following ablative removal of tumors of the aerodigestive tract. Therefore restoration of both speech and swallowing is critical and must be considered in treatment selection and reconstruction in order to ultimately ensure a satisfactory quality of life.

Speech and swallowing are dependent on the precise coordination and temporal organization of a series of complex neuromuscular movements and actions. Intelligible speech production requires articulatory contacts of structures of the oral and oropharyngeal cavities specifically placed and rapidly executed. Swallowing includes a series of four stages or phases in hierarchical arrangement: the oral preparatory, oral, pharyngeal, and esophageal stages. Each phase takes place based on the movement patterns and timely occurrence of neurologic triggers from the previous stage. Any interruption in movement resulting from alteration to the oropharyngeal and/or laryngeal structures or supporting framework will cause some degree of speech and swallowing difficulties.

In general, current data demonstrate that surgical procedures resulting in larger surgical defects produce more severe speech and swallowing deficits. Reconstructive procedures that utilize flaps that are adynamic, are bulky, and overfill the surgical defect will be associated with a poorer functional outcome. In some oropharyngeal reconstructions, primary closure of the defect may best preserve function postoperatively.[45,48,63]

OPERATIONS

The interrelationship of general health with functional status and its impact on quality of life provides the basis for surgical intervention and serves as a guide to help determine a reconstructive endpoint. Since the reestablished level of function in the reconstructed patient is highly predictive of the overall success of surgical rehabilitation, and functional disability is dependent on the site and size of the surgical defect, the recovery potential is determined by the methods chosen for repair.

MANDIBULECTOMY

Oral cavity malignancies that extend into the mandible require composite resections of bone and soft tissue. These defects can nutritionally cripple patients, leaving them with marked deformities influencing deglutition, mastication, speech, and salivary retention. Continuity of the mandible and soft tissue reconstruction can be accomplished in a single stage with composite osteocutaneous flaps. Osseointegrated dental implants are placed in the reconstructed mandible to complete oral rehabilitation.

We have found it helpful to classify mandibular defects by the location and extent of resection. Lateral and posterior defects involving the ramus and temporomandibular joint may be reconstructed with soft tissue alone in selected patients.[36,37] The added complexity of osseous reconstruction for lateral and posterior defects may be of little benefit in older patients, those with a poor prognosis, or those who are edentulous. Soft tissue reconstruction adequately replaces bulk and restores facial contour. The remaining bony defect interferes little with oral opening; however, mandibular deviation and alterations in dental occlusion may occur. Bony reconstruction of segmental defects of the body or ramus is justified in younger patients and in those patients in good medical condition. Anterior segmental and angle-to-angle defects of the mandible result in collapse of the mandibular arch and loss of support for the tissues of the floor of the mouth, and allow both remaining lateral segments to float freely (Figure 71-1, A). These defects can lead to oral incompetence and interfere with both speech

and nutrition. Reconstruction of these defects requires bone.

During mandibular resection, condylar removal is frequently not required. The remaining 1 to 2 cm of condylar bone at the temporomandibular joint is frequently adequate for plate fixation. If condylar support is lacking, temporomandibular joint reconstruction can be performed; however, the loss of the pterygoid insertions may still cause lateral deviation. Furthermore, despite condylar replacement, radiotherapy may cause severe ankylosis. If required, reconstruction of the temporomandibular joint is possible with one of several methods. When vascularized bone grafts are used, the end can be shaped to resemble an articular surface that fits into the glenoid fossa. If histologically proven to be disease-free, the patient's own condyle can be replaced as a nonvascularized graft; however, caution should be employed with this method. Good functional

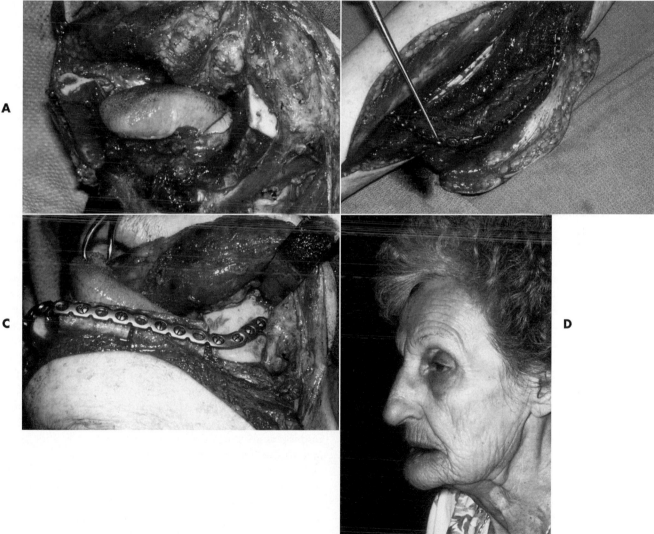

Figure 71-1. **A,** A 63-year-old woman with squamous cell carcinoma along the anterior gingival buccal sulcus of the left mandible. The patient underwent anterior mandibulectomy. The defect is demonstrated with the tongue and remaining mandibular segments in view. **B,** Free fibula flap harvest and plating in situ on the lower extremity. **C,** The osteotomized fibula is placed into the mandibular defect after bending the plate prior to mandibulectomy. The microvascular anastomosis proceeded to the external carotid artery and internal jugular vein in an end-to-side fashion following insetting. **D,** Postoperative view of the patient following resection and reconstruction.

results are possible in selected patients with all of these methods. Prosthetic condylar heads are also available and can be screwed to the vascularized bone graft or are positioned on the plate. Again, good results are possible, but infection, extrusion, and superior migration can occur in as many as 15% of patients. The main function of the reconstructed condylar head is to act as a spacer, which helps decrease horizontal translation of the mandible during opening. In general, we have not been enthusiastic about condylar reconstruction, and would advocate its use for younger patients with a good prognosis or in situations where postoperative radiation is not planned.

A variety of flaps have been described for mandibular reconstruction. Flap selection should take into consideration the need for soft tissue as well as the bony requirements. Our donor site of choice has traditionally been the fibula, which can provide up to 25 cm of sturdy, uniform bone with a circumferential cortex (Figure 71-1, B). The periosteal blood supply is segmental, and the endosteal blood supply is usually preserved so multiple osteotomies are possible without jeopardizing the viability of the bone. Skin can be harvested with bone to replace oral mucosa. The skin derives its blood supply from the septocutaneous and musculocutaneous perforators originating from the peroneal vessels. These perforators are highly variable and inclusion of a portion of the soleus muscle can increase the viability of the skin paddle. The donor vessels are of good quality; however, they may be adversely affected by either atherosclerotic disease or venous hypertension. Long-term lower extremity morbidity is not frequently seen with the use of the fibula flap.

Dental restoration can be achieved in mandibular reconstruction with osseointegrated implants.[28,61] The osseous portion of the implant is screwed into the reconstructed mandible initially, and prosthetic teeth are attached later. This technique allows for dental reconstruction that closely matches the patient's preoperative state. Implant placement can be performed concurrently with mandibular reconstructions or can be delayed, with the implants placed at the time of bone grafting. Implants must be precisely positioned to ensure proper occlusion. This may be easier in the more controlled setting of the dental oncologist's office rather than in the operating room. Proper positioning may be achieved when soft tissue swelling has resolved and necessary revisions have been performed. However, immediate insertion of osseointegrated implants allows for more rapid restoration of oral function. Placement of implants in irradiated bone is controversial, and inadequate purchase and delayed wound healing may be encountered. An interval of at least 3 months between insertion of the implants and radiotherapy should be observed to allow for bony union.

Several plating systems are available for mandibular reconstruction, and selection is generally based on surgeon's preference. Once the ablative surgeon has determined the extent of resection, the borders are permanently marked on the mandible with an oscillating saw. Before any bone is removed, a fixation plate is temporarily secured and contoured to the mandible. At least three bicortical screw holes are placed on each side of the defect prior to plate removal and osteotomy placement. The bone graft can then be shaped to fit the plate and is secured by a series of unicortical screws while still being perfused (see Figure 71-1, B). The plate/bone graft construct is then transferred to replace the resected mandible, and an accurate fit is ensured by the pre-drilled screw holes (Figure 71-1, C). Maintenance of an occlusal plane is critical during the placement of fixation points for the mandibular bone. The fibula is mobilized by placing a hip roll underneath the patient on the side of the anticipated harvest. The extremity is flexed and bent at the knee. The head of the fibula and the lateral malleolus are identified. One should plan harvest of the bone in such a way that approximately 8 to 10 cm of bone is preserved proximally and distally to avoid impairing function at the ankle and knee joints. It is possible to tailor the bone to fit the defect appropriately by preserving the periosteum and the connections with the vasculature proximally. The periosteum may be stripped from the bone and the bone cut to the desired size. This maneuver also lengthens the vascular pedicle, allowing for easier inset. Fixation is advisable prior to revascularization if possible. This ensures that the vascular anastomosis will not be disrupted during fixation of the flap. After the flap is inset and revascularized, care is taken during skin closure. If skin closure is too tight, the vascular pedicle may be compromised. It is better to place a skin graft on an exposed area rather than compromise the vascular pedicle. The skin graft will contract postoperatively and can be excised later, if necessary. If a skin paddle has been harvested, it provides a suitable means for flap monitoring. Furthermore, if placed intraorally, skin provides fill for a floor of the mouth defect and prevents tongue tethering. If a skin paddle is not used, a percutaneous point for Doppler examination is identified. Alternatively, an implantable device may be employed; our practice is to use the 20 MHz ultrasonic Doppler to monitor buried bone flaps (Figure 71-1, D).[32]

Speech and swallowing deficits associated with mandibular resection are relatively minor following surgical reconstruction. Although oromandibular reconstruction has been shown to significantly improve masticatory function, dental rehabilitation, and bite force, mandibular resection versus preservation has not been found to be predictive of either speech or swallowing efficiency in head and neck cancer patients.[47,72]

The mandible provides the foundation for the tongue and muscles of the floor of the mouth and periodontal support for the teeth. The horizontal orientation of the bone provides the platform for the soft tissue, which allows greater control during speech and swallowing.[2] Together with the lips and teeth it contributes to the articulation of some sounds and helps prevent the anterior loss of food from the mouth during the oral preparatory phase of swallowing. The degree of speech and swallowing impairment will largely depend on the amount of resection and possible involvement of the floor of mouth and tongue. The patient who has had the upper marginal mandibulectomy and/or a portion of the floor of the mouth resected and closed primarily will have relatively little change in swallowing following surgery. Lingual propulsion and control of the material in the oral cavity will be good because the remaining tongue segment is mobile and the inferior rim of the mandible has been left to maintain the mandibular contour.[56]

Musculature forming the floor of mouth, including the mylohyoid, geniohyoid, and anterior belly of the digastric, attaches to the body of the mandible anteriorly and the hyoid bone posteriorly. Because the hyoid bone is embedded in the tongue and also suspends the larynx, movement in one of these structures moves other structures attached to it. When the suprahyoid musculature is resected, the elevation and anterior tilting action of the larynx is lost, resulting in aspiration during swallowing. Therefore disruption to the muscular complex of the floor of mouth and upper neck may result in significant functional morbidity due to the close anatomic relationship between the mandible and its associated musculature and the hyolaryngeal complex.

Probably more important to speech and swallowing is the impaired sensation that often occurs following mandibular resection. The lower lip is often permanently insensate due to sacrifice of the alveolar nerve. A reduction in the strength of the labial seal may interfere with the production of some sounds. Air escape and sound distortion often occur during production of those sounds that require oral air implosion or bilabial or labiodental articulatory placement (e.g., *p, b, f,* and *v*).

Swallowing is also likely to be impaired when the lower lip is insensate. Oral manipulation and movement patterns vary, depending on the viscosity of the material to be swallowed. A labial seal becomes increasingly difficult to maintain, depending on the consistency of the material. This will result in loss of food from the mouth while eating. Additionally, attempts to drink from a cup or straw are often frustrating because of the proprioceptive loss of labial sensation and the functional inability to maintain oral competence.

Discontinuity of the mandible after surgical resection destroys the balance and symmetry of mandibular function specifically during mastication. The rotary action of the jaw crushes the food in order to help formulate it into an appropriate consistency so that when mixed with saliva and shaped into a cohesive bolus, it is ready to be swallowed. Patients who have had surgery to the lower jaw will experience difficulty aligning the mandible for proper occlusion while chewing. Patients in whom the normal maxillary mandibular relationship has been disrupted will not only experience problems chewing and swallowing but will also suffer significant cosmetic deformity. Following resection and reconstruction, few or no mandibular teeth may be left. The degree to which prosthetic and dental restoration may be accomplished will depend on the extent of the surgical procedure, the amount of soft tissue loss, and the presence or absence of teeth.[30]

GLOSSECTOMY

Speech, or the ability to articulate words intelligibly, is greatly dependent on oropharyngeal competence and tongue mobility. As with speech, deglutition is dependent on an intact oropharyngeal mechanism. Reconstructive strategies must account for these functional relationships. In addition to its obvious role in speech, the oral tongue is important for propulsion of food and liquid through the mouth. Adequate soft tissue bulk is

necessary to prevent pooling in the lateral buccal recess, as well as to decrease intraoral volume, which will facilitate oral transit and swallowing. The base of the tongue has been specifically identified as a major generator of pressure in the pharynx and is responsible for transit of food into the esophagus. Both tongue mobility and bulk therefore are essential for proper oral cavity function. Although a variety of free flaps are available for repair of any given glossectomy defect, the size of the resection helps dictate flap selection. Two workhorse flaps in our institution for glossectomy reconstruction include the radial forearm and the rectus abdominis free flap. If 30% or greater of native tongue remains (Figure 71-2, *A* and *B*), a thin pliable flap to ensure mobility should be employed (radial forearm). If, however, less tongue remains, replacement of bulk by the use of a thicker, less pliable flap is appropriate (rectus abdominis).

The radial forearm flap not only has the optimal characteristics to ensure tongue mobility, but is highly reliable due to the large diameter of its recipient vessels.[19,54,66,73] An additional advantage to the radial forearm flap is its potential for sensation.[58] A sensate flap may assist with oral competence and prevent the patient from biting the flap while eating; however, currently no prospective randomized trials have proved its efficacy over noninnervated controls. The anatomic basis of the radial forearm free flap lies with the vascularity supplied by the radial artery. This artery runs longitudinally along the volar aspect of the forearm and gives off perforating branches to the skin, subcutaneous tissue, muscle, and bone. The flap's septocutaneous perforators lie between the flexor carpi radialis and the brachioradialis muscles. The entire flap may be raised on this septal stalk with preservation of vascularity.[68] Reconstruction of the radial artery with interposition vein grafts is usually not required. However, if necessary due to insufficient flow to the radial side of the hand through the palmar arch, radial artery replacement can be achieved by using one of the many forearm veins.

Three separate venous systems provide drainage for the flap. These systems are the cephalic vein, the basilic vein, and the venae comitantes that run adjacent to the artery. The venae comitantes are the veins most frequently utilized for flap transfer, but are occasionally too small. Consequently, it is advisable to elevate a cephalic or basilic vein with the flap for use as an alternative venous drainage pathway if required (Figure 71-2, *C*).

Sensory innervation of the flap is provided by the medial and/or lateral antebrachial cutaneous nerves of the forearm and sensory branches of the radial nerve. If a sensate flap is desired, one of these branches can be harvested with the flap and sutured to the lingual nerve or other cutaneous nerves in the neck. The lateral antebrachial cutaneous nerve is a continuation of the musculocutaneous nerve. It passes deep to the cephalic vein at the elbow and then descends along the radial border of the forearm to the wrist. Innervation is provided to the skin over the lateral half of the anterior surface of the forearm. The medial antebrachial cutaneous nerve pierces the deep fascia with the basilic vein at about the middle of the forearm and divides into anterior and posterior branches. The anterior branch supplies the skin over the medial half of the

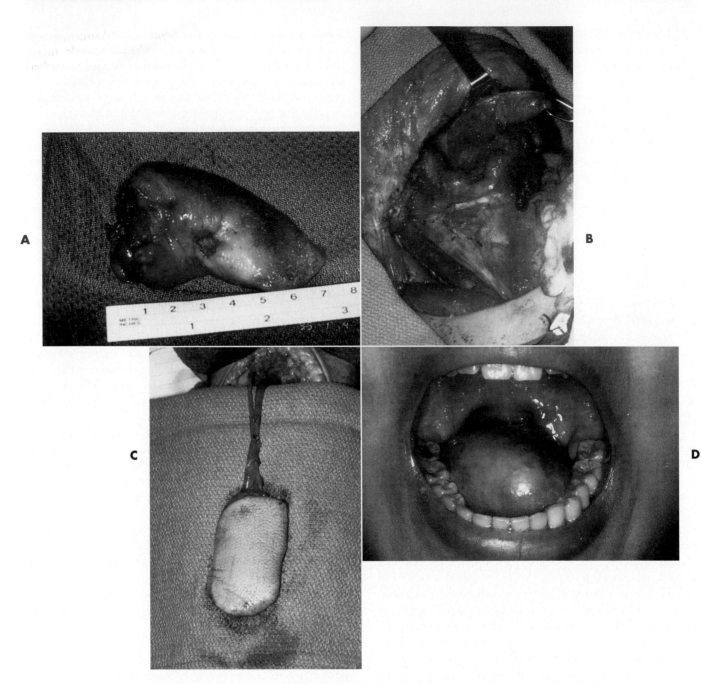

Figure 71-2. **A,** Resected partial glossectomy defect in a 23-year-old woman with squamous cell carcinoma. **B,** The defect following surgical ablation. **C,** Reconstruction proceeded with the radial forearm flap. The radial artery and cephalic vein were utilized for the revascularization. **D,** Six months following reconstruction with the radial forearm flap for a hemiglossectomy. The patient did well functionally, but succumbed to systemic disease.

anterior surface of the arm. The posterior branch lies anterior to the medial epicondyle of the humerus and supplies the skin over the medial third of the posterior surface of the forearm. In dissecting the radial forearm flap, division of the lateral or medial antebrachial cutaneous branches is frequently required. Patients should be advised of the potential for sensory loss when this flap is used. Nerve ends should be buried into muscle to prevent the potential for painful neuromas.

The radial forearm flap offers a highly mobile three-dimensional reconstruction. Portions of the skin may be deepithelialized to allow for fill in areas under mucosa. The flap is ideal for reconstruction of portions of the tongue and floor of mouth with its ability to create a sulcus for retention of food and fluid (see Figure 71-2, *B*). Consideration must be taken when designing the flap to allow for excess skin for sulcus formation (Figure 71-2, *D*). Placement of too small a flap can cause tethering and subsequent speech alterations.

In contrast, total glossectomy defects result from the resection of a large volume of tissue. These patients are at high risk for recurrent aspiration. The goal of reconstruction is to replace the tissue volume (Figure 71-3, *A*). The rectus abdominis is a good choice for this defect. The flap has a long pedicle with

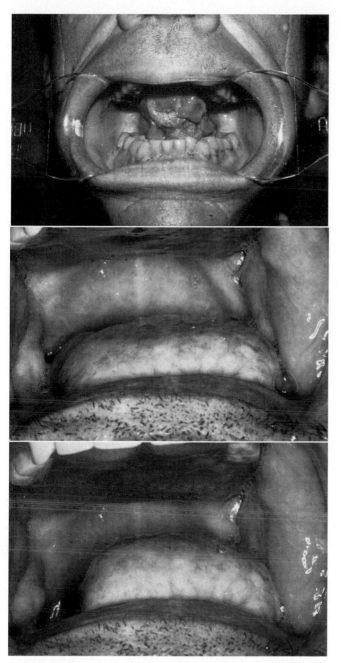

Figure 71-3. A, A 43-year-old man with squamous cell carcinoma to the anterior tongue. **B,** Reconstruction proceeded with a rectus abdominis flap. This photograph demonstrates the inset of the rectus flap. **C,** Remaining musculature allowed partial elevation of the reconstructed tongue.

large-caliber vessels, and the donor site can be easily hidden by clothing. The flap can be folded onto itself to provide a continuous closure of the anterior pharynx with an intraoral defect, or for the formation of a neotongue. Because of the bulk that the flap provides, it is ideal for the elimination of dead space. Furthermore, the well-vascularized, hardy muscle brings vital tissue into areas that are frequently prone to poor wound healing.

Since the arterial system of the rectus abdominis muscle has an extensive circulation, the well-vascularized tissue is available for coverage of exposed structures. The muscle provides bulk,

decreases dead space, and can conform around structures and prosthetic devices. The richly vascularized muscle brings chemotherapy and antibiotics into the tumor field. Furthermore, well-vascularized muscle tolerates irradiation, as well as enhances wound healing in areas treated preoperatively with adjuvant therapy.

Occasionally the flap may provide too much bulk. In this instance, the skin paddle can be excised and muscle and fascia alone used for closure of the defect. The exposed intraoral tissue may then be skin grafted, or alternatively allowed to remucosalize.

Previous abdominal surgery may preclude the use of the rectus muscle flap. If upper abdominal surgery has been performed, the inferior epigastric pedicle may be viable and flap transfer can proceed. If lower abdominal surgery has been performed, however, the inferior epigastric vascular system may have been injured. In both of these instances, exploration of the vessels should proceed before flap elevation to assess if flap transfer is possible.

Muscle function allows flexion of the vertebral column. The rectus muscle is enclosed by a fascial sheath, except below the arcuate line where a posterior fascial cover is absent. There are a variable number of tendinous insertions, but three are consistently present. The average muscle is 30 cm long, 6 cm wide, and 0.5 cm thick. Variations exist depending on the physical status of the patient. Arterial supply arises from two sources, the superior and inferior epigastric vessels. The inferior epigastric artery usually divides into a lateral and medial branch. Consequently, the rectus abdominis free flap can be raised on either lateral or medial branches, thus leaving the remaining muscle intact. Alternatively the flap can be raised and transferred without muscle, based on the perforators alone. The average arterial diameter is 2.7 mm, with a pedicle length of up to 15 cm. This artery also carries two venae comitantes, which occasionally join prior to their origin from the external iliac vein. The cutaneous paddle above the rectus abdominis muscle is classically supplied by a lateral and medial row of perforators. These perforators tend to be concentrated around the umbilicus, and despite their constancy in anatomic dissections, variations can occur that alter the reliability of the cutaneous paddle. The innervation of the rectus abdominis muscle is supplied by the ventral rami of the lower six or seven segmental thoracic spinal nerves. Consequently, the ability of transferring the rectus abdominis muscle for functional recovery is limited due to this segmental innervation.[49]

The rectus abdominis flap can be harvested either in the vertical, oblique, or transverse orientation. Additionally, flap harvest can proceed during surgical extirpation and subsequently can be tailored to fit the defect. Revision with liposuction is possible at a later date. By adding excess bulk, especially in the area of the base of tongue, the risk of aspiration is minimized.

During oral cavity reconstruction, one should make an effort to restore the gingival buccal sulcus inferior to the alveolar ridge. Failure to do so will lead to drooling and difficulty with oral competence. Portions of the flap can be anchored to the underlying bone to achieve this result (Figure 71-3, *B* and *C*). Alternatively if the mucosa on the lingual side of the mandible is sparse, the flap may be sutured around the teeth. Palatal splints may be useful, but will not overcome an ill-designed reconstruction. Late sulcus reconstruction with local tissue rearrangement and skin grafting is difficult due to tissue scarring and contracture, especially if postoperative irradiation has been administered. The orbicularis oris muscle function must be maintained in order to preserve oral competence.

The tongue and tongue movement are the most critical features to swallowing and speech production. The goals of reconstruction after partial glossectomy are to preserve mobility of the residual segment of tongue, to restore the shape and volume of the tongue, and, more recently, to recover normal sensation. However, the ability of new surgical techniques to restore normal sensation and function with innervated cutaneous free flaps remains controversial.

During the oral preparatory stage of swallowing, the tongue, in combination with the rotary action of the jaw, moves the food onto the teeth for chewing. Subsequently, it pulls the food into a semicohesive bolus or ball prior to the initiation of the oral phase, during which it lifts and propels the material posteriorly through the oral cavity. Sensory receptors in the oropharynx and tongue itself are stimulated and trigger the swallow reflex to initiate the pharyngeal stage of the swallow. Tongue base retraction and contraction of the posterior pharyngeal wall contribute to the inferior propulsion of the material through the pharynx. Structural alterations of the tongue following surgical resection will therefore affect both the oral and pharyngeal stages of swallowing. The presence of food alone will not provide the neural stimulation of the swallow reflex to trigger the pharyngeal phase of swallowing and will result in a premature loss of material over the base of tongue with aspiration.

Likewise, intelligible speech production depends primarily on the precise coordination of movements of the tongue in conjunction with the other structures of the oropharyngeal cavity including the lips, jaw, teeth, hard and soft palate, and pharynx. In general, reconstructions of the oral cavity that preserve neural innervation and that allow the greatest residual tongue movement, especially the back and base of tongue, will result in the best function for both swallowing and speech production.

Partial tongue resection, 50% or less, without any other tissue involvement and primary closure will usually result in the best swallowing outcomes.[13,48,70] However, there have been many reports of adequate swallowing abilities after major tongue resection.[22,69] Generally, the extent of resection has dictated functional outcome in nonreconstructed glossectomized patients. Following reconstruction, the degree of speech and swallowing impairment has been determined by the quality of the reconstruction rather than the extent of resection in some patients.[2]

Any reconstruction that tethers or limits the movement of the tongue will be associated with a poorer functional outcome than those in which no tongue is used in the surgical closure. Patients with total glossectomy have been shown to speak and swallow better than those with composite resection of the tongue, floor of the mouth, and mandible.[2] When total glossectomy defects require replacement of large soft tissue volumes,

biologic success of the reconstruction does not always ensure functional success.

When tongue involvement is minimal, swallowing difficulties are usually temporary and the tongue is initially clumsy, most likely from edema. Patients may have difficulty triggering the swallow, and speech may be slurred and imprecise. Usually exercises to improve lingual range of motion and control are helpful early in the recovery process and will expedite a return of swallowing function in the first 3 to 4 weeks postoperatively.[41] Logemann and Bytell reported that the extent of tongue resection did not affect long-term swallowing until over 50% was resected.[44]

Mechanisms for articulatory compensation may include exaggeration of lip, jaw, and laryngeal movements. Pharyngeal widening may be used for the articulation of high vowels (i, e, and u) and a narrowing or compression of the pharynx for low vowels (a and o).[76]

Preservation of a tongue remnant may improve verbal communication as long as the remaining portion of the tongue is able to contact the palate. This is one reason why the rectus flap has an advantage in total glossectomy. Lingual sounds in the reconstructed total glossectomy are created by the patient attempting to move the jaws to position the flap as close as possible to the palate to simulate the normal position of the tongue. A palatal reshaping or augmentation prosthesis is often beneficial for patients who remain unable to make these contacts following reconstruction. Additionally, palatal augmentation often prevents stasis or collection of food in the palatal arch when the tongue is unable to contact the palate during swallowing. Nevertheless, too much bulk to the palatal prosthesis will impede both swallowing and speech production.

LARYNGOPHARYNGECTOMY

As with other areas of the head and neck, pharyngoesophageal reconstruction is often complicated by previous cancer therapy, multiple medical problems, poor nutrition, and a history of alcohol and tobacco abuse. Circumferential resection of the cervical esophagus and/or oropharynx is most often required for advanced laryngeal cancer, but similar defects may result from lye ingestion or trauma. Speech and oral nutrition are lost without reconstruction. All current methods of reconstruction require isolation of the airway from the digestive tract. Gastric pullup and pectoralis major flaps have been used for reconstruction of proximal defects, but are associated with prolonged recovery, operative mortality rates of up to 20%, and fistula formation in as many as 40% of patients. Furthermore, thoracotomy may be required for exposure, and pedicle length can limit flap position. Following gastric pullup, lower esophageal sphincter function is altered and may lead to chronic reflux.

Although there are many surgical alternatives for functional reconstruction of the pharynx, larynx, and cervical esophagus after extirpative tumor resections, the free jejunal transfer is probably the method of choice for reconstruction of complete circumferential defects (Figure 71-4, A and B). At our institution, the free jejunal transfer is preferred for reconstruction

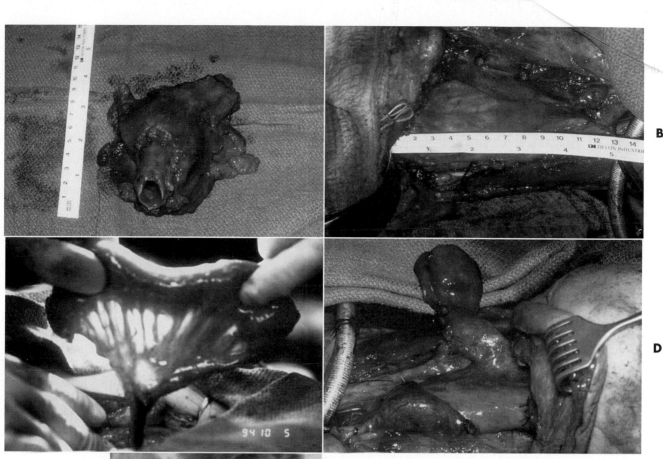

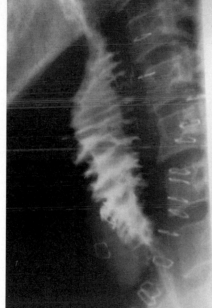

Figure 71-4. **A,** A 42-year-old woman with recurrent squamous cell carcinoma to the larynx. Photograph demonstrates resected specimen. **B,** Surgical defect of the cervical esophagus measuring 13 cm. **C,** Reconstruction proceeded with free jejunal transfer. **D,** Segment of jejunum sewn to the neck skin used to monitor flap perfusion. **E,** Barium swallow following jejunal transfer. The patient proceeded to tolerate a regular diet but succumbed to her disease 2 years later.

because it allows for a reliable, single-stage procedure useful for almost any size defect.[57] Flap survival has been reported ranging from 80% to 100%, but has been at least 95% since 1988 at our institution. If necessary, salvage of a failed free jejunal transfer with a second segment of jejunum is usually successful. Overall operative mortality has been documented between 0% and 6%. Fistula and stenosis remain the most common complications, each occurring in about 20% of patients, similar to other free tissue transfer techniques and pedicled flaps for pharyngoesophageal reconstruction. Distal defects near the gastroesophageal junction, or when thoracotomy is required for resection, demand the use of a gastric pullup.

The jejunum constitutes the first two fifths of the 7-meter-long small bowel from the ligament of Treitz to the ileocecal valve. Its diameter is about 4 cm and the mesentery is fan-shaped, with its vertebral root 15 cm long. There is an average of 12 to 15 branches to the jejunum and ileum. They run almost parallel to one another between the mesenteric layers. The vessels form a series of arcades in which the upper portion of the jejunum contains a single arcade giving off long vasa recta and the lower portion contains 2 to 3 arcades giving off shorter vasa recta. The first intestinal branch is usually not selected as a vascular pedicle for free jejunal transfer because the pedicle length is short and its origin much too high and deep. Furthermore, it may give off a common stem with the inferior pancreatic duodenal artery. Thus, the second through fourth intestinal branches are preferred. The main application of free jejunal transfer is the reconstruction of defects following extensive excision of the hypopharynx and cervical esophagus (see Figure 71-4, B). The length of the jejunum is selected to fill the defect and to provide a flap monitor. An additional 3 to 5 cm may be taken if the defect is longer than anticipated. Splaying of the jejunum to fit the proximal anastomosis may also require further length. The jejunal segment is harvested (Figure 71-4, C) and the flap is positioned in the neck in the isoperistaltic direction. Because of the size discrepancy between the lumen of the jejunal segment and the pharyngeal defect, it is often necessary to spatulate the proximal end of the segment along the antimesenteric border. The proximal bowel anastomosis is performed first, which allows the more difficult part of the procedure to be completed without peristalsis, mucus production, and bleeding. It has been our practice to perform the anastomosis in two layers using an inner 3-0 absorbable suture and an outer serosal Lembert suture of 4-0 silk. The microvascular anastomosis is then constructed in an end-to-side fashion utilizing the external carotid artery and the internal jugular vein. After the jejunum is revascularized, the distal bowel anastomosis is performed. Redundancy may be avoided by applying slight traction on the jejunum in a caudal direction while marking the flap for the distal anastomosis. It should be remembered that the neck is in the extended position during dissection and that redundancy may occur once the neck is restored to normal. The distal anastomosis may be performed with a single- or double-layer anastomosis. The antimesenteric side should be enlarged by 1 to 2 cm to prevent potential stricture formation. A monitor segment is developed from the remaining jejunum by resection of an intervening segment of bowel on a mesenteric pedicle (Figure 71-4, D). This monitor is sutured to the neck and split open to avoid mucus accumulation. The monitor can be removed in clinic after 2 to 3 weeks.

Since speech restoration is not critical to patient survival, the majority of early reports on oropharyngeal reconstruction have focused on the restoration of alimentation. Recent attention to issues of postoperative quality of life has resulted in greater consideration of speech restoration in the choice of surgical reconstruction following laryngopharyngectomy.

Anatomically, the jejunal graft serves as a conduit for food passage from the oral cavity to the esophagus (Figure 71-4, E). Physiologically, studies have suggested that with optimal lumen diameter, mucus secretion and intrinsic peristalsis of the jejunal graft enhance food passage through the segment. In fact, a majority of data confirm near-normal swallowing function following reconstruction with jejunal transfer.[5,7,27]

Our experience has shown that swallowing will be enhanced when jejunal redundancy is avoided. Excessive length will result in marked difficulties in bolus transit through the segment, stasis of material, and in some instances, a retrograde flow of food upward into the nose or mouth. Even when reconstruction has been optimal, patients may continue to experience delayed transit through the segment and difficulty swallowing more solid foods. Alternating liquid and solid swallows often facilitates passage through the segment.

Conversely, successful alaryngeal speech restoration following radical surgical resection such as laryngopharyngectomy may be more complicated. Three major contemporary approaches are used to restore oral communication following laryngectomy. They include the artificial larynx, esophageal speech production, and surgical-prosthetic alternatives such as tracheoesophageal voice restoration. Although the final choice for alaryngeal speech production should always be that of the patient's, our experience has shown that only two, the artificial larynx and surgical-prosthetic voice restoration, are truly viable alternatives following removal of both the larynx and pharynx with jejunal reconstruction. The traditional method of esophageal speech production via oral implosion has not proven to be easily achievable for most patients with jejunal interposition. Several authors have suggested that the major functional problem with the jejunal autograft has been the failure to develop adequate neoesophageal speech. The failure has been attributed to the large lumen of the jejunal segment, which limits effective vibration for speech production by standard techniques of oral air implosion.[20,33,59] The additional bulk of the jejunal mucosa also inhibits efficient air charging and vibration of the jejunal wall.

Although the artificial larynx has the advantage of providing immediate verbal communication with relative ease and little if any medical complications, many patients find it unacceptable because of its mechanical sound quality. Therefore tracheojejunal puncture (TJP) has become a popular alternative for patients who undergo treatment of more advanced tumors that involve the hypopharynx or cervical esophagus. TJP, like tracheoesophageal puncture (TEP) following simple laryngectomy, can be done as a primary procedure at the time of surgery or later as a secondary procedure. The advantages of primary TJP remain the same as the advantages of primary TEP; the psychologic benefits and quick restoration to a quality lifestyle are the payoffs of a single operation with simultaneous voice restoration.

In spite of the benefits, there are several disadvantages and conditions that have been cited as contraindications to TJP as a primary procedure. The few studies that have examined tracheojejunal voice restoration have generally reported restored sound production and a potential for communication but a lack of acceptability of the sound quality. Laryngopharyngectomized patients consistently score lower in fundamental frequency, intensity, intelligibility, and social acceptability than both laryngectomized and normal subjects.[50,51] Postoperative vocal quality has often been described as "wet," most likely a result of the increased mucus secretions, which most patients find equally unacceptable. Therefore the long-term use of tracheojejunal voice for daily conversational needs may be limited for aesthetic reasons as opposed to problems producing sound.

It has been our experience that it is often better to wait until healing has occurred and consider TJP as a secondary procedure. When TJP is performed as a secondary procedure, it has the advantage of allowing preoperative examination of postoperative tracheojejunal sound quality and speech potential. Insufflation of the jejunum can be performed similar to the preoperative insufflation testing that has been used to evaluate and predict postoperative tracheoesophageal speech production.[6,39] The patient has the ability to refuse the alternative if the predicted speech results are unacceptable.

Other objections to primary TJP include surgical contraindications. Some authors have suggested that the only contraindication to primary puncture is an interposition flap such as a gastric pullup or jejunum following complete cervical esophagectomy because the retrotracheal space is opened.[23]

No current method of reconstruction following laryngopharyngectomy permits the same quality of speech and swallowing function as that which can be obtained following total laryngectomy. Nevertheless, successful speech and swallowing outcomes are not limited to simple laryngectomy alone. The goal of restoration must not be to simply restore a conduit that does not leak. Postoperative rehabilitation will be optimized when consideration of both speech and swallowing function is given to the selection of the technique that results in functioning that is as close to normal as possible.

OUTCOMES

FUNCTIONAL EVALUATION

Although there are numerous reports regarding reconstructive methods for the oral cavity, pharynx, and larynx, there are relatively few reports that objectively assess and compare the functional results of each. Most are subjective reports with little objective data, thus making comparison of different methods problematic and decisions as to how to modify surgical procedures for improved function difficult. Various evaluative techniques for swallowing and speech production provide a more objective assessment of functional outcome and success.

A number of imaging and nonimaging instrumentation procedures have been used to evaluate swallow physiology. Each procedure provides specific and often unique information on oropharyngeal anatomy and swallowing physiology. Perhaps the most widely utilized tool to evaluate swallowing is the videofluoroscopic examination or modified barium swallow (MBS).[17,42,43] The videofluoroscopic study provides information regarding bolus transit times, motility deficits, and the presence and etiology of aspiration. It allows visualization of activity during mastication, the occurrence of the swallow reflex, and the movement of the structures involved in the pharyngeal stage of swallowing including the larynx, hyoid, tongue base, pharyngeal walls, and cricopharyngeal region. The study is usually performed in lateral and anteroposterior planes with relatively minimal radiation exposure. Various food consistencies are given in measured increments and when mixed with barium can be evaluated during the swallow. Additionally, the study is designed to evaluate the optimal eating strategies to enable possible continuation of oral alimentation.[40]

Fiberoptic endoscopic examination of swallowing (FEES) has become increasingly more popular as a videoendoscopic tool for the examination of the pharynx and larynx before and after swallowing.[38] Endoscopic examination has several advantages. It is portable and can be brought to the bedside or performed in the office when the patient cannot be easily moved or positioned on the fluoroscopy platform or table. It does not require the extensive effort and expense involved in the radiographic examination with a radiologist, a technician, and a speech pathologist. It can be done immediately and can be repeated as often as necessary without the hazard of radiation exposure to the patient. Most important, it affords a highly sensitive evaluation of aspiration through direct visualization. The tool also has the advantage of providing biofeedback to the patient while learning various swallowing maneuvers. Two of the criticisms of the technique are that the visual image is blocked during the swallow and the oral stage of swallowing cannot be visualized. Therefore oral physiology must be inferred.

Intelligible speech is produced by articulatory movements of the structures of the oropharyngeal cavity. The movement of these structures and the shape of the oropharyngeal cavity determine the shape of the resonating chambers of the vocal tract. The sound produced in the larynx is shaped by the articulators into various consonants and vowels with varying distinctions such as plosives, continuants, and nasals. Via spectrography, these sounds can be further broken into component frequencies and patterns.

Glossectomy and composite resection change the properties of the vocal tract by altering the shape of the sound chamber as the tongue changes in relationship to the rest of the articulators of the oropharyngeal cavity. The changes in shapes will have new movement patterns. In essence, the more closely the pattern resembles normal, the more intelligible the vowel or consonant will be.

The speed with which the tongue moves from consonant position to vowel position will also affect intelligibility. Acoustic studies and perceptual analyses of articulation and intelligibility demonstrate that although there is loss of certain speech sounds, compensatory movements substitute approximations for the impaired sound. Speech increases in intelligibility as the reconstructed tongue makes better contact with the other structures of the oral cavity, specifically the palate.

QUALITY OF LIFE ASSESSMENT

The management philosophy for head and neck patients with defects in the upper aerodigestive tract has expanded to fine tuning of aesthetic detail, and an approach to reconstruction that focuses on specialization of function. From a practical standpoint, the surgical head and neck patient must be approached with function in mind.

One method of assessing the impact of disease and the effectiveness of treatment is to consider the patient's quality of life. Although difficult to precisely define,[18] quality of life can be conceptualized as an appraisal of a person's overall well-being.[9] This appraisal should reflect the patient's own viewpoint on the effectiveness of therapy.[1,64] Several definitions have been proposed depicting the multidimensional and complex nature of quality of life.[10,14,67] Quality of life has been described as dynamic, in that it changes over time.[11] Factors determined to influence the perception of a person's sense of well-being include psychologic and emotional stability, behavioral independence, social adaptability, and economic security. General health status and functional rehabilitative potential have also been identified as having a particularly notable impact on the quality of life.[46] Quality of life issues are especially important when determining treatment options.

Cancer-related disability, particularly in the head and neck region, affects all aspects of a patient's life.[3,60] From a general health standpoint, the disease is chronic and often terminal. The impact of health status and the perceived threat by the patient has been assessed by determining general health measures.[21,52,65] These measures include a global assessment of the patient's overall health, and its effect on the ability to cope with illness. Examples of general health domains utilized to measure the effect of health on illness include the systemic effects of the disease, with the resulting physical limitations; treatment side effects; and the psychologic distress resulting from the threat of personal loss and impending death. From a comprehensive standpoint, these general health measures directly influence the patient's quality of life.

More precise head and neck specific measures have also been identified that relate to the site-specific effect the disease process has on a patient's well-being.* In the cancer patient, this may involve gross disfigurement from major resections, with attendant body and self-image problems. Whereas general health measures describe the global impact of health status on physical well-being, head and neck specific measures relate to site-specific functional disability.[4,55] Loss of specialized functions such as taste, deglutition, and speech subjects the patient not only to a compromised general health status, but also to a reduced ability to perform important activities for daily living. The importance of functional status therefore is paramount.

Several methods or instruments have been developed to quantitatively measure quality of life and related issues. These instruments are primarily derived from patient and clinician interviews and questionnaire-based patient responses. Two tested and proven general health surveys as they relate to life quality include the Medical Outcomes Studies Short-Form 36 (SF-36) and the Functional Assessment of Cancer Therapy (FACT) Scale.[12,75] Each survey is designed to measure variable conditions such as pain perception, energy level, feelings of nausea, depression, and ability to interact with others. A composite score is generated and treatment efficacy is analyzed as related to physical, emotional, functional, and social well-being.

Disease-specific multiple-domain instruments have also been developed to determine the effect a particular disease site has on overall quality of life.[15] Examples include the University of Washington Quality of Life Scale (UW-QOL), the FACT Head and Neck Subscale (HNS), the Performance Status Scale for Head and Neck Cancer (PSS-HN), and the Head and Neck Cancer-Specific Quality of Life Instrument (HNQOL).[71] These methods determine specific functional limitations resulting from the disease process, such as difficulties with speech and swallowing and the influence on a patient's ability to communicate, eat, and tolerate physical and emotional discomfort.

Unlike the general health surveys in which overlapping domains influence the overall score, site-specific surveys separate out each domain as it relates to outcome. For example, within the domain of eating, difficulty in swallowing could be a chemotherapy-related side effect or the result of a structural deficit from an oropharyngeal tumor. Both would be reflected in the general health survey score. Utilizing head and neck–specific measures, however, the final score better reflects the functional limitation as it relates to the specific site and not to adjuvant therapy. These scores represent a precise measurement of functional deficit on quality of life, and yield more accurate information regarding rehabilitative outcome.

SUMMARY

Upper aerodigestive tract reconstruction mandates a team approach. Working together, the surgeon, the speech pathologist, and the medical oncologist can identify structural and functional deficits, formulate a treatment plan, and subsequently assist in the reconstructive needs of the patient.

REFERENCES

1. Aaronson NK: Quality of life: what is it? How should it be measured? *Oncology* 2:69-74, 1988.
2. Allison GR, Rappaport I, et al: Adaptive mechanisms of speech and swallowing after combined jaw and tongue reconstruction in long-term survivors, *Am J Surg* 154:419-422, 1987.
3. American Cancer Society: Cancer facts and figures, New York, 1986, American Cancer Society.
4. Baker C: A functional status scale for measuring quality of life outcomes in head and neck cancer patients, *Cancer Nurs* 18(6):452-457, 1995.
5. Biel MA, Maisel RH: Free jejunal autograft reconstruction of the pharyngoesophagus: review of a 10-year experience, *Otolaryngol Head Neck Surg* 97(4):369-375, 1987.
6. Blom ED, Singer MI, et al: An improved esophageal insufflation test, *Arch Otolaryngol* 111:211-212, 1985.

---

*References 24, 25, 31, 53, 74, 77.

7. Bradford CR, Esclamado RM, et al: Monitoring of revascularized jejunal autografts, *Arch Otolaryngol Head Neck Surg* 118(10):1042-1044, 1992.

8. Breitbart W, Holland J: Psychological aspects of head and neck cancer, *Semin Oncol* 15:61-69, 1988.

9. Calman KC: Quality of life in cancer patients: a hypothesis, *J Med Ethics* 10:24-127, 1984.

10. Cella DF: Quality of life: concepts and definition, *J Pain Symptom Manage* 9:186-192, 1994.

11. Cella DF, Tulsky DS: Measuring quality of life today: methodological aspects, *Oncology* 4:29-38, 1990.

12. Cella DF, Tulsky DS, et al: The Functional Assessment of Cancer Therapy scale: development and validation of the general measure, *J Clin Oncol* 11(3):570-579, 1993.

13. Conley JJ: Swallowing dysfunction associated with radical surgery of the head and neck, *Arch Surg* 80:602-612, 1960.

14. Croog SH: Current issues in the conceptualization and measurement of quality of life. Paper presented at the National Institutes of Health (Office of Science Policy and Legislation) Special Workshop on Quality of Life Assessment: Practice, Problems, and Promise, Bethesda, Md, October 15-17, 1990.

15. D'Antonio LL, Zimmerman GJ, et al: Quality of life functional status measures in patients with head and neck cancer, *Arch Otolaryngol Head Neck Surg* 122:482-487, 1996.

16. David DJ, Barritt JA: Psychological implications of surgery for head and neck cancer, *Clin Plast Surg* 9:327-335, 1982.

17. Dodds WJ, Stewart ET, et al: Physiology and radiology of the normal oral and pharyngeal phases of swallowing, *Am J Roentgenology* 154:953-963, 1990.

18. Drettner B, Ahlbom A: Quality of life and state of health for patients with cancer in the head and neck, *Acta Otolaryngol (Stockh)* 96:307-314, 1983.

19. Evans GRD, Schusterman MA, Kroll SS, et al: The radial forearm free flap for head and neck reconstruction: a review, *Am J Surg* 168:446-450, 1994.

20. Fisher SR, Cole BC, et al: Pharyngoesophageal reconstruction using free jejunal interposition grafts, *Arch Otolaryngol* 111:747-752, 1985.

21. Flanagan JC: Measure of quality of life: current state of the art, *Arch Phys Med Rehabil* 63:56-59, 1982.

22. Frazell EL, Lucas JC: Cancer of the tongue: report of the management of 1,554 patients, *Cancer* 15:1085-1099, 1962.

23. Freeman SB, Hamaker RC: In Blom ED, Singer RI, Hamaker RC, editors: *Tracheoesophageal voice restoration following total laryngectomy,* San Diego, 1998, Singular Publishing Group, pp 19-25.

24. Gliklich RE, Goldsmith TA, et al: Are head and neck specific quality of life measures necessary? *Head Neck* 19:474-480, 1997.

25. Gotay CC, Moore TD: Assessing quality of life in head and neck cancer [Review], *Qual Life Res* 1:5-17, 1992.

26. Graham WP, Rosillo RH: Social rehabilitation of the patient with head and neck cancer. In Anderson R, Hoopes JE, editors: *Symposium on malignancies of the head and neck,* St Louis, 1975, Mosby, pp 215-220.

27. Gullane P, Havas T, et al: Pharyngeal reconstruction: current controversies, *J Otolaryngol* 16(3):169-173, 1987.

28. Gürlek A, Miller MJ, et al: Functional results of dental restoration with osseointegrated implants after mandible reconstruction, *Plast Reconstr Surg* 101:650-655, 1998.

29. Hardesty RA, James NF, et al: Microsurgery for macrodefects: microvascular free tissue transfer for massive defects of the head and neck, *Am J Surg* 154:399-405, 1987.

30. Hurst PS: The role of the prosthodontist in the correction of swallowing disorders, *Otolaryngol Clin North Am* 21(4):771-781, 1988.

31. Jones E, Lund VJ, et al: Quality of life of patients treated surgically for head and neck cancer, *J Laryngol Otol* 106:238-242, 1992.

32. Jones NF: Intraoperative and postoperative monitoring of microvascular free tissue transfer, *Clin Plast Surg* 19:783-797, 1992.

33. Juarbe C, Shemen L, et al: Tracheoesophageal puncture for voice restoration after extended laryngopharyngectomy, *Arch Otolaryngol Head Neck Surg* 115:356-359, 1989.

34. Khouri R: Practice patterns and outcome data in a prospective survey of 495 microvascular free flaps, Abstract *ASRM,* Tucson, 1996.

35. Khouri RK, Cooley BC, Kunselman AR, et al: A prospective study of microvascular free-flap surgery and outcome, *Plast Reconstr Surg* 102:711-721, 1998.

36. Komisar A: The functional result of mandibular reconstruction, *Laryngoscope* 100:364-373, 1990.

37. Kroll SS, Robb GL, et al: Reconstruction of posterior mandibular defects with soft tissue using the rectus abdominis free flap, *Br J Plast Surg* 51:503-507, 1998.

38. Langmore SE, Schatz K, et al: Endoscopic and videofluoroscopic evaluations of swallowing and aspiration, *Ann Otol Rhinol Laryngol* 100:678-681, 1991.

39. Lewin JS, Baugh RF, et al: An objective method for prediction of tracheoesophageal speech production, *J Speech Hear Dis* 52(3):212-217, 1987.

40. Logemann JA: In Berman D, editor: *Evaluation and treatment of swallowing disorders,* Austin, Tex, 1998, Pro-Ed, pp 53-70.

41. Logemann JA: Swallowing disorders after treatment for oral and oropharyngeal cancer. In Berman D, editor: *Evaluation and treatment of swallowing disorders,* Austin, Tex, 1998, Pro-Ed, pp 251-279.

42. Logemann JA: Imaging the oropharyngeal swallow, *Adm Radiol* 3:20-24, 43, 1993.

43. Logemann JA: In Hyams H, editor: *Manual for the videofluoroscopic study of swallowing,* ed 2, Austin, Tex, 1993, Pro-Ed.

44. Logemann JA, Bytell DE: Swallowing disorders in three types of head and neck surgical patients, *Cancer* 44(3):1095-1105, 1979.

45. Logemann JA, Rademaker AW, et al: Speech and swallow function after tonsil/base of tongue resection with primary closure, *J Speech Hear Res* 36:918-926, 1993.

46. Long SA, D'Antonio LL, et al: Factors related to quality of life and functional status in 50 patients with head and neck cancer, *Laryngoscope* 106:1084-1088, 1996.

47. McConnel FMS, Logemann JA, et al: Surgical variables affecting postoperative swallowing efficiency in oral cancer patients: a pilot study, *Laryngoscope* 104:87-90, 1994.

48. McConnel FMS, Pauloski BR, et al: Functional results of primary closure vs flaps in oropharyngeal reconstruction, *Arch Otolaryngol Head Neck Surg* 124:625-630, 1998.

49. McCraw JB, Arnold PG: *McCraw and Arnold's atlas of muscle and musculocutaneous flaps,* Norfolk, Va, 1986, Hampton Press.

50. Medina JE, Nance A, et al: Voice restoration after total laryngopharyngectomy and cervical esophagectomy using the duckbill prosthesis, *Am J Surg* 154:407-410, 1987.

51. Mendelsohn M, Morris M, et al: A comparative study of speech after total laryngectomy and total laryngopharyngectomy, *Arch Otolaryngol Head Neck Surg* 119(5):508-510, 1993.

52. Morris J: Life after treatment—quality of life, *Head Neck* 13:554-556, 1991.

53. Morton RP, Witterick IJ: Rationale and development of a quality of life instrument for head-and-neck cancer patients, *Am J Otolaryngol* 16(5):284-293, 1995.

54. Muldowney JB, Cohen JI, et al: Oral cavity reconstruction using the free radial forearm flap, *Arch Otolaryngol Head Neck Surg* 12:1219-1224, 1987.

55. Olson ML, Shedd DP: Disability and rehabilitation in head and neck cancer patients after treatment, *Head Neck Surg* 1:52-58, 1978.

56. Rappaport L, Swirsky A, et al: Functional considerations after resection of the hyomandibular complex, *Am J Surg* 116:581-584, 1968.

57. Reece GP, Bengtson BP, Schusterman MA: Reconstruction of the pharynx and cervical esophagus using free jejunal transfer, *Clin Plast Surg* 21:125-136, 1994.

58. Santamaria E, Wei F, et al: Sensation recovery on innervated radial forearm flap for hemiglossectomy reconstruction by using different recipient nerves, *Plast Reconstr Surg* 103:450-457, 1999.

59. Schecter GL, Baker JW, et al: Functional evaluation of pharyngoesophageal reconstructive techniques, *Arch Otolaryngol Head Neck Surg* 113:40-44, 1987.

60. Schliephake H, Neukam FW, et al: Long-term quality of life after ablative tumor surgery, *J Craniomaxillofac Surg* 23:243-249, 1995.

61. Schmelzeisen R, Neukam FW, et al: Postoperative function after implant insertion in vascularized bone grafts in maxilla and mandible, *Plast Reconstr Surg* 97:719-725, 1996.

62. Schusterman MA, Horndeski G: Analysis of the morbidity associated with immediate microvascular reconstruction in head and neck cancer patients, *Head Neck* 13:51-55, 1991.

63. Sessions D, Zill R, et al: Deglutition after conservative surgery for cancer of the larynx and pharynx, *Otolaryngol Head Neck Surg* 87:779-796, 1979.

64. Slevin ML, Plant H, Lynch D, et al: Who should measure quality of life, the doctor or the patient? *Br J Cancer* 57:109-112, 1988.

65. Smart CR, Vates JW: Quality of life, *Cancer* 60:620-622, 1987.

66. Song R, Gao T, Song Y, et al: The radial forearm flap, *Clin Plast Surg* 9:21, 1982.

67. Spilker B: Introduction. In Spilker B, editor: *Quality of life assessments in clinical trials,* New York, 1990, Raven, pp 3-9.

68. Strauch B, Yo HL: *Atlas of microvascular surgery,* New York, 1993, Theime Medical.

69. Summers GW: Physiologic problems following ablative surgery of the head and neck, *Otolaryngol Clin North Am* 7:217-250, 1974.

70. Teichgraeber J, Bowman J, et al: Functional analysis of treatment of oral cavity cancer, *Arch Otolaryngol Head Neck Surg* 112(9):959-965, 1986.

71. Terrell JE, Nanavati KA, et al: Head and neck cancer—specific quality of life, *Arch Otolaryngol Head Neck Surg* 123:1125-1132, 1997.

72. Urken ML, Buchbinder D, et al: Functional evaluation following microvascular oromandibular reconstruction of the oral cancer patient: a comparative study of reconstructed and nonreconstructed patients, *Laryngoscope* 101(9):935-950, 1991.

73. Urken ML, Weinberg H, Vickery C, et al: The neurofasciocutaneous radial forearm flap in head and neck reconstruction: a preliminary report, *Laryngoscope* 100:161-173, 1990.

74. Van Knippenberg FCE, Out JJ, et al: Quality of life in patients with resected oesophageal cancer, *Soc Sci Med* 35(2):139-145, 1992.

75. Ware JE: SF-36 health survey: manual and interpretation guide, Bolton, Mass, 1993, The Health Institute.

76. Weber RS, Ohlms L, et al: Functional results after total or near total glossectomy with laryngeal preservation, *Arch Otolaryngol Head Neck Surg* 117:512-515, 1991.

77. Wilson KM, Risk NM, et al: Effects of hemimandibulectomy on quality of life, *Laryngoscope* 108:1574-1577, 1998.

CHAPTER

Benign Tumors and Conditions of the Head and Neck

Bruce S. Bauer

INTRODUCTION

Benign conditions of the head and neck can be grouped into congenital and acquired lesions, as pediatric or adult, based on embryologic origin of the involved tissues, and by the region of the head and neck involved. By knowing the embryology and germ layer involved, one can generally recognize the path of development, the location of the lesion, and the anatomy of the structures adjacent to the lesion or, in the case of branchial sinuses, through which the structure passes. This chapter will cover pediatric as well as adult conditions, concentrating on understanding many of the lesions based on their embryology and germ cell layer of origin and then moving on to acquired lesions.

For many of these conditions, once a diagnosis is made and there is an indication for treatment, the operation is straightforward, with the desired outcome one of elimination of the problem. For some conditions like neurofibromatosis, the outcome is a function of the often slow but relentless progression of the disease, being as varied as the disease in its presentation. Given the wide range of conditions to be discussed, it is hoped that this chapter will lay the groundwork for an organized approach to the evaluation and treatment of any lesion that may be encountered.

INDICATIONS

BENIGN PEDIATRIC TUMORS AND CONDITIONS

Hamartomas

Many tumors and conditions seen in both pediatric and adult populations have their origin in "errors" occurring during development of the varied germ layers and movement of the facial processes during formation of the head and neck. The hamartomas embrace a heterogenous group of congenital malformations comprising normal tissue found in a particular location either in excessive numbers or in an abnormal relationship to the surrounding structures. Unlike true neoplasms, the cells within the hamartoma usually retain their normal histology and function, growing and maturing in proportion to the surrounding tissue. However, they demonstrate the capacity for enlargement as a result of distention of vascular, ductal, or cystic components.[3]

With the exception of the hemangiomas, which manifest true neoplastic qualities (with disproportionate cellular proliferation in the postnatal period), hamartomas do not show evidence of cell alteration and unrestrained growth. Nonetheless, malignant degeneration of cells within a hamartoma is well recognized, and even without a loss of cellular growth restraints, the excessive growth of "normal cells" and disturbance of surrounding structure, function, and appearance will prompt surgical intervention.

The fact that these lesions may arise from any of the three germ layers, either singly or in combinations, and that they exhibit varied growth potential has resulted in an equally varied terminology, classification, and approach to treatment.

HAMARTOMAS OF ECTODERMAL ORIGIN. The hamartomas of purely ectodermal origin are typically referred to as nevi, with their name modified to indicate the epidermal structures that predominate in the lesion. The most common are epidermal nevi, sebaceous nevi, and nevoid basal cells. Although the first two of these may exist as an isolated lesion or group of lesions, each also exists as a cutaneous manifestation of a systemic disease involving multiple organ systems. In the latter condition, the presence of benign odontogenic cysts, a common associated manifestation of the syndrome, is particular pertinent to the current discussion.

Since the indications, operations, and outcomes for the congenital nevi have been discussed in Chapter 65, the discussion will not be repeated here; however, it is worth mentioning that from an indication standpoint, this group of benign cutaneous conditions manifests varying degrees of risk of malignant degeneration. Therefore many are addressed surgically. Mandibular cysts, associated with Gorlin's syndrome (basal cell nevus syndrome), have been discussed at greater depth elsewhere in this text, and the reader is referred to Chapter 77.

HAMARTOMAS OF NEUROECTODERMAL ORIGIN. Hamartomas of neuroectodermal origin arise embryologically from the neural crest and can involve all tissues of neural crest

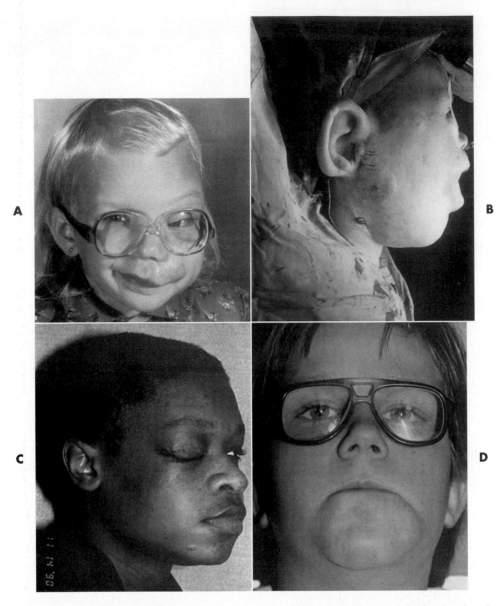

Figure 72-1. The varied "facies" and manifestations of neurofibromatosis of the head and neck. **A** to **D,** Varied degrees of involvement of the orbit and face, macrotia secondary to overgrowth of the ear, involvement limited to the orbit, and involvement limited to the chin and lower lip.

origin, although typically they involve abnormalities of the skin and nerve tissue. There are two primary disorders, neurofibromatosis and melanocytic nevi; since melanocytic nevi have been discussed in depth in Chapter 65,[3] we will concentrate on neurofibromatosis.

Neurofibromas and Neurofibromatosis. Neurofibromas may occur as solitary lesions without associated café au lait spots or as evidence of a neurocutaneous syndrome, von Recklinghausen's disease. Neurofibromatosis is an autosomal dominant inherited syndrome of multiple neurofibromas, café au lait spots, and other associated findings (NF I). This disorder generally manifests itself in infancy or childhood with the appearance of the café au lait spots (the presence of six or more lesions 0.5 cm or greater in size is a strong indicator of the disorder in an infant). It may also present with freckling in the axilla and may have Lisch nodules that can be seen on slit

lamp examination. In general neurofibromatosis progresses to adulthood, affecting skin, soft tissue, nerve, and bone to varying degrees.[20]

Neurofibromas are typically flesh-colored papules or nodules with soft consistency. Occasionally the lesions may be pedunculated, and large masses with numerous palpable thickened nerves (plexiform neurofibromas) may grow to massive proportion. These hanging masses of tissue, common on the face as well as the trunk, have been termed *pachydermatoceles*. The indications for treatment of neurofibromatosis include correction of the aesthetic disfigurement and the functional disruption caused by the enlarged and distorted tissue (Figure 72-1).[9,10]

From an aesthetic standpoint, as the affected tissues gradually enlarge, show surface pigment change, and gradually lose connective tissue support, the facial features can be grossly distorted. Correction is often limited by the slow but relentless

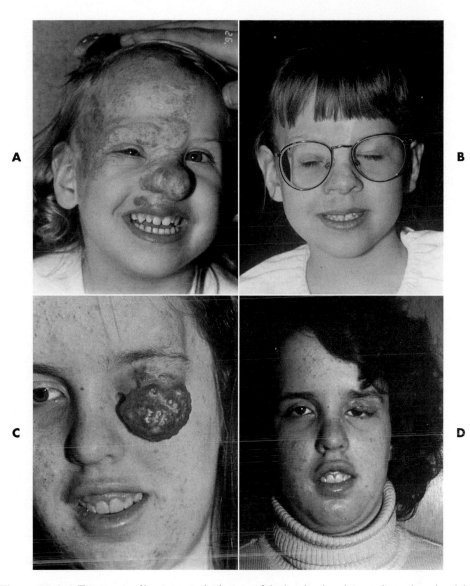

Figure 72-2. Treatment of benign vascular lesions of the head and neck is predicated on the ability to assess the lesion by appearance and history and determine its nature and expected behavior. **A** and **B,** Preoperative and postoperative appearance of an extensive hemangioma of the face and nose. Surgery began at age 4½ years with reduction of the residual lesion and fibrofatty tissue of the nose, while the upper facial lesion was left to involute further. **C** and **D,** Preoperative and postoperative views of a venous malformation of the upper eyelid. *Continued*

progress seen in many patients and is rarely definitively successful with one stage. Areas commonly addressed are the eyelids and orbit, cheek, and ear. These can be daunting and discouraging procedures for both the surgeon and the patient, but the patient is often grateful for whatever improvement can be gained.

Since areas requiring both aesthetic and functional improvement must be addressed, many procedures deal with the eyelid and orbital manifestations of the disease. Not only are the tissues of the eyelid, periorbita, and orbit affected, but commonly the vision is also affected by compression or optic nerve involvement. As the disease progresses a decision may need to be made concerning whether to sacrifice the globe for optimal aesthetic correction, removing what at this stage may be a sightless eye. One must also address the orbital defect, which most typically exhibits both enlargement of the orbit

and a defect in the greater wing of the sphenoid bone. The latter, in combination with the soft tissue overgrowth about the globe, may lead to a pulsatile exophthalmos.[13,15,29]

HAMARTOMAS OF MESODERMAL ORIGIN. Vascular malformations, including those of capillary, venous, arteriovenous, and lymphatic vessels, are hamartomas of endothelial cells that vary primarily in the type of vasoformative tissue that has overgrown.[9] Although there is still considerable controversy regarding the most appropriate classification for "lumpers" and "splitters," Mulliken and Glowacki's[19] classification based on cellular growth characteristics is most helpful in both understanding and explaining an appropriate approach to treatment. Although hemangioma was once considered a vascular hamartoma, its origin and cellular behavior warrant its designation as a true neoplasm (Figure 72-2).

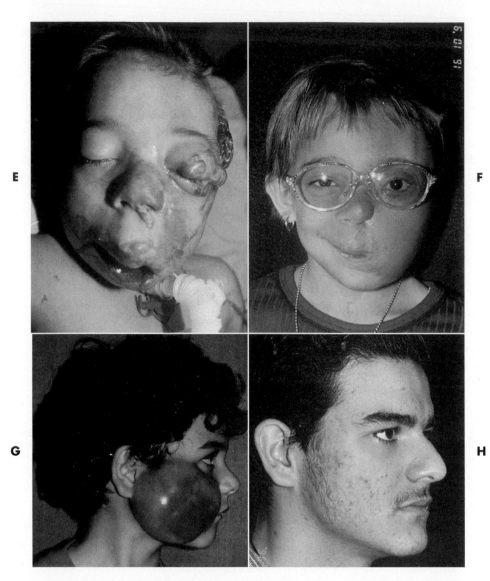

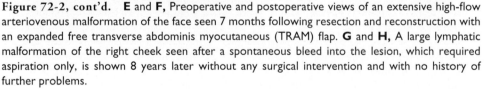

Figure 72-2, cont'd. **E** and **F,** Preoperative and postoperative views of an extensive high-flow arteriovenous malformation of the face seen 7 months following resection and reconstruction with an expanded free transverse abdominis myocutaneous (TRAM) flap. **G** and **H,** A large lymphatic malformation of the right cheek seen after a spontaneous bleed into the lesion, which required aspiration only, is shown 8 years later without any surgical intervention and with no history of further problems.

The hamartomas of mesodermal origin present three different indications for treatment: aesthetic disfigurement associated with the hamartomas; functional impairment related to their presence, including pain or chronic infection; and potentially life-threatening consequences of either encroachment on vital organs, cardiac decompensation related to shunted blood flow, or bleeding associated with them. These indications will vary, depending on the type of vessels making up the malformation.

Any of the vascular malformations may present disfigurement due either to the size of the lesion and its distortion of the facial appearance or to the surface lesion's color or abnormal surface texture. The capillary vascular malformations, being primarily superficial lesions, are amenable to treatment with laser. Venous malformations that may discolor the surface of the skin but primarily affect the subcutaneous and deeper

layers of the face may be amenable to combined treatment with laser and sclerosing agents.

Functional impairment requiring treatment may come about in a variety of ways. The location of the lesion may affect function, such as compression or distortion of the globe with expansion of a venous malformation into the orbit. Movement of the jaw and chewing may be affected by a vascular malformation involving the temporalis muscle or a malformation affecting the buccal lining, with the mass of the lesion both distorting and interfering with the occlusion. Pain may occur from either of these effects or may occur if there has been bleeding into the lesion following incidental trauma, or on occasion from small thrombosis within low flow venous malformations. Some of these problems may be amenable to conservative management; some will require intervention. Lymphatic malformations, if superficial (lymphangioma circumscripta),[4] may require excision because of chronic infection and drainage from superficial vesicles. Deeper lymphatic malformations may be approached either with observation alone or with occasional need for oral antibiotics if the lesion flares up (not uncommon in the presence of upper respiratory infections), may be amenable to sclerosis, or may require excision. Impairment of vital functions, with potentially life-threatening effects, may come as a consequence of either a "steal" effect due to high flow in an arteriovenous malformation (AVM),[18] encroachment on vital structures such as the airway, or massive blood loss also from an AVM. AVMs may require combined treatment with embolization and wide surgical extirpation.

Although not hamartomas, hemangiomas still fall within the group of benign conditions of the head and neck discussed in this chapter. The indications for treatment of hemangiomas are mentioned along with the treatments for other vascular lesions in the operations section of this chapter. Hemangiomas are the most common neoplasms in the head and neck region in neonates and children. They occur in approximately 10% of all children under 10 years of age. By definition, hemangiomas are proliferative lesions that may or may not be present at birth (approximately 30%), go through a varied proliferative period of growth, and then reach a stage of growth arrest and involution. With the exception of lesions of the eyelid and orbit with associated obstruction of the visual axis or pressure on the globe (with possible late anisometropic amblyopia) and lesions compromising the airway, most hemangiomas of the head and neck can be treated with expectant observation. Rapidly growing lesions may require treatment with systemic steroids and, for extensive function or life-threatening lesions, alpha interferon. Some superficial lesions have been encouraged to involute early with laser treatment, but this is most effective for relatively small, thin lesions.

There are still varied opinions on the timing of surgical intervention. Although some surgeons have advocated early excision of hemangiomas, it is rarely necessary. It has been this author's experience, in evaluating a number of patients who had early procedures, that the amount of tissue excised and the consequent scarring (not to mention nerve injury) were far greater than would be required had the surgeon waited for the normal involution process. This waiting period does not always mean delaying treatment until the lesion has totally involuted. It is often possible to excise the excess crepe-like abnormal skin left in the wake of the lesion by school age without compromising the final result. The surgical procedures required for treatment of a hemangioma are as varied as the lesion's presentation. Some of these will be discussed below.

HAMARTOMAS OF MIXED ORIGIN. Hamartomas of mixed origin include a varied mix of cyst and cystlike structures that make up a large portion of the benign lesions of the head and neck.[8,27] An understanding of the anatomy, histology, and "geography" of these lesions requires one to be well versed in the embryology of the region. Many of these lesions present in the neonatal period and exhibit "classical" signs and symptoms that will direct the physician toward an understanding of their natural history so he or she can appropriately recognize the indications for and timing of

treatment. Other cystic masses may not become apparent until later in life, even though they may be derived from similar embryologic remnants. We will look at these by both age at and site of most common presentation.

CYST AND CYSTLIKE LESIONS OF SKIN AND SUBCUTANEOUS TISSUE—PEDIATRIC AGE GROUP

Scalp
DERMOID CYSTS. Cysts of the scalp in an infant or young child must be examined carefully for their proximity to an underlying cranial suture, because most of these lesions are dermoid cysts. Regardless of location, dermoid cysts are slow-growing congenital hamartomas that occur along embryonic "fault lines" where developing ectodermal tissue becomes sequestered. Lesions overlying the anterior and posterior fontanel or lamboid suture may extend intracranially, whereas those over the coronal and squamous sutures generally do not (Figures 72-3 and 72-4).[21,27]

The lesion overlying the anterior fontanel may sit in a trough in the bone and attach to the sagittal sinus through this bone defect (part of the defect being the fontanel itself). The cyst over the posterior fontanel may extend through the patent fontanel and down to the roof of the third ventricle. A computed tomographic (CT) scan is imperative in evaluating these lesions before attempting excision.

Histologically, dermoid cysts are true cysts with moderately well-defined epidermoid structures including sebaceous, eccrine, and apocrine glandular elements and rudimentary hair follicles. Anterior fontanel dermoids will, upon sectioning, often have clear sweat inside. Posterior fontanel dermoids can on occasion be intermixed with neural elements when examined histologically.[20,27]

Generally dermoid cysts are excised because of their potential for continued growth, because of erosion of adjacent bone if they are in contact with it, and on occasion because of a risk of infection.

Face
DERMOID CYSTS. Whereas a superficial sequestration of ectoderm during development appears to explain the origin of the more common external (or lateral) angular dermoid (and the unusual dermoids along cranial sutures and at the columellar base), a cranial origin best explains the lesions of the frontonasal midline. An understanding of the differences between the lesions arising by these two different embryologic errors is essential to their diagnosis and treatment.

Dermoids of the Lateral Brow. Often seen from as far medially as the midthird of the brow to superolateral to the brow, dermoids of the lateral brow are generally asymptomatic and slow growing (Figure 72-5). They rarely grow larger than a few centimeters, but may get as big as 4 cm. They may in some cases appear to fluctuate in size. Although these cysts may be mobile and extend down onto the eyelid, in many cases they are firmly fixed to the periosteum of the

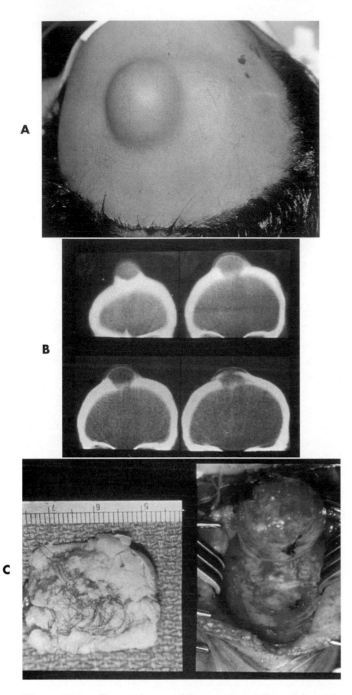

Figure 72-3. Dermoid cysts of the anterior midline of the scalp should be investigated for extension through the anterior fontanel. **A** to **C,** The typical appearance of an anterior fontanel dermoid with the coronal CT scans showing extension through the fontanel. The intraoperative view shows the small defect in the bone where the cyst attaches over the sagittal sinus and the presence of hair inside the cyst on cut section.

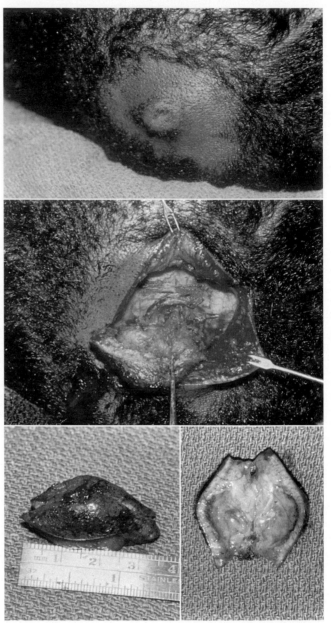

Figure 72-4. **A** to **D,** The somewhat different appearance of a posterior fontanel dermoid from the lesion involving the anterior fontanel. The lesion may lie slightly off of midline and may have other components (neural) than the typical dermoid. It may extend through the fontanel to the roof of the third ventricle. (**A** and **D,** From Spira M, Stal S: *Clin Plast Surg* 14:2, 1987.)

orbital rim, particularly in the area of the frontozygomatic suture. A firm, rounded swelling in the lateral brow in a child is pathognomonic of this lesion. Large cysts may lie in a depression in the bone, split the lateral orbit wall, or extend back into the temporal fossa. Of the hundreds of dermoid cysts excised by the author, only three have been seen to be both intraosseous and, due to growth in the bone, eroded through the inner table and in contact with the dura. In each

case, slight variations from the typical presentation and physical examination led to a preoperative CT scan. In all other cases, a CT scan is unnecessary prior to treatment of these lateral dermoids.

With the exception of the rare cysts of the columellar base (which extend only to the area of the nasal spine), dermoids of the frontonasal area, from glabella to nasal tip, arise following incomplete obliteration of a tract from the foramen cecum to

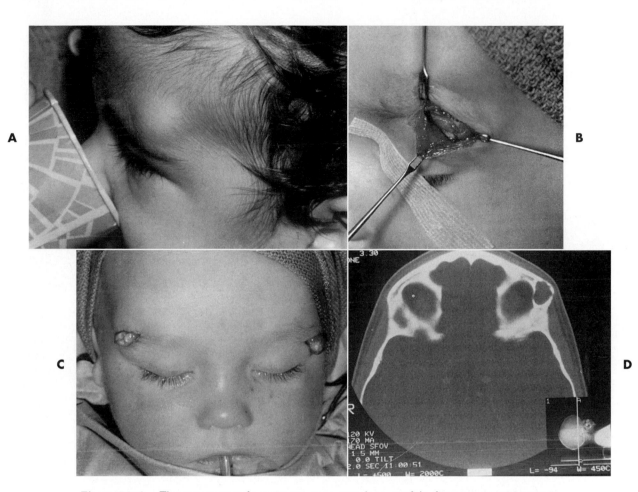

Figure 72-5. The appearance of a cystic structure near the area of the frontozygomatic suture in a child pathognomonic for an external angular dermoid cyst. **A** and **B,** The cyst in this location will frequently sit in a trough in the underlying bone. **C,** The occasional bilateral appearance of the dermoid. **D,** The rare occurrence of an intraosseous external angular dermoid on axial CT view.

the nasal tip or foramen cecum through the frontonasal suture (Figure 72-6). The fact that the dermoid cyst and sinus, glioma, and encephalocele represent a continuum of lesions of like origin in this region is understood embryologically by recognizing that this tract (or prenasal space) contains a dural projection prior to closure of the foramen cecum that extends in close continuity to an ectodermal tract at the surface. Any failure of normal obliteration may leave both ectodermal and glial tissue in its midline path (Figure 72-7). Therefore it should be clear that a CT scan (or magnetic resonance imaging [MRI]) is essential prior to surgery. CT scans in the axial, coronal, and sagittal planes will clearly demonstrate the extent of the tract, allowing prior planning in those cases that require a combined intracranial and extracranial approach for complete excision.[21,23,24]

The presence of a frontonasal dermoid may be noted at birth or in early infancy as a midline pore, possibly with protruding hair and possibly with associated widening of the nasal dorsum (Figure 72-8). Some children may initially present at the time of an infection in the cyst with swelling and erythema anywhere from the glabella to the nasal tip (Figures 72-9 and 72-10). On rare occasions, a child may present with brain abscess without previous recognition of the cyst or sinus opening from which the infection arose (Figure 72-10).

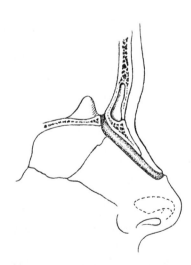

Figure 72-6. The common embryologic pathway through which dermoid cyst, glioma, and encephalocele develop. There is a pathway through the foramen cecum, down through the prenasal space (between the nasal cartilaginous capsule and the skin). Under normal circumstances this pathway, in which an early dural evagination retracts back from its close proximity to the skin, is obliterated as the foramen cecum closes. The second possible path of development of both dermoid cyst/sinus and glioma is through the area of the frontonasal suture and then through the foramen cecum.

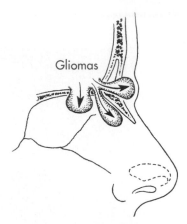

Gliomas

Figure 72-7. The varied path of development of intranasal and extranasal gliomas. Depending on the timing and extent of tissue left behind as the embryologic processes of normal obliteration of the prenasal space, tissue will be left behind that is either ectodermal or neural.

A, B 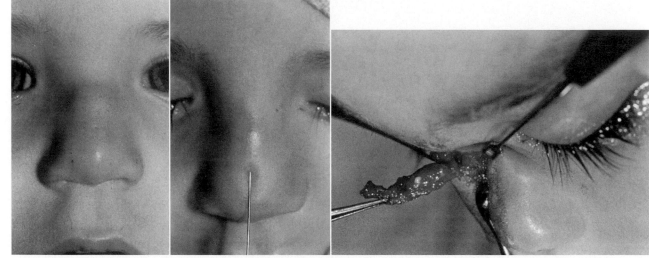 C

Figure 72-8. **A** and **B,** A frontonasal dermoid cyst and sinus may present with both fullness in the area of the nasal dorsum and with a sinus opening. The sinus tract will extend a variable distance through the underlying septum, with the lesion **(C)** being dissected from the surrounding tissues.

A, B 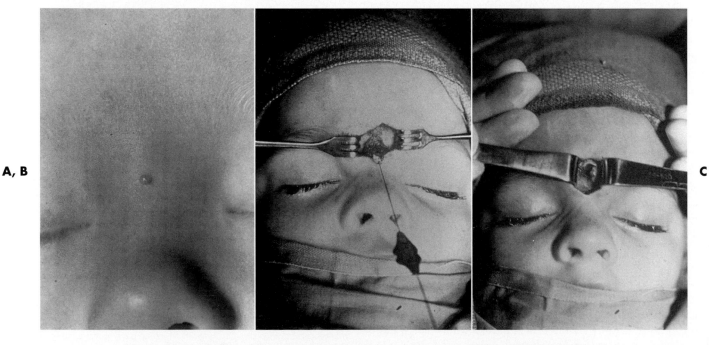 C

Figure 72-9. **A,** This child presented with a chronic draining sinus in the glabellar area. **B** and **C,** At the time of resection the extension of the sinus and cyst through the frontonasal suture is evident with erosion of the bone secondary to chronic infection.

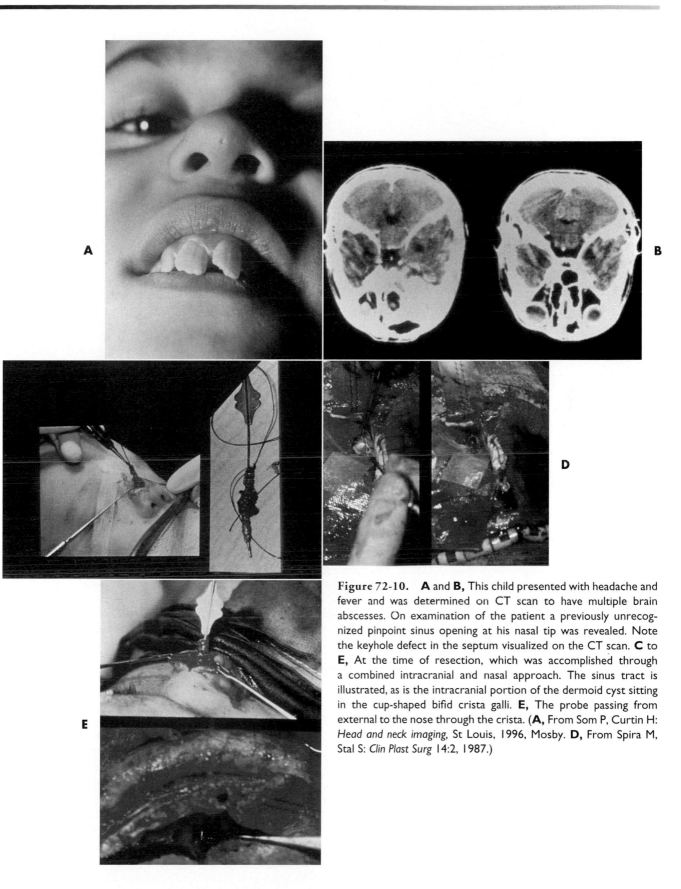

Figure 72-10.   A and **B,** This child presented with headache and fever and was determined on CT scan to have multiple brain abscesses. On examination of the patient a previously unrecognized pinpoint sinus opening at his nasal tip was revealed. Note the keyhole defect in the septum visualized on the CT scan. **C** to **E,** At the time of resection, which was accomplished through a combined intracranial and nasal approach. The sinus tract is illustrated, as is the intracranial portion of the dermoid cyst sitting in the cup-shaped bifid crista galli. **E,** The probe passing from external to the nose through the crista. (**A,** From Som P, Curtin H: *Head and neck imaging,* St Louis, 1996, Mosby. **D,** From Spira M, Stal S: *Clin Plast Surg* 14:2, 1987.)

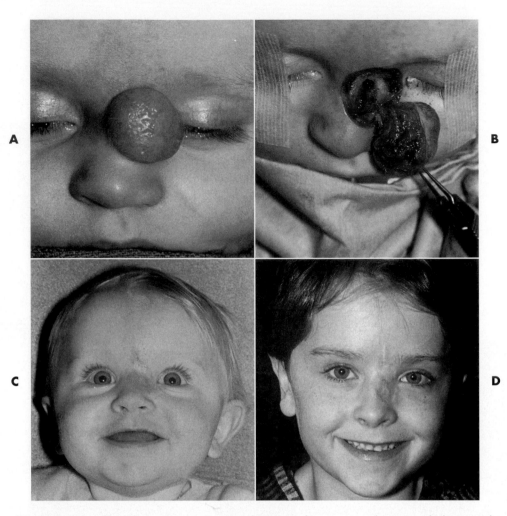

Figure 72-11. This infant was noted at birth to have a firm mass on the nose, which on work up was demonstrated to be an extranasal glioma. **A** and **B,** The mass prior to and during the resection, which extended down onto the nasal bone. **C,** The reconstruction was accomplished with a galeal flap for vascular coverage of the exposed nasal bone covered with a full-thickness skin graft. **D,** The child is seen 7 years after resection presenting for further reconstruction. Examination demonstrates some growth disturbance with deviation of the nasal pyramid as well as a soft tissue contour defect. (**A** and **B,** From Som P, Curtin H: *Head and neck imaging,* St Louis, 1996, Mosby.)

Lesions with intracranial extension will course either beneath the nasal bones through a widened septum (look for a keyhole appearance to the septum on axial CT views [Figure 72-10, *B*]) and then through the foramen cecum, or through a widened frontonasal suture and then through the foramen cecum. In both cases a bifid crista galli is usually noted on the CT scan (particularly on the coronal view), and an intracranial portion of the dermoid may lie between the leaves of the falx. Evaluation and treatment of these lesions is best done with the cooperative efforts of a plastic surgeon and a neurosurgeon using a craniofacial approach.[23,24]

NASAL GLIOMAS. Nasal gliomas are uncommon, smooth, firm, noncompressible masses that typically present at birth or in early childhood. They are seen in either extranasal or intranasal position. The former are generally readily visible at birth, whereas the latter may not present until there is some evidence of chronic nasal obstruction (Figures 72-11 and 72-12). For the visible ones, the lack of fluctuation in size during the child's crying or straining may help to distinguish this lesion from a frontonasal encephalocele.[21,27]

Gliomas in an extranasal location may still penetrate the bone in the frontonasal suture area and are often associated with broadening of the nasal root and increased intracanthal distance. Continued extension through the widened foramen cecum and attachment to the dura in the area of the falx are ruled out by CT or MRI. Dural continuity may be ruled out by positive contrast cisternography. Those gliomas presenting intranasally are usually first noted on physical examination in association with complaints of nasal airway obstruction, chronic nasal discharge, or evidence of distortion of the nasal bones secondary to an expanding lesion. Once the diagnosis is

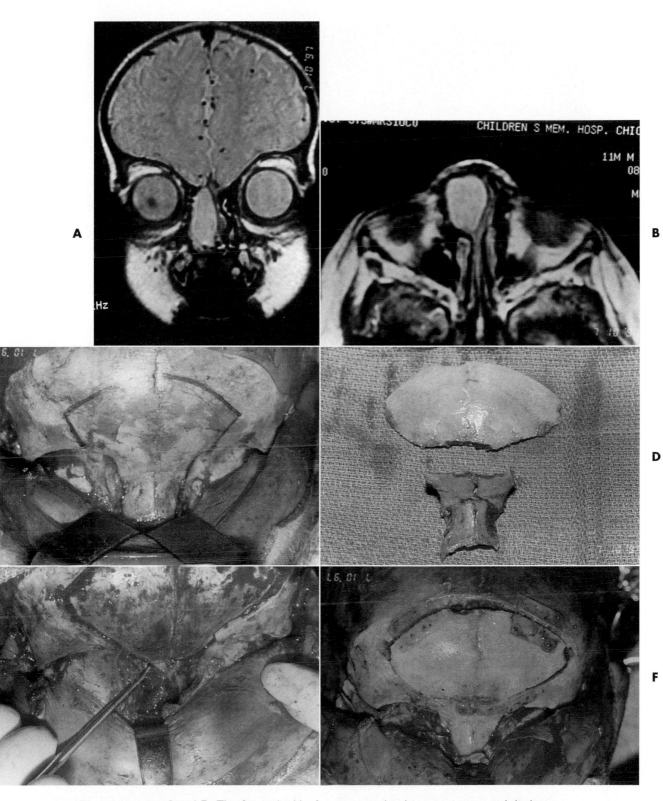

Figure 72-12. **A** and **B,** This 9-month-old infant was noted to have persistent nasal discharge, with examination revealing an obstructing nasal mass on the right side despite no visible distortion of the nasal bones. On both coronal and axial MRI the intranasal glioma is readily evident. **C** to **F,** The planned osteotomy for direct visualization of the glioma, the removed frontal and nasal bone flaps, the attachment of the mass to the dura without CSF continuity, and the replaced bone fixed with absorbable plates and screws.

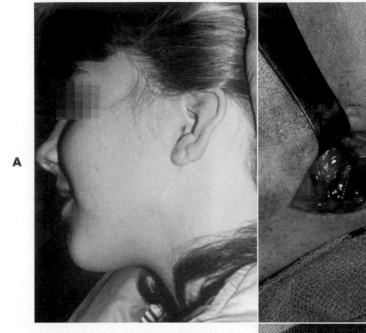

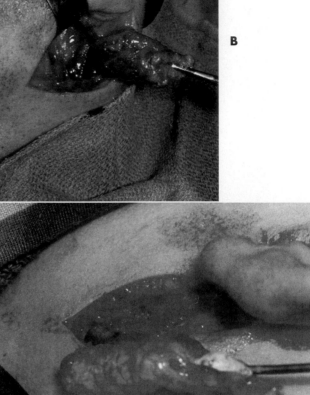

Figure 72-13. **A,** This young woman presented with a recurrent mass at the angle of the mandible. **B** and **C,** The first branchial cleft (cervicoauricular cyst) during the resection, which includes a small segment of cartilage of the external auditory canal and the resected specimen with attached cartilage.

made and the extent of the lesion determined, excision is carried out. Generally, excision requires a craniofacial approach for full visualization.

Histologically, these lesions comprise benign glial tissue, primarily astrocysts and fibrous tissue in an extradural location.

FRONTONASAL ENCEPHALOCELES. Frontonasal encephaloceles, midline or paramedian cystic masses, present at birth and can attain enormous proportions. Fluctuation in size can be noted during crying and straining. In general, much of the dural sac is cerebrospinal fluid (CSF) filled, but it may contain herniated frontal lobe along with amorphous glial tissue. Again the most common path of herniation is through the open foramen cecum and the widely patent frontonasal suture, but they may also be seen to herniate caudally through defects in the sphenoid and ethmoids with presentation in the mouth (and are associated with a widely cleft palate and possible midline cleft lip). The latter lesion falls beyond the scope of the current discussion. CT and MRI with and without contrast (and possibly positive contrast cisternography) will delineate the full extent of the lesion. Arteriography may be necessary to determine the best surgical approach and the

presence or absence of functional brain tissue. Again a craniofacial team is essential in planning and treatment of these lesions. Histologically, the sac is lined by arachnoid with possible heterotopic glial tissue.[21,24]

Lateral Cervical Masses

BRANCHIAL CLEFT ANOMALIES. Branchial cleft anomalies are the most frequently occurring masses of the lateral neck. An understanding of branchial cleft anomalies, which may include cysts, fistulas, or sinus tracts, requires an understanding of branchial arch embryology. Branchial cleft anomalies and/or sinus tracts occur because of a failure of the first and second branchial arch to attain maturity. The residual remnant is trapped in the neck.[6,8,20,23,27]

Anomalies of the first arch may be manifest (1) in the preauricular area, (2) posterior to the angle of the mandible, and (3) in the upper cervical area. First branchial cleft cysts, which are extremely rare, usually present as a small asymptomatic-dimple or fistulous tract that is in close proximity to the parotid gland, is also intimately associated with the facial nerve, and may extend to the external auditory meatus (Figure 72-13).[14,23] Anomalies of the second branchial

A　　　　　　　　　**B**　　　　　　　　　**C**

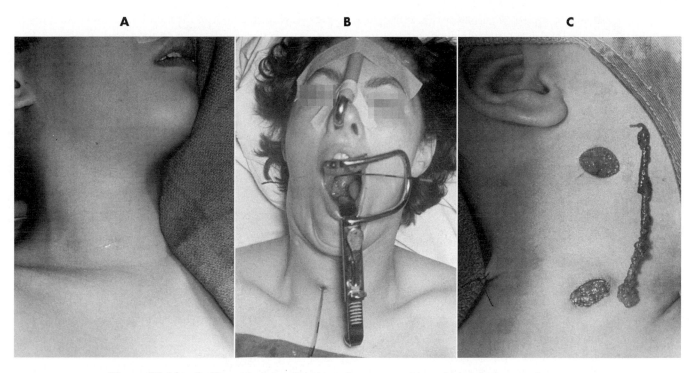

Figure 72-14. **A,** The typical site of drainage from a second branchial cleft sinus can be seen at the anterior border of the sternocleidomastoid at the junction of the upper two thirds and lower third of the muscle. **B** and **C,** The full extent of this type of cyst and sinus through the neck into the pharynx and the stair-step incision used in the resection.

arch, particularly the second branchial cleft cysts, are more common. They are manifested as fistulas, cysts, or sinuses in the lower midthird of the sternocleidomastoid muscle (Figure 72-14). The cystic mass may appear anywhere along the anterior border of the sternocleidomastoid muscle from the hyoid bone to the sternal notch. The tract, if present, may extend through the platysma muscle and follow superiorly along the carotid sheath, extending deep to the posterior belly of the digastric muscle, and superficial to the hypoglossal nerve below the hyoid bone, with its internal opening at the base of the tonsillar fossa or lateral pharyngeal area (the Rosenmuller pouch). The occurrence of third branchial cleft cysts is rare and the fourth branchial cleft anomaly extends deep to the platysma muscle posterior to the internal carotid artery and along the hypoglossal nerve, and then descends beneath the subclavian artery on the right and aortic arch on the left, with its internal opening in the region of the upper esophagus or pyriform sinus.[6,8,14,27]

Branchial cleft anomalies may present at any age. Sinus openings may be visualized at birth or on an early examination by the pediatrician. The cysts usually present by 8 years of age, with most appearing by the second or third decade (Figure 72-15). There is no sex predominance, nor is one side more common than the other. When they present, the cysts appear as soft, nontender, smooth, round lesions along the border of the sternocleidomastoid muscle, usually deep to the muscle. They may be located in sites extending from the region of the external auditory canal to the midclavicular area. These cysts increase in size when there is a concomitant upper respiratory infection due to lymphoid tissue that has become trapped within the cyst. They often become infected and will then exhibit associated inflammation.[6,14]

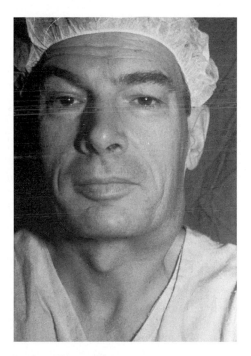

Figure 72-15. This patient presented with a cystic mass in the upper lateral neck, which on resection was confirmed to be a branchial cleft cyst. (From Spira M, Stal S: *Clin Plast Surg* 14:2, 1987.)

Although preoperative diagnosis in the face of a sinus opening is straightforward, the diagnosis of the cysts may be difficult. An attempt should be made to delineate the extent of the anomaly before attempted excision. This may be aided by CT scan, ultrasonography, or MRI.[2,6,14,23] If the cysts become infected, they should be treated vigorously with antibiotics after culture is obtained and, if necessary, incision and drainage performed. Every effort should be made to resolve the inflammation before surgery. At the time of excision, the many adjacent structures should be kept in mind in order to avoid inadvertent nerve or vessel injury.

Histologically, the cyst and tract are typically lined with a stratified squamous or low columnar epithelium. Treatment consists of surgical excision, with effort being made to keep the neck incisions small; use "stepladder" incisions if necessary.[6,8,14,23]

LYMPHATIC MALFORMATIONS OF THE LATERAL NECK.

Most discussions of lateral cervical masses include "cystic hygroma" as one of the more common lesions of the lateral neck in a child; however, this is more appropriately termed a *lymphatic malformation* and will be described in detail in Chapter 64. These lesions arise as a developmental anomaly of the lymphatic channels. Large endothelial-lined spaces are displaced from the venous system during development. These may be found along the branches of the jugular vein, around the esophagus and larynx, and throughout the mediastinum and interdigitate with cervical vessel, nerves, and muscle, making excision arduous and difficult. Large masses may cause respiratory compromise.[9,19]

It is well recognized, however, that not all of these malformations need to be excised. Reports of "spontaneous involution" have varied between 16% and 70%, with Grabb et al[9] reporting 41% complete involution and 29% partial involution, during the first 20 years of life.[9] What exactly occurs is still unclear, since this is not the same involution process that hemangiomas go through. The lymphatic cysts may collapse with subsequent fibrosis. It is certain that macrocystic lymphatic malformation rarely is seen in adulthood. Many of them can be observed without surgery, at the very least until the child is old enough to minimize the risk of facial nerve injury during the excision. Total excision is not required and conservative surgery should be considered when the "cure is worse than the disease."

PAROTID GLAND AND OTHER SALIVARY GLAND LESIONS.

These lesions, which occur at all ages, are classified according to their primordial cell derivation and histological appearance. They may present as painless, firm to cystic, slow growing, and solitary swelling, and can be located in the preauricular area or in the region of the angle of the mandible. For this reason they must be included in the differential diagnosis of lateral neck masses in both children and adults. The parotid tumors will be discussed in detail in another section of this text. Submaxillary gland tumors occur in the upper mid to midlateral neck and midsubmandibular area. They present as firm, nonmobile masses that are occasionally tender to palpation. The mass is usually a benign adenoma or may be a glandular enlargement secondary to a large calculus. The latter is associated with pain and tenderness, particularly with chewing and eating. Diagnostic differentiation between the two entities can be made with a suitable intraoral radiograph of the floor of the mouth or a sialogram. Surgical excision of the gland is the treatment of choice for both problems.[8]

CERVICAL LYMPHADENOPATHY.

When evaluating cystic masses in the neck in both the pediatric and adult age groups, cervical lymphadenitis must be included in the differential diagnosis. Cervical lymphadenitis is frequently secondary to a regional infectious process within the head and neck region and is associated with inflammatory changes occurring within the reactive lymph node. These symptoms will respond to appropriate treatment of the underlying problem. Obviously in the absence of any underlying etiology, or with history more suggestive of a neoplastic process, the work up should proceed accordingly. This subject is discussed elsewhere.

Midline Neck Masses

THYROGLOSSAL DUCT CYSTS.

The most common midline neck mass in the pediatric age group is the thyroglossal duct cyst.[1,5,25] The formation of this mass is intimately related to the embryologic development of the thyroid gland anlage (Figure 72-16). This commences during the third week of gestation from a diverticulum in the floor of the pharynx whose oral opening is the foramen cecum linguae. As the embryo continues to mature, the thyroid gland descends into its final location in the neck in close proximity to the hyoid bone and anterior to the trachea still maintaining its connection to the tongue for a short time by a narrow isthmus. This usually disappears, but on occasion it persists. The persistent remnant can develop into a thyroglossal duct cyst. It may present as a cyst and/or sinus anywhere along the course of the descent. The most common location is at the level of the thyrohyoid membrane close to the midline deep to the deep cervical fascia and just inferior to the hyoid bone, where it represents about 70% of all congenital abnormalities of the neck.[1,5,8,25,27]

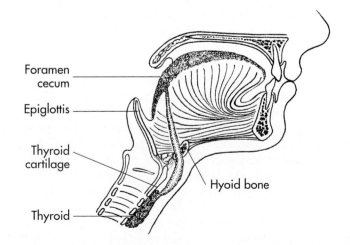

Figure 72-16. The typical course of descent of the developing thyroid from its origin at the foramen cecum of the tongue down through the midhyoid and into the neck. A thyroglossal duct cyst is the remnant of this process having been incompletely done.

The thyroglossal duct cyst usually presents as an asymptomatic slow-growing mass in the anterior midline of the neck (Figure 72-17). There have been case reports, however, of thyroglossal duct cysts occurring away from the midline. The patients may describe dysphagia or a feeling of fullness in the neck, a fluctuation in size, or even spontaneous regression, and usually do not seek medical attention until the cysts become infected, inflamed, tender, or markedly increased in size. On physical examination, these cysts will move up and down with swallowing and protrusion of the tongue with the neck hyperextended. External fistulous openings, originating from the thyroglossal duct or tract, are usually considered a secondary feature because normally the duct does not communicate with the outside. Such openings are marks of previous surgical drainage or incomplete removal.

These cysts/sinuses should be excised because of their propensity to grow, become infected, and occasionally cause the above-mentioned symptoms. Before excision of a suspected thyroglossal duct cyst, the neck mass should be evaluated with ultrasonography to delineate its consistency and with thyroid scans to confirm the presence of normal functioning thyroid tissue or persistent lingual thyroid.

The procedure synonymous with the treatment of thyroglossal duct cysts was reported in 1928 by Sistrunk (see Figure 72-17).[25] The incision should be marked in a horizontal skin crease in the infrahyoid region over the cyst. After infiltration with the appropriate hemostatic agent, the platysma is incised and the strap muscles identified and retracted laterally to obtain adequate exposure for careful dissection. Some surgeons inject the cyst with methylene blue to outline its contents, although many find this more hindrance than help. The infrahyoid strap muscles are then transected in order to clear the junction of the greater cornu and body of the hyoid bone, enabling the surgeon to excise the tract from the pharyngeal wall in continuity with the involved midportion of the hyoid. As the surgeon approaches the tongue, an index finger is placed in the area of the foramen cecum at the base of the tongue to delineate the tissue to be removed in association with the sinus tract. This dissection may be extremely difficult if there were antecedent infections. The intraoral incision should be closed with chromic sutures and the remaining surgical incisions closed in layers, usually with a drain placed.[1,5]

Histologically, although these cysts rarely involve thyroid gland parenchyma, there may be associated retention cysts and small accumulations of thyroid tissue. Thyroglossal duct cysts are true cysts with epithelial lining of either columnar, squamous, transitional, or mixed cell type. The cavity is often filled with a mucinlike material. There have been a number of case reports of these cysts being the site of malignancy, with the most common being papillary carcinoma.[8]

"ACQUIRED" CYSTS OF THE SKIN—PEDIATRIC AND ADULT POPULATION

Epidermal Cysts

Epidermal cysts are the most common form of cysts encountered in adults, although they can on occasion be seen in adolescents as well. They can occur in any area of the body, but most commonly occur in areas of increased pilosebaceous activity like the head and upper trunk.[20,28] They may present in either an intradermal or subcutaneous position, growing as large as 5 cm in diameter. It is believed that they arise from the infundibular portion of the pilosebaceous unit as epithelial cells become trapped and form a cystic structure. They may present singly or, in some cases, as multiple cysts. Multiple

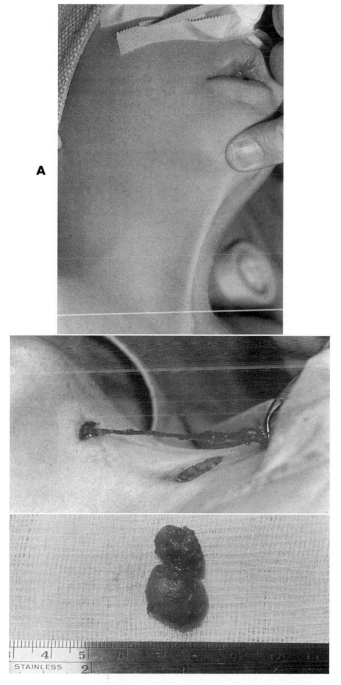

Figure 72-17. **A** to **C,** The "cord" of thyroglossal duct cyst and sinus, the excision through a stair-step incision, and the bilobed cyst constricted by the excised central portion of the body of the hyoid bone following the technique described by Sistrunk.

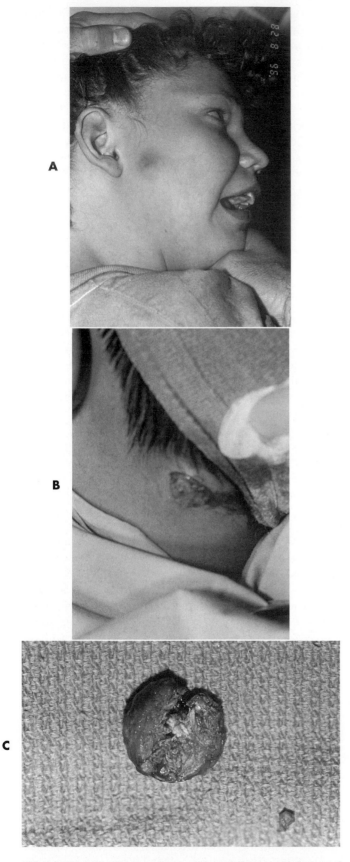

Figure 72-18. Two patients with calcifying granuloma of Malherbe. **A,** The discolored skin with overlying telangiectasia and thinning of the skin. **B,** A cyst as it is excised from the occipital region, with the calcium granules evident on cut section of the cyst in **C.**

epidermal cysts can be seen as one manifestation of Gardner's syndrome. The other findings of Gardner's syndrome include polyposis coli, osteomas of the jaw, and intestinal desmoid tumors.[30]

Histologically, epidermal cysts are lined with true epidermis that forms a granular layer and keratin. The keratin forms in laminated layers within the cyst. The rupture of these cysts with extrusion of the keratin debris into the dermis or subcutaneous tissue may incite intense foreign body reaction associated with pain, erythema, and drainage of purulent material. Although typically benign, cases of malignant degeneration to squamous cell carcinoma have been described in the literature. Long-term history of recurrent infection, drainage, surface skin changes, and possible ulceration should raise suspicion of this possible change in the character of the lesion.

Tricholemmal Cysts

The commonly occurring tricholemmal cysts have been described in the literature under a variety of other names, including sebaceous cysts, wens, and pilar cysts.[12,27] They are distinguishable clinically from epidermal cysts because of their unique distribution, with over 90% of them occurring within the scalp. They are derived from the outer hair sheath. Histologically, they are true cysts that characteristically consist of a cell wall with epithelial cells that appear to lack intercellular bridges or desmosomes. Other distinctive microscopic features include a palisading arrangement of the lining squamous cells. They also lack a true granular layer and therefore appear to undergo an abrupt process of keratinization. The cavity is filled with a homogeneous eosinophilic material that has focal calcification approximately 25% of the time.

"ACQUIRED" SKIN APPENDAGE TUMORS—LESIONS OF FOLLICULAR DIFFERENTIATION

Pilomatrixoma

The pilomatrixoma, or calcifying epithelioma or granuloma of Malherbe, is perhaps the most common cyst after dermoid cysts of the head and neck of children, usually arising before age 21 and rarely seen in adults. Occasionally these cysts are seen elsewhere in the body and may be single or multiple, usually presenting as yellowish, calcified, deep-seeded nodules with stone-hard consistency.[11,20,27,28] They are firmly fixed to the overlying skin, which may be normal, and often show telangiectasia, bluish discoloration, and on occasion pronounced thinning, particularly in the setting of recurrent inflammation and infection (Figure 72-18). They rarely obtain a size greater than 2 cm.

Excision of a pilomatrixoma should include a portion of the overlying skin in those patients presenting with recurrent inflammation and skin surface changes. Typically the cysts will shell out of the surrounding tissue and appear as a very thin-walled structure with prominent calcium granules within. On histologic examination these are sheets of epithelial cells with basophilic shadow cells arranged in irregular bands. Masses of keratin are found interspersed between cells with calcification. The latter finding is a late manifestation of cellular degeneration.

Trichoepithelioma, Trichofolliculoma, and Tricholemmoma

Three other lesions of follicular differentiation, trichoepitheliomas, trichofolliculomas, and tricholemmomas, occur as either solitary or multiple papular lesions in the head and neck. They are 2 to 8 mm in size, and single ones may be difficult to distinguish clinically, but can be differentiated by their varied histologic architecture. They are more common in adults but occur in childhood, especially in the multiple forms where two of the three exist as part of a syndrome.[20]

Multiple trichoepitheliomas are inherited as an autosomal dominant trait, with their onset in adolescence, increasing in size and number through adulthood. The most common locations are the nose, nasolabial folds, and central face. Usually the lesions do not ulcerate, although larger lesions may have telangiectasias. Multiple tricholemmomas have been described with Cowden syndrome, which is an inherited condition with fibroepithelial polyps of the oral mucosa, keratoses of the palms and soles, multiple tricholemmomas, and an increased risk of breast cancer. The skin lesions are typically seen first on the face, around the mouth, nose and ears.

Treatment of these lesions is surgical. Biopsy of the multiple lesions of Cowden syndrome may be helpful to distinguish tricholemmomas from verrucae.

LESIONS OF SEBACEOUS DIFFERENTIATION

Sebaceous Hyperplasia

Sebaceous hyperplasia occurs as small 2 to 4 mm papules on the face of middle-aged adults. The lesions are pale yellow with central umbilication and telangiectasias. Lesions do not show tendency to ulcerate. Histologically, the lesions are collections of sebaceous glands with enlarged lobules located around a central enlarged sebaceous duct. Some patients will also demonstrate ectopic sebaceous glands on the vermillion border of the lips and oral mucosa, known as Fordyce's spots.[17,20]

These lesions can be treated with a full spectrum of modalities, from excisional biopsy to destruction by cryotherapy, electrodesiccation, and laser therapy.

Sebaceous Adenoma

Sebaceous adenomas are rare lesions that present most commonly on the face and scalp of older adults. Typically they are small, flesh-colored papules. Histologically, the lesion is an incompletely differentiated sebaceous lobule with irregular shape and size. Lobules contain undifferentiated germinating sebaceous cells and more mature sebaceous cells. Simple excision is the treatment of choice.[17]

Sebaceous Epithelioma

Sebaceous epitheliomas may resemble basal cell epitheliomas as pale or yellow papules with ulceration centrally. Typically

there is a solitary lesion located on the face or scalp. Excisional biopsy is usually appropriate and may be necessary to distinguish it from basal cells. Histologically, sebaceous epitheliomas are not well circumscribed. Lesions are differentiated toward sebaceous cells, but many are undifferentiated. They appear in clusters with peripheral palisading. Mature sebaceous cells may be located in the center of most cell masses.[17]

OTHER MISCELLANEOUS TUMORS OF THE SKIN

Juvenile Xanthogranuloma

Juvenile xanthogranulomas are self-limited benign papules that occur from early infancy into adulthood.[7,20] Some may be present at birth. The typical lesion is papular and red to yellow. They occur as single or multiple lesions in the head and neck, with possible involvement of the iris or epibulbar area (the former may lead to glaucoma). Lesions generally involute spontaneously, but may be present for up to a year or longer before this occurs. When excised and examined they show accumulation of histiocytes with few lymphocytes and eosinophils. A granulomatous infiltrate may be present that contains foam cells, foreign body giant cells, and Touton giant cells. The latter is the hallmark of juvenile xanthogranuloma.[7]

OPERATIONS AND OUTCOMES

Despite the desire to make the distinction between operations and outcomes in this text, for the discussion of this heterogeneous group of benign head and neck lesions, the separation would tend to confuse what in most cases should be a simple discussion. Provided that the nature of the lesion being treated is understood, excision is definitive and recurrence rare. Therefore the outcome, with few exceptions, is elimination of the lesion. That being the case, it is perhaps best to discuss the procedures that may not be straightforward and, within that context, also discuss areas in which either the nature of the lesion or the "wrong" approach to the lesion may increase the likelihood of a recurrence or a poor outcome.

NEUROFIBROMATOSIS

Beyond the reasonably direct excision of smaller neurofibromas, the surgical approach to the tissue ravages of this disease process is frequently less than satisfying for both surgeon and patient. The surgical approach is determined by the area of involvement and by whether the surgeon is dealing with soft tissue alone or trying to correct both a soft and hard tissue problem.

This is a highly vascular lesion and the surgeon must be prepared in any large resection for significant blood loss. This loss can be minimized, as in most other resections, with initial injection of a vasoconstricting agent combined with the use of bipolar cautery. If available, the newly marketed combined bipolar/cautery scissors have in our experience significantly cut blood loss in this setting. Since skin, as well as the deeper tissues, is pathologically involved, extensive thinning of skin flaps can be dangerous. Swelling is often prolonged following surgery for neurofibromatosis and there may be some benefit in intraoperative and early postoperative use of steroids.

Many approaches have been described for treatment of neurofibromatosis of the orbit and periorbital area. Discussions by Jackson,[13] Marchac,[15] and Van der Meulen[29] are among the better descriptions of both the problem and the surgical approach. The debulking of the lid and periorbita may be effective in the early deformity, but as the disease process progresses treatment must be directed at the correction of the expanded orbit and the classic orbital defect in the greater sphenoid. The surgical approach may be through combined lid incisions, with lateral canthotomy alone or in combination with a craniofacial approach (Figure 72-19). Preoperative assessment of the degree of orbital expansion will aid in matching orbit size during the reconstruction, but will be limited in success as long as there is extensive involvement of the periorbita. If the eye is sightless and the decision made to enucleate the eye and place a prosthesis, the final aesthetic outcome may be significantly improved.

Debulking of the lid should be combined with a lateral canthopexy, and more severe cases require wedge resections of a portion of the lids, as well as typical debulking procedures.

As with many other areas of neurofibromatosis surgery, reduction of the cheek and lips may require a staged surgical

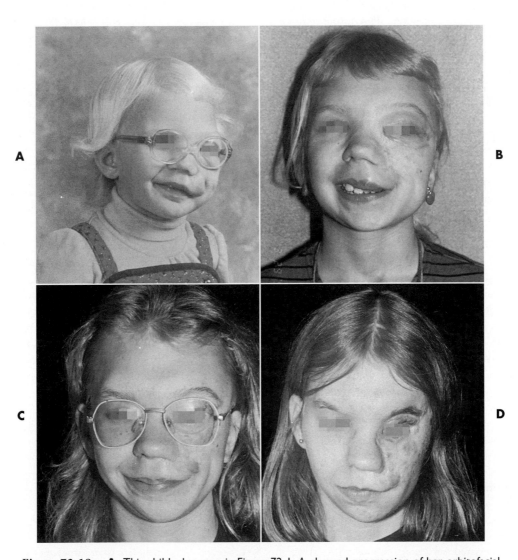

Figure 72-19. **A,** This child, also seen in Figure 72-1, A, showed progression of her orbitofacial neurofibromatosis from 2 years of age on. **B** and **C,** She underwent multiple excisions through both preauricular rhytidectomy approach and excision with a direct approach through the lateral nasal and nasolabial approach. She had repeated excisions in the orbital area limited by the extensive involvement of the periorbita. **D,** The early result after enucleation of her sightless eye and placement of a prosthesis. This last procedure allowed correction of the proptosis and orbital distortion, as well as repair of the defect in the sphenoid.

approach. Lateral fullness in the cheek typically requires dissection of the facial nerve (which on the affected side may be markedly enlarged) with resection of all involved tissue superficial to it; however, often much of the bulk of the cheek lies medially and may require a separate stage direct wedge excision along the newly proposed nasolabial fold, with reduction and suspension of the lip carried out simultaneously. We have found that suspension of the tissue to the underlying bone with Mitek anchors may give more prolonged retention than other forms of fixation.

Mitek suspension in combination with soft tissue debulking and varied wedge excisions has been relatively effective in treatment of the macrotic and often ptotic ear in neurofibromatosis (Figure 72-20). One can reduce the ear in a similar fashion to that described for other forms of macrotia, or suspend the ear by debulking any involved tissues above the ear and securing the suspension sutures to the temporal bone, but these procedures should be staged in order to prevent potential vascular compromise. Unfortunately, even the best suspension of the ear seems to be followed long term by a gradual continued drift of the ear; however, the improvement gained is usually viewed very favorably by the patient, even if repeated surgery is required.

In our experience, the outcomes of the above procedures vary as widely as the procedures discussed. In some cases where the disease is either more localized or slower growing, improvement may be dramatic and long term. In others, the slowly insidious growth of the lesion may continue to undo the gains of the previous reduction, and continued surgical assaults must be mounted throughout the life of the patient, timed to

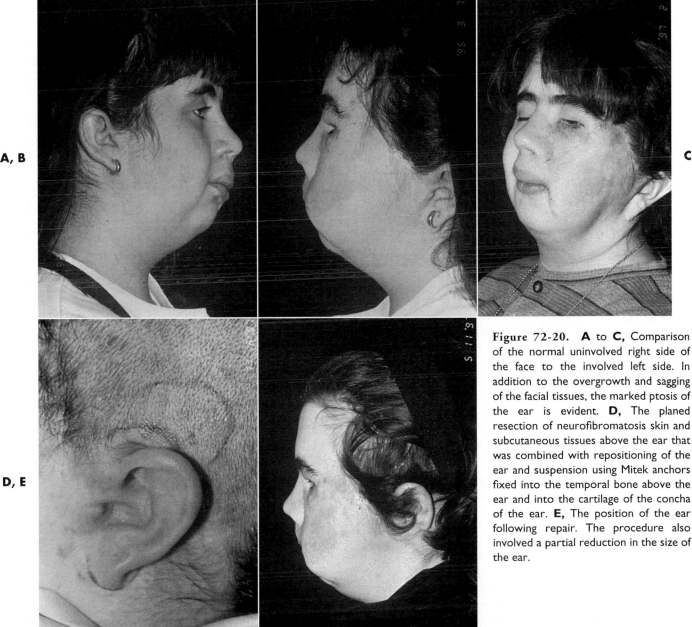

A, B

C

D, E

Figure 72-20. **A** to **C,** Comparison of the normal uninvolved right side of the face to the involved left side. In addition to the overgrowth and sagging of the facial tissues, the marked ptosis of the ear is evident. **D,** The planed resection of neurofibromatosis skin and subcutaneous tissues above the ear that was combined with repositioning of the ear and suspension using Mitek anchors fixed into the temporal bone above the ear and into the cartilage of the concha of the ear. **E,** The position of the ear following repair. The procedure also involved a partial reduction in the size of the ear.

meet the patient's desires and directed at his or her specific concerns. In some cases, where patients with particularly complex problems present with a litany of previous failed procedures, the surgeon must recognize that the patient may not be a candidate for further surgery.

DERMOIDS, GLIOMAS, AND ENCEPHALOCELES

The successful surgical approach to each of these lesions is dependent on a clear understanding of the varied anatomy of the lesion, in each area of involvement, combined with the appropriate preoperative radiological assessment.[21,24,27] It is perhaps easiest to discuss the surgical approach to the "lateral" lesions first followed by the "midline" lesions.

Dermoid Cysts
As discussed previously these lesions are typically in the region of the lateral brow in the vicinity of the frontozygomatic suture, but may be seen along the whole supraorbital rim in more medial positions. They vary in depth of position from the mobile lesion to those in a shallow trough in the bone to those that are interosseous. They do not extend intracranially except in the latter case.

Excision can be approached through the upper lateral lid skin incision or immediately below the brow in most cases (see Figure 72-5). Where in the past we occasionally placed the incision just above the upper hairs of the lateral brow, the lower incision seems to result in a less visible scar (although I have never been asked to revise either of these scars). Some surgeons prefer a transconjunctival approach to this lesion, which obviously eliminates the scar. This may be more effective below the brow but more difficult for lesions lying 1 cm or more above the brow. Others have more recently used an endoscopic approach, but having heard of two temporal branch frontal nerve traction injuries using this approach, we would recommend against it. The rare intraosseous lesion, presenting as a fullness in the bone, appears on approach as a yellow lesion in the bone, possibly with only an eggshell of bone overlying it (see Figure 72-5, C). This eggshell can be gently lifted or burred off and the cyst lifted out. Care must be taken to assess if the inner table has eroded, and the cyst should be gently separated from the dura. The "cavity" does not need to be filled in since the bone will remodel.

FRONTONASAL DERMOID CYSTS. The surgical approach to frontonasal dermoid cysts is dependent on whether they present as a cyst alone without intracranial extension, a sinus and cyst without intracranial extension, or with intracranial extension.

Cysts of the nasal dorsum are usually approached through a vertical midline incision, as are those of the glabellar region. Care is taken to dissect closely along the cyst wall to not inadvertently pick up tissue that appears to be a connected stalk. Most cysts alone are as easily excised as the external angular dermoids (see Figures 72-8 to 72-10).

Although the vertical midline scar in the glabellar region generally heals well, those on the nasal dorsum have tended to widen a bit over time. Some have benefited late from revision with excision or, more commonly, dermabrasion. Recently we have used a small crescent-shaped incision curving just below the medial brow in the shadow of the orbital rim to approach isolated glabellar cysts, with the scar being even less visible than the midline one.

Excision of a frontonasal dermoid cyst and sinus is best accomplished with a direct approach placing a lacrimal probe into the sinus, circumscribing the sinus opening with a vertical ellipse and enlarging the ellipse enough to follow the tract upward. At the point that it dives beneath the nasal bones it may be necessary to remove a small segment of the bone. Meticulous hemostasis and care not to stray out from the immediate cyst and sinus will most readily reveal the anatomy and allow accurate total excision. In the rare occasions where preoperative CT or MRI were unclear in delineating a possible narrow stalk of tissue extending intracranially, this "ribbon" of tissue may be examined with frozen section to determine whether or not it contains epithelial remnants. If only fibrous tissue is noted, then the excision is complete.

Lesions with intracranial extension typically present no differently than those frontonasal lesions without extension, although we have had one case present with intracranial abscess who during work-up, was noted to have a previously unrecognized sinus opening on his nasal tip (see Figure 72-10). Typically we have approached the excision of an intracranial dermoid through a "small" frontal bone flap; this allows isolation of the intracranial lesion before beginning the excision of the extracranial portion, which is a potential source of contamination. The intracranial segment typically sits in a cup-shaped bifid crista galli with the mass of the dermoid between the leaves of the falx. On occasion a lacrimal probe can be passed through the full extent of the tract. Once the surface portion of the nasal excision is completed, the remainder is completed from the underside with good exposure, thereby limiting the size of surface incision required.

Although other approaches have been described and used by other surgeons for excision of frontonasal dermoids, including open rhinoplasty and intraoral labial sulcus incisions with nasal degloving, their limited visibility and therefore inaccurate excision predispose to recurrence. With the approach we describe and follow, we have not had a single recurrence.

The single frontonasal dermoid cyst and sinus following a different path of resection is the cyst and sinus at the columellar base. This lesion tracts toward the nasal spine only. Its excision is accomplished by circumscribing the sinus opening, freeing the sinus opening from the surface subcutaneous tissue, then completing the excision through an incision in the labial sulcus (where the cyst is easily visualized).

Gliomas
EXTRANASAL. The approach to excision of an extranasal glioma is dependent on whether the lesion involves the surface

skin or lies at a subcutaneous level. Obviously surface involvement requires resection of all involved skin and dissection in a similar fashion to the frontonasal dermoid, following the lesion below the nasal bones if necessary (see Figure 72-11).

The defect that remains following excision may require flap coverage with choices including a forehead flap or a galeal flap with full-thickness skin graft coverage if the periosteum is resected with the lesion. (If the surface involvement is limited, primary closure is possible.) One of our early cases involving both a large intraosseous segment of the nasal dorsum and a portion of the nasal bones was closed with the latter approach. The late contour defect and disruption of normal nasal bone architecture required later coverage with a forehead flap and also required osteotomy and correction of the distorted nasal pyramid.

INTRANASAL. Intranasal gliomas are addressed with a craniofacial approach (see Figure 72-12). The best visualization of this lesion is accomplished through a bicoronal approach, frontal craniotomy, and osteotomy with removal en bloc of the frontonasal portion of the bandeau and nasal bones. With this accomplished, the anatomy of the intranasal lesion is widely and easily visualized and accurate expansion possible.

Encephaloceles

A full discussion of frontonasal encephaloceles is beyond the scope of this chapter. A craniofacial approach is required and follows accurate preoperative assessment of the extent of involvement. Since many of these involve the overlying skin or present with considerable excess skin overlying, a direct approach from the surface is possible for part of the resection. The intracranial dissection may be accomplished through a limited craniotomy in many cases (as described by Barone[2a]). The medial nasal walls may be osteotomized and the infraorbital distance reduced, in some cases simultaneously. Some will require late correction. The bony defect can be repaired with a cranial bone graft.

Two patients in our series of frontonasal encephaloceles demonstrated late "trigonocephalic-like" frontal distortion that required correction of both frontal and supraorbital bone distortion in a similar manner to that used for treatment of the deformity seen with craniosynostosis. Each case showed excellent stable postoperative correction.

BRANCHIAL CYSTS AND SINUSES

Auricular/Preauricular Sinus and Cyst

The common auricular sinus with opening at the junction of the first arch contribution to the ear (helical crus and tragus) and second arch contribution (remaining helical rim, antihelix, and lobule) may be one of the "easier" sinuses/cysts to excise if properly addressed; however, we have seen a considerable number where prior excision failed, and a history of recurrent infection and drainage is common. This is also the case for the

preauricular cysts that present either as a palpable fullness anterior to the helical root or with history of infection.[6,14,23]

The sinus/cyst excision follows the same approach described for others above. A lacrimal probe is passed into the sinus, the opening elliptically circumscribed, and the tract followed. The incision is extended just anterior to the helical crus and tragus. However, in this region the course of the sinus and cyst may be circuitous, wrapping around or under the helical crus cartilage or, at times (particularly in recurrent cases), adherent to it. When delineation of the tract is difficult, one must dissect directly on the cartilage surface and, if necessary, include a portion of cartilage with the specimen. The course of this particular group of lesions has no proximity to the facial nerve, so this is not a concern.

Again, if properly approached, recurrence of even recurrent lesions can be avoided, which has been our experience.

CERVICOAURAL SINUS AND CYST

First Branchial Arch

Every effort should be made to accurately complete these resections on the first attempt. Meticulous hemostasis with initial injection of a vasoconstricting agent plus bipolar cautery is essential. In treating a recurrent lesion, or a lesion with history of recurrent bouts of inflammation and swelling, the lesion should be as quiescent as possible at the point of excision (this may require prolonged antibiotic coverage during the time between treatment of acute inflammation and excision). The patient should be covered with broad-spectrum antibiotics.

As with the above case, the intimate relation of this cyst and the cartilage of the external auditory canal must be understood if complete excision is to be attained (see Figure 72-13). The incision can wrap around the lobule as in a facelift or remain preauricular as a parotidectomy-type incision. This cyst/sinus can track between branches of the facial nerve, the patient must not be paralyzed, and the nerve must be monitored during excision. Dissection must stay intimately close to the cyst wall and then immediately on the cartilage surface. At the point of cartilage attachment, a button of cartilage is removed, ensuring complete excision of all epithelial remnants.

Second Branchial Cleft

The embryonic path followed by these lesions has been described in detail above. While the length and extent of the tract varies from case to case, a clear understanding of the adjacent anatomy is critical for both complete and safe excision without injury to nerves or vessels.

The same approach is used in these excisions as in treatment of lesions in the first branchial arch, but here a stair-step incision may be required (see Figure 72-14). We have found absolutely no benefit in injecting the tract with either methylene blue or lucent green, although some surgeons "swear" by this approach.

In cases of the complete fistulous tract, a long catheter can be passed from skin surface to pharyngeal area and the track followed staying immediately on its surface, pulling it from lower to upper incision, then completing the removal with the intraoral excision around the upper limit of the fistula.

When working in the vicinity of the ear, the best adage is if in doubt of where to cut, "stay on the cartilage surface," and understand the relationship of the lesion to the adjacent fascial planes.

THYROGLOSSAL DUCT CYSTS

As with the lateral group of "embryonic" cysts and sinuses, the understanding of the embryologic path and defect leading to the lesion formation is the key to successful treatment of thyroglossal duct cysts (see Figures 72-16 and 72-17). The Sistrunk procedure has been well described in many texts of head and neck surgery and need not be repeated here.[5,25] The well-recognized need to excise a segment of the hyoid bone with the cyst and tract is critical. With that fact understood, recurrence following excision should be unheard of.

SUMMARY

This chapter has attempted to address a wide assortment of benign head and neck lesions, many of congenital origin, others acquired. We have tried to emphasize that proper diagnosis and detailed work-ups (as in other areas of surgery), an understanding of the embryonic pathways along which some of these lesions arise, and recognition of the pathophysiology and maternal history will make the outcome for most a successful one, with only a single procedure required. Early recognition and high index of suspicion will prevent repeated episodes of infection, which might decrease the likelihood of primary surgical success and increase overall cost of treatment.

For the vascular lesions and the neurofibromatosis lesions, the timing of procedures commensurate with the lesions' growth, characteristics, or potential functional effects will help to optimize the outcome of the approach chosen and possibly limit the number of procedures required over the lifetime of the patient. Timing should address not only present morbidity but hopefully mitigate future functional complications that would necessitate further surgery and decrease the patient's social productivity. Obviously, genetic counseling of the families and young adult patients with neurofibromatosis will be an important feature in decreasing the future impact of this disease. Similarly, knowledge of the high likelihood of involution of hemangiomas and the ability to transfer such information to patient and family will limit unnecessary aggressive early surgical intervention that may result in permanent deformity or the need for more extensive future reconstruction than would a cautious watch-and-wait regimen.

REFERENCES

1. Alland RD: The thyroglossal duct cyst, *Head Neck Surg* 5:134, 1982.
2. Badoni J, Athey P: Sonography in the diagnosis of branchial cysts, *Am J Roentgenol* 137:1245, 1981.
2a. Barone C, Jimenez D, Guevarra M, et al: Evaluation and treatment of sincipital encephaloceles: report of 27 consecutive cases. In Whitaker LA, editor: *Craniofacial surgery*, ed 7, Bologna, Italy, 1997, Monduzzi Editore, p 171.
3. Bauer BS: The hamartoma, In Vistnes LM, editor: *Procedures in plastic and reconstructive surgery*, Boston, 1991, Little Brown, pp 291-315.
4. Bauer BS, Kernahan DA, Hugo NE: Lymphangioma circumscriptum: a clinico-pathologic review, *Ann Plast Surg* 7:318, 1981.
5. Brown PM, Judd ES: Thyroglossal duct cysts and sinuses: results of radical (Sistrunk) operation, *Am J Surg* 102:494-501, 1961.
6. Buckingham JM, Lynn HB: Branchial cleft cysts and sinuses in children, *Mayo Clin Proc* 49:172, 1974.
7. Cohen BA, Hood AF: Xanthogranuloma: report on clinical and histological findings in 64 patients, *Pediatr Dermatol* 6:262-266, 1989.
8. Georgiade GS, Georgiade NG: Cervical masses. In Georgiade GS, Riefkohl R, Levin LS, editors: *Plastic, maxillofacial, and reconstructive surgery*, Baltimore, 1997, Williams & Wilkins, pp 521-528.
9. Grabb WC, Dingman RO, Oneal RM, et al: Facial hamartomas in children: neurofibroma, lymphangioma, and hemangioma, *Plast Reconstr Surg* 66:509-527, 1980.
10. Griffith BH, McKinney P, Monroe CW, et al: Von Recklinghausen's disease in children, *Plast Reconstr Surg* 49:647, 1972.
11. Hawkins DB, Chen WT: Pilomatrixoma of the head and neck in children, *Int J Pediatr Otorhinolaryngol* 8:215, 1985.
12. Headington JT: Tumors of the hair follicles, *Am J Pathol* 85:480, 1976.
13. Jackson IJ, Laws ER, Martin RD: The surgical management of orbital neurofibromatosis, *Plast Reconstr Surg* 71:751-758, 1983.
14. Karmody CS: Anomalies of the first and second branchial arches. In English G, editor: *Otolaryngology*, Philadelphia, 1986, Harper & Row, pp 1-8.
15. Marchac D: Intracranial enlargement of the orbital cavity and palpebral remodeling for orbitopalpebral neurofibromatosis, *Plast Reconstr Surg* 73:534-541, 1984.
16. McClatchey K, Batsakis JG, Van Wieren CR: Odontogenic keratocysts and nevoid basal cell carcinoma syndrome, *Arch Otolaryngol* 101:613-616, 1975.
17. Mehregen AH, Rahbari H: Benign epithelial tumors of the skin. II. Benign sebaceous tumors, *Cutis* 19:317-320, 1977.
18. Mulliken JB: Diagnosis and natural history of hemangiomas. In Mulliken JB, Young AE, editors: *Vascular birthmarks—hemangiomas and malformations*, Philadelphia, 1988, WB Saunders, 41-62.

19. Mulliken JB, Glowacki J: Hemangiomas and vascular malformations in infants and children: a classification based on endothelial characteristics, *Plast Reconstr Surg* 69:412, 1982.

20. Murray JC, Vollmer RT, Georgiade GS. Benign skin tumors: clinical aspects and histopathology. In Georgiade GS, Riefkohl R, Levin LS, editors: *Plastic, maxillofacial, and reconstructive surgery,* Baltimore, 1997, Williams & Wilkins, 138-149.

21. Naidich TP, Zimmerman RA, Bauer BS, et al: Midface: embryology and congenital lesions. In Som PM, Curtin HD, editors: *Head and neck imaging,* St Louis, 1996, Mosby, 3-60.

22. Paller AS: Epidermal nevus syndrome, *Neurol Clin* 5:451, 1987.

23. Randall P, Royster HP: First branchial cleft anomalies, *Plast Reconstr Surg* 31:497-506, 1963.

24. Sessions RB: Nasal dermal sinus—new concepts and explanations, *Laryngoscope* 92(Suppl 29):1, 1982.

25. Sistrunk WE: Technique of removal of cysts and sinuses of the thyroglossal duct, *Surg Gyne Obstet* 46:109, 1928.

26. Solomon LM, Esterly NB: Epidermal and other congenital organic nevi, *Curr Probl Pediatr* 6:3, 1975.

27. Thaller SR, Bauer BS: Cysts and cystlike lesions of the skin and subcutaneous tissue, *Clin Plast Surg* 14:327, 1987.

28. Thomson HG: Common benign pediatric cutaneous tumors: timing and treatment, *Clin Plast Surg* 17:49-64, 1990.

29. Van der Meulen JC, Moscone AR, Vandrachen M, et al: The management of orbitofacial neurofibromatosis, *Ann Plast Surg* 8:220, 1982.

30. Weary PE, Linthicum A, Cawlwy EP, et al: Gardner's syndrome, *Arch Dermatol* 90:20-30, 1964.

CHAPTER 73

Nonepidermoid Cancers of the Head and Neck

Mark R. Sultan

INDICATIONS

THE PROBLEM

The anatomic, physiologic, and aesthetic complexity of the head and neck poses significant challenges to the management of all neoplasms arising in this compact region. The rare but highly diverse nature of nonepidermoid cancers (sarcomas) in the head and neck raises these challenges to even higher levels. Sarcomas are those malignancies that arise from bone and connective tissues. They are classified according to their line of differentiation toward normal tissue, and include such tumors as osteogenic sarcoma and angiosarcoma. In general, they are far less common than their epidermoid carcinoma counterparts. In the United States there are 6,000 new cases of sarcoma each year, leading to 4,000 deaths. Approximately 15% of sarcomas arise in the head and neck. Therefore sarcomas account for only 1% of all head and neck neoplasms. This low incidence has prevented any one physician or medical center from accumulating sufficient experience to develop a comprehensive treatment plan.

The difficulties in management created by the rarity of head and neck sarcomas are further exacerbated by their heterogeneity. More than 20 histologic types have been described. Although the type of sarcoma does offer some predictive value of its local aggressiveness and metastatic potential, the pathophysiology of any one lesion is also determined by the patient's age, the location and size of the primary mass, and, most important, the degree of differentiation of the tumor.[24,27] The evaluation and treatment of all patients with head and neck sarcomas must therefore be highly individualized, taking all of these factors into account and stratifying their importance appropriately.[10]

Sarcomas are characterized by aggressive growth at the primary site (Figure 73-1) and by local recurrence. Therefore the mainstay of therapy remains adequate surgical extirpation.[20,24] In a landmark 1981 paper about sarcomas of the trunk and extremities, Enneking et al introduced the concept of a "compartment" containing the tumor and proposed that a complete "compartmentectomy" should be performed whenever possible.[12] This approach dramatically lowered local recurrence rates and, consequently, cure rates. In the uniquely restricted confines of the head and neck, however, "compartmentectomy" has little application because at presentation the majority of these infiltrative tumors have extended well beyond their origin.[23] Also, many lie adjacent to vital neurovascular or functional structures, preventing their complete resection without risk of unacceptable morbidity. In recent years advances in reconstructive techniques have greatly expanded the gamut of what tumor is "resectable" and have helped reestablish surgery as the primary treatment modality for sarcomas of the head and neck. Still, in a great number of cases curative extirpation cannot be achieved. Therefore a multidisciplinary approach to these tumors, including radiation therapy and chemotherapy, must often be utilized to obtain superior results.[25]

ETIOLOGY

For most nonepidermoid cancers no definite predisposing cause can be identified. However, associated etiologic agents or conditions have been implicated in many instances. For example, a prior history of radiation therapy is well recognized as being an etiologic factor in the development of secondary malignancies, and the majority of these are sarcomas.[28,29,37] The incidence is believed to be between 0.2% and 0.7% of all patients receiving radiation therapy. The criteria for radiation-induced tumors were established by Cahan et al in 1948.[5] These include tumor developing in the radiation field, evidence of nonmalignancy in affected tissues, a long latency period (>5 to 10 years), and a different histology for the new tumor. It is believed that sarcomas are likely to develop at the periphery of the prior radiation fields where less devitalized tissue exists. The risk of secondary malignancy begins with a prior history of as little as 500 to 1000 rads.[37] These dosages were used commonly decades ago for benign conditions such as acne and are used rarely today as, for example, in the treatment of keloid scars. The latency period for sarcoma genesis in these cases is quite long, approximately 50 years. In the more common situation of prior high-dose radiation (greater than 5000 rads) for cure of a malignancy, the average latency interval is 10 to 15 years. It is generally believed that

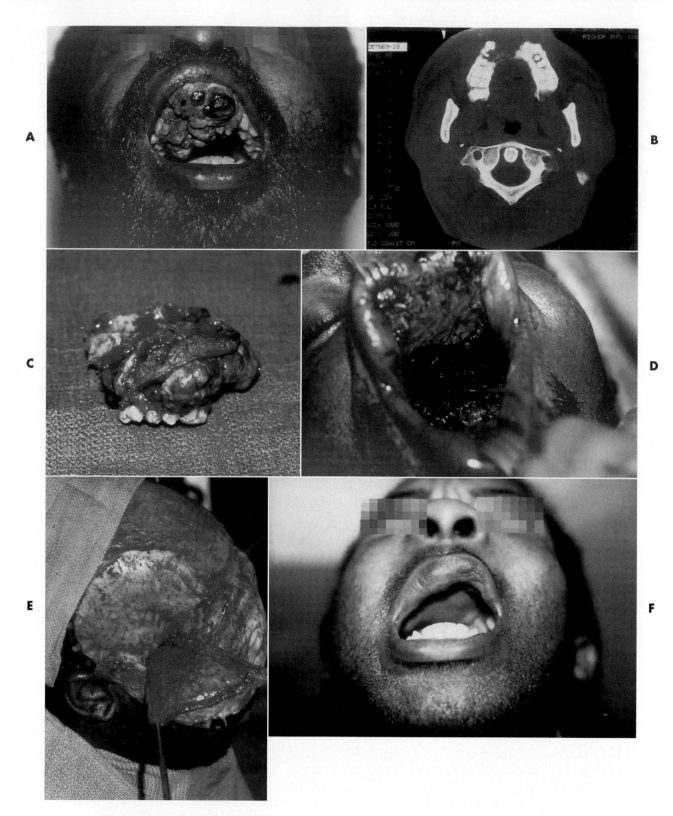

Figure 73-1. **A** and **B,** Rapidly growing leiomyosarcoma of the palate showing exophytic growth into the mouth as well as invasion of the bony maxillary alveolus. **C** and **D,** Resected specimen includes palate and maxillary sinus leaving extensive defect in the roof of the mouth. **E** and **F,** Reconstruction was performed with a temporalis muscle flap transposed beneath the zygoma and through the buccal mucosa and covered with a split-thickness skin graft.

the secondary cancer risk increases at higher radiation doses. The most common types of sarcoma to arise in the head and neck as a result of prior radiation are osteogenic sarcoma and fibrosarcoma. Their course and prognosis may be slightly worse than nonradiation-induced tumors of the same type. For example, a recent report of 13 cases from UCLA reported a 5-year survival rate of 19%.[27,28]

A number of malignant neoplasms including retinoblastoma and Wilms' tumor are associated with subsequent sarcoma formation. A chromosomal anomaly (on the 13q chromosome) is believed to be responsible.[16] The germ line mutations of the p53 tumor suppressor gene are also associated with a high risk for the development of sarcomas and other malignancies. In addition, several benign conditions such as neurofibromatosis (von Recklinghausen's disease), fibrous dysplasia, and Paget's disease of the bone can degenerate into sarcomas late into their course with or without a prior history of radiation therapy.[28] Exposure to chemicals such as polyvinyl chloride, arsenic, and dioxin or to alkylating chemotherapeutic agents is known to be sarcomagenic.[31] Recently, surgical trauma such as prior sinus surgery has also been associated with sarcoma development following a long latency period.[7] Finally, acquired immunodeficiency syndrome (AIDS) is linked to Kaposi's sarcoma. This is a subtype of an angiosarcoma that most commonly presents as papules or nodules in the oral cavity.

PRESENTATION

Typically, a sarcoma of the head and neck presents as a painless mass. The more advanced or more deeply invasive lesions may cause pain, epistaxis, nerve deficits, or functional disturbances such as a change in vision or voice. The most common sites include the neck (28%), face and forehead (20%), maxilla (15%), scalp (10%), mandible (10%), paranasal sinuses (<10%), and oropharynx and larynx (>10%). The size of the lesion at presentation tends to vary with location. Those lesions that arise in functionally "quiet zones" such as the supraclavicular fossa or posterior neck tend to be larger (>5 cm), whereas those that develop in functionally sensitive sites such as the nasal cavity are generally detected at a smaller size (<3 cm).[23] This correlation of size and location was recently confirmed by the Head and Neck Sarcoma Registry.[38] Some 10% to 20% of head and neck sarcomas arise in children and adolescents.[26] The majority of these are rhabdomyosarcomas. The remainder occur in adults with a median age of 45 to 50 years.

DIAGNOSIS AND EVALUATION

The evaluation of any patient with a suspicious mass of the head or neck must begin with a complete history and physical examination. A careful assessment of the patient's cranial and sensory nerve status and of the cervical lymph nodes should be performed. Indirect laryngoscopy or direct endoscopy of the oropharynx and hypopharynx is carried out whenever direct or secondary involvement is suspected. The primary mass is then evaluated clinically to analyze its size and degree of invasiveness, important factors needed to help stage the disease and to formulate treatment plans.

Following clinical evaluation, fine-needle aspiration (FNA) cytology using a 20-gauge needle should be performed. FNA can correctly distinguish between benign, malignant, and inflammatory lesions in over 95% of cases. FNA alone is not sufficient to diagnose the specific type of sarcoma; however, in a recent series of 52 patients the FNA correctly suggested the diagnosis of sarcoma in 88.4%.[6] This high specificity, coupled with its ease and low cost, makes FNA an extremely useful screening tool for any patient with a suspicious mass of the head or neck, including those who ultimately prove to harbor sarcomas.

Definitive diagnosis of sarcomas requires an open, incisional biopsy. The incision must be planned carefully so that it will subsequently lie well within the boundaries of a wide excision and will not interfere with a local flap potentially needed for reconstruction.[2] A direct approach without undermining skin or fascia is preferable. Areas of hemorrhage or necrosis within the tumor should be avoided, since these are often "nondiagnostic." Instead, solid areas of the tumor are biopsied. Frozen section analysis can be performed to confirm that representative tissue for diagnosis has been obtained. Careful hemostasis and wound closure are important. A generous sample of the tumor should be obtained because the histologic diagnosis of nonepidermoid cancers can be extremely difficult. Therefore, in addition to standard hematoxylin and eosin techniques, electronmicroscopy and special immunostains are often needed to allow the pathologist to complete characterization of the tumor subtype and, importantly, of the grade. A preoperative discussion regarding the site and extent of the biopsy should be held with the involved pathologist to coordinate efforts whenever possible.

Once the diagnosis of head and neck sarcoma is established, further staging of the patient's lesion is obtained. A computed axial tomography (CAT) scan and magnetic resonance imaging (MRI) of the region for this purpose are roughly equivalent. A CAT scan generally provides a more well-defined view of bony erosion, whereas an MRI, with its excellent image contrast, more accurately detects smaller tumors. In cases where significant scar formation such as from prior surgery may be intertwined with tumor, dynamic MRI scanning with intravenous contrast to enhance the tumor image is the study of choice.[22] Use of the contrast agent gadolinium in conjunction with surface coils has increased the accuracy of staging for sarcomas of the skull base. A method that holds promise for the evaluation of sarcomas is positron emission tomography (PET) scan.[2] Since sarcomas generally have increased glucose metabolism, they are therefore amenable to detection with a high degree of sensitivity by the PET scan, which utilizes radiolabeled glucose to obtain these images.

Table 73-1.
TNM Staging for Sarcoma

STAGE	DESCRIPTION	DIFFERENTIATION	TUMOR	NODAL INVOLVEMENT	METASTATIC DISEASE
I	Low-grade, small, superficial, and deep	G 1-2	T 1a-1b	No	Mo
	Low-grade, large, superficial	G 1-2	T 2a	No	Mo
II	Low-grade, large, deep	G 1-2	T 2b	No	Mo
	High-grade, small	G 3-4	T 1a-1b	No	Mo
	High-grade, large, superficial	G 3-4	T 2a	No	Mo
III	High-grade, large, deep	G 3-4	T 2b	No	Mo
IV	Any metastasis	Any G	Any T	Ni	Mo
		Any G	Any T	No	Mi

G 1, Well differentiated; G 2, moderately differentiated; G 3, poorly differentiated; G 4, undifferentiated.
Tumor <5 cm: T 1a, superficial; T 1b, deep. Tumor >5 cm: T 2a, superficial; T 2b, deep.
No, No nodal involvement; Ni, any nodal involvement; Mo, no metastatic disease; Mi, any metastatic disease.

For small, low-grade sarcomas the metastatic work-up should include a chest x-ray and liver enzymes. In more advanced or higher grade lesions, a more complete evaluation including CAT scans of the chest and abdomen to rule out pulmonary or hepatic metastases is indicated.

STAGING

The most important factors utilized in staging sarcomas of the head and neck and determining their prognosis are the size of the primary lesion (>5 cm or <5 cm) and the histologic grade of malignancy.[36] The presence of regional lymphade-nopathy or distant disease is also noted. The TNM classification is available for staging these tumors (Table 73-1). However, few authors adhere strictly to this system when reporting their data because of the tremendous diversity of sarcomas by histologic type and biologic activity and the multitude of prognostic factors. Therefore authors generally list the number of each type of sarcoma treated, for instance fibrosarcoma or angiosarcoma, and then stratify their results according to staging criteria within each type.[35] A separate and unique method has proved useful for staging of rhabdomyosarcomas in children. In this system, staging takes place after surgical intervention and is based on the completeness of surgical resection.

RHABDOMYOSARCOMA

In children only 5% of all primary malignant tumors arise in the head and neck. The most frequent are lymphomas (45%). Sarcomas account for 17% of the total, with 60% of these rhabdomyosarcomas.[8,9,26,41] There are three major variants of rhabdomyosarcomas: embryonal, alveolar, and pleomorphic. The embryonal subtype predominates. These lesions tend to arise in young children between 3 and 5 years of age. They most often involve the orbit and usually do not metastasize. Therefore, they carry a distinctly better prognosis than the alveolar and pleomorphic variants. The latter more commonly arise in the neck or parameningeal spaces of older children and have a high incidence of regional lymph node and distant metastases.

In the 1960s multimodality therapy of children with rhabdomyosarcoma was introduced. The Intergroup Rhab-domyosarcoma Study has since shown that the combina-tion of surgery, irradiation, and chemotherapy (Adriamy-cin, cyclophosphamide, dacarbazine [DTIC]) improved 5-year survival to 55%, markedly better than any single modality was previously able to achieve.[30] Recently, how-ever, there has been a renewed interest in the role of surgical excision as the primary mode of controlling local disease, since 50% of treatment failures occur because of local recurrence.[39] Complete extirpation of the rhabdo-myosarcoma with negative surgical margins improves local control dsand survival and obviates the need for adjuvant radiotherapy, thereby avoiding its potential long-term se-quelae. The development of more sophisticated craniofacial and infratemporal approaches to the cranial base, along with more reliable reconstructive techniques, is expanding the potential to fully excise these lesions with acceptable morbidity.

MALIGNANT FIBROUS HISTIOCYTOMA

Malignant fibrous histiocytomas (MFH) are among the most common of the head and neck sarcomas. Their reported

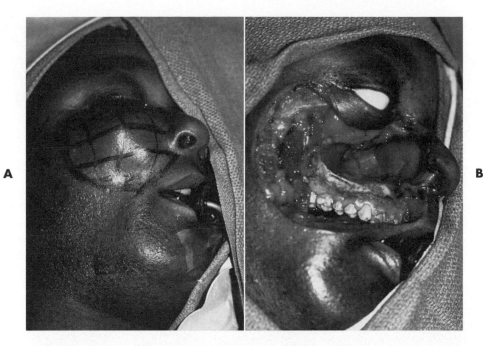

Figure 73-2. A, Recurrent malignant fibrous histiocytoma of the midface in a 42-year-old man. **B,** Defect after radical excision involving skin, maxillary bone and sinus, and orbital floor. *Continued*

incidence has risen in recent years because lesions previously classified as high-grade fibrosarcomas are now designated as MFH. The pathologic diagnosis of this lesion can be difficult, and although no one reliable marker for the disease exists, histochemical analysis for alpha-1-antitrypsin and alpha-1-antichymotrypsin can be helpful. In its classic form it is composed of fibroblast-like (spindled) and histiocyte-like (circular) cells arranged in a storiform pattern. These are most often accompanied by pleomorphic giant and inflammatory cells. Mitotic activity is usually rapid. Two major histologic variants exist, myxoid and inflammatory, with the latter carrying a worse prognosis.[31] MFH has been associated with several other disease entities including leukemia, neurofibromatosis, Paget's disease, thyroid disease, and prior radiation therapy.

The most common sites of head and neck involvement include nasal and paranasal sinuses (32%), craniofacial bones (20%), soft tissues of the neck (10% to 15%), major salivary glands (10%), and oral cavity (10%). These are aggressive lesions. The local recurrence rate approaches 70% unless widely negative margins can be achieved (Figure 73-2). For this reason, adjuvant radiation therapy is included in the treatment regimen in the majority of cases. MFH is also unique among the head and neck sarcomas in its propensity for regional nodal metastases. These occur in at least 50% of cases. Therefore full neck dissections must be performed for clinically positive neck disease and modified dissections considered for the clinically negative (No) neck. Overall 5-year survival is approximately 50%.

ANGIOSARCOMA

Angiosarcomas are rare malignancies of the head and neck that generally arise in the skin of the scalp or face and secondarily invade the underlying soft tissues.[19] The typical presentation is a soft, violaceous, painless, and compressible mass arising in a middle-aged or elderly man (Figure 73-3). The subsequent growth can be explosive, with rapid development of deep invasion, ulceration, and regional or distant metastasis. Definitive extirpation, when possible, offers the most realistic chance for cure, although sporadic reports citing the efficacy of radiation therapy and/or chemotherapy have appeared in the literature. Prognosis is most closely tied to the size of the primary at presentation as well as the status of regional or distant disease. Overall, 5-year disease-free survival is rare.

OSTEOGENIC SARCOMA

Osteogenic sarcoma is the most common primary malignancy of bone; however, only 4% arise in the head and neck. Known etiologic factors include long-standing bone disease such as Paget's disease of the bone, fibrous dysplasia, enchondromas, and prior radiation therapy. There is a male predominance and a mean age at detection of 31 years. X-ray examination may reveal an osteoblastic or osteolytic appearance (Figure 73-4). By physical examination the lesions are hard and, although they may appear to be well circumscribed, often extend into adjacent soft tissues. This

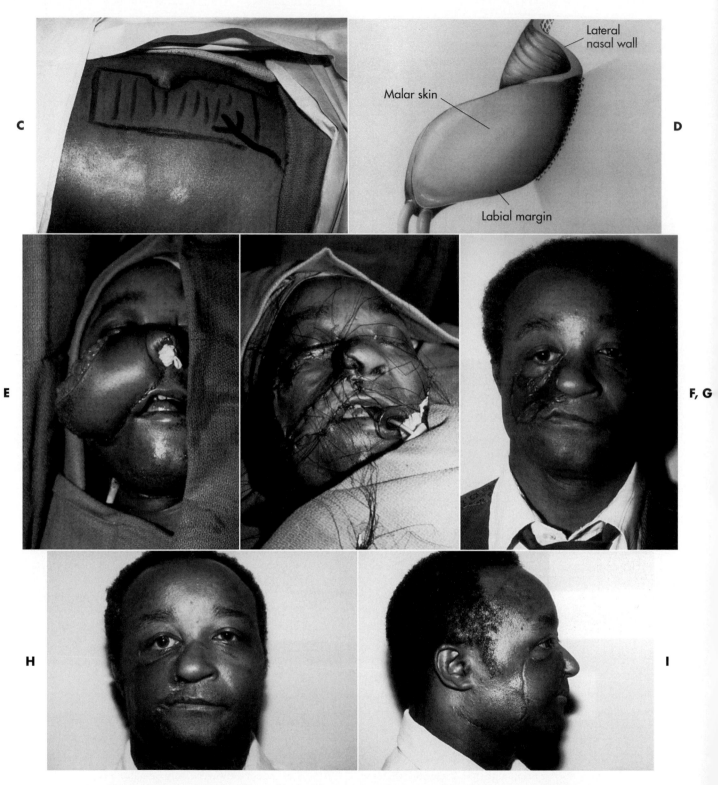

Figure 73-2, cont'd. C to **E,** Initial reconstruction was done with rectus abdominis musculocutaneous flap inset to obturate the three-dimensional defect. **F** and **G,** Revision of the overcorrection and subsequent atrophy of the denervated muscle and hypopigmentation of the skin graft gave an unsatisfactory result. **H** and **I,** This was improved by an iliac bone graft to replace the orbital floor and a radial forearm free flap for contour, improvement, and coverage.

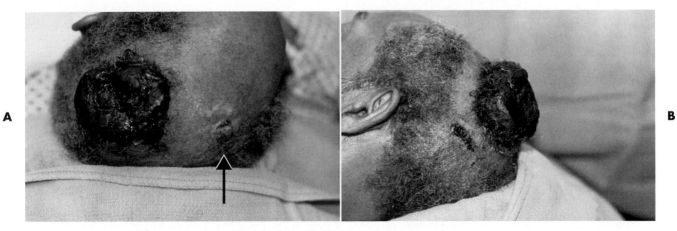

Figure 73-3. **A** and **B,** Angiosarcoma in elderly man. Note metastatic nodule (arrow).

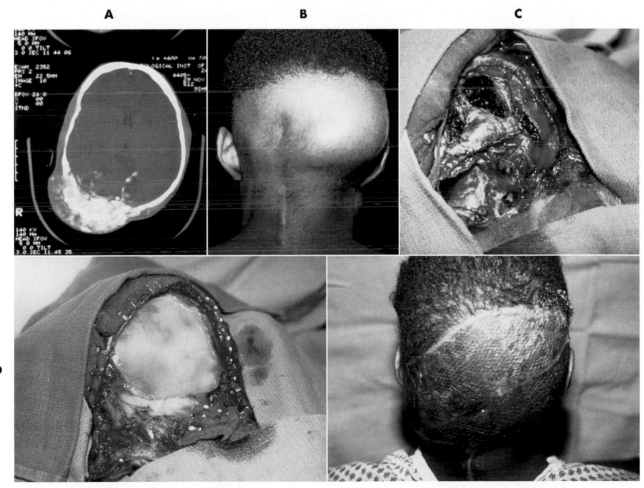

Figure 73-4. **A,** Extensive involvement of posterior scalp documented by osteogenic sarcoma CAT scan. **B,** Preoperative clinical appearance. **C,** Intraoperative appearance following composite resection and reconstruction of the confluence of the venous sinuses by fascia lata. **D,** Protection of the brain with a methyl methacrylate cranioplasty. **E,** Postoperative appearance following coverage with a latissimus dorsi muscle free flap and skin graft.

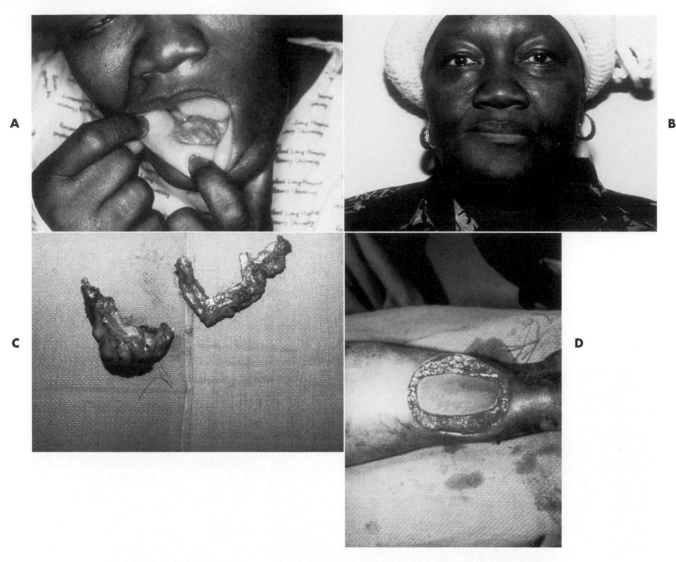

Figure 73-5. **A** and **B,** Osteogenic sarcoma of the mandible in a 35-year-old woman. This tumor did not respond to preoperative chemotherapy. **C,** Resected tumor and mandible from left angle to right mid-ramus. Reconstruction of the bony mandible was performed with fibula free flap. **D,** Because the skin of her leg was so thick, a radial forearm free flap was also used to create intraoral lining. *Continued*

underscores the fact that, once a diagnosis is established by incisional biopsy, a careful assessment of the extent of the osseous and soft tissue involvement with an MRI or CT scan should be carried out because definitive excision must include not only adequate bony margins but generous soft tissue margins as well. Regional lymph node dissections are not often indicated since metastasis is generally by the hematogenous route to the lungs.[31] Common areas of involvement in the head and neck include the bones bordering the paranasal sinuses and the mandible (Figure 73-5). Those lesions arising toward the anterior segment of the jaw carry a better prognosis than those located in the ramus or condyle, most likely due to the ability to achieve negative surgical margins in the former. Overall, the 5-year survival is approximately 30%.[36] Therefore chemotherapy (Adriamycin, methotrexate) is frequently used postoperatively.

ESTHESIONEUROBLASTOMA (OLFACTORY NEUROBLASTOMA)

Esthesioneuroblastoma is a rare low-grade sarcoma that arise from the epithelial lining surrounding the olfactory bulb at the apex of the nasal cavity. This tumor has been reported in a wide age range of patients, from the first to eighth decade, with a peak incidence in the second or third decade. It has a slight male predominance. In its earlier stages it may present as a fleshy upper nasal mass causing epistaxis, unilateral nasal obstruction, or rhinorrhea. In its later stages it can extend directly through the cribriform plate into the overlying anterior cranial fossa and frontal lobe,[14] at which time possible signs and symptoms include anosmia, rhinorrhea, headaches, or personality changes. This tumor is highly vascular, and when suspected on the basis

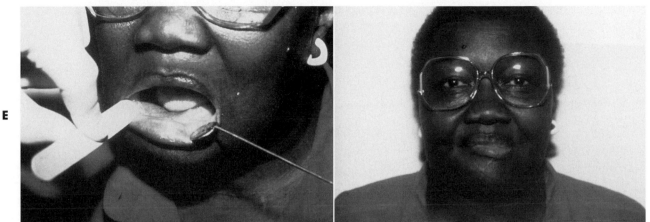

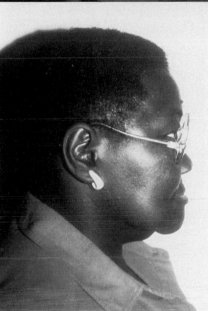

Figure 73-5, cont'd. **E** to **G**, Postoperative result demonstrating reasonable appearance and good postoperative intraoral anatomy and function.

of the history, endoscopic appearance, or CT findings (showing erosion of the cribriform plate), the biopsy should be performed in the operating room. Once the diagnosis is confirmed, careful staging of the lesion should be performed to assess the extent of local invasion, to rule out the 20% chance of regional neck adenopathy, and to rule out distant metastases that most commonly occur to lungs and bone.

Esthesioneuroblastomas have a relatively slow growth rate and a 5-year survival rate of approximately 50%. However, the disease-free 5-year survival rate is only 20%, and the majority of patients eventually do succumb to aggressive intracranial extension. This underscores the need for definitive local control whenever possible. For early lesions a lateral rhinotomy and complete ethmoidectomy may suffice. More advanced lesions require a combined neurosurgical-craniofacial effort to fully expose the anterior cranial base. This allows complete resection of the cribriform plate and ethmoid sinuses from a superior and transfacial approach. Dural resections are often required to obtain negative margins, and an extended galeal-myofascial flap can be utilized for dural repair. With large or complicated defects, however, free tissue transfer, such

as the rectus abdominis muscle, may be required to securely separate the brain from the paranasal sinuses. Due to the high local recurrence rate, adjuvant radiation therapy is routinely utilized postoperatively. Inoperable lesions may be treated by radiation therapy alone.

DERMATOFIBROSARCOMA PROTUBERANS

Dermatofibrosarcoma protuberans (DFSP) is a low-grade sarcoma that tends to arise on the trunk of young adults. Less commonly it occurs on the head and neck. These tumors present as plaquelike dermal masses that raise the overlying, normal-appearing skin into a "protuberant" nodule (Figure 73-6). Although generally painless, they may also cause tenderness, ulceration, and hemorrhage when their rate of growth is rapid, causing necrosis of the overlying skin. The clinical differential diagnosis can include hypertrophic scar, keloid, dermatofibroma, localized scleroderma, or nodular fasciitis. A generous biopsy is necessary to establish the diagnosis. Histologically, these tumors display spindle cells in a cartwheel or storiform pattern. Few mitoses are seen and yet

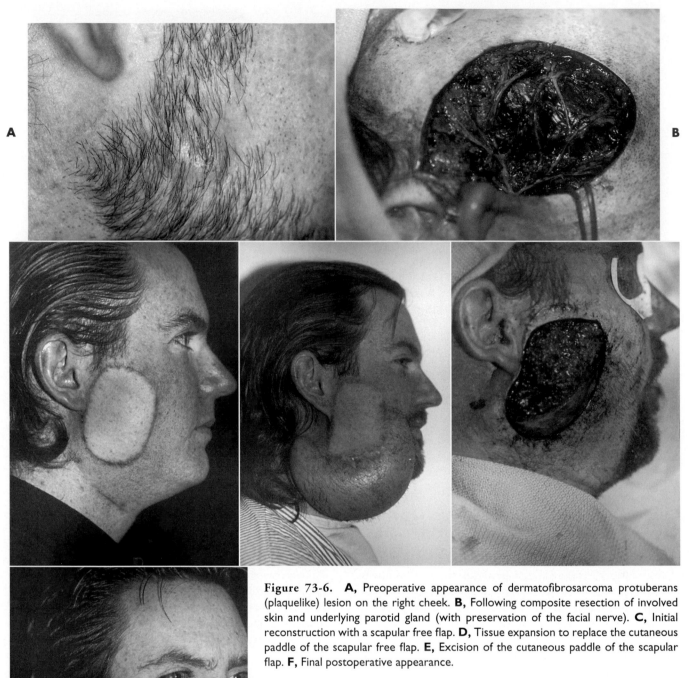

Figure 73-6. **A,** Preoperative appearance of dermatofibrosarcoma protuberans (plaquelike) lesion on the right cheek. **B,** Following composite resection of involved skin and underlying parotid gland (with preservation of the facial nerve). **C,** Initial reconstruction with a scapular free flap. **D,** Tissue expansion to replace the cutaneous paddle of the scapular free flap. **E,** Excision of the cutaneous paddle of the scapular flap. **F,** Final postoperative appearance.

these lesions can be highly infiltrative of adjacent adipose tissue, fascia, or musculature. This explains the high local recurrence rate of 32% to 76%. Regional distant nodal involvement and distant metastases are rare, but the few cases that have been reported have most often been associated with recurrent tumors. The same is true of degeneration of DFSP into high-grade fibrosarcomas. Therefore definitive local control is imperative. Recently, the use of Mohs' micrographic surgery has been proposed as an alternative to conventional wide local excision to better map and eradicate the primary lesions.[18] Preliminary reports using this technique are encouraging.

OPERATIONS

PRINCIPLES OF THERAPY

Extirpative Surgery

For most cases of head and neck sarcomas the primary determinant of successful therapy is the adequacy of local excision.[1,36] The definition of "adequate" for soft tissue sarcomas was first delineated by Bowden and Booher in 1958 for tumors of the extremities and included a wide margin of what appeared to be normal tissue around the primary tumor; resection of the entire muscle involved by the tumor, including its origin and insertion; ligation of major points of venous egress early in the procedure; and the use of sharp rather than blunt dissection. They stated that when those criteria could not be met, amputation of the affected limb should be considered. Of course, the latter cannot literally be applied to the head and neck. However, the principles of a "wide excision," as well as those of a "compartmentectomy" advocated by Enneking et al, can be utilized to the patient's advantage by appreciating the regional anatomy of the head and neck. When a sarcoma is found to arise within the anterior neck, for example, a complete radical or modified radical neck dissection may be the most effective way to satisfy the requirements of an "adequate" local excision. In this way, resection of all involved musculature such as the sternocleidomastoid, control of venous tributaries, and widely negative margins can be achieved. Other sites amenable to approach as compartments include the maxilla (maxillectomy) and orbit (orbital exenteration). In other areas, when functional resections are not possible, compromises may be necessary as the balance between "adequacy" and morbidity is weighed.

Reconstructive Surgery

Recent advances in the management of head and neck sarcomas have in large part centered on improvements in both extirpative and reconstructive surgery. These, in turn, are due to multiple and intertwined factors such as improved localization of tumors by more sophisticated diagnostic studies, better selective embolization of tumors when needed, improved access to the skull base through lateral temporal and craniofacial approaches, and more reliable reconstructive procedures. The method chosen for reconstruction is, of course, dictated by the nature of the specific defect. Skin grafts or local flaps may suffice for small or superficial defects. More commonly, however, indecently vascularized tissue must be imported to counter the effects of prior or anticipated radiation therapy and/or to protect vital structures. Distant pedicled flaps such as the pectoralis major and deltopectoral are helpful in the management of some defects of the lower head and neck within their arc of rotation (below the zygomatic arch). Their main utility is for repair of defects in the neck itself or the lower oral cavity. The trapezius myocutaneous flap has particular utility in closure of lateral facial and skull base defects. However, in order to achieve sufficient pedicle length to reach these areas, the transverse fibers of the trapezius lying above the spine of the scapula must often be divided, potentially leading to a "shoulder drop." Therefore free flaps, unencumbered by limited arcs of rotation, have become the reconstructive tools of choice for many defects created by the extirpation of head and neck sarcomas, as they have for head and neck wounds in general. This is particularly true of midface, scalp, and forehead and skull base defects, as well as those requiring vascularized bone. Microvascular reconstruction has improved the quality of life for scores of patients requiring resection of head and neck sarcomas. It has also extended the gamut of what may be considered resectable. It should follow that survival would also be improved. This will hopefully be borne out by statistical analysis of patients treated in the next decade.

Panchal et al recently utilized free flaps in conjunction with early (within 5 days) postoperative brachytherapy using iridium-192 wires following resection of sarcomas in an attempt to maximize therapy to the primary site while preventing wound breakdown.[32] The flap healed well in 9 of 10 patients. Survival data have not yet been reported.

Radiation Therapy

In the past decade radiation therapy has emerged as an important adjunct to surgery for the treatment of head and neck sarcomas. Previously, sarcomas were often considered radioresistant, and some authors continue to hold this view. However, as extensive experience with sarcomas of the extremities has shown, selected lesions can be quite responsive to radiotherapy, behaving similarly to many squamous cell carcinomas.[40]

In the management of sarcomas of the extremities there has been a trend toward the use of preoperative radiotherapy.[3,4] This has not been the case in head and neck sarcomas. Here radiotherapy has been delivered postoperatively except for recurrent lesions. There are both major and minor indications for postoperative radiation therapy. Major indications include high-grade lesions, in particular when the surgical margins are positive or close. Relative or minor indications include all lesions greater than 5 cm in diameter or any recurrent lesion. The techniques utilized for delivery of the radiation to sarcomas of the head and neck are similar to those used for treatment of squamous cell carcinomas, with 6000 to 6500 cGy utilized. One important difference is that elective radiation of the clinically negative neck is rarely indicated, since the risk of subclinical nodal metastasis is only 2% to 4%. In addition to external beam radiation, adjuvant radiotherapy may also be administered in the form of brachytherapy.[17] Here thin tubes are placed directly into the tumor and subsequently "loaded" with radiation sources such as iridium-192 wires to maximize the dose of radiation delivered to the lesion itself. This technique is often chosen in situations where it has been determined preoperatively that due to anatomic constraints a complete excision of the sarcoma will not be possible or in the management of large recurrent lesions.

To date, there have been no prospective randomized data that prove the overall efficacy of adjunctive radiation therapy for head and neck sarcomas. Some authors have reported a 10% to 25% decrease in the local recurrence rate in high-risk lesions as opposed to 40% to 60% in comparably matched patients who underwent surgery alone. Because of the lack of prospective data, the precise role of radiation therapy remains somewhat controversial. More recent developments in the field of radiation therapy for head and neck sarcoma include its potentiation by hyperthermia[11,13] and "re-irradiation" of recurrent lesions.[15]

Chemotherapy

With the exception of rhabdomyosarcomas, and possibly angiosarcomas, there are little definitive data to establish a role for chemotherapy in the management of sarcomas of the head and neck. As with radiotherapy, the basic guidelines for chemotherapy have been extrapolated from experience gained in the treatment of sarcomas of the extremities. Therefore the backbone of most combination chemotherapy regimens utilized has been Adriamycin. DTIC appears to fortify the effect of Adriamycin to improve response rates and prolong remission. Cyclophosphamide has also been used, but it does not appear to contribute significantly to the results achieved by the other two agents. Ifosfamide, an analog of cyclophosphamide, and cisplatin are also being studied in various combination protocols.

As outlined previously, chemotherapy is a mainstay in the management of rhabdomyosarcoma. It may also prove vital in the cure of angiosarcoma because of its proclivity toward distant metastasis early in its natural history, unlike the more typical head and neck sarcoma where local infiltration and therefore local control are more important. For other types of sarcomas of the head and neck, chemotherapy is generally given only to patients with unresectable lesions and/or to those who have failed surgery and radiation therapy or have disseminated disease.

One recent and potentially beneficial development regarding chemotherapy for sarcomas is its direct delivery by superselective arterial infusion.[34] With this method, an agent such as cisplatin is infused directly into the head or neck lesion in very high doses utilizing angiographic techniques, while a neutralizing agent, sodium thiosulfate, is given systemically to rapidly inactivate the cisplatin that would otherwise reach the body as a whole. Although initial reports about this method have dealt predominantly with advanced squamous cell carcinomas of the head and neck, several have also mentioned modest experience but encouraging results with sarcomas, particularly recurrent lesions.

OUTCOME

The natural history and outcome of specific sarcomas of the head and neck are highly dependent on the histologic type and degree of differentiation.[20,21,33] The stage of disease at diagnosis is also critical. Some generalities regarding metastatic potential, recurrence rate, and overall survival are listed in Table 73-2.

Table 73-2.
Soft Tissue Sarcomas of the Head and Neck

SARCOMA	REGIONAL NODAL METASTASIS (%)	DISTANT METASTASIS (%)	RECURRENCE RATE (%)	5-YEAR SURVIVAL (%)
Dermatofibrosarcoma protuberans	<1	5	20	95
Malignant fibrous histiocytoma	50-60	40	70	50
Rhabdomyosarcoma	15-74	50	30-50	55
Osteogenic sarcoma	20	65	70	30
Angiosarcoma	28	55	85-90	20
Esthesioneuroblastoma	20	10-20	80	50

SUMMARY

Once a definitive diagnosis of sarcoma is established, a complete and informative explanation of biology and natural history of the particular sarcoma should be carried out with the patient and their family. Although it is not advisable to quote specific recurrence and cure rates, patients must understand that advanced stage disease and high-grade lesions carry a higher recurrence rate and a worse prognosis. It should be explained that the goal of surgery is the complete extirpation of the neoplasm, but that this may not be possible. Therefore the potential role for radiation therapy and chemotherapy should be introduced; when indicated, involvement of the radiation oncologist and medical oncologist should be arranged prior to surgery. The risks of the extirpative surgery obviously depend on the location and on the tumor extent. These may range from bleeding, infection, and unsightly scars to major nerve injury or loss of vision. A complete list of the risks should be outlined.

In cases requiring reconstructive surgery, a discussion regarding the options available should be held, along with their advantages and disadvantages and the rationale for the surgeon's choice. The limitations, as well as the risks, of the various procedures should be reviewed so that realistic expectations can be established.

No specific data exist on the cost of treatment for sarcomas of the head and neck. However, certain principles apply. The entire staging process can take place as an outpatient. When definitive therapy is rendered, a well-thought-out and orchestrated single-stage plan will be most cost-effective and most beneficial to the patient. For instance, immediate reconstruction of major head and neck defects in general has been shown to be advantageous from both an economic and therapeutic standpoint.

REFERENCES

1. Azzarelli A: Surgery in soft tissue sarcomas, *Eur J Cancer* 29A:618-623, 1993.

2. Balm AJM, Coevarden FV, Bos KE, et al: Report of a symposium on diagnosis and treatment of adult soft tissue sarcomas in the head and neck, *Eur J Surg Oncol* 21:287-289, 1995.

3. Barkley HT, Martin RG, Romsdahl MM, et al: Treatment of soft tissue sarcomas by pre-operative irradiation and conservative surgical resection, *J Radiat Oncol Biol Phys,* 14:693-699, 1988.

4. Bujko K, Suit MD, Springfield DS, et al: Wound healing after pre-operative radiation for sarcoma of soft tissues, *Surg Gynecol Obstet* 176:124-134, 1993.

5. Cahan WG, Woodard HQ, Higinbotham NL, et al: Sarcoma arising in irradiated bone—report of 11 cases, *Cancer* 1:3-29, 1948.

6. Costa MJ, Campinan SC, Devis RL, et al: Fine needle aspiration cytology of sarcoma: retrospective review of diagnostic utility and specificity, *Diagn Cytopathol* 15:23-32, 1996.

7. Dijkstra MD, Balm AJM, Gregor RT, et al: Soft tissue sarcomas of the head and neck associated with surgical trauma, *J Laryngol Otol* 109:126-129, 1995.

8. Dillon PW, Whalen TV, Azizkhan RG, et al: Neonatal soft tissue sarcomas: the influence of pathology on treatment and survival, *J Pediatr Surg* 30:1038-1041, 1995.

9. Dillon P, Mauer H, Jenkins J, et al: A prospective study of nonrhabdomyosarcoma soft tissue sarcomas in the pediatric age group, *J Pediatr Surg* 27:241-245, 1992.

10. Eeles RA, Fisher C, A'Hern RP, et al: Head and neck sarcomas: prognostic factors and implications for treatment, *Br J Cancer* 68:201-207, 1993.

11. Engin K, Tupchong L, Waterman FM, et al: Thermoradiotherapy for superficial tumor deposits in the head and neck, *Int J Hyperthermia,* 10:153-164, 1994.

12. Enneking WF, Spanier SS, Malawer MM: The effect of the anatomic setting on the results of surgical procedures for soft parts sarcoma of the thigh, *Cancer* 47:1005-1022, 1981.

13. Feyerabend T, Steeves R, Wiedemann GJ, et al: Local hyperthermia, radiation, and chemotherapy in locally advanced malignancies, *Oncology* 53:214-220, 1996.

14. Freedman AM, Reiman HM, Woods JE: Soft tissue sarcomas of the head and neck, *Am J Surg* 158:367-372, 1989.

15. Graham JD, Robinson MH, Harmer CL: Re-irradiation of soft tissue sarcoma, *Br J Radiol* 65:157-161, 1992.

16. Hansen M, Koufos A, Gallie B, et al: Osteosarcoma and retinoblastoma: a shared chromosomal mechanism revealing recessive predisposition, *Proc Natl Acad Sci U S A* 82:6216-6220, 1986.

17. Harrison LB, Franzese F, Gaynor JJ, et al: Long term results of prospective randomized trial of adjuvant brachytherapy in the management of completely resected soft tissue sarcomas of the extremity and superficial trunk, *Int J Radiat Oncol Biol Phys* 27:259-265, 1993.

18. Haycox CL, Odland PB, Olbricht SM, et al: Dermofibrosarcoma protuberans (DFSP): growth characteristics based on tumor modeling and review of cases treated with Mohs' micrographic surgery, *Ann Plast Surg* 38:246-251, 1997.

19. Holden CA, Spittle MF, Jones EW: Angiosarcoma of the face and scalp: prognosis and treatment, *Cancer* 1046-1057, 1987.

20. Kowalski LP, Chen IS: Prognostic factors in head and neck soft tissue sarcomas: analysis of 128 cases, *J Surg Oncol* 56:83-88, 1994.

21. Kraus DH, Dubner S, Harrison LB, et al: Prognostic factors for recurrence and survival in head and neck sarcoma, *Cancer* 74:697-702, 1994.

22. Kraus DH, Lanzieri CF, Wanamaker JR, et al: Complementary use of computed tomography and magnetic resonance imaging in assessing skull base lesions, *Laryngoscope* 102:623-629, 1992.

23. Lawrence W Jr: Operative management of soft tissue sarcomas: impact of anatomic site, *Semin Surg Oncol* 10:340-346, 1994.

24. LeVay J, O'Sullivan B, Catton C, et al: An assessment of prognostic factors in soft tissue sarcoma of the head and neck, *Arch Otolaryngol Head Neck Surg* 120:981-986, 1994.

25. Lise M, Rossi CR, Alessio S, et al: Multimodality treatment of extra-visceral soft tissue sarcomas MO: state of the art and trends, *Eur J Surg Oncol* 21:125-135, 1995.

26. Lyos AT, Goepfert H, Luna MA, et al: Soft tissue sarcoma of the head and neck in children and adolescents, *Cancer* 77:193-200, 1996.

27. Mandard AM, Petiot JF, Marnay J, et al: Prognostic factors in soft tissue sarcomas, *Cancer* 63:1437-1451, 1989.

28. Mark RJ, Bailet JW, Ben J, et al: Postirradiation sarcoma of the head and neck, *Cancer* 72:887-893, 1993.

29. Mark RJ, Poen J, Luu MT, et al: Postirradiation sarcomas, *Cancer* 73:2653-2662, 1994.

30. Maurer HM, Beltangady M, Gahan E, et al: The Intergroup Rhabdomyosarcoma Study—a final report, *Cancer* 61:209-220, 1988.

31. Odell P: Head and neck sarcomas: a review, *J Otolaryngol* 25:7-13, 1996.

32. Panchal JI, Agrawal RK, McLean NR, et al: Early postoperative brachytherapy following free flap reconstruction, *Br J Plast Surg* 46:511-515, 1993.

33. Rao BN, Santana VM, Fleming ID, et al: Management and prognosis of head and neck sarcomas, *Am J Surg* 158:373-377, 1989.

34. Robbins KT, Storniolo AM, Kerber C, et al: Rapid superselective high-dose cisplatin infusion for advanced head and neck malignancies, *Head Neck* 14:364-371, 1992.

35. Russel WO, Cohen J, Enzinger F, et al: A clinical and pathological staging system for soft tissue sarcomas, *Cancer* 40:1562-1570, 1977.

36. Tran LM, Mark R, Meier R, et al: Sarcomas of the head and neck, *Cancer* 70:169-177, 1992.

37. Van der Laan BF, Baris G, Gregor RT, et al: Radiation-induced tumors of the head and neck, *J Laryngol Otol* 109:346-349, 1995.

38. Wanebo HJ, Koness RJ, MacFarlane JK, et al: Head and neck sarcoma: report of the Head and Neck Sarcoma Registry, *Head Neck* 14:1-7, 1992.

39. Weiss SW, Enzinger FM: Malignant fibrous histiocytoma: an analysis of 200 cases, *Cancer* 41:2250-2266, 1978.

40. Willers H, Hug EB, Spiro IJ, et al: Adult soft tissue sarcomas of the head and neck treated by radiation and surgery or radiation alone: patterns of failure and prognostic factors, *Int J Radiat Oncol Biol Phys* 33:585-593, 1995.

41. Xue H, Horowitz JR, Smith MB, et al: Malignant solid tumors in neonates: a 40 year review, *J Pediatr Surg* 30:543-545, 1995.

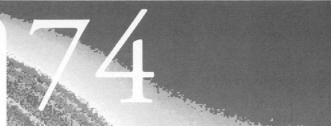

CHAPTER 74

Local Flaps for Closure of Facial Defects

Sean Lille
Robert C. Russell

INTRODUCTION

Soft tissue defects of the face most commonly arise from trauma (e.g., from dog bites or motor vehicle accidents) or following surgical extirpation of cutaneous malignancies. Many of these defects are small and can be closed primarily by local undermining of the adjacent tissue edges with good cosmetic results. Mobile structures of the face, however, such as the lower eyelids, lips, and alar base may be significantly distorted when primary closure is attempted. Larger defects covered with a split-or full-thickness skin graft often heal with a depression and leave a noticeable contour deformity (Figure 74-1). Skin grafts from outside the head and neck are often poor color matches to the surrounding facial skin, especially in young dark- or fair-complexioned patients. Thin split-thickness grafts, however, can be used as an initial closure method to facilitate wound contracture. The graft contracts during healing and can then be serially excised to help minimize the final scar. The disadvantages of this approach, however, include the necessity of multiple procedures depending on the size of the skin graft and the potential for distortion of adjacent mobile facial structures. Mohs' surgical excisions, allowed to heal by secondary intention, can also produce scarring, resulting in suboptimal aesthetic outcomes and/or significant distortion of mobile facial features.[6,25,31]

Local flaps elevated from adjacent or regional facial tissue provide composite tissue of similar color and texture and allow optimal contour restoration. Wound closure is performed in one stage and mobile lid and lip structures can be supported by flap advancement or rotation, minimizing residual scar contracture and distortional deformity.

The head and neck skin and subcutaneous tissues have an abundant blood supply derived from both the external and internal carotid systems. This allows the reconstructive surgeon to design a variety of random and, in many areas of the face, local axial pattern skin flaps. The donor sites of local flaps can usually be closed primarily. The total length of the scar is larger compared to primary closure, but there is a reduced risk for scar hypertrophy or contour irregularity, and because scars often can be placed in normal facial wrinkle lines, it is possible to close most facial defects with local tissue to provide the most aesthetic result and to preserve facial harmony and balance. The reliability of local skin flaps utilized for closure of small and intermediate-size defects, however, requires a thorough knowledge of facial anatomy including the mechanical properties of the skin, precise surgical technique, and, most important, sound judgment.

SKIN FLAP ANATOMY AND PHYSIOLOGY

The epidermis is the most superficial skin layer, composed of keratinizing stratified squamous epithelium with four distinct cell types—keratinocytes, melanocytes, Merkel cells, and Langerhans' cells. The dermis is a fibrous connective-tissue matrix made up of collagen, elastin, and ground substance. It contains dispersed adnexal structures such as hair follicles, sebaceous glands, sweat glands, immune cells, nerves, and blood vessels that are responsible for many of the skin's physiologic properties. The dermis is divided into a relatively thin, superficial papillary layer and the thicker, deep reticular layer. There is regional variation in the thickness of the dermis and the type and concentration of adnexal structures in different areas of the face. The eyelid dermis, for example, is 1 to 1.5 mm thick, whereas the scalp dermis is 2.5 mm thick.[2] The dermis is thin at birth, but progressively thickens through the age of 40 to 50, after which it again becomes progressively thinner.[2] Some areas on the face, such as nose skin, have a high concentration of adnexal structures compared with the neck or cheek skin. These structures can hypertrophy with age or associated medical conditions such as rhinophyma, making reconstruction by any technique more difficult.

The face has an extensive blood supply arising from branches of both the external and internal carotid arteries (Figure 74-2). The forehead is supplied by the supratrochlear and supraorbital arteries exiting the supraorbital rim. They are easily visualized and preserved in this region when dissection is performed between the frontalis muscle and the pericranium. These vessels become superficial to the frontalis muscle as they ascend toward the scalp. The superficial temporal artery supplies the temporal scalp and lateral forehead. It is the

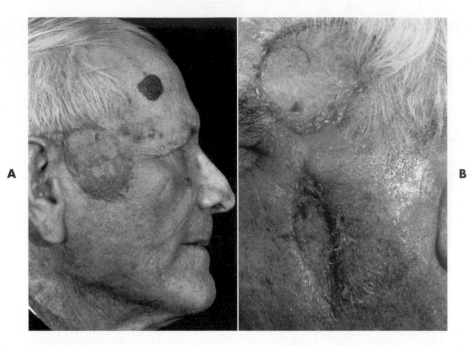

Figure 74-1. **A** and **B,** Skin grafts used to close facial defects can cause visible color and/or contour irregularities.

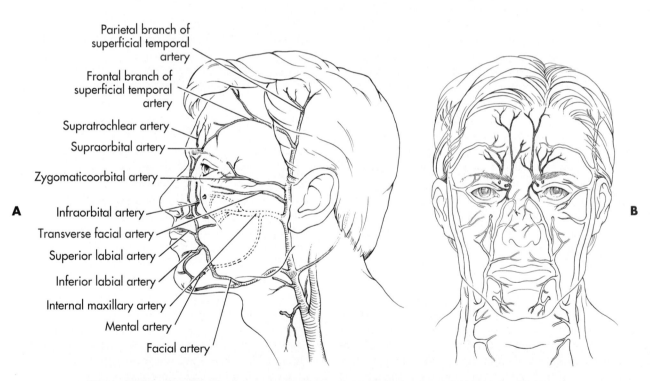

Parietal branch of superficial temporal artery

Frontal branch of superficial temporal artery

Supratrochlear artery

Supraorbital artery

Zygomaticoorbital artery

Infraorbital artery

Transverse facial artery

Superior labial artery

Inferior labial artery

Internal maxillary artery

Mental artery

Facial artery

Figure 74-2. **A** and **B,** The face is supplied by numerous branches from the internal and external carotid arteries with numerous vascular connections between branches, creating overlapping angiosomes accessible from several directions. Areas shaded black represent internal carotid branches. Nonshaded areas are derived from branches of the external carotid system.

terminal branch of the external carotid artery and emerges from the parotid gland to become superficial just anterior to the tragus of the ear. The artery bifurcates into the frontal branch anteriorly and the parietal branch posteriorly at a point approximately 2 cm above the zygomatic arch. The frontal branch anastomoses in the subcutaneous plane with the branches of the supraorbital and supratrochlear vessels.

The blood supply to the cheek arises from branches of the facial and internal maxillary artery. Contributions to the face from the internal maxillary artery include the infraorbital artery, which divides into branches to supply the lower eyelid, cheek, and upper lip. The lips are supplied by the inferior and superior labial arteries, which branch off the facial artery and travel tangentially just deep to the orbicularis oris muscle at the juncture of the dry and wet mucosa. The facial artery continues cephalad after giving off the labial arteries and a lateral nasal branch to supply the nasal wall and becomes the angular artery, which travels along the base of the nose toward the medial canthus. The angular artery anastomoses with the palpebral and dorsal nasal branches of the ophthalmic artery and establishes a communication between the external and internal carotid systems. This rich vascular plexus of the face supplied by both the external and internal carotid arteries allows the creation of dependable flaps that can be based in almost any direction.

The nerves that supply the anterior scalp and forehead include the supraorbital and supratrochlear nerves, terminal branches of the ophthalmic division of the fifth cranial nerve (V1 of CN V). They exit from the supraorbital foramen at the junction of the middle and medial one third of the supraorbital rim. The temporal region is supplied by the auriculotemporal nerve, a branch of the mandibular division of the trigeminal nerve (V2 of CN V), which travels with the superficial temporal artery just above the zygomatic rim. The great auricular nerve provides sensation to the posterior auricular region, ear lobe, and angle of the mandible. The cheek and lip area receive sensory innervation by branches from the maxillary (V2) and mandibular (V3) division of the trigeminal nerve through the infraorbital and mental nerves, respectively. Most local facial flaps are elevated under local anesthesia. We use a 50/50 mixture of 0.25% Marcaine and 0.5% lidocaine with 1:2,000,000 epinephrine. Local anesthesia can be injected around the major cutaneous nerves of the face, producing the required anesthesia. Care should be taken, however, to avoid injecting epinephrine into the base of random pattern flaps.[35]

Motor innervation to the frontalis muscle is provided by the frontal branch of the facial nerve, which exits the parenchyma of the parotid gland approximately on a line from the tragus of the ear to a point 1.5 cm from the lateral canthus.[29] It consists of two to five rami, which course just beneath the superficial musculoaponeurotic system (SMAS) layer until they become superficial to innervate the frontalis muscle. It is unlikely that a local flap in this area will require elevation of the SMAS layer, but whenever exposure of the zygomatic arch is required, dissection must be performed deep to the superficial layer of the deep temporal fascia to avoid injury to the temporal branch of the facial nerve. The remainder of the motor branches of the facial nerve (zygomatic, buccal, marginal mandibular, cervical) lie deep to the mimetic muscles. The surgeon must have a detailed knowledge of the cutaneous, vascular, and neural anatomy of the face to design and move local flaps without risk of vascular compromise or nerve injury.

The blood supply to the skin provides nutritional support and is a thermoregulatory mechanism for the body.[21] The amount of blood flow to a facial skin flap after transfer is determined by the arteriolar pressure, the sympathetic innervation, local hypoxemia, or the presence of metabolic byprod-

ucts. The amount of blood flow through the skin, under normothermic conditions, is approximately 10 times the flow required for nutritional support.[15] This may increase by as much as sevenfold, as part of the thermoregulatory response to cool the body, for example, during heavy exercise in a warm environment.[15] The overlapping angiosomes of the facial arterial system can be accessed from many directions and allow a greater freedom of flap design and movement than in any other area of the body. The surviving length of a particular flap depends on the relationship between the intravascular perfusion pressure and the critical closing pressure of the arterioles, which is influenced by several factors at different time intervals following the elevation and inset of a skin flap. The release of catecholamines during the first 48 hours in the subdermal plexus from divided sympathetic nerves and inflammatory mediators such as O_2 radicals, cytokines, complement factors, and eicosanoids (prostaglandins and thromboxane) all contribute to tissue edema and local vasoconstriction resulting in a redirection of blood flow.[20,27,28] There are various physiologic interventions that have been used to enhance flap viability such as surgical delay,[14] tissue expansion,[14] vasodilators,[22] free radical scavengers,[26] agents that alter red blood cell (RBC) rheology,[24] and angiogenic growth factors.[16] Appropriate flap design, however, is the most critical factor in the maintenance of adequate intravascular perfusion pressure and the avoidance of tissue necrosis.[8] It is presently impossible to pharmacologically overcome a flap design error that results in terminal flap necrosis due to a lack of nutritional blood flow.

Neovascularization from adjacent skin edges begins at 3 to 5 days after flap transposition.[27,34] Tobacco use and/or previous radiation have been shown to have an effect on the microcirculation that may adversely affect the survival of local flaps designed without the benefit of a central arterial, axial blood supply.[13] Patients who smoke should be asked to stop prior to any elective procedure that will require local flap elevation and movement. Flaps that are required for patients with previously radiated skin should, if possible, include an axial vessel to ensure survival.

The surgeon familiar with the various flap closure options should also consider a number of other factors in choosing the method of closure. The natural skin tension lines, which usually run perpendicular to the underlying muscle fibers, can sometimes be difficult to determine in some areas of the face, such as the cheeks, where mimetic muscles travel in several directions. Other areas, such as the forehead or neck, have vertically oriented muscles that produce transverse skin creases. Flaps should be designed whenever possible to take advantage of these natural skin creases. Incisions placed within or parallel to these skin creases are less visible after healing and, because the underlying muscle contraction pulls the wound edges together, are less likely to produce a thick or hypertrophic scar.[1]

The surgeon should anticipate the size of the defect, for example after a planned excision of a skin cancer, and plan various options for flap closure. The final decision, however, should not be made until the full extent of the defect has been determined, in the case of a malignancy, until frozen sections have confirmed the adequacy of the resection. The initial plan may sometimes have to be slightly altered to create a larger flap or, in some cases, completely changed to a new closure method when the surgical deficit is much larger than initially anticipated. In areas of the face where the skin tension lines are less clear, such as the cheek, the defect can be excised in a circle and the skin edges undermined slightly to determine in which direction the skin retracts. A circular skin excision will become an oval and can be closed in this direction primarily for small lesions or used to plan the best method of flap closure.

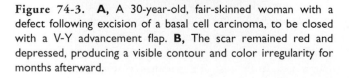

Figure 74-3. **A,** A 30-year-old, fair-skinned woman with a defect following excision of a basal cell carcinoma, to be closed with a V-Y advancement flap. **B,** The scar remained red and depressed, producing a visible contour and color irregularity for months afterward.

The very mobile structures of the face, such as the lower eyelids, the lips, and the alar bases, often require a reconstruction that will provide support as well as wound coverage. A flap reconstruction that places even minimal tension on the lower eyelid or lip, for example, can easily produce an ectropion or lip eversion, which will create a cosmetic and sometimes functional deformity after surgery.[17,25]

Finally, the surgeon should consider the patient's skin type and quality when choosing a method of local flap closure. Most local facial flaps are used to close a surgical defect following the excision of cutaneous malignancy. These patients typically have a fair complexion, are over 50, and have a long history of sun exposure. Their skin will usually show evidence of sun damage such as thinning, loss of elastic collagen, actinic keratoses, and many rhytides, which must all be considered when planning a flap closure. Younger patients with good skin quality and few wrinkles or fair-or dark-skinned individuals may not be good candidates for local flap closure because the resulting scars are more difficult to hide and are more prone to scar hypertrophy (Figure 74-3).[13] Local flaps in such patients are also more prone to contract circumferentially, producing a noticeable contour irregularity by elevating the flap above the plane of the face, producing a so-called "trapdoor deformity."[17,30]

CLASSIFICATION

Local flap classifications can be based on three criteria: blood supply, flap composition, or the method of tissue movement. Flaps categorized by blood supply can be referred to as either axial or random pattern flaps. Random skin flaps are those supplied by the subdermal vascular plexus, whereas axial pattern flaps include a dominant arterial and venous pedicle coursing through the flap. Flaps classified by tissue composition include skin, fascia, fasciocutaneous, muscle, musculocutaneous, bone, and finally bone flaps in combination with other tissues. Local facial flaps are best described by their design or method of movement and whenever possible should include an axial vessel in their design.

Advancement Flaps
Advancement flaps are designed to slide in a single direction and advance directly into a soft tissue defect (Figure 74-4 and 74-5). Rectangular and V-Y advancement flaps are commonly employed examples of these flaps. The donor defect is closed primarily. The movement of rectangular advancement flaps is limited by the elasticity of the skin and subcutaneous tissues. The V-Y advancement flap does not have an intact skin bridge and its movement is dependent on the mobility of the subcutaneous tissue and the degree of underlying muscle dissection.[3]

Transposition/Rotation Flaps
Transposition (Figure 74-6) or rotation (Figures 74-7 and 74-8) flaps are those that are designed adjacent to a soft tissue defect and are then transposed or rotated to cover the defect.

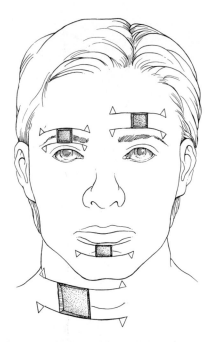

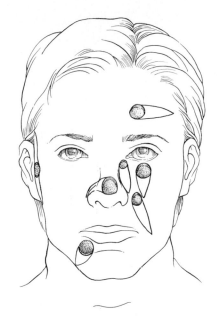

Figure 74-4. Rectangular advancement flaps are best designed in skin tension lines and can be more easily advanced by excision of Burow's triangles at their base.

Figure 74-5. V-Y advancement flaps are best designed along facial planes and are most advantageous in the region of the central face.

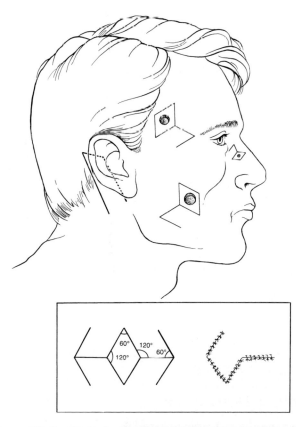

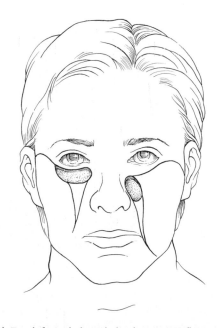

Figure 74-6. A classic rhomboid (Limberg) transposition flap, designed as a parallelogram from the soft tissue adjacent to a defect, which has been shaped into a rhomboid with 60- and 120-degree angles. The flap shares one side with the rhomboid defect, with four potential flaps possible.

Figure 74-7. Inferiorly based cheek rotation flaps are useful to close medium- to large-sized cheek and lower eyelid defects.

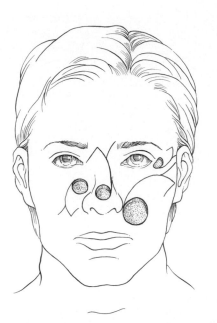

Figure 74-8. Sickle-shaped rotation flaps are useful to provide coverage of small- to medium-sized defects in the central portion of the face and lower eyelids. The Marchac dorsal nasal flap is a variation of this technique.

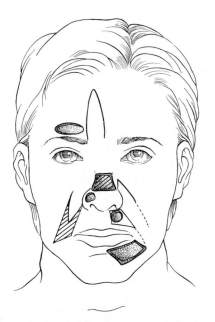

Figure 74-9. Interpolation flaps can be designed from the forehead, nasolabial fold, or neck skin and mobilized to close regional defects.

The classic Limberg (rhomboid) transposition flap is designed as a parallelogram using 60- and 120-degree angles to achieve a primary wound and donor site closure (see Figure 74-6).[11,18] Smaller Z-plasties or opposing Z-plasty flaps are used to flatten scar bands or to close small defects. Local rotation flaps are designed in an arc and are rotated as much as 90 degrees to cover adjacent soft tissue defects. Cheek or neck rotation flaps (see Figure 74-7), sickle-shaped flaps (see Figure 74-8), and the

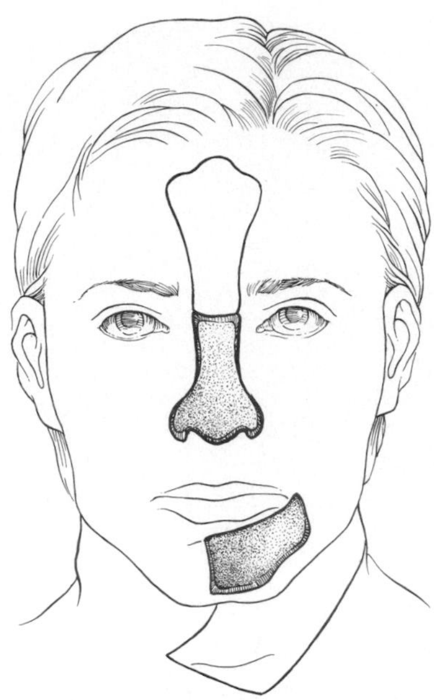

Figure 74-10. Transverse cervical and midline forehead flaps can be used to close large defects. The forehead flap can be designed to resurface a portion or the entire nose.

Marchac glabella flap are examples of local rotation flaps. The donor defect is usually closed by the rearrangement of local tissue, with a Z-plasty or a skin graft.

Interpolation Flaps

Interpolation flaps transfer a segment of tissue on an intact vascular pedicle over or under an adjoining bridge of normal skin to provide coverage for a nonadjacent defect (Figure 74-9). The midline forehead (Figure 74-10), nasolabial, or other island fasciocutaneous flaps can be elevated as interpolation flaps. The donor site of these flaps is either closed primarily or with a skin graft for larger flaps. Occasionally, pedicled interpolation flaps can be modified or extended prior to wound coverage by a delay procedure, with tissue expansion,[19] or modified by the addition of lining or cartilage tissue as a first-step procedure prior to transfer.[5] Flaps elevated on a pedicle may be returned to the donor area after division and insetting of the terminal portion of the flap over the defect or may be discarded, depending on which gives the superior aesthetic result.

INDICATIONS

ADVANCEMENT FLAPS

Rectangular Advancement Flap

Rectangular advancement flaps are elevated on one or both sides of a soft tissue defect in a subcutaneous plane and are advanced centrally to close the defect (see Figure 74-4). The skin flap(s) is incised by making parallel incisions away from

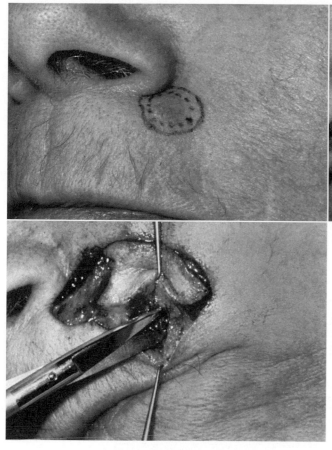

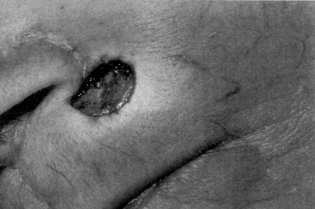

Figure 74-11. **A,** A patient with a basal cell carcinoma along the alar groove. The margins of the tumor are identified with dotted lines and the planned resection marked with a solid line. **B,** A V-Y flap designed following tumor excision and frozen section analysis demonstrates clear margins in the nasolabial fold, 1.5 to 2 times as long as the diameter of the defect. **C,** The skin is sharply incised, and blunt scissor dissection is used to mobilize the flap.

Continued

the defect, and it receives a blood supply from the subdermal plexus through the base of the flap. Rectangular advancement flaps are best designed on the forehead and neck and occasionally are useful in the temporal area to restore the hairline or in the periorbital area to support the lip. Advancement of the flap(s) can be improved by excision of Burow's triangle(s) away from the base of the flap (see Figure 74-4). Rectangular advancement flaps in the neck can be elevated to include the platysmal muscle, which will augment their blood supply. Advancement of these flaps is largely dependent on the elasticity of the flap and surrounding skin and should therefore not be closed under excessive tension to prevent compromise of the subdermal vascular plexus.[3] Relatively long flaps are usually required to close a small defect, and therefore these flaps are seldom appropriate. They are best utilized on the forehead or in the brow area where the parallel flap incisions can be hidden in the forehead wrinkles or used to advance a section of eyebrow following a traumatic loss or surgical resection.[3,17]

Cheek Advancement Flap

The skin and soft tissue of the cheek can also be elevated as a large advancement flap to close central facial defects along the side of the nose (see Figure 74-7). Surgical defects from cancer excision commonly occur along the junction between the lateral nose and the medial cheek.[28] The cheek flap is based laterally, incised over the orbital rim below the eye laterally and, if needed, toward the ear at the level of the lateral canthus. The medial incision borders the defect and extends into the nasolabial fold inferiorly. This flap is undermined in the subcutaneous plane and advanced medially without tension to close large, medial cheek defects. Any lateral skin irregularities created by advancement of the cheek skin can be corrected by excising Burow's triangles away from the base of the flap.

V-Y Advancement Flap

The V-Y advancement flap is one of the most useful flaps for reconstructing facial defects and can be used in almost all areas of the face.[9,10,25,37] The nasolabial fold, the medial canthal area, the glabellar area, the cheek, and the sides of the nose are all good areas to design V-Y advancement flaps[9] (see Figure 74-5). The flap is designed from the edge of the defect and is planned to be 1.5 to 2 times as long as the diameter of the defect (Figure 74-11, *A* and *B*). The skin is sharply incised and the subcutaneous tissues are bluntly dissected by spreading the scissor tips perpendicular to the skin edges (Figure 74-11, *C*). The fibrous septa connecting the skin to the underlying fascia can be identified and divided, preserving small perforating vascular branches into the flap. The flap is gently advanced without tension, using skin hooks, into the defect (Figure 74-11, *D*). Spreading and

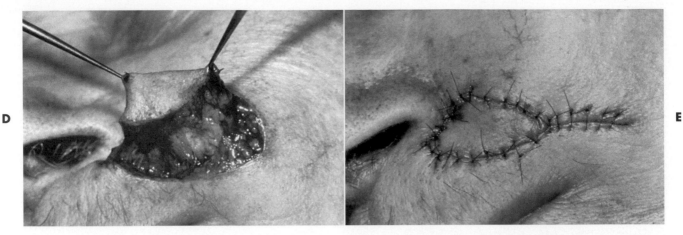

Figure 74-11, cont'd. **D,** The flap is easily advanced into the defect with skin hooks. **E,** The Y-shaped closure after flap advancement.

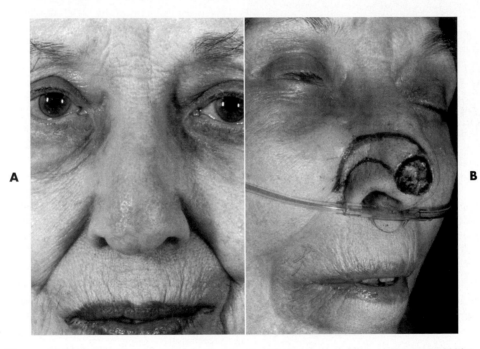

Figure 74-12. **A,** A female patient with a basal cell carcinoma on the nasal tip. **B,** A V-Y flap designed in the alar groove is based on a consistent perforating branch of the angular artery.

Continued

dissection into the underlying facial muscles are sometimes necessary to obtain flap advancement without tension. The donor site is closed primarily in a **Y** by undermining the lateral skin edges (Figure 74-11, *E*). The corners of the flap must sometimes be excised to create a semicircle along the forward edge when advancing it into a round defect. The leading edge of the flap can be thinned, if necessary, to accommodate a shallow defect, creating the best final contour. The flap is sutured with buried 5-0 absorbable sutures and interrupted 6-0 nylon.

The mobility of these flaps varies in different areas of the face, depending on the laxity of the subcutaneous tissues, which must be considered when planning the flap.[17] Flaps designed in skin that is closely adherent to the underlying cartilage on the nasal dorsum, ala, or ear are much harder to dissect and advance and should be avoided whenever possible. Ideally, these flaps should be designed along facial contour junctions, such as the nasolabial fold, nasofacial junction, or between forehead wrinkles. Nasal tip lesions can be closed using a curved **V-Y** flap design in the

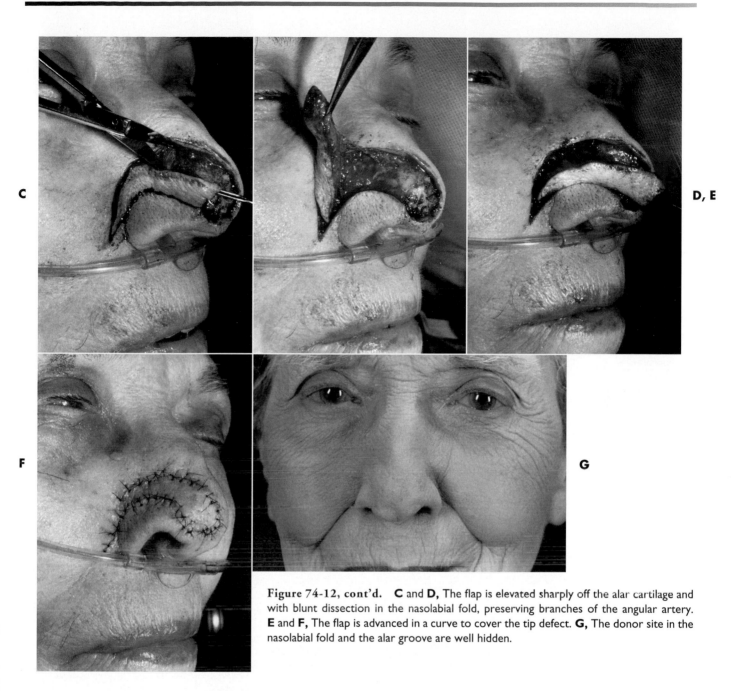

Figure 74-12, cont'd. C and **D,** The flap is elevated sharply off the alar cartilage and with blunt dissection in the nasolabial fold, preserving branches of the angular artery. **E** and **F,** The flap is advanced in a curve to cover the tip defect. **G,** The donor site in the nasolabial fold and the alar groove are well hidden.

skin along the upper margin of the lateral alar cartilage by advancing the flap in an arch toward the nasal tip (Figure 74-12, *A* to *D*). If portions of the flap are designed over the alar cartilage, this section must be elevated completely off the cartilage by sharp dissection, leaving the flap based on the loose areolar tissue on the side of the nose (see Figure 74-12, *C* and *D*). Blunt dissection of the remaining portions of the flap centered over the nasalis muscle and alar branches of the angular artery is performed to preserve the blood supply. Arterial branches are often visible at this junction and should be preserved. Once sufficient dissection of the muscle and fibrous septa is achieved, the flap

is pulled gently around the ala into the defect and closed without tension (Figure 74-12, *E* and *F*). The curved shape of the final scar blends nicely with the natural lines of the ala (Figure 74-12, *G*).

The V-Y advancement flaps can be used around the eye to support or reconstruct the lower lid (Figure 74-13). The flap should be sutured to the orbital rim at the desired height to eliminate the possibility of an ectropion.

Designing opposing V-Y flaps is useful to preserve the beard line on the cheek in men (Figure 74-14) or to prevent distortion of the lips when closing larger defects (Figure 74-15).

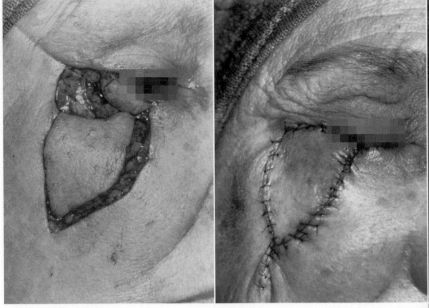

A, B   **C**

Figure 74-13. **A** and **B,** A patient requiring a composite lower lid reconstruction with conchal cartilage used to restore the tarsal plate and a V-Y flap advanced from the cheek to reconstruct the lid. **C** and **D,** The flap and ear cartilage graft provide good lid support and appearance.

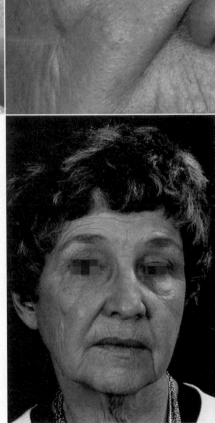

D

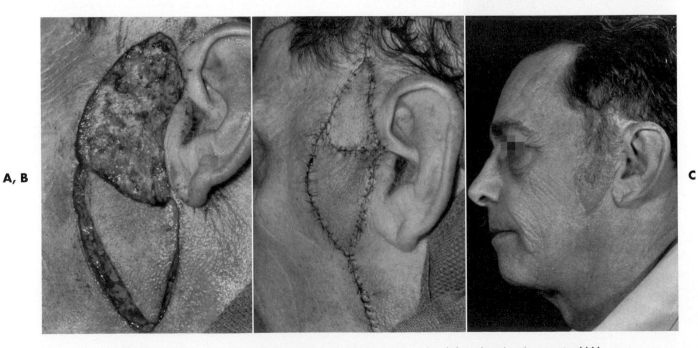

A, B   **C**

Figure 74-14. **A** to **C,** A male patient with a large preauricular defect closed with opposing V-Y advancement flaps, preserving the sideburn and beard line.

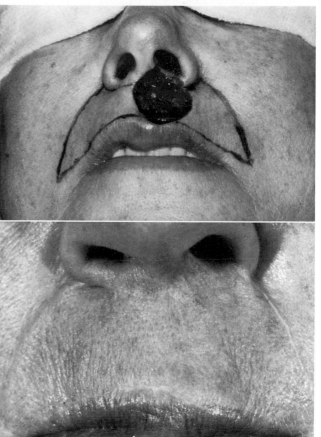

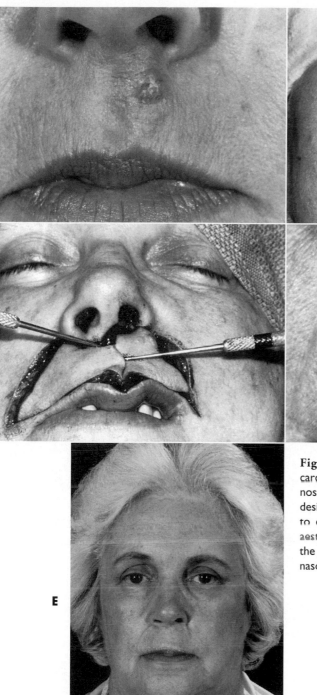

Figure 74-15. A to **D**, A female patient with a basal cell carcinoma of the upper lip, including a portion of the columella and nostril floor. Double opposing V-Y advancement flaps were designed as aesthetic units of the upper lip and advanced medially to close the defect. **E**, The patient's final result preserves the aesthetic appearance of the lip without distortion and places the donor site scars along the vermilion border and in the nasolabial fold.

ROTATION FLAPS

Rhomboid (Limberg) Flap

The rhomboid flap is extremely versatile and can be used to close a variety of defects in all areas of the body including the face (see Figure 74-6). The facial defect is converted to a rhomboid shape consisting of a parallelogram with opposing angles of 60 and 120 degrees.[18] Two 60-degree equilateral triangles are placed side by side, one pointing up and one pointing down to create a parallelogram with 60- to 120-degree angles. The Limberg flap is elevated from tissue adjacent to the defect by designing the leading edge away from the 120-degree angle of the defect for a distance equal to the length of one side of the defect. The flap is then created by a second incision parallel to the side of the defect at a 60-degree angle from the first incision. All limbs of the flap and defect should be equal in length. A rhomboid-shaped defect may therefore have four potential adjacent flaps for closure (see

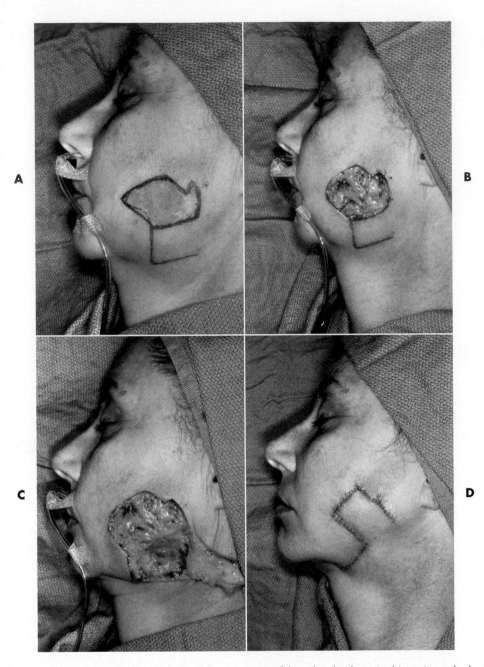

Figure 74-16. **A** to **D,** The rhomboid flap is most useful on the cheeks as in this patient who had a facial defect following excision of a lentigo malignant melanoma closed with an adjacent rhomboid flap.

Figure 74-6). It is important to understand the resultant tension vector in planning a flap on the face to avoid distortion of surrounding mobile facial structures. The rhomboid flap donor site is closed primarily after flap rotation by advancing adjacent skin. The problem with the rhomboid flap when used in the face is that more than half of the resulting scar does not fall within or parallel to the natural skin lines.[18] It is therefore less useful in the forehead region where the multiple directions of the resulting scar fail to complement the horizontal forehead creases. A rhomboid flap designed for up to 2.5-cm defects in the temporal region will maintain the distance between the lateral eyebrow and the anterior hairline and avoid distortion of the lateral eyebrow or webbing of the lateral canthus. Two flaps can be transposed, one inferiorly and one superiorly, to close larger defects and the flaps sutured together over the defect. It is also helpful for defects in the cheek, lateral nose, jawline, inferior orbital region, and lower lip (Figure 74-16). It can be used to close defects up to 6 cm in diameter on the cheek due to the inherent laxity of the skin in this area.[13] Flaps designed to close defects that extend to the lower eyelid margin should usually be elevated with the base laterally and closed by advancing cheek skin under the lid with little or no flap tension on the lower lid. Small defects up to 2 cm in diameter can be closed with a rhomboid flap in this area. Because of the thick texture and relative inelasticity of the skin on the nose only smaller defects, up to 1.5 cm, can be closed with this technique. Flaps should be designed on the cheek to provide a tension-free closure and align the scar along the nasolabial fold.

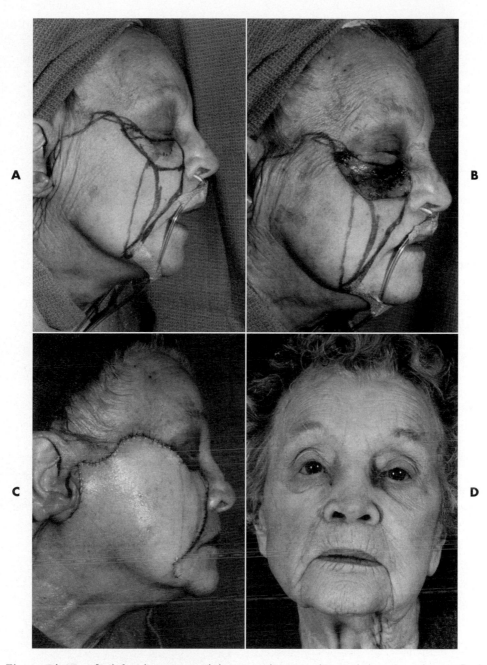

Figure 74-17. **A,** A female patient with lentigo malignant melanoma below the right eye. **B,** A large inferiorly based cheek rotation flap extending above the lateral canthus, designed and elevated to include the SMAS layer. **C,** The flap is rotated medially as an aesthetic unit to close the defect below the eye and to place the scar in the nasolabial fold. **D,** The patient's final appearance 3 months later.

A good method to determine in which direction to create the flap before the defect is reshaped into a rhomboid is to pinch the skin adjacent to the defect in several directions to determine where it appears most lax. The 60-degree angled defect left after flap elevation and rotation must be closed primarily and is therefore best designed with the leading edge parallel to the skin wrinkles.

Cheek Rotation Flap

Cheek rotation flaps can be used anywhere on the face and may be based superiorly or inferiorly (see Figure 74-7). The optimal design of these flaps ensures that the resulting scars reside along the borders of the facial aesthetic units.

Large cheek rotation flaps can be designed in the preauricular region in women or along the beard line in men. An inferiorly based flap can be extended superiorly to just above the zygomatic arch in the temporal region and curved inferiorly along the nasofacial sulcus. Cheek rotation flaps lined with mucosal or chondromucosal grafts have been used to reconstruct the lower eyelid as described by Mustarde,[21] but are also very useful to cover large defects lateral to the nose and below the eyelid (Figure 74-17). The flap is best elevated in a plane beneath the SMAS layer with careful attention to include the platysma muscle in its base. It is rotated toward the nose with a Burow's triangle excision of skin at the point of rotation along the nasolabial groove. The remaining preauricular donor defect can be closed by using a posterior auricular skin flap rotated in the front of the ear or closed primarily, depending on the extent of the defect and laxity of the facial skin. The posterior auricular flap is designed to share a common base with the cheek rotation flap and can be as wide as 2 to 3 cm and still allow primary donor site closure behind the ear. The skin in the posterior auricular area has no beard hair and is therefore most suitable in women or to close narrow preauricular defects in men.

Sickle Flap

Sickle- or scimitar-shaped skin flaps are also useful to close small- to medium-sized facial defects (see Figure 74-8).[13] These flaps are a variation of a local rotation flap, which includes a Z-plasty in the tail of the flap that allows primary donor site closure. The flaps are designed adjacent to the defect in an arc for a distance of 1.5 to 2 times the diameter of the defect. The arc of the flap extends away from the outer edge of the defect and then is cut back to create a tail. The base of the flap, adjacent to the defect, should be left wide enough to provide sufficient subdermal vascular plexus blood flow into the entire flap, which is elevated in a subcutaneous plane. The flap is rotated over the defect and its tail becomes one limb of a Z-plasty, which is transposed by cutting a second small triangular flap from the skin beneath the rotated tail. This limb of the Z-plasty is advanced into the donor defect to provide primary donor site closure. Small sickle-shaped flaps can be used on the cheeks, in the area of the medial or lateral canthus to provide lid support, or to close perioral defects. They are ideal for closing lower lid defects, and allow cheek skin to be rotated under the lid for support and wound coverage (Figure 74-18). Larger cheek or lateral lip defects can also be closed with large sickle-shaped flaps from the cheek (Figure 74-19). The Marchac dorsal nasal flap, when extended onto the forehead, is a large version of the sickle-shaped flap, which can be rotated toward the tip of the nose, and the forehead donor site closed with a Z-plasty. Most sickle flaps have a random blood supply and should therefore be rotated and closed without tension.

Marchac Dorsal Nasal Flap

Soft tissue defects over the nasal dorsum can be closed with an axial pattern nasal dorsum rotation flap described by Marchac[19] (see Figure 74-8). This flap is best suited for closure of defects of the distal nasal dorsum that are 2.5 cm or less in diameter. The flap is based on cutaneous perforating branches of the lateral nasal artery in the area of the medial canthus. The angiosomes of the facial and lateral nasal arteries of the external carotid system overlap those of the internal carotid system from the supraorbital and supratrochlear arteries. The vascular pedicle is located on one side of the nose and can be back-cut to the level of the medial canthal ligament. This allows elevation of a large flap of dorsal nasal skin extending onto the

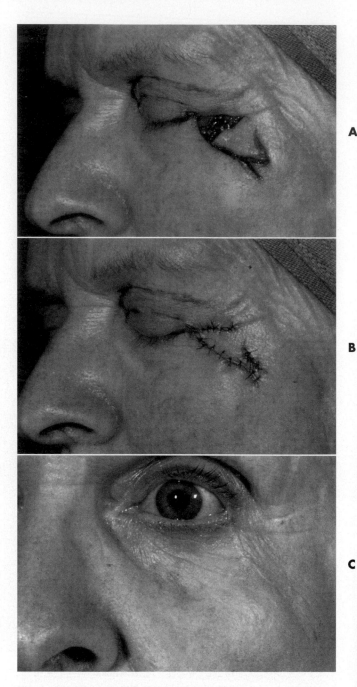

Figure 74-18. **A** to **C,** A patient with a small lower lid/lateral canthal defect closed with a sickle flap that includes a Z-plasty in the tail to provide lower lid support and primary donor site closure.

glabellar area and/or forehead. The laxity of the glabellar and dorsal nasal skin, especially in the elderly, allows closure of the defect after flap rotation without distorting the nasal tip or alar margin (Figure 74-20).

The design of the flap begins at the medial canthal region on the opposite side of the defect. A line is directed superiorly toward the upper glabella and a 30- to 45-degree angled back-cut is then created from the highest glabellar point toward the contralateral medial canthus to ensure incorporation of the vascular pedicle. The higher the V extends onto the

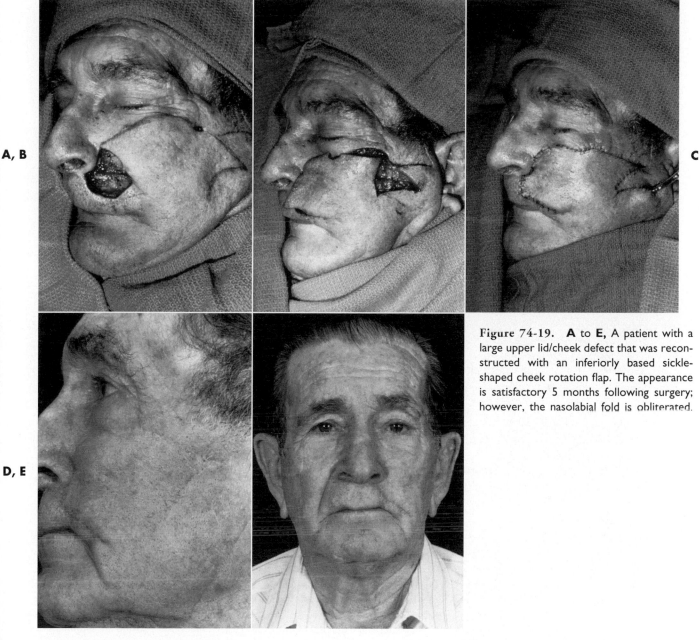

A, B

C

D, E

Figure 74-19. **A** to **E,** A patient with a large upper lid/cheek defect that was reconstructed with an inferiorly based sickle-shaped cheek rotation flap. The appearance is satisfactory 5 months following surgery; however, the nasolabial fold is obliterated.

forehead, the greater the length of the rotation flap and the easier it will be to close the secondary defect. The distance from the base of the glabellar portion of the flap to the tip should be approximately 1.5 to 2 times the diameter of the nasal defect to ensure adequate tissue movement. The lateral incision of the flap should be placed within the nasofacial sulcus to include the entire nasal skin. Local anesthesia is infiltrated along the edges of the flap and around infraorbital nerves bilaterally. The flap is incised and elevated at the level of the perichondrium and nasalis muscle and at the level of the frontalis muscle on the forehead. The pedicle of the flap must also be carefully undermined and dissected to permit unrestricted movement without injury. Wide undermining along both sides of the lateral nasal wall and medial cheek is necessary to close the secondary defect. Once the flap is completely mobilized, the

flap is rotated distally to cover the nasal defect. It is imperative to design the flap in such a manner that the leading edge extends beyond the defect. This flap has an axial blood supply and can be back cut inferiorly to eliminate the dog-ear at the angle of the rotation. Closure is achieved with deep dermal absorbable sutures and 6-0 nylon skin closure. The secondary defect on the forehead can be closed primarily or by using a Z-plasty.

Nasolabial Flap

The nasolabial flap based either superiorly or inferiorly includes the skin and subcutaneous tissue along the nasolabial fold[4-6] (see Figure 74-9). The flap is designed to include perforating branches of the facial or angular artery, which course through the underlying muscle into the base of the flap.

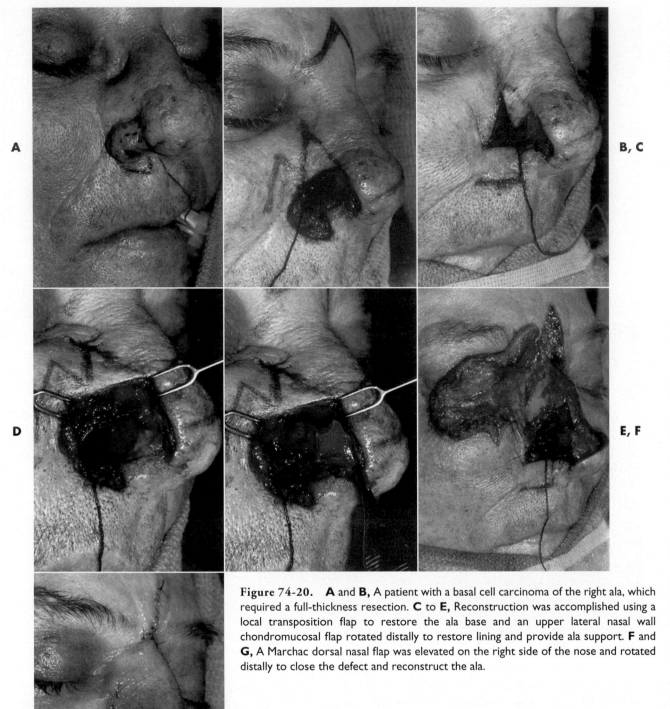

Figure 74-20. **A** and **B,** A patient with a basal cell carcinoma of the right ala, which required a full-thickness resection. **C** to **E,** Reconstruction was accomplished using a local transposition flap to restore the ala base and an upper lateral nasal wall chondromucosal flap rotated distally to restore lining and provide ala support. **F** and **G,** A Marchac dorsal nasal flap was elevated on the right side of the nose and rotated distally to close the defect and reconstruct the ala.

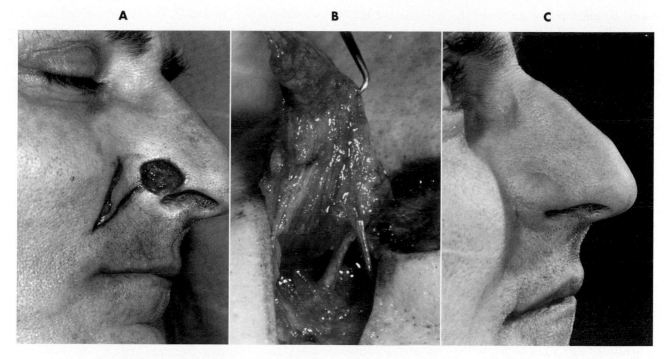

Figure 74-21. **A,** A male patient with a right alar defect to be closed with a small nasolabial flap. **B,** The flap is elevated with preservation of vascular branches derived from the angular artery. **C,** The patient's appearance 1 year after surgery.

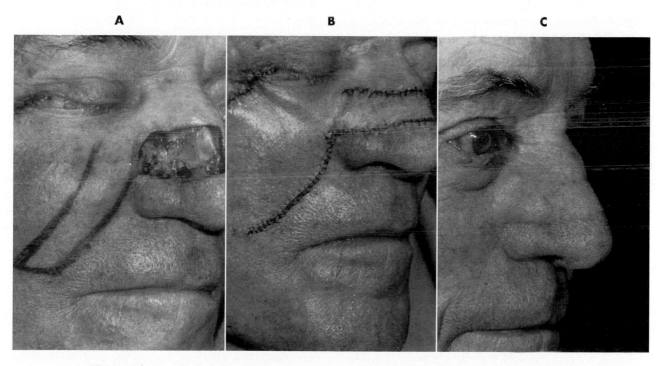

Figure 74-22. **A,** A male patient with a defect on the dorsum of the nose that will be closed using a superiorly based nasolabial flap. **B** and **C,** The immediate result following closure and 1 year after surgery.

Small defects of the nasal ala (Figure 74-21), nasal tip, and dorsum (Figure 74-22) are easily reconstructed with a superiorly based flap. An inferiorly based flap is ideally suited to close defects of the lips that do not involve the vermilion. One side of the upper lip subunit can be restored with an inferiorly based flap designed from a template made from the contralateral lip subunit. Inferiorly based flaps can be partially de-epithelized and tunneled through the cheek to reach the intraoral cavity to close defects along the alveolar ridge, or in the floor of the mouth.[12] The donor site can be closed primarily by undermining the lateral cheek skin in the line of the previous nasolabial fold, creating a donor site that is very hard to detect. The maximum width of the flap varies between individuals but can be as wide as 3 to 4 cm and still allow primary donor site closure. The width of a flap used for upper lip reconstruction is roughly calculated to be equal to the height of the defect. It is important to make the flap slightly wider than the actual height of the defect to prevent distortion of the lip due to a tight closure following flap rotation.

The medial incision for a superiorly based flap should be along the nasolabial fold and should be continued no higher on the cheek than the most superior part of the defect to be reconstructed. The lateral incision should be placed at approximately the end of the inferior margin of the defect. The flap is elevated at the level of the underlying facial muscles. Blunt scissor dissection is used near the base of the flap to enhance rotation and advancement. Perforating branches from the angular artery through the muscles should be preserved, but dissected to permit rotation without tension (see Figure 74-21, B). The flap can be extended distally below the lateral commissure. The inset portion of the flap may be thinned distally to improve the final contour of a nasal defect. The flap is usually inset, using a deep dermal closure of 5-0 absorbable suture followed by 6-0 nylon skin approximation. The final appearance can be improved by excision of a Burow's triangle away from the base of the flap at the medial pivot point to prevent a dog-ear at the angle of rotation.

Occasionally, nasolabial flaps are used as an interpolation flap to close a nasal tip or columellar defect.[23,36] The flap is inset for 2 to 3 weeks and is then divided, with the residual portion discarded and the wound closed so that the final scar line lies along the nasolabial and/or alar facial plain. Superiorly based nasolabial flaps can also be turned upside down into a full-thickness midline nasal defect to provide lining as part of a total nasal reconstruction, or folded on themselves for total alar reconstruction.[23]

The pivot point for inferiorly based flaps is located adjacent to the oral commissure. It is often necessary to perform a secondary procedure to re-create the nasolabial sulcus in this area, since it is often obliterated by transposition of an inferiorly based flap.

Periauricular Flap

The relatively hairless skin in front of and behind the ear is ideally suited for creation of rotation flaps for closure of defects on and around the ear (Figure 74-23). The amount of preauricular skin available for elevation of a flap increases in older patients with lax skin, while the more adherent skin over the mastoid bone behind the ear remains less mobile, even with advancing age. These flaps can be based superiorly or inferiorly and behind the ear posteriorly to close defects on the anterior or posterior surface of the ear. Preauricular flaps can be as wide as 3 to 4 cm in women without much facial hair, but are limited to the width of the

nonbearded skin in males. The donor site can usually be closed primarily by advancing the cheek or posterior scalp skin. These flaps can be folded on themselves, for example, to reconstruct the helical rim, or brought through the ear from the back to close anterior surface defects.[33] The base can be de-epithelized when passing the flap from the posterior to the anterior surface to permit primary donor site and defect closure or divided in a second stage 2 to 3 weeks later when used, for example, to complete a rim reconstruction. The three-dimensional shape and location of the flap can be planned before surgery with a piece of glove paper to determine the length, width, and arc of flap rotation. We use a moist cotton dressing on the anterior surface of the ear placed within the ear folds and covered with a soft gauze dressing, all held with a Surgiflex elastic net. This creates light pressure on the ear after surgery, which helps mold the flap to the irregular cartilaginous surface of the ear and helps prevent the accumulation of blood or serum beneath the flap. A small suction drain made from a 23-gauge butterfly connected to a 10-cc red-cap vacuum tube is also useful to evacuate blood and serum from beneath the flap and the donor site. The skin thickness, texture, and color closely match the ear skin, resulting in a cosmetically superior reconstruction.

Transverse Cervical Flap

The supple skin of the anterior upper neck is ideally suited for creation of a transverse cervical flap, which can be used to close medium- to large-sized lower facial defects (see Figure 74-10). This flap is based posteriorly over the sternocleidomastoid muscle and is elevated in a plane beneath the platysma muscle, and above the external jugular vein (Figure 74-24). A myocutaneous flap with an improved blood supply is created by inclusion of the platysmal muscle within the flap. The flap is designed in a rhomboid shape distally, which allows primary closure of the donor site for flaps as wide as 8 to 10 cm by flexing the patient's neck. The design can be extended safely for a short distance across the midline of the neck, but this area of the skin has a random blood supply. Any perforating arterial or venous branches near the base of the flap entering the platysmal muscle should be dissected and preserved during elevation.

Transverse cervical neck flaps are best used to resurface the lower lip to the vermilion border, the chin, and the lower cheek areas. They provide good support to the lower lip and prevent an eversion deformity after surgery (Figure 74-25). The donor site transverse scar on the neck is usually quite good, and the remaining neck skin stretches with time, permitting normal neck range of motion after surgery. The skin of the neck is also bearded in males, providing a good reconstruction for the cheek and chin area. A "dog-ear" may be created along the superior margin at the pivot point of the flap, which can be improved by excision of a Burow's triangle away from the base of the flap or resected in a secondary procedure.

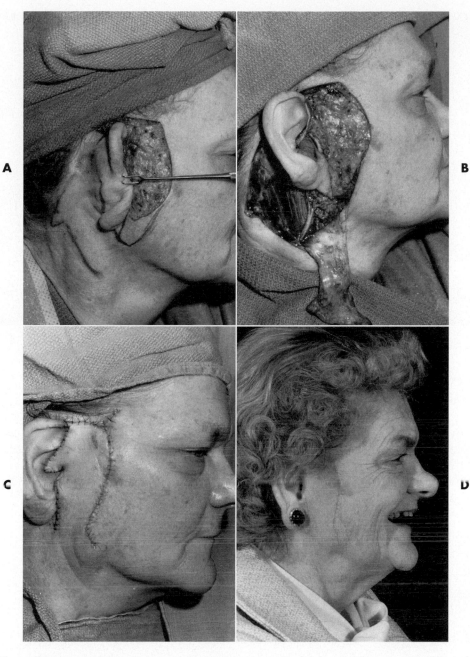

Figure 74-23. **A,** A female patient with a large preauricular defect to be closed with an inferiorly based postauricular flap. **B** and **C,** The flap elevated with exposure of the great auricular nerve and transposed into the preauricular defect. The donor site is closed primarily. **D,** The result 1 year after surgery.

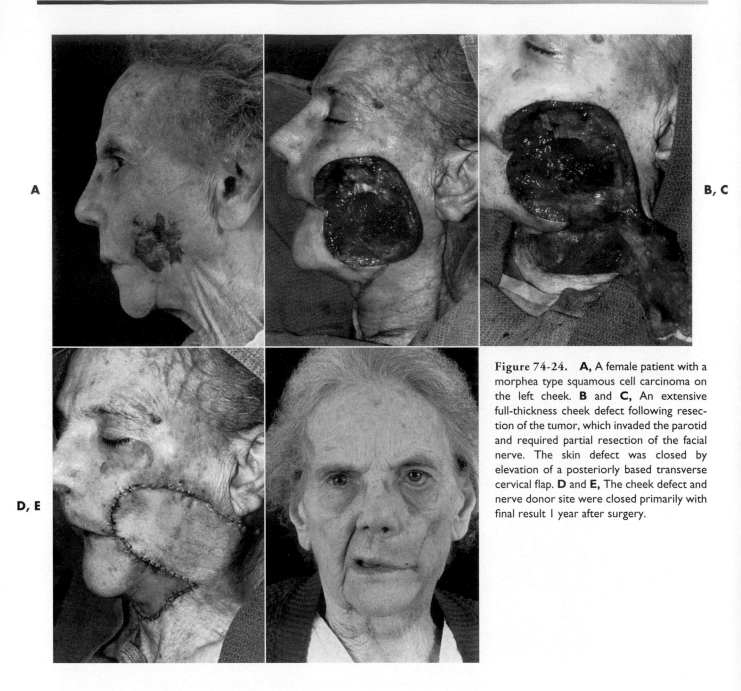

A

B, C

D, E

Figure 74-24. **A,** A female patient with a morphea type squamous cell carcinoma on the left cheek. **B** and **C,** An extensive full-thickness cheek defect following resection of the tumor, which invaded the parotid and required partial resection of the facial nerve. The skin defect was closed by elevation of a posteriorly based transverse cervical flap. **D** and **E,** The cheek defect and nerve donor site were closed primarily with final result 1 year after surgery.

INTERPOLATION FOREHEAD FLAPS

Forehead Flap

A number of flap options are available from the forehead skin for closure of nasal, eyelid, and adjacent forehead defects (see Figures 74-9 and 74-10). The supraorbital and supratrochlear vessels exiting the superior orbital rim and coursing below the frontalis muscle, for most of the height of the forehead, make it possible to design and pattern flaps in a variety of shapes to close medium- to large-sized nasal defects or smaller forehead and upper eyelid defects. The forehead skin can be modified prior to transfer as part of a staged reconstruction by placing tissue expanders beneath the flap, which serves to enlarge and thin the skin prior, for example, to total nasal reconstruction.[19] Expansion also serves as a delay procedure,

further enhancing the blood supply to the elevated skin flap. Burget et al[4,5] and others have performed complex nasal reconstruction using a combination of nasolabial turn-over flaps for nasal lining, cartilage grafts from the ears and nasal septum for stable contour reconstruction, all covered with a forehead skin flap (Figure 74-26). Smaller central forehead flaps can be rotated laterally to close brow and/or upper eyelid defects (Figure 74-27), although this technique is not ideal for the upper eyelid because the flap is thicker than normal eyelid skin.[13] The donor site for flaps as wide as 3 to 4 cm can be closed primarily by wide undermining of the lateral skin edges. The donor site of larger/irregular-shaped forehead flaps may require a skin graft for closure. The flap can be elevated as a transposition flap for forehead defects or as a pedicled interpolation flap for

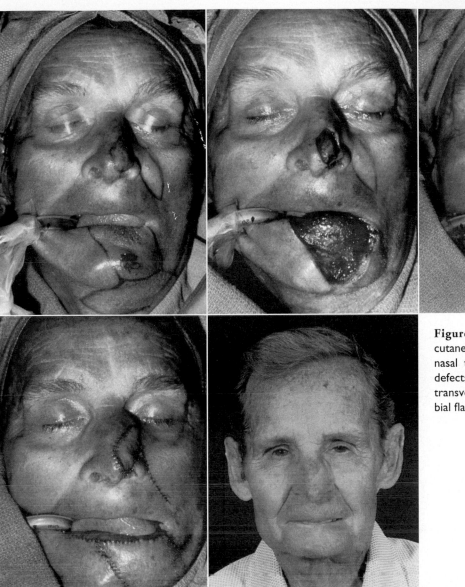

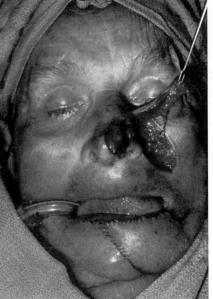

Figure 74-25. **A,** A male patient with cutaneous malignancies on the left side of the nasal tip and lower lip area. **B** to **D,** Facial defects following excision were closed with a transverse cervical and superiorly based nasolabial flap. **E,** The result 1 year later.

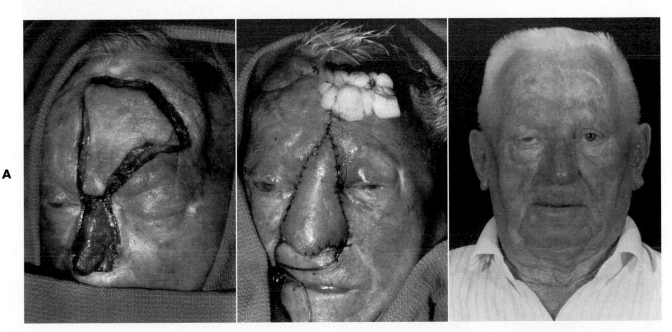

Figure 74-26. **A,** The design and incision of a midline forehead flap to resurface the entire nose. **B,** The results following inset of the flap with a skin graft applied to part of the forehead donor defect. **C,** The patient's appearance 1 year after surgery.

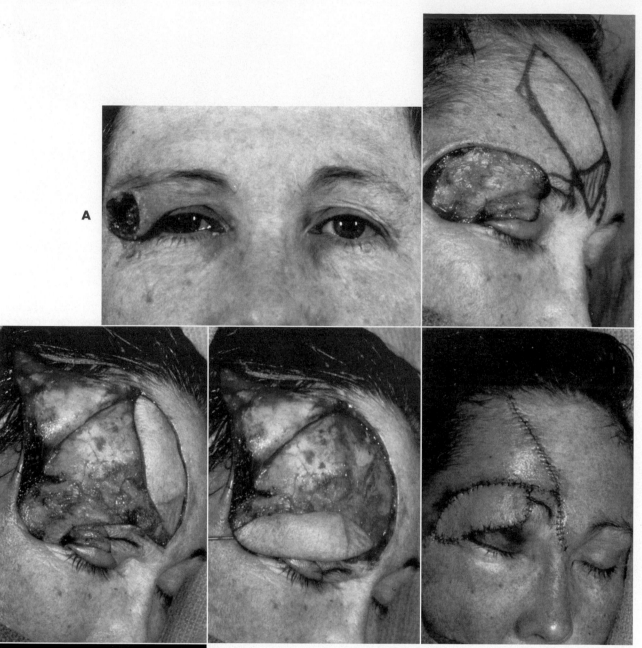

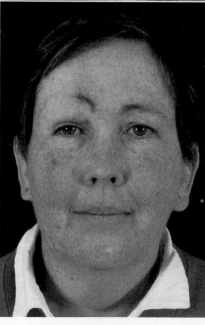

Figure 74-27. **A,** A female patient with a lateral brow cutaneous malignancy. **B,** A large lateral brow and upper lid defect following excision with a planned forehead flap. The striped area at the base of the flap represents the area that will be de-epithelized. **C,** The flap incised with intervening tissue elevated superiorly deep to the frontalis muscle. **D** and **E,** Mobilization of the flap directly into the defect with primary closure. **F,** The patient's result 1 year after surgery.

nasal defects (Figure 74-28). The base of the flap should be left wide enough to capture the venous and arterial branches of the supratrochlear and supraorbital vessels and may require a secondary revision. The base of interpolation flaps can be replaced on the forehead to restore a normal width of forehead skin between the medial eyebrows after the distal portion of the flap has been inset on the nose or discarded, depending on which gives the superior aesthetic result.

A design of the defect to be covered is first made from glove paper or sterile aluminum foil and then transferred to the appropriate position over the forehead (see Figure 74-28, *B*). The pattern must be positioned, for example, during nasal reconstruction, far enough to reach the surgical defect after elevation and rotation of the flap without tension or excessive twisting of the pedicle. The flap can be elevated above the frontalis muscle to about the midforehead but should be dissected from beneath the frontalis muscle to the level of the superior orbital rim. The supraorbital nerve may sometimes need to be sacrificed, resulting in a numbness of the anterior scalp. Blunt spreading dissection is required at the base of the flap to facilitate rotation and advancement while preserving vascular branches into the base of the flap. Wide undermining of the adjacent skin edges, usually in a plane beneath the frontalis muscle, is often necessary to close the donor site defect. Larger flaps elevated without a delay may suffer from venous congestion after rotation inferiorly into a dependent position. Congested flaps can be returned to the donor site for a couple of days and then returned to cover the defect or can be treated by medical leeches.

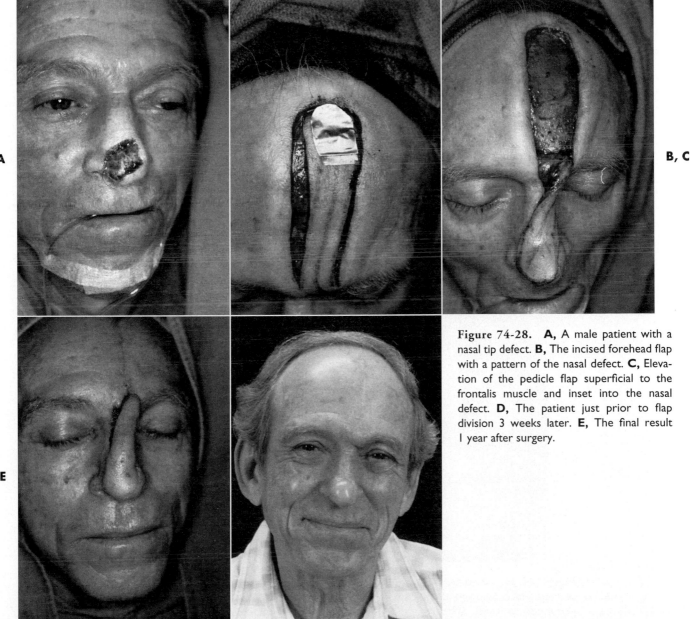

A

B, C

D, E

Figure 74-28. A, A male patient with a nasal tip defect. **B,** The incised forehead flap with a pattern of the nasal defect. **C,** Elevation of the pedicle flap superficial to the frontalis muscle and inset into the nasal defect. **D,** The patient just prior to flap division 3 weeks later. **E,** The final result 1 year after surgery.

OUTCOMES

The use of local flaps has many distinct advantages, but the potential complications must also be considered. The risk of performing a more complex operative procedure, such as a facial flap, compared with primary closure was prospectively studied by Syliadis et al.[32] They found the rate of wound infections was increased to 6.5% in the nasal area and 5% in the auricular area compared with 1.5% for the rest of the face. Patients treated with complex procedures, such as skin grafts or local flaps, and those who had surgery performed for skin cancer were found to have a significantly higher risk of postoperative infection. Skin cleansing in this series was performed with aqueous chlorhexidine and the authors used subcutaneous Vicryl sutures, both of which may have contributed to their infection rate. We use a 3- to 5-minute facial scrub with pHisoHex soap containing 3% hexachlorophene and use chromic or Monocryl absorbable sutures, which are less likely to extrude or produce a stitch abscess after surgery. The nose and ear skin contain abundant sebaceous glands, which are known to harbor bacteria and are more

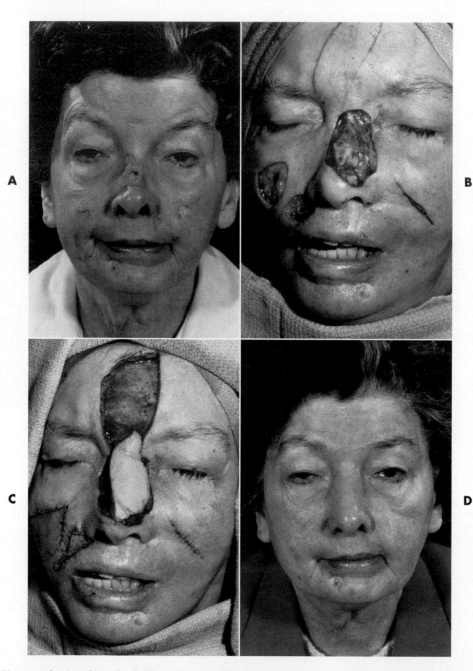

Figure 74-29. **A** to **D,** Different kinds of flaps may be required in the same patient to close several defects following the excision of multiple skin malignancies. This patient had a primary closure on the cheek, and a forehead, rhomboid, and V-Y advancement flap closure of the other defects, all performed during a single operative procedure.

difficult to cleanse adequately before surgery. The authors conclude that perioperative antibiotics are indicated in patients undergoing skin graft or flaps for closure of facial defects in the regions of the ear and nose and in patients with cutaneous malignancies. We routinely use antibiotics in patients undergoing local facial flap coverage.

The outcome, as judged by the preservation of a normal appearing face, is better in older patients with appropriately designed and executed local flaps than can be achieved with skin grafts or healing by secondary intention.[7,13] Several types of flaps may be required to close multiple defects in the same patient (Figures 74-25 and 74-29). Younger patients with few facial rhytides and the potential for active collagen synthesis may not be good candidates for use of local facial flaps because the resulting scar takes longer to mature and may remain visible for a much longer time (see Figure 74-3). The use of facial flaps to cover defects following the resection of cutaneous malignancies has been debated in the older literature because of fears that a potential recurrence could be masked by flap closure. Proper identification of the resected margins to be free of tumor by meticulous frozen section technique has all but removed this problem as a potential complication. Zook et al[37] studied the results of 76 patients treated with a total of 107 V-Y flap closures for 86 facial defects for a cutaneous malignancy with an average follow-up time of 9 months. There was only one case of flap necrosis and not a single case of tumor recurrence. Other investigators have corroborated these findings.[9,10,30]

Poorly designed flaps may result in local anatomic distortion, producing asymmetry. More problematic is the occurrence of functional impairment such as ectropion or nasal obstruction. The decision-making process for designing a local flap must include a knowledge of anatomy, a consideration of surrounding tissue laxity, the placement of incisions relative to existing rhytides or the junction of facial plains, and the estimated long-term effects of wound healing and scar maturation on the final result. The final decision to use a local flap to close a facial defect requires a knowledge of the various options available, sound surgical judgment, and, finally, meticulous technique to restore the optimal in final form and symmetry.

REFERENCES

1. Borges AF: Relaxed skin tension lines, *Dermatol Clin* 7:169, 1989.
2. Braverman IM, Fonterleo E: Studies in cutaneous aging: II. the microvasculature, *J Inver Dermatol* 78:444, 1982.
3. Brown MD: Local flaps in facial reconstruction. In Baker SR, Swanson NA, editors: *Advancement flaps,* St Louis, 1995, Mosby, p 91.
4. Burget GC, Menick FJ: The subunit principle in nasal reconstruction, *Plast Reconstr Surg* 76:239, 1985.
5. Burget GC, Menick FJ: *Aesthetic reconstruction of the nose,* St Louis, 1993, Mosby Year Book.
6. Cameron RR, Latham W, Jawling JA: Reconstruction of the nose and upper lip with nasolabial flaps, *Plast Reconstr Surg* 52:145, 1973.
7. Cuono CB, Ariyan S: Versatility and safety of flap coverage for wide excision of cutaneous melanomas, *Plast Reconstr Surg* 76:281, 1985.
8. Cutting CA: Critical closing and perfusion pressures in flap survival, *Ann Plast Surg* 9:524, 1982.
9. Doerman A, Hauter D, Zook EG, et al: V-Y advancement flap/or tumor excision defects of the eyelids, *Ann Plast Surg* 22(5):929-936, 1988.
10. Doerman A, Hauter D, Zook EG, et al: V-Y advancement flaps for closure of nasal defects, *Plast Reconstr Surg* 84(6):916-920, 1989.
11. Fee WE, Gunter JP: Rhomboid flap principles and common variations, *Laryngoscope* 86:706, 1976.
12. Gewwirtz HD, Eilber FR, Zarem HA: Use of nasolabial flap for reconstruction of the floor of the mouth, *Am Journ Surg* 136:508, 1978.
13. Goldiminz D, Bennett RG: Cigarette smoking and flap and full thickness graft necrosis, *Arch Dermatol* 127:1012-1015, 1991.
14. Guba A: Study of the delay phenomenon in axial pattern flaps in pigs, *Plast Reconstr Surg* 63:550, 1979.
15. Guyton A: *Textbook of medical physiology,* ed 5, Philadelphia, 1993, WB Saunders.
16. Ham D, Asseta G: The effects of endothelial cell growth factor on vascular comprised skin flaps, *Arch Otolaryngol Head Neck Surg* 118:624, 1992.
17. Jackson IT: *Local flaps in head and neck reconstruction,* St. Louis, 1985, Mosby Year Book.
18. Limberg AA: Design of the local flaps. In Gibson T, editor: *Modern trends in plastic surgery,* Sevenoaks, England, 1979, AGG Butterworth.
19. Marchac D, Toth B: The axial frontonasal flap revisited, *Plast Reconstr Surg* 76:686, 1985.
20. McKee PH: Normal physiology of the skin. In Lowell M, Smillie L, editors: *Physiology of the skin,* Philadelphia, 1989, JB Lippincott.
21. Mustarde JC: *Repair and reconstruction in the orbital region,* New York, 1971, Churchill Livingstone.
22. Nichter L, Sobieski M: Efficacy of verapamil in salvage of failing random skin flaps, *Ann Plast Surg* 21:242.1, 1988.
23. Rawat SS, Sharma K: One-stage repair of full thickness alar defects, *Br J Plast Surg* 28:317, 1975.
24. Roth A, Briggs P, Jones E, et al: Augmentation of skin flap survival by parenteral pentoxifylline, *Br J Plast Surg* 41:515, 1988.
25. Russell RC: *Flaps for closure of facial defects.* Instruction Vol. 6. St Louis, 1993, Mosby Year Book.
26. Sagi A, Fender M, Levens S: Improved survival of island flaps after prolonged ischemia by perfusion with superoxide dismiltose, *Plast Reconstr Surg* 77:639, 1986.
27. Sasaki G, Pang C: Pathophysiology of skin flaps raised on expanded pig skin, *Plast Reconstr Surg* 74:59, 1984.
28. Sellke FW, Boyle EM, Vertur E: The pathophysiology of vasomotor dysfunction, *Annals Thoracic Surg* 64:510-515, 1997.

29. Stuzin JM, Wagstrom L, Kawamoto HK, et al: Anatomy of the frontal branch of the facial nerve. The significance of the temporal fat pad, *Plast Reconstr Surg* 83:265, 1989.

30. Summers BK, Seigle RT: Facial cutaneous reconstructive surgery: general aesthetic principles, *J Amer Acad Derm* 29:669-683, 1993.

31. Swanson NA, Grekin RC, Baker SR: Mohs' surgery: applications in head and neck surgery, *Head Neck Surg* 6:683, 1983.

32. Syliadis P, Wood S, Murray DS: Postoperative infection following clean facial surgery, *Ann Plast Surg* 39:342-346, 1997.

33. Tanzer RC, Converse JM, Brend B: Deformities of the auricle. In Converse JM, editor: *Reconstruction plastic surgery*, ed 2, Philadelphia, 1977, WB Saunders.

34. Tsur H, Danviller A, Strauch B: Neovascularization of skin flaps: route and timing, *Plast Reconstr Surg* 66:85, 1980.

35. Wu G, Calamel PM, Schedd DP: The hazards of injecting local anesthetic solutions with epinephrine into flaps, *Plast Reconstr Surg* 62:396, 1978.

36. Yanai A, Nagata X, Tanaka H: Reconstruction of the columnella with bilateral nasolabial flaps, *Plast Reconstr Surg* 77:929, 1986.

37. Zook EG, VanBeek AL, Russell RC, et al: V-Y advancement flap for facial defects, *Plast Reconstr Surg* 65:786-797, 1980.

Reconstructive Lip Surgery

Ramin A. Behmand
Riley S. Rees

INTRODUCTION

In most societies, the lips are recognized as a measure of personal beauty and charm, constituting the most important anatomic and aesthetic unit of the lower face. The upper and lower lips together form a muscular ring that determines the fine motor movements of the mouth. The vermilion registers delicate sensory stimuli and the lips confine solids and liquids to the oral cavity. The orbicularis oris muscle makes up the body of the lips and facilitates the precise mechanical functions of the soft tissues of the mouth. Several muscles attach to the outer border of the orbicularis oris muscle to govern articulation of speech and animation of the lips. Together these muscles determine facial expression via selective contraction, affecting modifications in the shape and configuration of the lips. The sensations conveyed by the lips, namely contact, temperature, texture, and pain, permit regulation of materials about to enter the oral cavity.

Such a combination of aesthetic and functional roles makes reconstructive lip surgery uniquely challenging to the surgeon since the loss or impediment of any of these functions bears a profound effect on the patient's daily existence. Reconstructive lip surgery aims to restore basic function, maintain sensation, and avoid cosmetic deformity. It requires a fundamental knowledge of cutaneous and oral pathophysiology and functional anatomy, as well as the ability to measure the significance of any resulting deformity.

Numerous techniques and procedures have evolved to reconstruct the lips, suggesting no clear advantage or disadvantage of one method over another. An algorithmic approach to the problem using several basic principles may provide a better functional and cosmetic outcome.

INDICATIONS

LIP CANCER

The overwhelming majority of lip reconstruction is performed following resection of lip carcinoma. Of all noncutaneous head and neck cancers, 12% are lip cancers.[10] The American Joint Committee on Cancer defines lip carcinoma as those malignancies arising within the vermilion portion of the lip. In addition, from a reconstructive standpoint, the lip can frequently be involved with contiguous spread of mucosal or cutaneous lesions. Often adequate resection of the lesion involves not only the vermilion, but also areas of the lip outside the vermilion.

Squamous cell carcinoma is the most common neoplasm of the lip. Basal cell carcinoma, salivary gland carcinoma, and other rare tumors are much less frequently encountered. The male to female ratio is 6 to 1 for all lip cancers, but the margin narrows to 2 to 1 for the upper lip.[7] The lower lip is the site of approximately 95% of all lip cancers, with the upper lip involved only 5% of the time. The commissures are involved in less than 2% of all cases. Solar radiation damage may explain this distribution. Exposure of the lower lip to the sun renders it most susceptible to formation of neoplastic lesions.

The typical patient is a fair-skinned, white male in the sixth decade of life, often with a history of outdoor occupations with prolonged sun exposure. Factors of less significance are tobacco use, poor oral hygiene, alcoholism, and syphilis.[14] Lesions of the lip that are nonhealing or ulcerating, areas of persistent erythema, and verrucous changes must be biopsied to rule out malignancy.

Most lip cancers remain localized and grow slowly, with a propensity for lateral rather than vertical spread. The great majority are histopathologically of low grade, and the lesions are well differentiated. The lymphatic drainage of the upper lip and the lateral third of the lower lip are to the submandibular nodes. The central third of the lower lip may drain into the submental lymph nodes on either side. Cervical metastasis is seen in less than 8% of patients at the time of presentation. The likelihood of metastasis may be higher if the squamous cell carcinoma originates at the commissure or on the upper lip.[14] When cervical lymph nodes are clinically palpable, a functional neck dissection is performed in addition to resection.

Although recommendations on the margin of normal tissue necessary for adequate cancer resection have varied, a 10-mm margin is generally preferred. Intraoperative use of frozen sections prior to reconstruction provides added support to the adequacy of the resection. Despite the presence of numerous diagrams in the texts showing a tapering wedge excision, such as a V or W, this may result in inadequate resection. The tumor should be excised with a shield type resection and a 1-cm margin of normal tissue.

TRAUMA

Traumatic lip injury is only rarely an indication for major reconstructive lip surgery and almost never in the acute setting. Primary repair and closure are often achievable. When significant lip tissue loss does occur, it is frequently in conjunction with other facial injuries and may be addressed concurrently. The principles of reconstruction, however, remain the same in that function takes precedence over aesthetic outcome.

OPERATIONS

LIP ANATOMY

Knowledge of the surgical anatomy of the lips and perioral region is crucial to satisfactory outcomes in lip reconstruction. Both the functional and aesthetic roles of the different components determine the choice of the reconstructive technique (Figure 75-1). The orbicularis oris muscle is solely responsible for the closure of the lips, and thus it is responsible for oral competence. Its fibers are predominantly horizontally oriented (Figure 75-2) and extend from one commissure to the other with some fibers inserting into the opposite philtral column. The oblique fibers, which also arise from the commissures, insert medially at the anterior nasal spine and septum, where they contract to evert the upper lip. Serving as a template onto which other supporting muscles insert, the orbicularis oris muscle controls the sphincteric function of the mouth. Together these muscles control the fine motor movements of the mouth.

The modiolus is a functional anatomic region at each commissure where several muscles converge and affect oral animation. The functional significance of the modiolus is evident by the difficulty involved in the reconstruction of the commissures. In this area, the upper and lower orbicularis oris integrate with muscle fibers from the zygomaticus major, levator anguli oris, depressor anguli oris, and risorius muscles. The zygomaticus major muscle arises from the zygomaticotemporal suture and inserts into the orbicularis oris at the modiolus. The muscle functions to elevate the commissures laterally and is the "smiling" muscle. The levator anguli oris arises below the inferior orbital rim and inserts into the modiolus region, pulling the angle of the mouth upward. The risorius inserts from a lateral position in the cheek soft tissues into the modiolus and pulls the angle of the mouth laterally. The depressor anguli oris arises between the symphysis and mental foramen, at the lower border of the mandible. It inserts superiorly into the modiolus region and draws the angle of the mouth downward and laterally.

The orbicularis muscle is manipulated by five sets of superiorly positioned elevator muscles. The two major lip elevators, levator anguli oris and zygomaticus major, are complemented by levator labii superioris, which originates from the medial orbital margin. Its fibers travel around the alar

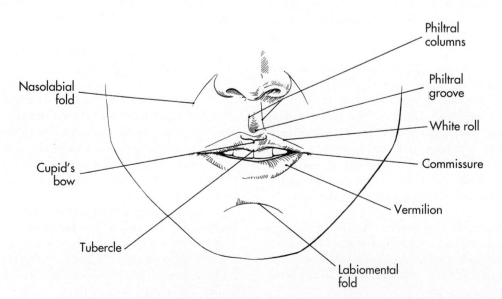

Figure 75-1. Surface anatomy of the mouth. (Courtesy Evelyn K. Mohalski.)

base and insert more medially into the orbicularis oris and the ipsilateral lower philtral columns. Less significant elevator functions are attributed to the levator labii superioris alaeque nasi and zygomaticus minor.

There are three nasolabial muscles with notable functions. The depressor septi is medial and arises from the periosteum over the central and lateral incisors. It travels upward to insert into the medial crura and, on occasions, the nasal tip. This forms the upper philtral columns, and functions to depress the nasal tip and provide secondary lift of the medial upper lip. The nasalis and nasalis transversus muscles arise from the alar base and insert into the ala and nasal dorsum, respectively. They elevate the alar base.

The muscles acting on the lower lip include the mentalis, depressor labii inferioris, and depressor anguli oris muscles. The mentalis muscle arises from the alveolar periosteum and inserts inferiorly into the skin of the chin. When it contracts the lower lip elevates and the central portion of the lip protrudes. The depressor labii inferioris originates at the lower border of the mandible, medial to the mental foramen, and inserts superiorly into orbicularis oris, functioning to pull down the lower lip.

The facial arteries supply the lips through the superior and inferior labial arteries. The labial arteries run tangentially to the orbicularis oris muscle laterally and parallel to its fibers medially along their deep surface. The upper and lower labial arteries from each side of the face are in continuity with the opposite side, forming collateral blood flow to the lip. The anatomic position of the arteries relative to the orbicularis muscle and the dual blood supply to each lip are unique features that form the basis for reconstructive lip surgery.

Motor innervation of the lip muscles is from the buccal and marginal mandibular branches of the facial nerve. The orbicularis oris muscle is supplied by the nerve endings of the buccal branch on each side of the face. The marginal mandibular branch alone innervates the depressor muscles;

injury results in abnormal elevation or lack of eversion of the affected lower lip with smiling. The nerves run deep to the muscles and insert on their deep surfaces, so surgical dissection in a plane superficial to the muscle will prevent injury to them.

The superior labial nerve provides sensation to the upper lip. It arises from the infraorbital branch of the trigeminal nerve. The inferior alveolar branch of the trigeminal nerve provides sensation to the lower lip through the mental nerve. Lymphatic drainage of the upper and lower lateral lips is via the submandibular nodes. The central portion of the lower lip, however, drains into the submental nodes bilaterally.

EVOLUTION OF LIP SURGERY

Many of the earliest procedures in plastic surgery were methods to restore the contour of the lips, approaching appearance much more vigorously than function. Mazzola and Lupo[9] have compiled a comprehensive record of the techniques in lip surgery, an abbreviated version of which is presented here to demonstrate the historical evolution of major concepts in lip reconstruction.

In 1597, Tagliacozzi produced one of the earliest and most famous sets of illustrations in plastic surgery, in which he described the use of a distant pedicle skin flap from the arm for the repair of upper and lower lip defects. In 1768 Louis reported the surgical wedge excision of a labial lesion with immediate primary repair. The late eighteenth century also witnessed Chopart's pioneering attempt to utilize a local advancement flap for lower lip repair, which was unsuccessful because of flap retraction. In 1834, Dieffenbach moved inferior-based cheek flaps lined with mucosa medially to repair a midline defect.

The modern era in lip surgery commenced in 1838. A number of concepts developed in the mid-nineteenth

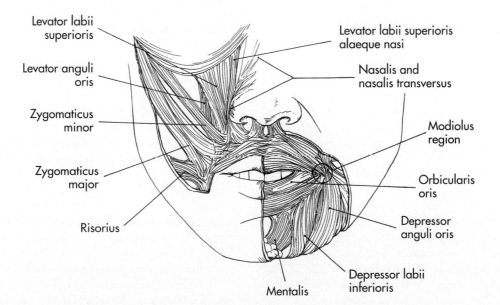

Figure 75-2. Muscular anatomy of the mouth. (Courtesy Evelyn K. Mohalski.)

century form the basis of techniques employed today. In 1838, Sabattini introduced the lip switch flap from the middle of the lower lip to repair an upper lip defect. This operation was later perfected by Abbé (1898) and still bears his name. Von Burow, in order to facilitate the advancement of local flaps, excised a triangular portion of adjacent tissue at the base of the flap to provide room for adequate movement of the cheek skin. Although initially performed in 1838, this revolutionary concept was not published until 1855 and remains in use today. Von Bruns (1857) reported the use of nasolabial flaps for lower lip repair using a curvilinear incision to maintain the oral sphincter, the precedent of the more functional dissection of the Karapandzic flap today.

Two other operations described in the middle of the nineteenth century, the Bernard procedure and the Estlander flap, played an influential role in shaping the future of lip surgery. Bernard's operation (1853) was similar to von Burow's because he excised full-thickness triangles lateral to the upper lip on both cheeks to provide relief space for advancing lower cheek flaps. This accommodation allowed closure of large central lower lip defects, although functional results were poor because the reconstructed lip was insensate and only acted as a dam. Subsequently, Webster et al added the use of buccal mucous membrane for vermilion reconstruction and incorporated the Schuchardt principle to provide innervated muscle for the new lip, maintaining oral continence and function.[12]

Estlander described his operation in 1872. He outlined a full-thickness triangular flap on the lateral side of the upper lip, and used it to repair a lower lateral lip and commissure defect. The Gillies' modification preserved the continuity of the orbicularis oris muscle (1957). Karapandzic (1974) further changed the Gillies' fan flap to reconstruct larger lower lip defects using von Bruns' circumoral incision. The Karapandzic design preserves the neurovascular supply and the sphincteric function of the mouth.[5]

LIP REPAIR AND RECONSTRUCTION

Tumor resection and traumatic injuries require the same general principles of lip reconstruction. Both appearance and function are crucial. A functional repair involves a three-layer closure, including the inner mucosal layer, the intervening muscle layer, and the outer skin layer. Motor and sensory innervation must be preserved to the greatest degree possible. Proper realignment of the orbicularis oris fibers maintains the sphincteric function and minimizes distortion during facial animation.

The most important aesthetic landmark is the white roll. Very small discrepancies in the skin vermilion junction at the white roll produce a noticeable deformity, thus mandating maximal attention to its accurate realignment. To avoid malalignment, it is prudent to mark both the inferior and superior limits of the white roll with blue dye before using a local anesthetic.

ANESTHESIA

Surgical procedures on the lips range from minor repairs to large oncologic tumor resections. In either case, local anesthesia may be very effective and safe to use. To achieve regional anesthesia of the upper lip the infraorbital nerves are blocked. A small gauge needle is passed intraorally over the canine eminence to a position just lateral to the alar base. The infraorbital nerve exits the infraorbital foramen 5 to 8 mm below the inferior orbital rim, in the axis of the pupil. Anesthesia of the lower lip is similarly achieved using transmucosal injection in the area of mental nerve bilaterally. The mental nerve exits the mental foramen between the first and second bicuspid teeth, and injection at the root of the lower canine or the first bicuspid tooth will anesthetize the lower lip. However, if more extensive surgery is planned and the area below the labiomental fold is involved, one must also block the inferior alveolar nerve bilaterally. The inferior alveolar nerve enters the mandibular foramen in the midportion of the mandibular ramus. Anesthesia is achieved by injecting the anesthetic along the medial border of the mandibular ramus bilaterally. Once regional block anesthesia is obtained, the site of surgical incisions may be injected directly with epinephrine containing local anesthetic for hemostasis.

The use of electrocautery or laser in the presence of a nasal cannula carrying oxygen in or near the operative field requires extreme caution. A distressing situation of oxygen ignition causing burn injury to the patient or the surgeon can occur if the oxygen flow is not turned off when using electrocautery. When laser is in use, the field should be draped with moist towels. Corneal protectors or moist pads should always protect the patient's eyes. Although adequate anesthesia is easily obtained with relatively innocuous blocks, keeping the oral cavity free of blood during lip surgery can be problematic and must be carefully addressed to keep the patient calm and immobile.

TRAUMA

When there is traumatic injury to the lips it can be difficult to assess the viability of the damaged tissue. Therefore the goal of lip repair in trauma is to preserve all the lip tissue with potential to survive and to reapproximate the wound edges with minimal tension. Debridement may be necessary but is kept to a minimum and limited to obviously devitalized tissue. The involved area is irrigated meticulously to remove debris and foreign objects. Meticulous examination is then carried out to identify all structures involved. In many cases, primary closure can be undertaken. The critical landmark structures, the white roll, philtral columns, the mucosa-vermilion junction, and the commissures are realigned first with key sutures before the lip is repaired. The muscle layer is repaired first with absorbable suture. The mucosa is then reapproximated with absorbable sutures to create a watertight seal. The skin is closed with fine monofilament suture that is removed after 3 to 5 days.

A difficult management problem is that of lip avulsion injuries. With a small avulsion injury a primary closure of the wound edges may be carried out. When the defect includes more than one third of the lip, primary closure is often not possible unless the patient is elderly with significant skin laxity. The type of flap used is determined by the size and location, as well as the functional and aesthetic deficit created. In cases where a rather large and difficult-to-reconstruct portion of the lip has been avulsed and does not appear to have sustained significant tissue trauma, one may consider microvascular reanastomosis of the facial vessels supplying the lip. Crush injuries, traumatized vascular pedicle, significant ischemia time, or other life-threatening injuries to the patient would preclude an attempt at a microvascular reanastomosis.

VERMILION RECONSTRUCTION

A modified mucosal surface forms the vermilion. The color causes it to be the most visible component of the lips with significant functional and cosmetic roles. As the sensory unit of the lips, the vermilion has a high degree of sensitivity to temperature, light touch, or pain. Scars are well hidden in the vermilion. Whenever possible, resection and repair should be confined to the vermilion to avoid crossing the vermilion-cutaneous junction. Incisions should be designed along the natural vermilion fold lines in the vertical plane, avoiding horizontal incisions. When the incision traverses the vermilion-cutaneous border, the white roll should always be crossed with a perpendicular incision.

The lower vermilion is far more frequently the site of neoplastic lesions since it is the target of solar radiation injury. Small malignant lesions may be treated with a shield excision (see Figure 75-9, *D*) or by laser ablation for squamous cell carcinoma in situ. However, when a premalignant lesion is present with extensive and severe actinic injury to the rest of the vermilion, total vermilionectomy, also known as a "lip shave" operation, is indicated (Figure 75-3). In this operation the vermilion is resected from the white roll to the contact area of the upper and lower lip.[2] Vermilionectomy is reserved for extensive premalignant lesions of the lip, such as severe actinic injury or leukoplakia. Following vermilionectomy, primary closure of the labial mucosa to the skin edge may be possible, but excessive tension may result in dehiscence or flattening of the lip, making a buccal mucosa advancement flap preferable[13] (Figure 75-4). The mucosa is released with an incision in the deep sulcus, then elevated in a plane deep to the

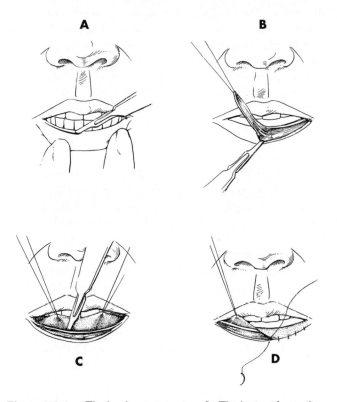

Figure 75-3. The lip shave operation **A**, The limits of vermilion excision are from the wet-dry border to the white roll. **B**, Vermilion and subcutaneous tissues are excised, leaving the muscle layer intact. **C**, Buccal mucosa is undermined and advanced. **D**, The advanced buccal mucosa is sutured at the cutaneous junction. (Courtesy Evelyn K. Mohalski.)

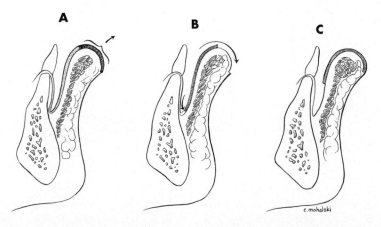

Figure 75-4. Vermilion reconstruction with buccal mucosa. **A**, Resection of the affected vermilion. **B**, Buccal sulcus relaxing incision and undermining of the anterior portion of the mucosal flap in a plane just deep to the minor salivary glands. **C**, Advancement of the mucosal flap. Buccal sulcus incision is allowed to heal secondarily. (Courtesy Evelyn K. Mohalski.)

salivary glands, and just superficial to the orbicularis muscle. The mucosal bipedicle flap is then advanced forward over the free margin of the lip and brought over to the anterior vermilion line. This decreases the inward retraction of the lip, which occurs with primary closure, avoiding irritation by the lower lip hairs, and producing a better contour.

Two-stage tongue flaps have significant disadvantages. The neovermilion created from the anterior tongue mucosal surface is red, resulting in a poor cosmetic match and an undesirable feminizing effect in men. The lateral and dorsal glossal mucosa has many fine papilla, making it unsatisfactory.[1] Generally, the tongue mucosal flap is an unpleasant experience for the patient and should rarely be chosen.

When the defect is limited to less than one third of the lower vermilion, a vermilion-muscle advancement flap based on the axial labial artery may be used to resurface the area of the defect[4] (Figure 75-5). To repair the notch and whistle deformity of the lower lip it is often necessary to excise the involved scar. Reapproximation is achieved with a Z-plasty closure in the area of deformity to avoid recurrence secondary to scar contracture. Alternatively, when the notch deformity is secondary to vermilion volume deficiency and not a scar band, a triangular musculomucosal V-Y advancement flap may better correct the defect. A V-shaped musculomucosal flap is designed and advanced forward. Only a superficial layer of the orbicularis oris muscle is included (Figure 75-6).

Kawamoto described a vermilion lip switch flap for correction of cases involving a large area of vermilion volume deficiency, as may be seen in hemifacial atrophy.[6] A transverse, centrally based flap is designed on the lower lip, which includes both vermilion and a thin layer of muscle. The flap is elevated and turned upward 180 degrees and sutured into an incisional space created in the deficient portion of the upper lip. The flap is later divided and inset at 10 to 14 days (Figure 75-7). This flap is generally not suitable for cancer reconstruction.

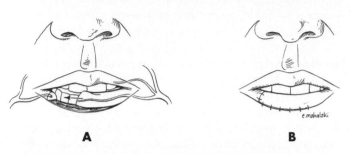

Figure 75-5. Axial musculovermilion advancement flap. **A,** The flap is elevated deep to the labial artery. The position of the labial artery can be identified at the time of the resection of the lesion. **B,** Forward advancement of the flap permits primary closure of the defect. (Courtesy Evelyn K. Mohalski.)

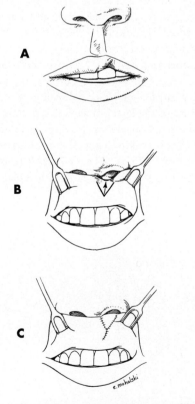

Figure 75-6. Musculomucosal V-Y advancement flap. **A,** Focal upper lip vermilion deficiency. **B,** V design of the musculomucosal advancement flap. **C,** Local volume increase following V-Y advancement flap. (Courtesy Evelyn K. Mohalski.)

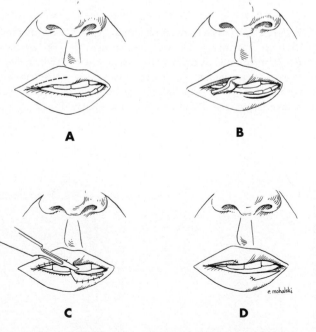

Figure 75-7. Vermilion lip switch flap. **A,** Left upper and lower lip volume deficiency. **B,** Right upper lip random vermilion pedicle flap is elevated. The transverse incision in the deficient left lower vermilion prepares the recipient bed. **C,** The pedicle is divided at 14 days. **D,** The flap adds volume to the left lower lip vermilion and the donor site is closed primarily. (Courtesy Evelyn K. Mohalski.)

LOWER LIP RECONSTRUCTION

When dealing with lower lip defects two anatomic properties provide a distinct advantage in contrast to the upper lip. The lower lip has greater soft tissue laxity and lacks a dominant central structure such as the philtrum and nose. These properties allow for better mobilization of tissues adjacent to the defect without causing obvious distortion (Figure 75-8).

Small Defects (less than one third of the lower lip)

Defects up to one third of the lower lip may be closed primarily. The patient's age, elasticity, and redundancy of adjacent soft tissues determine the size of the defect that can be closed primarily. The resection must completely remove all neoplastic tissue with adequate margin of uninvolved tissue using intraoperative frozen sections. Where possible, the incision should conform to the natural skin lines of the lower face (Figure 75-9). Often, wedge resections in the form of a V or W may provide an inadequate margin at the lower portion of the resection. Therefore a shield excision is used to ensure complete removal of the tumor. Alternatively, a single or double barrel excision may be used. The "barrel" is excised in full thickness. The Burow's triangle at the base of the barrel involves resection of skin and subcutaneous tissue only. This is sufficient to allow medial advancement of the lip tissue.

Crossing of the labiomental fold is avoided to reduce the risk of unfavorable scar formation.

Medium Defects (one third to two thirds of the lower lip)

Four operations have been described that provide adequate tissue to reconstruct a medium defect of the lower lip while producing aesthetically acceptable results. These are the Abbé switch flap, Karapandzic flap, modified Bernard-Burow's procedure, and the Estlander switch flap. To achieve the best reconstructive outcome, the technique must suit the problem.

THE ABBÉ FLAP. The Abbé lip switch flap may be used to partially fill a medium-size defect. By so doing, the defect is converted to a small one, which may then be closed primarily. The use of this flap is limited to defects not involving the commissure and to cooperative patients who are able to understand the two-stage nature of this procedure and can tolerate 14 to 21 days with their lips apposed. The main complication is total flap loss, either intraoperatively or postoperatively, which must be discussed with the patient prior to the procedure. A defect that necessitates new lip tissue to create a functionally adequate oral aperture is unsuitable for the Abbé flap, because new lip tissue is not formed in this

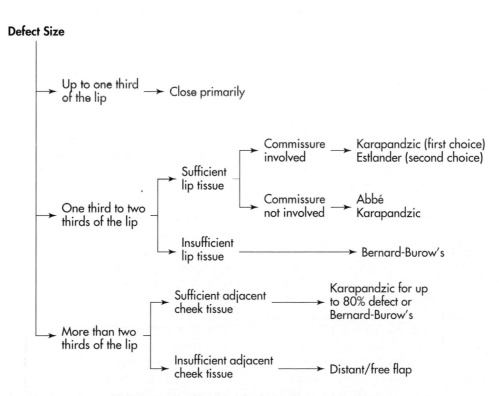

Figure 75-8. Algorithm for lower lip reconstruction.

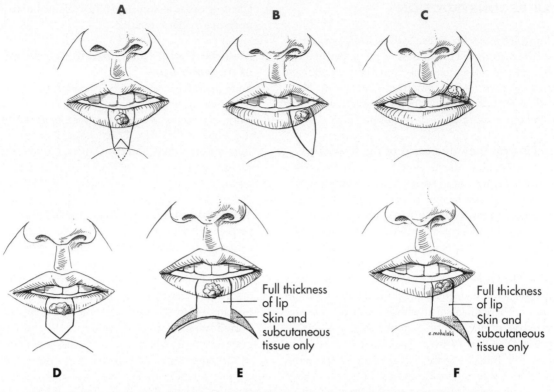

Figure 75-9. Wedge excision of lesions. **A,** W-shaped excision. **B,** V-shaped excision of the lower lip. **C,** V-shaped excision of upper lip lesion, tapered into the nasolabial fold. **D,** Shield excision. **E,** Double barrel excision. The lesion is excised in full-thickness of the lip. Burow's triangles involve only excision of skin and subcutaneous tissue. **F,** Single barrel excision. (Courtesy Evelyn K. Mohalski.)

procedure. Electromyographic studies have shown return of muscle function to the transferred flap at its recipient site.[11] Microstomia is rarely a problem, but must be considered preoperatively in patients who use dentures. The cosmetic outcome is generally better than that seen with the Bernard-Burow's procedure or Karapandzic flap. If necessary, minor revisions of the white roll and vermilion may be undertaken at the time of pedicle takedown. The flap is designed at the junction of the middle and lateral thirds of the upper lip so that neither the philtral columns nor the commissure is affected. A paper template of the defect is made and rotated along the axis of the vascular pedicle to the recipient site in order to ensure proper design of the donor flap. Since the remaining upper lip segment must be advanced medially to close the donor site defect, the pedicle may be designed on the medial or lateral side of the flap. The distal portion of the flap can be tapered into the nasolabial fold or designed as a rectangle. Because the average span of the upper lip is 8 cm, the maximum size of the flap should not exceed 2 to 3 cm to allow primary closure of the donor site without dysfunction.[8] The donor site defect may require crescentic excisions to facilitate primary closure (Figure 75-10). Because the labial artery is supplied from both sides of the face, the flap may be based on either side. The white roll is properly marked, both in the area of the defect and donor tissue to avoid discrepancies. Full-thickness division of

the nonpedicle side of the flap can locate the exact position of the labial artery within the flap, allowing more precise dissection of the pedicle side. It is crucial to leave enough soft tissue around the pedicle to provide support and prevent tension or twisting of the vascular pedicle. The flap is then rotated into position. The musculovermilion bridge spanning between the upper and lower lips carries the blood supply. The white roll is approximated first, then the rest of the flap is sutured in place. During the 3 weeks in which the pedicle remains attached, liquids and soft foods constitute the greater portion of the patient's diet. Oral hygiene must be maintained, with frequent antiseptic rinses. The pedicle is divided at 2 to 3 weeks and any discrepancies between the flap and recipient vermilion are corrected at that time (Figure 75-11).

KARAPANDZIC FLAP. Indications for the Karapandzic flap are defects that do not require new lip tissue for reconstruction and that are either located centrally or more laterally where they involve a portion of the commissure. This flap provides the ideal reconstruction for such situations because it preserves the neurovascular supply and the integrity of the oral sphincter, allowing the mouth to remain sensate with complete sphincteric function after reconstruction. The intact oral sphincter and normal sensation resulting from the Karapandzic repair make it preferable to the

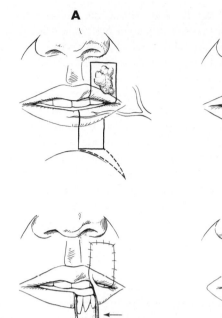

A   **B**

C   **D**

Figure 75-10. Abbé flap. **A,** An example of a rectangular design of a lip switch flap that fills an upper lip defect. The continuity of the labial artery is maintained in the pivoting portion of the flap. **B,** The flap is elevated in full thickness of lip tissue and rotated into the upper lip defect. **C,** Excision of a Burow's triangle at the base of the donor site allows medial advancement of the lower lateral lip flap and primary closure of the donor site in much the same fashion as the single barrel excision. **D,** The pedicle is divided and inset at 14-21 days. (Courtesy Evelyn K. Mohalski.)

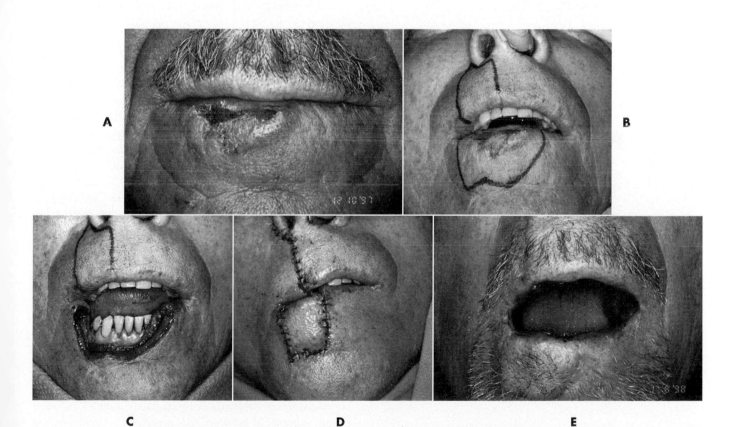

A   **B**

C   **D**   **E**

Figure 75-11. Upper lip Abbé flap for lower lip reconstruction. **A,** Lower lip squamous cell carcinoma. **B,** Design of W excision of lesion and upper lip Abbé flap. **C,** Excision of lesion with 1-cm margins. **D,** Flap transferred to lower lip and the use of perialar crescentic excision for primary closure of the upper lip donor site. The pedicle holds lips together. **E,** Four weeks postoperative and one week after division of pedicle. Some flap edema is present in the early postoperative period. (Courtesy Dr. Theodoros N. Teknos.)

Bernard-Burow's repair. The microstomia, however, is more pronounced with the Karapandzic repair for the same size defect, because new lip tissue is not imported. When compared with the Abbé flap, a two-stage procedure is avoided, as is the risk of flap loss, but the aesthetic outcome may be inferior. Potential complications of this procedure are unsightly scarring and microstomia, which can be particularly troublesome to patients who use dentures. The circumoral scarring is more noticeable because the incisions do not follow the normal pattern of facial aging. Older patients who have more tissue laxity and who are likely to have only moderate scars are excellent scarring candidates for this operation.

The vertical height of the defect determines the width of the Karapandzic flap. This width is maintained as the incision is carried circumorally to the alar base bilaterally (Figure 75-12). The incisions are made full thickness through skin, muscle,

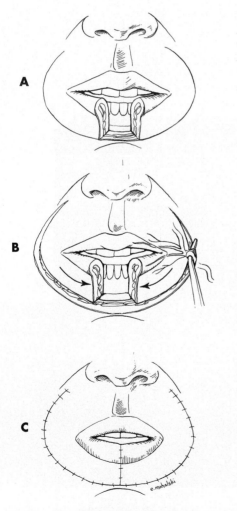

Figure 75-12. The Karapandzic flap. **A,** The width of the circumoral incision must be equal to the height of the defect at all points of the flap. **B,** The labial arteries and buccal nerve branches are identified and preserved bilaterally. **C,** Three-layer closure following medial advancement of the flaps. (Courtesy Evelyn K. Mohalski.)

and mucosa medially. Laterally, at the level of the commissures the skin is incised only down to subcutaneous tissue. Careful dissection is required to identify the labial arteries and buccal nerve branches and preserve them prior to mobilizing the flap further (Figure 75-13). The flaps are rotated inward to fill the defect. If the defect is central, the flaps must be advanced equally from both sides to avoid unilateral commissure distortion. When the defect has a lateral position, more advancement must be obtained from the contralateral lower lip, thus minimizing upper lip distortion. Reapproximating the orbicularis muscle, mucosa, and skin edges in separate layers closes the defect. Oral animation is significantly improved by reattachment of the muscles of the modiolus into the orbicularis template.

THE BERNARD-BUROW'S PROCEDURE. The need for new lip tissue and the necessity to avoid microstomia are the best indications for the Bernard-Burow's procedure. The potential complications include incomplete recovery of sensation and mobility in the new lip tissue, scar contracture at the commissure causing an unnatural "smiley face," color mismatch of the reconstructed vermilion with adjacent vermilion, and drooling. That part of the reconstructed lip that is advanced cheek tissue lacks sensation and sphincteric function, contributing to postoperative oral incontinence and drooling.

In the original operation, full-thickness triangles of cheek tissue were excised on each side of the upper lip, providing relief room for the lower cheek flaps to be advanced medially (Figure 75-14). Following this repair, the lower lip was insensate and acted much the same as a dam. This original operation has undergone multiple modifications aimed at improved function and cosmetic result. Through modifications by Freeman[3] and Webster et al,[12] full-thickness excision of Burow's triangles was abandoned. Instead, skin and subcutaneous tissue are excised in a more lateral position, placing the scar in the nasolabial fold and resulting in improved postoperative sensation of the reconstructed lip. Furthermore, the double barrel excision of the lower lip lesion has been incorporated into the repair, and buccal mucosa is used for vermilion reconstruction (Figure 75-15).

The initial step in the modified Bernard-Burow's procedure involves excision of the lesion as a full-thickness block of lip tissue extending from the vermilion down to the mental fold. Adequacy of resection is confirmed intraoperatively with the use of frozen sections. Isosceles triangles of skin are excised at the labiomental fold to advance the adjacent tissue. Triangles of skin and subcutaneous tissue are excised on both sides adjacent to the upper lip, at the nasolabial fold, and superficial to the orbicularis oris muscle (Figure 75-16). The buccal mucosa is undermined superficially, avoiding the buccal nerve branches and the orbicularis muscle. At this stage, the skin and mucosa have been released from the orbicularis muscle and are advanced medially. The lower cheek flaps make up the deficiency in the lower lip. Skin, muscle, and mucosa are individually reapproximated. Ad-

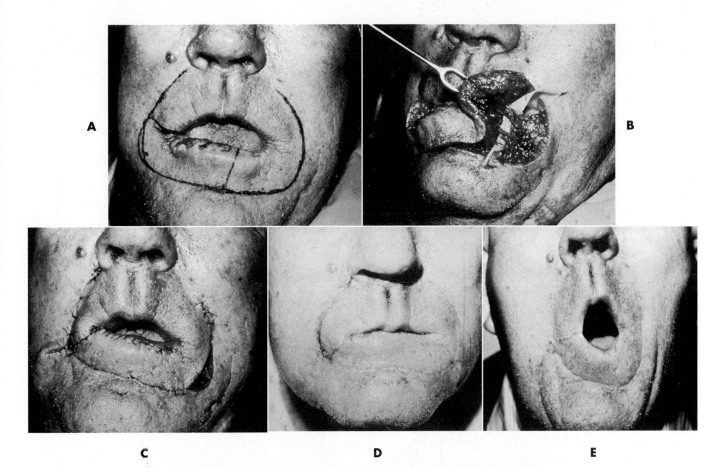

Figure 75-13. The Karapandzic flap. **A,** Lower lip squamous cell carcinoma involving two thirds of the lip. **B,** Dissection of the neurovascular pedicle. **C,** Reconstitution of the oral sphincter with primary closure. **D** and **E,** Three weeks postoperative with intact oral continence.

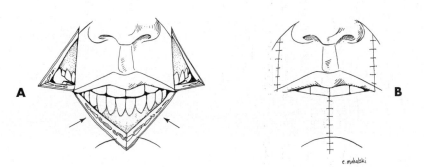

Figure 75-14. The original Bernard procedure. **A,** Triangular excision of the lower lip lesion involved the full thickness of the lip and extended beyond the labiomental fold. Full-thickness Burow's triangles were excised lateral to the upper lip bilaterally. **B,** Lower cheek flaps were advanced medially to reconstruct the lower lip. (Courtesy Evelyn K. Mohalski.)

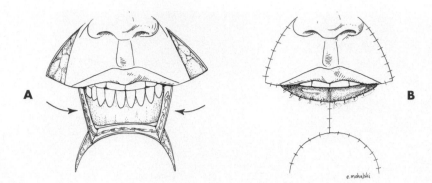

Figure 75-15. Modified Bernard-Burow's procedure. **A,** Excision of lesion does not violate the labiomental fold, but improved resection of the lesion is achieved by widening the base of the resected area. Burow's triangles are resected more laterally, along the nasolabial fold, and only involve the resection of skin and some subcutaneous tissue. Along the labiomental fold skin and subcutaneous Burow's triangles are excised to give way for the medial rotation of the lower cheek flaps. **B,** Medial advancement of the lower cheek flaps is followed by three-layer closure at the midline and vermilion reconstruction with buccal mucosa. The nasolabial fold defects are closed in a single layer. (Courtesy Evelyn K. Mohalski.)

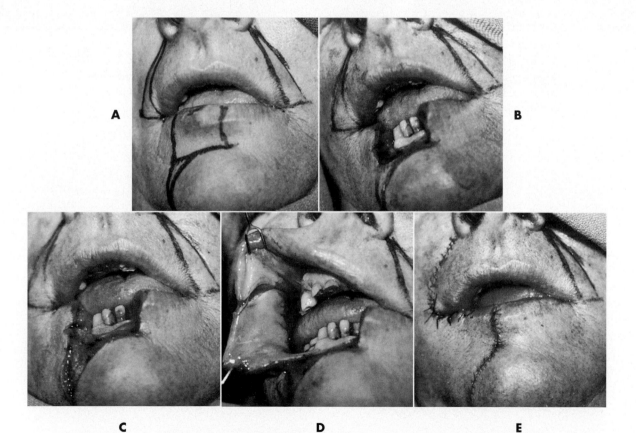

Figure 75-16. Modified Bernard-Burow's procedure. **A,** Lower lip squamous cell carcinoma. **B,** Full-thickness barrel excision of the lesion including skin, muscle, and mucosa. **C,** Excision of Burow's triangle, including only skin and subcutaneous tissue. **D,** Release of buccal mucosa. **E,** Closure with the excision of only one Burow's triangle at the nasolabial fold and partial vermilion reconstruction.

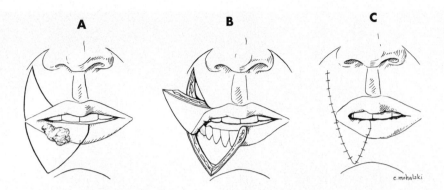

Figure 75-17. Estlander flap for lower lip reconstruction. **A,** The flap is designed to be one third to one half the size of the defect. The commissure must be involved. **B,** Full-thickness upper lateral lip flap is rotated into the lower lip defect. Blood supply to the flap is at the pivoting point by the contralateral upper labial artery. **C,** The flap is inset and the donor site is closed primarily. (Courtesy Evelyn K. Mohalski.)

vancing and reapproximating the previously undermined buccal mucosa with the skin edge completes reconstruction of the vermilion.

THE ESTLANDER FLAP. The Estlander flap is a laterally based lip switch flap, pivoting around the corner of the mouth. Indications for this flap are a defect that involves the commissure and is not amenable to repair by the Karapandzic method. This is a one-step procedure, although attempts have been made to reconstruct the rounded commissure as a delayed secondary procedure. This type of commissureplasty leads to poor results and is not practiced by the authors. The complications of the Estlander flap are similar to the Abbé flap with one main exception, the rounded appearance with poor angle definition of the commissure. The Estlander flap maintains continuity of the orbicularis oris muscle with acceptable postoperative oral competence. Oral animation, however, will be somewhat altered because the commissure and modiolus functional region are distorted.

The flap is designed as a full-thickness medially based flap of the lateral lip. The vascular pedicle is within the pivoting point and is supplied from the contralateral side labial artery (Figure 75-17). The flap is designed on the upper lateral lip at a size equivalent to one half of the lower lip defect. The distal edge of the flap is tapered into the nasolabial fold. It is rotated around the vermilion pivoting point into the defect and the donor site is closed.

Large Defects (more than two thirds of the lower lip)

Total or near-total lower lip tissue loss is a challenging problem. The main goal in this type of reconstruction is to provide a reasonable degree of oral function and competence. Because of the large size of the defect, adjacent tissue must be used to reconstruct the new lip. The Bernard-Burow's procedure is often the method of choice since it provides new lip tissue, and is well suited for the large lower lip defects. After this type of a large reconstruction the return of lip sensation is often less than desirable and drooling can be a problem. The Karapandzic flap may be used for the reconstruction of larger central lower lip defects measuring up to about 80% of the lower lip. The oral sphincter remains intact and functional after this procedure. Microstomia must be considered when planning the operation and may require lip stretching or oral splinting in the postoperative period. This problem is especially important to consider in edentulous patients who use dentures. In the older patient, there is a tendency for the tissues of the reconstructed mouth to relax and increase the oral aperture.

In massive lip defects where there is insufficient remaining lip or cheek tissue, free flap reconstruction of the lip, chin, and often mandible defect provides the most consistent results. If the mandible is not involved, a radial forearm free flap is useful to reconstruct the lower lip and chin. The palmaris longus tendon is taken with the flap and anchored to the modiolus on either side of the mouth. Thus the flap is suspended over the tendon like a curtain rod. This is necessary because the transferred flap will be immobile and insensate, generally functioning as a dam (Figure 75-18). The preoperative design of the flap on the patient's forearm is an important part of the operative plan. The design must ensure harvest of sufficient vascularized tissue for an adequate labial sulcus and, if necessary, skin of the mental area. By suturing the antebrachial cutaneous nerve of the flap into the stump of the mental nerve,[8] the flap may become sensate. In the event of a more extensive defect involving the mandible, a fibula free flap may be used to provide bony support for mandible, lip, and chin reconstruction.

Indications for free flap reconstruction are insufficient adjacent lip and cheek tissue for local flap reconstruction. The outcome often fails to achieve some of the main goals of reconstruction, the lip remaining immobile and insensate and functioning simply as a dam.

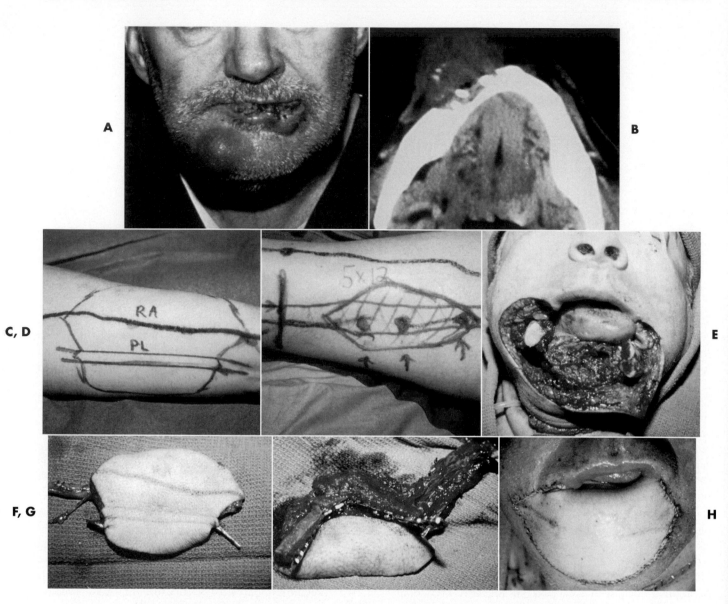

Figure 75-18. Composite lower lip free flap reconstruction. **A,** Lower lip squamous cell carcinoma with invasion of the mandible. **B,** CT scan demonstrates extent of the tumor. **C,** Design of the radial forearm free flap including the palmaris longus tendon for reconstruction of the lower lip. **D,** Design of the fibular free flap for the reconstruction of the mandible and anterior floor of the mouth. **E,** Resection of the tumor and bilateral neck dissection. **F,** Radial forearm free flap. **G,** Fibular free flap fashioned for mandibular and intraoral reconstruction. **H,** Immediately postoperative. Vermilion reconstruction is undertaken at a later date.

UPPER LIP RECONSTRUCTION

Upper lip defects are less common than lower lip problems. There are several features unique to the upper lip that must be considered in repair and reconstruction. The presence of central structures, namely the nose, columella, Cupid's bow, and philtrum, makes it more challenging to close defects without distortion of the mouth. The problem must be approached differently for men and women. In men, the upper lip is hairbearing and local nasolabial and cheek flaps provide cosmetically inferior results as the nonhairbearing area becomes more demarcated late in the day, virtually outlined by the hairbearing area. This is especially noticeable in dark-haired patients. On the other hand, men can hide upper lip reconstructive scars with a mustache. The upper lip's role in oral competence is significantly less than the lower lip. Thus regional and distant flap reconstructions of the upper lip may provide more acceptable functional results than comparable procedures for the lower lip (Figure 75-19).

Small Defects (less than one third of the upper lip)

Primary closure of small upper lip defects tends to yield the most satisfactory results. When more laterally positioned, the

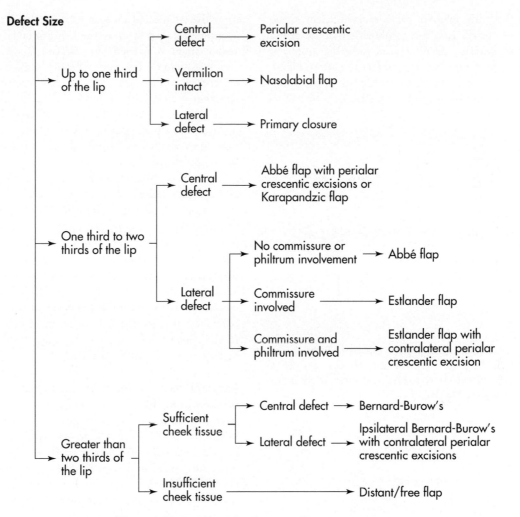

Defect Size

Up to one third of the lip
- Central defect → Perialar crescentic excision
- Vermilion intact → Nasolabial flap
- Lateral defect → Primary closure

One third to two thirds of the lip
- Central defect → Abbé flap with perialar crescentic excisions or Karapandzic flap
- Lateral defect
  - No commissure or philtrum involvement → Abbé flap
  - Commissure involved → Estlander flap
  - Commissure and philtrum involved → Estlander flap with contralateral perialar crescentic excision

Greater than two thirds of the lip
- Sufficient cheek tissue
  - Central defect → Bernard-Burow's
  - Lateral defect → Ipsilateral Bernard-Burow's with contralateral perialar crescentic excisions
- Insufficient cheek tissue → Distant/free flap

Figure 75-19. Algorithm for upper lip reconstruction.

incision may be tapered into the nasolabial fold (see Figure 75-9, *C*). The medially positioned philtral defect can be closed primarily but requires perialar crescentic skin excisions and release of upper buccal sulcus to allow medial advancement of the lip tissue (Figure 75-20). The principle of this operation is similar to that of excision of Burow's triangles: to create room for flap advancement. However, in this case the area to be excised is shaped such that it conforms to the alar base. The excision involves skin and subcutaneous tissue. The lip tissue is then advanced medially and repaired in three layers. Naturally, with a central defect the philtral groove is lost, and there is flattening of the vermilion centrally due to the absence of Cupid's bow. In men, this deficit may easily be concealed with a mustache.

When the defect involves only the upper lip tissue, not the vermilion, a nasolabial flap from the ipsilateral side is used to fill the defect. The flap is either superiorly or inferiorly based and is rotated into place from a position adjacent to the defect. The flap layers contain skin and subcutaneous tissue. The donor site is closed primarily along the nasolabial fold.

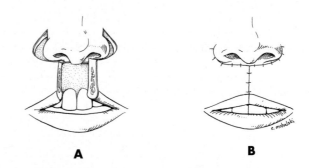

A   **B**

Figure 75-20. Perialar crescentic excisions. **A,** In continuity with the midupper lip defect, full-thickness perialar skin is resected. **B,** After the medial advancement of the upper lip flaps, three-layer closure is achieved. The site of the perialar crescentic excision is repaired in a single layer. (Courtesy Evelyn K. Mohalski.)

Medium Defects (one third to two thirds of the upper lip)

When located centrally, the medium-sized defect may be amenable to primary closure after perialar crescentic excisions. However, when the defect spans more than one half of the central upper lip, this method provides insufficient tissue mobilization. In such a case the combination of crescentic perialar excisions with a centrally placed Abbé flap from the lower lip would provide the best reconstructive option (Figure 75-21). Some surgeons use the Karapandzic flap of the upper lip as an alternative; in this method, it is generally sufficient to

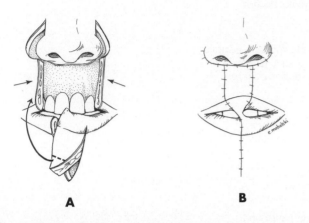

Figure 75-21. Combination of perialar crescentic excision and central Abbé flap. **A,** Flap elevation and perialar crescentic excisions. **B,** The flap pedicle is divided and inset at about 14 days. (Courtesy Evelyn K. Mohalski.)

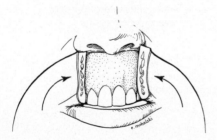

Figure 75-22. Upper lip Karapandzic flap. The incision allows medial mobilization of the flap, which must have the same width as the defect height. As with the lower lip Karapandzic flap, the neurovascular pedicle on either side must be identified and preserved. (Courtesy Evelyn K. Mohalski.)

carry the circumoral incision to the level of the commissures (Figure 75-22), preserving the neurovascular pedicle. If more advancement is needed, the incision is carried around the commissure to the lower lip. This method is less desirable than the combination of crescentic perialar excisions and the Abbé flap, which creates less distortion of the mouth and produces more acceptable scarring. Because of the laxity of the lower lip, relatively more tissue can be borrowed for upper lip reconstruction than is available where the upper lip is used to reconstruct lower lip defects.

Laterally positioned medium-sized defects must be considered in the context of presence or absence of commissure involvement. When the commissure is not involved, an Abbé flap from the lower lip may be rotated up into the defect. Thus the normal commissures are preserved. When the commissure is involved, an Estlander flap from the ipsilateral lower lip is designed, as described, and rotated up into the defect (Figure 75-23). If the defect involves the philtrum, then perialar crescentic excisions on the contralateral side may be used in combination to gain advancement of the remaining lip tissue. In the presence of the philtrum, this would be a distorting maneuver and should be avoided.

Large Defects (more than two thirds of the upper lip)

Reconstruction of large upper lip defects is associated with less functional morbidity than that seen with the same size defects of the lower lip. In part, gravity is responsible for this difference, since oral contents are in the lower half of the mouth. An insensate lower lip therefore is much more likely to result in drooling and inadequate oral competence.

In cases where the upper lip loss involves most or all of the upper lip tissue, new lip must be reconstructed. Use of the existing lip tissue alone for reconstruction would result in significant microstomia. When there is no deficiency of adjacent cheek tissue, the method of choice is an inverted Bernard-Burow's procedure (Figure 75-24). The upper lip defect is replaced with midcheek tissue. Burow's triangles are excised lateral to the lower lip, on both sides, and lateral to each alar base. The triangular excisions involve only skin and

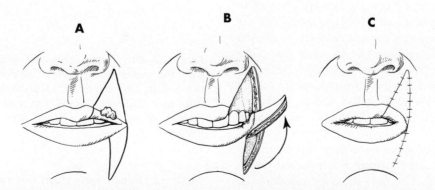

Figure 75-23. Estlander flap for upper lip reconstruction. **A,** The lower lip flap is designed to be no more than one half the size of the upper lip defect. **B,** The flap is rotated about the vermilion, which harbors its blood supply by the contralateral labial artery. **C,** Three-layer closure of the inset flap and donor site. The new commissure is rounded. (Courtesy Evelyn K. Mohalski.)

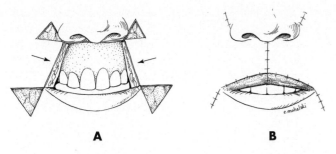

Figure 75-24. Upper lip Bernard-Burow's procedure. **A,** Burow's skin triangles are resected lateral to the alar bases and the lower lip. **B,** Upper cheek flaps are advanced medially to reconstitute the lip tissue, and vermilion is reconstructed from buccal mucosa. (Courtesy Evelyn K. Mohalski.)

subcutaneous tissue. The remaining orbicularis muscle is not violated. The cheek tissue is then advanced medially to create the new upper lip. Vermilion reconstruction is undertaken using mucosa from the advanced cheek flaps. If the defect is more lateral, a unilateral upper lip Bernard-Burow's procedure combined with contralateral perialar crescentic excision would provide adequate closure.

Rarely, major cancer ablation surgery or trauma may result in inadequate adjacent cheek tissue for reconstruction. In such cases, the option of a distant pedicle flap or free flap reconstruction must be considered.

OUTCOMES

The data on outcomes in reconstructive lip surgery remain limited. The greatest body of knowledge is scattered among various publications, with a heavy reliance on personal experience. Randomized prospective studies have not yet been undertaken to evaluate and compare the various techniques described for lip reconstruction. The greatest void in lip surgery outcome research is in the areas of functional limitations, patient's quality of life, and body image postoperatively. In addition, the long-term costs associated with each procedure have not been studied.

BIBLIOGRAPHY

1. Baker SR, Swanson NA: *Local flaps in facial reconstruction,* St Louis, 1995, Mosby-Year Book.
2. Esmarch F, von Kowalzig E: *Chirugische technik,* Kiel, 1982, Lipsius and Tischer.
3. Freeman BS: Myoplastic modification of the Bernard cheiloplasty, *Plast Reconstr Surg* 21:453, 1958.
4. Goldstein MH: A tissue expanding vermilion myocutaneous flap for lip repair, *Plast Reconst Surg* 73:768, 1984.
5. Karapandzic M: Reconstruction of lip defects by local arterial flaps, *Br J Plast Surg* 27:93, 1974.
6. Kawamoto HK: Correction of major defects of the vermilion with a cross lip vermilion flap, *Plast Reconstr Surg* 64:315, 1979.
7. Lindqvist C, Teppo L: Is upper lip cancer "true" lip cancer? *J Cancer Res Clin Oncol* 97:187-191, 1980.
8. Luce EA: Reconstruction of the lower lip, *Clin Plast Surg* 22:1, 109, 1995.
9. Mazzola RF, Lupo G: Evolving concepts in lip reconstruction, *Clin Plast Surg* 11:583, 1984.
10. Rice DH, Spiro RH: General management guidelines. In *Current concepts in head and neck cancer,* Atlanta, 1989, The American Cancer Society, pp 1-15.
11. Smith JW: The anatomical and physiologic acclimatization of tissue transplanted by the lip switch technique, *Plast Reconstr Surg* 26:40, 1960.
12. Webster RC, Coffey RJ, Kelleher RE: Total and partial reconstruction of the lower lip with innervated muscle-bearing flaps, *Plast Reconstr Surg* 25:360, 1960.
13. Wilson JSP, Walker EP: Reconstruction of the lower lip, *Head Neck Surg* 4:29, 1981.
14. Zitsch RP: Carcinoma of the lip, *Otolaryngol Clin North Am,* 26:2, 1993.

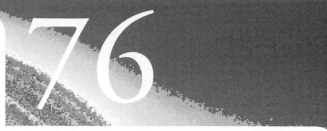

CHAPTER 76

The Oral Cavity

Mark D. DeLacure
M. Abraham Kuriakose

INDICATIONS

THE PROBLEM

The oral cavity is the most common site for malignancies of the head and neck region (about 30%), with the tongue and floor of mouth the most frequent primary sites. Squamous cell carcinoma is the most common histologic type of oral malignancy, representing over 90% of such cases. Over 30,000 new cases of oral cavity cancer and over 8,000 deaths due to disease occur each year. Due in large part to the changing demographics of our population (women >65 years now outnumber men >65 years) and to the increased incidence of smoking among women over the past 3 decades, a male : female ratio of 6 : 1 has become 2 : 1. The current popularity of cigar chic and the prevalence of smoking among teens will further impact these statistics for years to come.

Despite the oral cavity's relative accessibility to direct examination and the recognition of definite risk factors for the development of malignancy, failure to seek treatment and delay in diagnosis (averaging 5 months) are not uncommon due to the nonspecificity of signs and symptoms of disease. Nearly half of all patients will present with advanced disease and about one third will present with cervical metastasis. The successful treatment of an index oral cavity malignancy will be followed by a second primary upper aerodigestive tract cancer in up to one third of patients.

The structures constituting the oral cavity are diverse and represent a complex interplay of form and function. Mastication, deglutition, articulation of speech, respiration, special sensory function, and facial expression are all considerations because the components of the oral cavity are intimately organized in a confined space. Any therapeutic intervention therefore has the potential to profoundly disrupt these critically interrelated aspects of function and aesthetics with devastating impact. Refinements in reconstructive techniques, due in large part to the application of free microneurovascular tissue transfer, have revolutionized our ability to restore meaningful form and function for this historically challenging group of patients. Simultaneous advances in precise techniques of resection, access osteotomies, mandibular conservation, and selective modifications of classic neck dissection techniques have facilitated reconstructive progress.

ANATOMIC CONSIDERATIONS (Figure 76-1)

The oral cavity is subdivided into several subsites. The upper and lower *lips,* extending from the skin-vermilion junction to that portion of mucosa in direct contact with the opposing lip, are joined together laterally at the oral commissures. The *buccal mucosa* includes all of the mucosal surface covering the inner surface of the cheeks and lips from the line of contact of the opposing lips to the line of attachment of the mucosa to the alveolar ridges and pterygomandibular raphe. It is pierced by the Stensen's (parotid) duct adjacent to the second maxillary molar tooth. The *lower (mandibular) alveolar ridge* is formed by the alveolar process of the mandible and includes its attached gingival mucosa from the gingivobuccal gutter to the line of free mucosa of the floor of the mouth. Posteriorly, it ascends with the vertical ramus of the mandible, where it is subdivided into the retromolar trigone. The *retromolar trigone* is the attached mucosa overlying the ascending ramus of the mandible from the posterior aspect of the last molar tooth as its base to the apex at the maxillary tuberosity superiorly. The *upper (maxillary) alveolar ridge* is the attached mucosa overlying the maxillary alveolus from the gingivobuccal gutter laterally to the hard palate medially. The posterior limit is the maxillary tuberosity. The *hard palate* includes the mucosa covering the semilunar area bounded by the maxillary alveolar ridges and that which covers the palatine processes of the maxilla posteriorly, represented by the junction of the hard and soft palate. The *floor of the mouth* extends from the junction of the attached gingiva of the mandibular alveolus to the ventral surface of the tongue. It overlies the mylohyoid and hyoglossus muscles, which form a muscular diaphragm, and the sublingual glands and ducts. It is pierced in the midline by Wharton's or submandibular gland ducts, and is divided in the midline by the lingual frenulum. The *anterior (oral) tongue* (anterior two-thirds) is defined posteriorly by the V-shaped circumvallate papillae and extends anteriorly to the tip. It extends laterally around its border to join the floor of mouth mucosa ventrally. The dorsum of the tongue is villous, the ventral aspect nonvillous. This portion of the tongue is freely mobile and is also referred to as the mobile tongue.

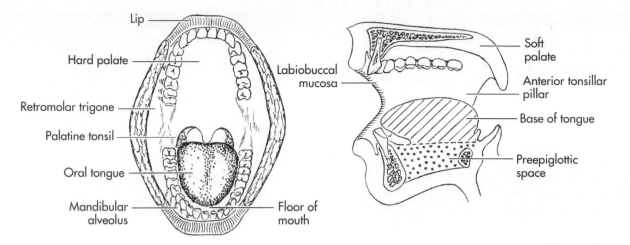

Figure 76-1. Anatomic subsites of oral cavity.

SPECIFIC SUBSITE CONSIDERATIONS

Hard Palate

Carcinoma of the mucosa overlying the hard palate is rare in the United States. Because of the variety of pathologic conditions that might mimic malignant tumors of this region and the different therapeutic approaches each entails, biopsy review is of particular importance. Necrotizing sialometaplasia and pseudoepitheliomatous hyperplasia may provide a diagnostic challenge. Early malignancy may present as a painless mass, progressing to a bleeding, painful, ulcerative one, with poor denture fit or loosening of native dental structures. Trismus may signify posterolateral extension into the pterygoid musculature. Primary T stage appears to be the determinant of long-term prognosis for this subsite.

Alveolar Ridge

Tumors of the alveolar ridge may result in change in denture fit or loosening of native teeth, associated with pain and bleeding, and are more common in the mandibular gingiva. Occult metastasis rate is low; therefore elective neck treatment is usually not indicated for early stage lesions, although advanced tumors will usually mandate neck treatment. A high level (up to 50%) of mandibular invasion has been noted and is more common in edentulous patients.

Retromolar Trigone

Primary tumors of the retromolar trigone may easily invade adjacent structures such as tonsil, soft palate, mandible, and tongue base, therefore behaving more like an aggressive pharyngeal primary. Direct extension into the pterygopalatine fossa may lead to failure at the skull base. Presentation is often that of a nonhealing ulceration associated with trismus, local pain, and referred otalgia. Local control is a significant problem with advanced tumors of this region.

Floor of Mouth

Primary tumors of the floor of mouth are often silent until assuming significant dimension. Extension onto the ventral surface of the tongue may result in restriction of motion and dysarthria. Extension through the sublingual space may allow advancement into the level I neck. The lingual nerve is at risk for direct involvement and perineural spread of disease. These tumors may abut the mandibular periosteum. The propensity for occult, and potential for bilateral, cervical metastasis warrants the consideration of elective treatment of the neck(s) more often than not in these cases.

Buccal Mucosa

Lesions of the buccal mucosa are noted for their aggressive metastatic potential and for the capability to extensively involve deeper structures. Posterior involvement may include parotid gland and pterygoid musculature. Extension onto the maxillary and/or mandibular alveolus is common. It is notable that cancers of this subsite more commonly arise from a background of leukoplakic change than other oral cavity sites.

Oral Tongue

The intrinsic musculature of the tongue provides little barrier to direct invasion and extension onto adjacent structures such as the floor of mouth, tonsillar pillar, and mandible. A nonhealing, painless ulcer progresses, often to considerable size, before becoming symptomatic with pain, referred otalgia, and dysarthria. A tendency to undertreat both the primary site and the necks must be resisted. Tumors requiring total glossectomy or its functional equivalent should be entered on organ preservation protocols. Neck failure, regardless of T stage, is common.

Lip

Lip cancers tend to present early due to their conspicuous location, typically as a nonhealing ulcerated mass remaining localized until advanced stage. The potential for mandibular invasion and for extension along the mental nerve into the inferior alveolar canal must be recognized in advanced lesions.

Miscellaneous

The entire mucosal lining of the oral cavity is stratified squamous epithelium. The submucosa has between 450 and

750 minor salivary glands scattered throughout the oral cavity, but concentrated in the palatal region. Malignant tumors of the minor salivary glands therefore may appear as submucosal swellings covered by a normal-appearing mucosa, in contrast to the more common ragged, ulcerative, and friable squamous cell carcinoma. Firm swellings of the hard palate and of the lingual aspect of the mandibular premolar region are normal variant hamartomas and are called torus palatinus and torus mandibularis, respectively. These are also covered by normal mucosa and are removed only to facilitate prosthodontic rehabilitation. The loss of vertical mandibular height as the alveolar process resorbs in the edentulous state brings the genial tubercles into palpatory range, and these are not to be confused with abnormality. This resorptive process also brings the inferior alveolar neurovascular bundle into a more submucosal position, allowing a route of mandibular entry for malignancies involving the overlying mucosa and rendering the structures vulnerable to surgical injury in other regional procedures. In the elderly atrophic mandible, blood supply is reversed in flow from the formerly physiologically dominant endosteal supply of the inferior alveolar vessels to periosteal perfusion from the multiple muscular attachments to the bone. Extensive periosteal dissection, especially in the irradiated edentulous mandible, may therefore significantly impair the healing of bone, lead to osteoradionecrosis, and/or pathologic fracture. Submucosal sialoliths may be palpable in the floor of mouth. The propensity for stone disease to present here is due to several factors including the ductal course superiorly (against gravity) around the posterior border of the hyoglossus muscle, and the different composition of its saliva (more mucus, higher mineral content, different pH). A desire to remove these stones per orally must be resisted because of the propensity for damage to the lingual nerve in such approaches.

Innervation

The intrinsic musculature is motored by the hypoglossal (CN XII) nerve. General sensation to the anterior two thirds of the tongue is via the lingual (CN V3) nerve, and special sensation (taste) by the chorda tympani (CN VII) nerve branches, which accompany the lingual nerve. Palatal sensibility is subserved by the greater palatine (CN V2) nerve. Sensory supply to the lips and anterior buccal mucosa is provided by the mental nerves (CN V3). Buccal sensory supply is via the long buccal nerves (CN V3). Dental structures and attached gingival mucosa are subserved by the anterior and posterior alveolar (CN V2) and inferior alveolar (CN V3) nerves.

Lymphatic Drainage

The oral cavity is subserved by a rich lymphatic drainage system. In previously untreated patients, a generally predictable and orderly pattern of spread is observed. First echelon drainage includes primarily levels I, II, and III, depending on subsite location of the primary lesion. Lesions of the lip, anterior floor of the mouth, oral tongue, and vestibule commonly drain first through this region. Level II is the primary target for more posteriorly located lesions within the oral cavity. Level III nodes include those between the carotid

bifurcation and the superior belly of the omohyoid muscle as it crosses the internal jugular vein. Bilateral lymphatic channels as well as direct pathways to the level IV and contralateral neck have been described and must be considered depending on T stage and subsite of tumor.[6] Level IV and, particularly, level V nodes tend to be involved, however, only with multiple levels of metastasis.[9] Ulcerated primaries in the septic oral environment may present diagnostic difficulty, with inflammatory adenopathy being a common and potentially confusing finding clinically and intraoperatively.

PATHOLOGY

Squamous Cell Carcinoma

Squamous cell carcinoma represents over 90% of all oral cavity malignancies. This distribution holds true for all subsites.

Nonsquamous Cancer

Extranodal non-Hodgkins lymphoma is the most common lymphomatous presentation in head and neck sites, yet it is a rarity. It may be associated with acquired immunodeficiency syndrome (AIDS) and must be differentiated from malignant melanoma and anaplastic carcinoma as well as benign lymphoepithelial processes. The palate and gingiva are the most commonly involved oral cavity sites, usually presenting as a painless mass.

Mucosal Malignant Melanoma

Mucosal malignant melanoma may represent up to 8% of all melanomas. Unlike its cutaneous counterpart, it is not related to actinic exposure. Preexisting benign melanosis is present in about one third of cases. In order of frequency of subsite involvement, the palate is followed by maxillary gingiva, buccal mucosa, mandibular gingiva, lip, tongue, and floor of mouth. Typical presentation includes swelling, ulceration, loosening of the teeth, and pain. Differential diagnosis includes metastatic *cutaneous* melanoma (tonsil, tongue, buccal mucosa), benign melanosis, amalgam tattoo, nevus, vascular malformation, and Kaposi's sarcoma. Structural differences between mucosa and skin do not allow prognostic histologic staging (Clark, Breslow).

About 80% of all minor salivary gland tumors of the oral cavity are malignant, with *adenoid cystic carcinoma* the most common histologic subtype (about 42%) (Box 76-1). Adenoid cystic carcinoma is characterized by its slow growth and a propensity for perineural invasion (trigeminal-inferior alveolar, lingual), which are associated with distant metastasis, long *apparent* disease-free interval, and ultimate skull base failure. *Mucoepidermoid carcinoma* is also observed in the oral cavity.

Half of patients with AIDS-related *Kaposi's sarcomas* will have oral cavity involvement. This tumor is slow-growing and begins as an asymptomatic discolored lesion, progressing to a bleeding, ulcerated tumor. Palatal involvement is followed by gingival and tongue sites.

Box 76-1.
Epithelial and Mesenchymal Tumors Affecting the Oral Cavity or Its Adnexa

---

SQUAMOUS CELL CARCINOMA
Undifferentiated carcinoma (transitional, spindle cell)
Differentiated carcinoma
Adenoid squamous carcinoma
Verrucous carcinoma

BASAL CELL CARCINOMA
MALIGNANT MELANOMA
CARCINOMAS OF GLANDULAR ORIGIN
Adenocarcinoma
Mucoepidermoid carcinoma
Adenoid cystic carcinoma
Acinic cell carcinoma
Undifferentiated carcinoma

SARCOMA
FIBROSARCOMA
Rhabdomyosarcoma
Osteogenic sarcoma
Chondrosarcoma
Neurogenic sarcoma
Angiosarcoma
Synovial cell sarcoma

HODGKIN'S AND NON-HODGKIN'S
 LYMPHOMAS
EXTRAMEDULLARY PLASMACYTOMA,
 MULTIPLE MYELOMA
LEUKEMIAS
METASTATIC CARCINOMA, SARCOMAS

ETIOLOGY

Lip malignancies are most related to actinic exposure (a pigmented layer is lacking in Caucasian races), although chronic irritation (pipe smokers–heat; cigars, smokeless tobacco) may also play a role. A classic promoter-initiator sequence is believed to underlie most oral cavity malignancies, with ethanol serving as a direct mucosal irritant (promoter or co-carcinogen) and tobacco carcinogens playing the initiator role. Nitrosamines intrinsic to tobacco act through point mutation of DNA molecules, creating malignant degeneration through alteration of tumor suppressor, oncogene, and autocrine growth factor expression. Areas of anatomic dependency—gingivobuccal and gingivolingual sulci and floor of mouth—concentrate these substances and may explain a higher frequency distribution of tumors in these areas through a prolonged direct contact mechanism. Subsite specificity may be observed for each agent, with smoking relatively more frequent in palate lesions, and alcohol more related to tongue and floor of mouth primaries.

A dose-response relationship has been observed in epidemiologic studies of carcinogenesis. About 90% of patients with cancer of the oral cavity are smokers, with an increased relative risk of about six times that of nonsmokers. The recent popularity of smokeless tobaccos, particularly among youth, has resulted in an increased prevalence of disease of the mandibular alveolus and buccal mucosa where the material is retained, and a four-times relative risk increase for the development of malignant oral cavity disease. About 80% of individuals presenting with oral cavity malignancy consume alcohol, with an observed six times increased relative risk. The combination of alcohol and tobacco consumption synergistically (not simply additively) increases relative risk of oral cavity malignancy to 15 times that of individuals with neither habit. Other factors *suggested* have included poor oral hygiene, poorly fitting dental appliances, viral infection, chronic mouthwash usage, nutritional deficiency, occupation, and ethnic custom (betel nut chewing, reversed smoking). The phenomenon of *field cancerization* or condemned mucosa, in which multiple synchronous or metachronous cancers develop in a background of dysplastic changes seen *throughout* the wide epithelial field of the upper aerodigestive tract, underlines principles of etiology.

Preexisting fields of leukoplakia and erythroplakia are common, with the latter believed to represent a more premalignant state. Leukoplakia is clinically defined as a white keratotic plaque that cannot be removed by rubbing. It may be confused with lichen planus and candidiasis. Histologically, these regions may represent hyperkeratosis, parakeratosis, acanthosis, or dysplastic change. An unjustified emphasis on leukoplakia (fewer than 6% are eventually diagnosed as cancer) persists and is confusing given the prevalence of such areas in this patient population. In fact, most lesions are mixed, the erythroplastic component the most significant. Erythroplasia must, however, be distinguished from obvious mechanical and inflammatory mucosal irritation. Verrucous hyperplasia is an irreversible leukoplakic condition virtually indistinguishable from verrucous carcinoma most commonly involving mandibular alveolar gingiva and mucosa, and less commonly buccal, lingual, and floor of mouth mucosa. Exophytic and endophytic tumor components are characteristic, particularly in larger squamous tumors.

Squamous cell carcinomas tend to grow along mucosal surfaces in early stages, typically extending into underlying musculature and bone in later stages. In the edentulous state, direct extension into the alveolus via tooth sockets is common. In contrast, minor salivary gland malignancies tend to present with intact overlying mucosa (unless traumatized or advanced), beginning as firm, painless masses.

Second primary malignancies occur most frequently in individuals with a history of an oral cavity index malignancy (14%). These geographically distinct cancers tie together the concepts of field cancerization, condemned mucosa, and the spectrum of premalignant mucosal change. The risk of development of such tumors is about 4% to 6% per annum, leveling off at about 5 years, with most second primaries detected within 2 years of discovery of the index lesion. Metachronous primary malignancies (hypopharynx, lung, larynx, oropharynx, esophagus) are the chief causes of treatment failure and death in patients who have presented with controlled index disease, and underline the need for continued surveillance of this population for an indefinite period. Ongoing risk factors (smoking, alcohol consumption) are *not* required for this phenomenon.

INFORMED CONSENT

The ability of the residual normal structures of the oral cavity to compensate for those removed in the treatment of malignant neoplastic disease is remarkable, so the surgical resection of small lesions (T1, T2) results in negligible functional derangement. It is difficult, however, for patients, particularly with advanced stage disease, to fully understand the profound impact of treatment on the structures of this region, despite the best efforts to prepare them. Those who are more motivated, youthful, and more highly educated seem to adapt best to such morbidity. Although major surgical resections most profoundly affect this region, primary curative-intent or postoperative adjuvant external beam radiotherapy may have a devastating impact on function because of xerostomia, fibrosis of the thin mucosa, and effect on the muscles of the oral cavity and pharynx, with significant resultant swallowing disability.

Access incisions, particularly midline lip-splitting and those of the soft palate, may cause problems with appearance or velopharyngeal incompetence. Submandibular incisions for submandibular gland and level I access may result in temporary or permanent lesions of the marginal mandibular branch of the facial nerve if not properly executed.

Loss of major *sensory* nerves such as the lingual and mental results in anesthesia of the anterior one third of the tongue and of the lower lip and chin, respectively. In general, sacrifice of the lingual nerve involves resection of the end organ, and this diminishes its impact over other considerations. Mandibulectomy or lateral mandibulotomy procedures that interrupt the inferior alveolar nerve in the mandibular canal on the mental nerve cause lower lip anesthesia and inability to sense and therefore control saliva, with resultant drooling. Both nerve lesions are the targets of refinements in functional restoration procedures such as the sensate radial forearm free flap for tongue (via medial and/or lateral antebrachial cutaneous nerves) and floor of mouth reconstruction, and the sensate fibula free flap (via the sural cutaneous nerve) for mandibular reconstruction. Despite our ability to restore touch, pressure, and thermal sensibility, the functional result is usually somewhat deficient.

Motor nerve lesions pertinent to surgery of the oral cavity include the facial and hypoglossal nerves. Damage to the marginal mandibular and buccal branch results from trauma or its resection for oncologic reasons. The impact of these lesions may be minimized through the postoperative use of chemo-denervative Botox injections into the normally functioning contralateral musculature for restoration of symmetry. Studies of the impact of lesions of the hypoglossal nerve[7] have shown that approximately 25% experience profound functional impact, 53% little impact, and 22% no notable functional deficit. This nerve may be injured in submandibular procedures and is a commonly excised structure in extended neck dissection procedures, particularly in previously treated patients.

Resection of the tongue usually causes profound derangement of articulatory and swallowing function. Resections of up to about one third of the oral tongue may be closed primarily with little functional loss. Larger lesions are addressed with skin graft or sensate radial forearm reconstructions, the key goals being the maintenance of mobility of the residual motored native tongue. Descriptions of elegant adaptations of tongue flaps to head and neck defects are largely of historical importance and are now generally to be avoided. Swallowing function can be remarkable even in those with three quarters of their tongue base and entire oral tongue resected. Studies of treatment of the tongue base have emphasized the role of combined brachytherapy and external beam radiotherapy in the achievement of superior functional outcomes.[15] Midline labiomandibulotomy incisions for access to the craniocervical junction should have little ultimate functional impact.

The disruption of mandibular continuity may affect occlusion in dentate patients despite the level of sophistication of current osteosynthesis systems. Despite the profound advancement in mandibular reconstruction provided by osteomyocutaneous free tissue transfer and the ability to achieve excellent skeletal results, function in patients requiring these techniques is still impaired. This is determined more by the associated soft tissue resection, particularly the amount of tongue, than the mandible section itself.[27] Only a minority of patients achieve full osseointegrated implant rehabilitation, and even they sometimes exhibit severe functional derangement. The role of subsequent refinement procedures (e.g., vestibuloplasty, implant exposure) must be understood to attain the best patient outcomes.

Postoperative reliance on prosthodontic devices in cases of maxillary surgery is significant in terms of both function and maintenance. Patients must be able to manipulate and clean these on a daily basis. These prosthetics represent large insensate areas in many and require considerable adaptation and acclimation.[8]

Donor site morbidity for individual grafts and flaps should receive equal emphasis in discussions of informed consent for oromandibular defects. Failure to adequately document informed consent may expose the practitioner to increased medical malpractice liability in this country. Time and effort invested here is critical not only for the development of the surgeon-patient relationship and the definition of reasonable treatment outcomes, but also to diminish threat of legal action. This is particularly true for patients with poor prognosis and significant treatment-related morbidity as compensatory capabilities of both patients and their families often unravel as complications mount and treatment failure and impending death approach.

NATURAL HISTORY

The natural history of untreated disease of the oral cavity typically begins as a small nonhealing exophytic and ulcerative lesion, which progressively increases in size and becomes exquisitely painful. *Fetor oris,* foul-smelling breath, follows as oral sepsis and necrotic tumor intermingle. Surface bleeding and the development of cervical adenopathy (inflammatory and/or metastatic) are also common. Referred pain to areas subserved by the same sensory afferent input can be confusing to patients and unsuspecting clinicians alike. This most commonly occurs via the auricular nerve of Arnold, a branch of CN X, and the tympanic nerve of Jacobson, a branch of CN IX, through irritation by malignant involvement of these branches, and is distributed at the level of the pharyngeal plexus. Despite lateralizing ear pain, the otoscopic examination is normal. Progression of disease is followed by mandibular involvement with exfoliation of teeth as bone destruction progresses.

Deep tumor invasion through the floor of the mouth and mylohyoid diaphragm may result in malignant nodules in the submental skin and/or malignant orocutaneous fistulization. Deep posterior involvement of tongue root musculature will result in restriction of mobility and dysarthria. As tumor volume increases posteriorly, a muffled or "hot potato" vocal quality ensues. The ability to maintain adequate peroral alimentation becomes severely compromised. With further increase in size, breathing becomes threatened. Intense and unremitting cranial neuropathic pain becomes a constant feature of this disease because it involves the many major afferent sensory nerves subserving the oral cavity. As neck disease progresses along with these features, ulceration and exposure of vital structures occur. Death is not uncommonly due to malnutrition, major vascular catastrophe, and/or airway obstruction and inability to handle one's own secretions. Although this end-stage presentation is rare, it is still not an infrequent occurrence in major medical centers in this country. Palliative-intent procedures aimed at securing a safe airway, the relief of bleeding and necrotic tumor and odor, the control of neuropathic pain, and the control of ulcerating, draining, and fistulizing soft tissues are humane and justifiable surgical endeavors, occasionally producing a long-term and grateful survivor.[4] Such efforts will undoubtedly profoundly impact *quality of life,* if not quantity of life, with the reliability of current reconstructive techniques minimizing days-of-life lost.

COMPLICATIONS

Complications must be distinguished from expected sequelae of resections involving this region. Soft tissue complications include dehiscence of closures, including flap interfaces that are generally handled conservatively with antibiotic mouth rinses[18] and secondary-intent wound healing. Fistulization may accompany any full-thickness procedure and is a significant morbidity. These are also managed conservatively, with only rare cases requiring surgical intervention. Time to closure may take months. Fistulas are more common in previously treated patients and in postradiotherapy contexts. Concern over vascular blowout catastrophes in the context of fistulization may be focused on those cases with active salivary flow over circumferentially dissected and exposed and potentially desiccated vessels. Loss of skin graft reconstructions are managed conservatively, since underlying muscle surfaces will

remucosalize,[1] often with a result superior to other alternative linings.

At the skeletal level, complications may include nonunion, which is a rare event when appropriate attention to detail is paid to the selection and application of contemporary osteosynthesis systems. This event is more common in patients with co-morbid medical conditions (diabetes) and previous radiation histories. Debridement, bone grafting, and redo osteosynthesis are recommended. Disruption of mandibular hardware can generally be traced to the misapplication of systems intended for lighter biomechanical demands. Malocclusion is avoidable in dentate patients through the adherence to basic principles of rigid internal fixation based in fracture and orthognathic work. Pathologic fracture may follow conservation mandibulectomy procedures due to unbalanced biomechanical forces despite resection of the depressor and elevator muscles and overlying teeth. This is more common in the elderly patient who is previously operated and irradiated and who has significant co-morbid disease. This is avoidable through the placement of a reconstruction type plate across the segment as a load-sharing type construct. Locking screw plate designs are ideal here. Intraoral plate exposure may be managed conservatively with hygiene, antibiotic rinses, and/or hardware removal at an appropriate interval if skeletal stability has been achieved. Extraoral plate exposure will generally require local flap coverage and debridement of exposed bone.

ALTERNATIVE THERAPY

The management of smaller lesions (T1, T2) of the oral cavity remains primarily a surgical endeavor except for lesions of the tongue base and soft palate, which are in the radiotherapeutic domain. One of the determinants for the use of radiation therapy in this region is the proximity of the lesion to bone and the attendant risk of osteoradionecrosis. Therefore lesions of the alveolus and those approaching or involving bone are *not* selected for radiotherapy. Where there appears to be equivalent possibilities and outcomes, surgical therapy has generally offered a more efficient, single-event treatment episode with equal outcome in terms of disease control. Although cryotherapy has intrigued some in the treatment of oral cavity lesions, it appears to offer little advantage, in practice, over more standard treatment approaches. Photodynamic therapy may become a modality of choice for the future treatment of superficial dysplastic and in situ lesions as more selective dyes diminish residual and systemic photosensitivity, and as photodiagnosis becomes increasingly applied.

Larger oral cavity lesions usually require the combination of surgery and postoperative radiotherapy for appropriate management. Tumors with a significant incidence of occult cervical metastasis (>3- to 5-mm thickness) require staging neck dissection (supraomohyoid) in order to determine the need for more comprehensive treatment of the neck.[24] Tumors with manifest adenopathy require modified or radical dissections.

Radiation therapy (RT) is most commonly administered as external beam photons (deeper penetrating particles) or electrons (superficially penetrating). Typical fractions of 180 to 200 Gy/dose are administered Mondays through Fridays for 5 to 7 weeks to total tumor doses of 55 to 65 Gy. Hyperfractionation schemes appear to offer some advantage in selected clinical contexts. The intent of treatment may be curative in the case of smaller volume primary tumors, or adjuvant following surgical management of the primary tumor and/or neck disease. Split combined modality treatment mixes the context of treatment (e.g., postoperative adjuvant RT after neck dissection for bulky cervical adenopathy from a small volume primary tumor for which RT is primary curative intent). Indications for therapeutic irradiation include close or involved surgical margins, multiple adenopathy, and extracapsular extension of metastatic disease. Here, the addition of postoperative adjuvant RT can significantly impact success in the locoregional control of disease. Similarly, patients found to have involvement of margins on intraoperative frozen section analysis, subsequently rendered "negative" by wider excision, will exhibit increased local recurrence and benefit from postoperative adjuvant RT as well.[19] Although radiation therapy rarely cures a recurrence after initial surgery, "salvage" surgery of radiation failures is a critical concept in head and neck oncology. Complications and sequelae of therapeutic radiation to the head and neck may be significant and are both dose-related and idiosyncratic, and acute and chronic. There is a dangerous tendency to minimize these aspects of treatment-related morbidity on both the part of the patient considering this alternative and on the part of many therapists delivering this modality of treatment.

Chemotherapy remains noncurative for head and neck malignancies and still has not demonstrated improvement in survival. Its role in oral cavity malignancy is generally third-line, reserved for the palliative-intent treatment of patients with failure of surgery and radiation to control disease. Chemotherapy may be rationally applied in combined concurrent chemoradiation protocols for its radiosensitizing effect and in organ sparing (tongue, larynx) protocols as a neoadjuvant modality to predict the radiosensitivity of particular tumors.

GOALS OF SURGERY

Control of disease while maximizing function is the ultimate therapeutic goal, with cure generally declared at 5 years. For some patients, however, the personal and psychologic cost of attaining this goal seems greater than succumbing to the malignant disease itself. This was particularly true of head and neck patients in the premyocutaneous flap era. These aspects of care must be combined with judgment, sensitivity, respect, and the responsibility to provide truly informed consent in treating these unfortunate patients. The mere ability to successfully plan and execute the technical tour de force that we are capable of providing in contemporary head and neck surgery and reconstruction, however, is not in and of itself justification for an aggressive approach to many of our patients. Indeed, flap survival, the avoidance of fistulization, and even cure itself

may all be "soft" endpoints and measures of success in the management of this problem.

OPERATIONS

Recent developments and refinements of both ablative and reconstructive surgical technique have considerably diminished the morbidity of oral cancer treatment. The reliability of advanced microsurgical reconstructive techniques has facilitated the resectability of many tumors. The concept of immediate reconstruction has replaced the preexisting historical surgical dogma that delayed reconstruction held advantages in terms of clinical surveillance for recurrent disease. Advances in diagnostic imaging techniques have allowed us to further the concept of immediate reconstruction as the imaging characteristics of flap reconstructions have been characterized. The surgical management of head and neck cancer represents a truly multidisciplinary endeavor in which excision and reconstruction go hand in hand as the foundation for the approach to management of these tumors. It is through this collaborative and collegial approach that efficiency is realized in the effective delivery of care to this group of unfortunate patients.

SURGICAL TREATMENT APPROACHES TO ORAL CAVITY TUMORS

1. *Peroral excision* (Figure 76-2) is the approach of choice for smaller lesions that are easily accessible.
2. The *upper cheek flap* (Figure 76-3) is best for larger lesions involving the hard palate, maxillary alveolus, cheek mucosa, and retromolar trigone. The *lower cheek*

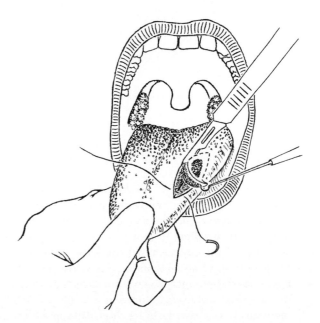

Figure 76-2. Peroral approach to partial glossectomy.

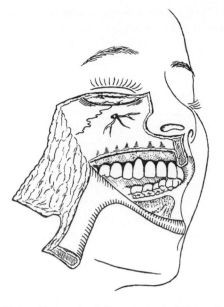

Figure 76-3. Upper cheek flap approach (Weber-Ferguson).

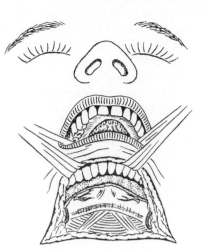

Figure 76-5. Visor flap.

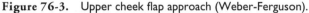

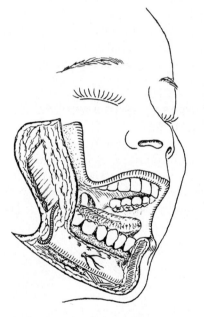

Figure 76-4. Lower cheek flap approach.

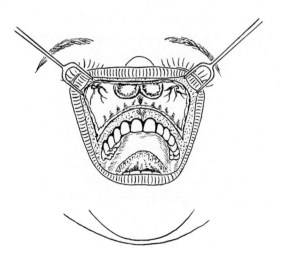

Figure 76-6. Midface degloving approach.

flap (Figure 76-4) is best for tongue, floor of mouth, mandibular gingiva, buccal mucosa, and retromolar trigone.

3. The *visor flap* (Figure 76-5) is most suitable for primary lesions of the anterior oral cavity, particularly floor of mouth, anterior mandibular alveolus, and anterior tongue with invasion of floor of mouth. The primary advantage of this approach over cheek flap techniques is the avoidance of an incisional scar over the lip and/or chin (lower). Both mental nerves are, however, sacrificed in the visor approach, rendering the lip and chin insensate. In contrast, the lower cheek flap approach will render only one side insensate. Relative devasculariza-

tion of the mandible is another important undesirable feature. The *midfacial degloving* (Figure 76-6) approach is visor type access for midfacial lesions, combining sublabial and intranasal rhinoplasty incisions without similar denervation issues to its lower counterpart.

4. *Mandibulotomy with paralingual extension* (Figure 76-7) is best suited to posteriorly located lesions that do not closely approximate or involve the mandible. Both mental nerves are spared. A lower lip and chin incision is requisite but usually is not of significant aesthetic impact in long-term follow-up. The lingual nerve should be identified and spared wherever possible. Refinements in technique have made paramedian osteotomies desirable

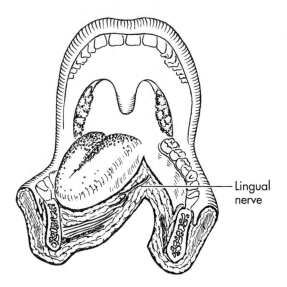

Figure 76-7. Mandibulotomy approach with paralingual extension.

Lingual nerve

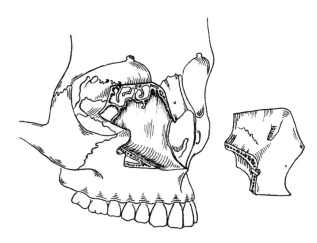

Figure 76-9. Subtotal maxillectomy.

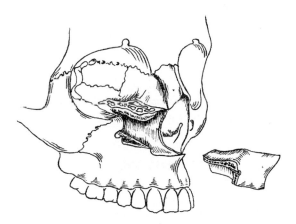

Figure 76-8. Medial maxillectomy.

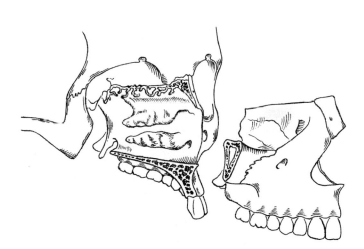

Figure 76-10. Total maxillectomy without orbital exenteration.

inasmuch as they cause less disruption to attached mandibular depressor and intrinsic tongue musculature. Reliable, low-profile, rigid internal osteosynthesis systems result in minimal occlusal complications and ensure primary bone healing.

5. In a *maxillectomy* (Figures 76-8 to 76-11), resection of the upper alveolus or hard palate tumors can be performed through a peroral or upper cheek flap approach.

Special considerations in the management of the mandible for cancer of the oral cavity have been recently reviewed by DeLacure.[10] The desire to limit the resection of bone to that which is absolutely required for oncologic reasons has prompted a number of studies on the patterns of tumor

invasion of the mandible. The selection of technique, however, remains heavily based in clinical assessment, experience, and judgment, despite recent advances in diagnostic imaging and reconstructive options. The two key factors that determine the pattern of invasion are dental status and previous therapeutic irradiation. Cases with frank bone invasion mandate segmental resection with margins of at least 1 cm proximally and distally. Marrow and/or inferior alveolar canal contents and periosteum should be submitted for intraoperative frozen section analysis of margins. Margins must be cleared prior to reconstruction. Specimen radiography is a simple and inexpensive adjunct to this technique for the assessment of margin adequacy. Contemporary microsurgical reconstructive techniques allow

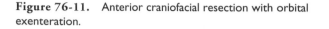

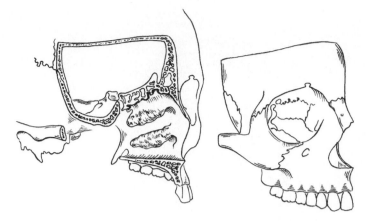

Figure 76-11. Anterior craniofacial resection with orbital exenteration.

surgeons to reconstruct even massive resections and should facilitate improved locoregional control and cure. Because locoregional recurrence frequently presents in associated soft tissues, particular attention should be paid to this aspect of the resective effort.

Lesions approaching the mandible with intervening normal-appearing mucosa, clinical mobility, and normal radiographic studies may be removed via conservation mandibulectomy. Any conservation technique must include the alveolus. Lesions more distant from the bone may be approached by stripping lingual periosteum as a lateral margin. With any technique, abnormal adherence of the periosteum or roughening of the cortical surface should be considered the bony response to malignant invasion, and more extensive bony and soft tissue resection is mandated. Previously irradiated mandibles demonstrate varied and unpredictable patterns of spread in terms of the surfaces involved and related soft tissue spread. In this context, the ability of the periosteum and attached musculature to resist malignant invasion is diminished considerably. Here there is no reliable way to assess early tumor invasion of bone, and segmental resections are appropriate. The dependence of such bone on its periosteal blood supply, in addition to chronic radiation damage, predisposes to later pathologic fracture when conservation techniques are applied.

The increased use of midline and subsequent paramedian mandibulotomy for resection of posteriorly located oral cavity, oropharyngeal, and skull base neoplasms parallels the development and application of techniques of rigid internal fixation osteosynthesis. Complex stairstep, dovetail joint, and zigzag osteotomy designs facilitated stability in the days of wire fixation, but are unnecessary today. Similarly, sagittal splitting techniques are unnecessarily complex.

Many incisional designs for the soft tissue lip-splitting aspect of the paramedian access mandibulotomy have been presented since the popularization of this technique.[22] It is, however, the authors' opinion that superior long-term aesthetic results are achieved through the use of a simple vertical midline incision with a vermilion junction or terminal horizontal zigzag to avoid retraction. Functional aspects of the soft tissue portion of lip-splitting incisional approaches include minimal disruption of the facial muscles and sensory nerve supply. This preserves orolabial competence, lip sensibility,

and mimetic function. Accurate reapproximation of incised tissues, preincisional marking of the vermilion-cutaneous junction, and resuspension of soft tissue components (chin pad, mentalis muscle) to avoid the "witch's chin" deformity and to provide adequate labial sulcular reconstitution all optimize functional results. Design of the intraoral mucosal component should avoid placing the suture line directly in the deepest aspect of the gingivolabial or gingivobuccal sulci where salivary pooling and local salivary contamination are maximal. Similarly, the development of limited mucosal flaps intraorally avoids placing suture lines directly over osteotomies and osteosynthesis hardware and preserves the sulcus anatomy to facilitate prosthetic dental rehabilitation and salivary retention. The vertical component of the lip incision is easily extended to join cervical incisions for neck dissection or vascular access. This aspect is best designed as a right angle joining the oblique submandibular incision at the level of the hyoid bone. Lower eyelid extensions of facial incisions for the performance of maxillectomy may be safely made transconjunctivally, minimizing the potential for lower eyelid malposition.

FACTORS INFLUENCING SELECTION OF THERAPY

Probability of Regional Metastasis

Overall, about 30% of patients with oral cavity malignancy will present with cervical metastasis on initial clinical examination, with some variation in frequency determined by primary site.

Lip, alveolar ridge, and hard palate primaries infrequently involve the neck (approximately 10% to 20% clinically), with a low occult rate of metastatic involvement. Elective treatment is usually unwarranted in early-stage disease in these subsites. The oral commissure is a more frequent site for subclinical metastasis, approximating 20%. The floor of mouth represents a more significant risk for nodal involvement (15% to 38%), as well as an increased potential for bilaterality. Lesions of the buccal mucosa and retromolar trigone are deceptively aggressive in metastatic potential and mandate neck treatment.

It is axiomatic that the oral tongue represents the most significant challenge in the treatment of oral cavity malig-

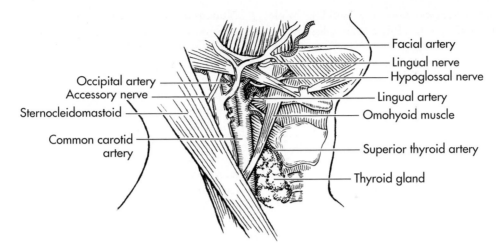

Figure 76-12. Supraomohyoid neck dissection.

nancy, with a distinctly different biologic behavior and capricious clinical course. The most common cause of treatment failure for this subsite is an underlying aggressive posture on the part of the initial therapist due to a failure to appreciate the predilection of oral tongue tumors to recur locally and metastasize regionally, despite *apparently adequate* initial therapy. Here, cervical metastasis occurs with a greater frequency than any other subsite within the oral cavity (up to 66% harbor occult disease and up to 50% eventually develop clinical neck involvement—even those presenting with low-stage lesions). Failure to control the neck is the most common cause of death from disease in this group. Traditional dogma that tumors more posteriorly located (base of tongue) are more aggressive than anteriorly disposed tumors (oral tongue) is incorrect.

Contemporary TNM staging fails to account for the "third dimension" or depth of tumor invasion, which has been correlated with likelihood of occult metastatic involvement of the neck. Although somewhat controversial, this parameter is sometimes used as a guideline for decision making with regard to elective neck treatment, a primary depth of 3 mm or greater (regardless of T stage) being the selection threshold. Vascular and perineural invasion may provide additional predictive information guiding treatment decisions. Studies of additional histologic parameters (differentiation, flow cytometry, cytogenetics, oncogene staining, photodynamic diagnosis) remain investigative, and hopefully the new era of molecular oncology will provide much needed tools to assist therapy design.

Survival rates for elective dissection of the clinically uninvolved, but pathologically positive, neck and for therapeutic dissection of the neck manifesting metastatic adenopathy discovered during surveillance are equivalent; therefore, *reliable* patients at low risk may be observed. Patients with moderate- to high-risk (some T2, all higher state primaries) necks should be sampled through ipsilateral or bilateral supraomohyoid neck dissection (Figure 76-12), which will clear regional lymph nodes at greatest risk (levels I to III), and if pathologically involved, will mandate additional therapy, usually adjuvant external beam radiotherapy or complete neck dissection. Clinically involved necks require comprehensive or modified radical neck dissection techniques.

SPECIFIC SUBSITE CONSIDERATIONS

Hard Palate
Peroral excision is possible for small primaries with secondary intention wound healing. Larger and more posterior tumors will require excision via formal maxillectomy. Skin graft, pedicled temporalis myofascial flap, or microvascular free tissue transfer reconstruction may be used to fill the ablative defect. Prosthodontic obturators have been historical reconstructive standards, although they are being increasingly scrutinized as methods of choice for large midface defects because of retention difficulty, unwieldiness, and large insensate surface area. Due to the relative sparsity of lymphatic drainage in this region, elective nodal treatment is unnecessary. Postoperative adjuvant external beam radiotherapy is indicated for advanced stage disease. Primary T stage appears to be the determinant of long-term prognosis for this subsite.

Alveolar Ridge and Retromolar Trigone
Peroral partial procedures may be used to remove the alveolar ridge, and traditional maxillectomy or mandibulectomy approaches may be chosen for larger tumors.

Floor of Mouth
Clinical attachment to the periosteum and the inability to otherwise achieve a satisfactory margin of resection are indications for marginal mandibulectomy. Although somewhat controversial, incontinuity resection with neck dissection is not absolutely necessary and discontinuity procedures offer a

potentially lower rate of complication and morbidity while simplifying reconstructive concerns. Bilateral neck dissection is appropriate for tumors approaching the midline. The propensity for occult, and potential for bilateral, cervical metastasis warrants elective treatment of the neck(s).

Buccal Mucosa

Poorly defined lesions on a background of abnormality may best be treated by primary radiotherapy. Larger lesions involving its deeper structures and bone, and/or full-thickness cheek skin, require composite resection and flap (temporalis, radial forearm) reconstruction.

Oral Tongue

Partial peroral resection is appropriate for selected lesions, and mandibulotomy approaches will be required for access to larger more posteriorly disposed tumors. Primary closure reconstruction is appropriate for smaller defects and skin grafts and local flaps for larger ones. Advanced tumors will require composite resection techniques with flap reconstruction. Laryngectomy may be required in total resections either because of tumor extension or to prohibit risk of aspiration. Neck failure, regardless of T stage, is common. Tumor thickness may provide the most rational basis for decision making with regard to treatment of the clinically uninvolved neck. Elective neck treatment as supraomohyoid neck dissection is generally advocated for all but the earliest tumors of the oral tongue.

Lip

In situ carcinomas and severe dysplasia may be treated by lip shave, vermilionectomy, with mucosal advancement reconstruction. Early-stage lesions may be resected with reconstruction via primary closure in defects up to about 30% of the lip length. Local flap options for larger defects are multiple. Sensate radial forearm free flap reconstruction has been recently described for total lip resections, with excellent cosmetic and functional results. Composite resection techniques are appropriate for advanced-stage lesions. Elective neck dissection is not warranted in most lip carcinomas but should be considered for larger tumors and for recurrent lesions. Tumors involving the oral commissure may be best treated with radiotherapy to provide a better cosmetic and functional result. Tumors of this area and of the upper lip drain to periparotid nodes, as well as to level I, as first echelon drainage, and may require superficial parotidectomy for an adequate surgical treatment.

Miscellaneous Considerations

Selective use of toluidine blue staining provides diagnostic control over subjective clinical impressions and control over false-negative clinical findings. This may confirm clinical suspicion and facilitate intraoperative decision making.

Because of the risk of osteoradionecrosis with subsequent adjuvant radiotherapy, careful dental evaluation is mandatory for every patient in this group, emphasizing prophylaxis, therapeutics, and maintenance. The oral and maxillofacial prosthodontist is a particularly critical member of the multidisciplinary team in maxillectomy procedures.

Nonsquamous Carcinomas

The role of surgery in *lymphoma* of the oral cavity is limited to the provision of adequate diagnostic material for accurate diagnosis. Combined surgery and postoperative adjuvant radiotherapy is the treatment of choice for *mucosal malignant melanoma,* with neck dissection generally reserved for clinical metastasis. Combined surgery with intraoperative control of neural margins followed by postoperative adjuvant external beam radiotherapy is the treatment of choice for *adenoid cystic carcinomas* of the oral cavity. *High-grade mucoepidermoid carcinoma* and *high-grade adenocarcinoma* should be similarly treated in a combined mode. Again, neck dissection is reserved for clinical metastasis. Treatment of oral cavity *Kaposi's sarcomas* is palliative-intent only, centering on radiotherapy, photodynamic therapy, and intralesional chemotherapy.

RECONSTRUCTIVE SURGERY OF THE ORAL CAVITY—INTRODUCTION AND HISTORICAL PERSPECTIVE

Reconstructive surgery of patients with oral cavity defects has undergone logarithmic advancement over the last 2 decades, fueled largely by the increased application of microneurovascular free tissue transfer techniques to ablative, traumatic acquired, and congenital defects. This era has been preceded by the fundamental contributions of many surgeons from the fields of plastic and reconstructive surgery, otolaryngology (head and neck surgery), neurosurgery, oral and maxillofacial surgery, and general surgery. The concept of immediate reconstruction[12] and the contribution of the deltopectoral fasciocutaneous flap[3] were followed by the application of the newly defined myocutaneous flaps of the mid-1970s, in particular, the pectoralis major myocutaneous flap.[2]

Despite the report of the successful microvascular transfer of a jejunal interposition flap in 1959, the modern era of clinical reconstructive microsurgery began in the early 1970s with increased refinement in instrumentation and technique, the description of new transfers, and the search for new applications of previously described flaps. This characterized the next decade with the reports of large series of the free jejunum interposition (1970s), the radial forearm fasciocutaneous flap for oral reconstruction (1983), and the fibula free flap for oromandibular reconstruction (1985) in particular. The recognition of the superiority of these techniques and the development of multidisciplinary teams and simultaneous two-team interdependent operative procedures have resulted in aesthetic and functional restoration of the head and neck patient to a heretofore unprecedented level.

The availability of an increased armamentarium of reliable reconstructive options has given the head and neck surgeon increased confidence in the application of radical ablative or intensive therapeutic approaches to advanced disease. It has also given him or her increased responsibility in planning the reconstructive requirements for a particular procedure and for choosing appropriate support teams to achieve the highest possible level of form and function in returning the patient toward his or her premorbid existence. General principles of defect analysis and of flap design, anatomy, and physiology apply across all techniques and must be emphasized.

The traditional concept of the *reconstructive ladder* begins defect analysis with a hierarchical approach to the suitability of a particular technique to a particular defect, emphasizing simplicity, and ascending from simple to complex. It begins at the bottom with primary closure reconstruction ascending to skin grafting to local flaps, through regional flaps, distant flaps, and on to the microneurovascular free tissue transfer of composite blocks of tissue at the top of the ladder. The surgeon must realize, however, that he or she is not obligated to push the patient through all or most of these steps and that many times the concept of the *reconstructive elevator,* advancing directly to microsurgical techniques from the initial preoperative planning phase, is most appropriate. Conversely, the surgeon must not be extravagant in the application of advanced techniques and must always have multiple contingency plans in place in the event of flap failure or recurrence of disease.

Defect considerations include volume, composition (soft tissue, bone), location (proximity to vital structures, need for external/internal surfaces), general status (previously operated, irradiated, infected), and need for oronasocranial or oropharyngocervical separation. Functional considerations include the provision of sensibility, bone stock for skeletal framework and osseointegration, secretory mucosal surface, and pliability. Flap donor sites have been largely well defined and chosen for acceptability of residual functional or aesthetic deficit.

SKIN GRAFTS

Skin grafts have primary application in small defects of the oral cavity, the maxillectomy cheek flap, temporalis fascia flap, and coverage of the radial forearm and fibula donor site. They allow the surgeon to overcome tethering and restriction of mobility, which can result from primary closure and can critically affect orolingual function. Skin grafts generally heal well over fat, muscle, perichondrium, and fascia. Although they will heal over periosteum, they afford neither adequate protection nor stable coverage in this context. Since such grafts are completely dependent on the recipient bed for survival via neovascularization, they are unsatisfactory for many previously operated, irradiated, or frankly infected sites that are characterized by ischemic scar tissue, relative soft tissue hypovascularization, and inflammatory response.

LOCAL SKIN FLAPS

Local skin flaps are primarily applied in the reconstruction of external facial defects and have little application in contemporary oral reconstruction. The forehead flap is of particular historical impact and interest.

REGIONAL FLAPS

As the distance of a required flap transposition increases, the incorporation of a defined axial blood supply becomes critical. This is further discussed in the section on myocutaneous flaps yet becomes a critical consideration in the Abbé, Abbé-Estlander (superior labial), and facial artery myomucosal (FAMM) flaps. Abbé designs transfer not only skin but also labial mucosa to compensate for soft tissue deficiency in lip reconstruction. The temporal fascias (superficial, or temporoparietal, and deep) may be transferred as a bilobed flap pedicled on the superficial temporal system and may be thought of as a transferable bed for split-thickness skin graft (STSG) placement. The layers are highly vascular and pliable, and may be transposed either prezygomatic or retrozygomatic for palate or cheek reconstruction. Accurate knowledge of facial nerve anatomy and of the nuances of the anatomy of this region is critical to confident surgery without complication.[25] The deltopectoral and forehead flaps are primarily of historical interest. The Karapandzic flap is a unique variation of a multiple-pedicle, innervated, local flap for major lip reconstruction.

MUSCLE AND MYOCUTANEOUS FLAPS

Descriptions of the axial arterial anatomy to major muscles and the recognition of defined territories of overlying skin, perfused by perpendicularly oriented myocutaneous perforating vessels, fueled many of the advances in head and neck reconstructive work through the 1970s. This vascular orientation allowed circumferential suture around skin islands transferred with such flaps without compromising viability. The pectoralis major myocutaneous, latissimus dorsi, and trapezius flaps have also been described for various oromandibular applications. Myocutaneous flaps allow the transfer of significant volumes of soft tissue (skin island, subcutaneous fat, and muscle) into major ablative head and neck defects and are usually reliable and versatile far in excess of their regional cutaneous and fasciocutaneous counterparts. Sinocranial, orocervical, and pharyngocutaneous separation can now be achieved. Single-stage major reconstructions have become the norm. Primary closure reduces donor site morbidity significantly in contrast to previous fasciocutaneous designs. The application of these flaps as vehicles for the transfer of vascularized segments of bone (trapezius-scapular, pectoralis-rib, latissimus-rib, sternocleidomastoid-clavicle) was an important historical step toward the microvascular transfer of bone.

The concept of angiosomes[26] challenged and extended the dogma that such flaps could reliably transfer only skin directly overlying the muscle component of a myocutaneous flap. The angiosome is a volume of tissue supplied by a single source artery and vein. Contiguous angiosomes are connected by a system of "choke" (oscillating) arteries. Adjacent angiosomes may be captured in tissue transfer after interruption of the adjacent source artery through the reversal of physiologic blood flow. Once harvested tissue is extended beyond adjacent angiosomes, the incidence of ischemic necrosis rises.

Pectoralis Major

The pectoralis major myocutaneous flap has persisted as the major myocutaneous pedicled tissue transfer in oromandibular reconstruction and remains a workhorse in selected application. Its ease of development and application remain fundamental parts of the armamentarium of the contemporary reconstructive head and neck surgeon. The flap is based on the pectoral branch of the thoracoacromial artery arising from the second portion of the axillary artery. The architecture of the axial supply follows that generally observed throughout the body, namely that the axial pedicle enters the muscle from its undersurface running in a fat plane up to its intramuscular course. Although traditional incisional designs have avoided crossing the horizontally disposed deltopectoral flap and required flap dissection beneath a bridge of uninterrupted skin, the increased difficulty of flap dissection is obviated by a continuous serpiginous incision (burning a historical bridge) joining the vertical limb of a neck dissection incision. (It is highly unlikely that a deltopectoral fasciocutaneous flap would be called on to salvage a failed pectoralis major flap, thus invalidating this carryover of dogma from the early and unproven days of the pectoralis flap.) The contribution of the lateral thoracic artery to this flap is insignificant in the final analysis of most transfers.

Refinements in technique include developing the entire flap as an island design allowing the transposition of a minimal amount of tissue over the clavicle, thus reducing external deformity. Section of the pectoral nerve branches to the muscle will ensure that the pedicle is not compressed against it when rotated into a defect and also that the flap muscle component will atrophy and contour to external defects more acceptably.

Transfer of the flap through the neck most easily follows radical lymphadenectomy procedures in which the sternocleidomastoid muscle is sacrificed, the transposed pectoralis muscle affording reliable coverage to exposed critical neurovascular structures. The arc of rotation of the flap allows it to usually reach the level of the hard palate. The flap may be applied to defects of nearly any configuration in structures inferior to this level. Simultaneous harvest without patient repositioning is a significant advantage.

A medially based curvilinear lunar skin paddle design facilitates primary closure of the donor site and minimizes the transfer of breast parenchyma and deformity in female patients. Preoperative marking should include the horizontal level of the contralateral nipple to minimize vertical deformity on closure. Flap dissection is based on the direct visualization of the pedicle, which is directed inferolaterally from its origin just medial to the insertion of the pectoralis minor muscle.

Disadvantages include the transfer of hair-bearing skin into the oral cavity and the bulkiness of this flap. Transposition of the flap, as with all pedicled designs, is limited by the arc of rotation of the flap pedicle. Inferiorly pedicled flaps all exhibit an often relentless tendency toward dehiscence and/or fistulization, particularly when inset superiorly. Moreover, the most distal aspect of the skin paddle (and most poorly perfused and vulnerable) is necessarily inset into the *most* distant portion of the defect. Partial flap loss, dehiscence, stricture (through the requirement for secondary wound healing and ischemic scar contracture), and fistulization are not uncommon phenomena despite the significant possibilities of myocutaneous flaps.

Latissimus Dorsi

The latissimus dorsi muscle flap is based on the thoracodorsal pedicle from the versatile subscapular system of flaps. It is a broad, thin muscle that can be transposed into the head and neck region either subcutaneously or via a transaxillary approach. Although its range of application as a pedicled flap and soft tissue volume are similar to the pectoralis, decubitus positioning, decreased reliability, and a high incidence of donor site morbidity make this a tertiary choice to the pectoralis and free tissue transfer techniques. As a free tissue transfer, it is characterized by a huge available surface area; thin, pliable consistency; a long, large caliber; and anatomically consistent vascular pedicle, allowing ease of anastomosis in the neck.

Trapezius

Both vertically and transversely oriented skin paddle designs may be taken with the trapezius flap, which is based on the occipital and descending cervical branches of the external carotid and transverse cervical vessels, respectively. Elegant anatomic studies have accurately documented variations in the vascular anatomy of these vessels.[20] Previous neck dissection status is an important consideration, since the exact status of the transverse cervical vessels is often unmentioned in the operative notes of previously treated patients. Although capable of reaching the midline neck, posteriorly situated defects are best suited to reconstruction with this method. Significant disadvantages are those of the pedicled latissimus transfer mentioned earlier in addition to the occasional requirement for donor site skin grafting.

OTHER FLAPS

Myocutaneous flaps based on the platysma and sternocleidomastoid muscles are occasionally useful, particularly the sternocleidomastoid muscle, superiorly pedicled, to bolster oral suture lines. Rotation is limited by the spinal accessory nerve's entry into the anterior border of the muscle. High-stage neck disease and extracapsular extension of metastatic disease are contraindications to this application. Similarly, the levator scapulae and posterior scalene muscles may be detached from their insertions as superiorly based muscle flaps for similar applications.

FREE MICRONEUROVASCULAR TISSUE TRANSFER

Clinical microsurgery has provided the single most important contribution to reconstruction of the head and neck patient in the last decade, restoring patients to a heretofore unprecedented degree of form and function. It is now possible to replace resected or missing tissues with nearly identical tissue types (e.g., mucosa, bone, sensate skin, composites), volumes, and character. Many of the most significant drawbacks inherent to pedicled myocutaneous transfers can be adequately addressed through the thoughtful selection of microsurgical techniques.

Properly executed flap design and development will usually produce a reconstruction with vascularity superior to traditional counterparts or alternatives, with a decreased incidence of dehiscence, fistulization, partial flap loss, and stricture. Microsurgery has allowed ablative surgeons to extend their resective techniques in more radical directions in both curative- and palliative-intent procedures by providing unprecedented reliability and versatility of design. Despite numerous papers on multiple simultaneous free flap reconstructions, such requirements are often avoidable through thoughtful flap design.[28] It is the responsibility of the head and neck surgeon to foster the development of the simultaneous two-team approach to the reconstruction of these unfortunate patients and to make such techniques available to this population. The preoperative planning, flap selection, flap development, and perioperative care of the microsurgical patient are as important as the actual microsurgical anastomosis.

PATIENT SELECTION

In general, most patients who are candidates for curative-intent resective procedures that produce defects that would benefit from free flap reconstruction are candidates for this technique. Numerous publications have documented the safety and efficacy of such procedures in elderly patients. The general principle of "keep it simple" must prevail, however, over the desire to reconstruct a posterolateral composite mandible defect with a fibula in an edentulous septuagenarian diabetic patient with severe coronary artery disease, just for the sake of reestablishing bony continuity! Prohibitive or prognostic co-morbid factors must be respected and considered in the planning phase. Age, chronic obstructive pulmonary disease (COPD), hypertensive vasculopathy and arteriosclerotic vascular disease, malnutrition, alcoholism, and active smoking, all common in the head and neck cancer patient population, contribute to a potentially compromised outcome regardless of technique. None are, however, absolutely prohibitive to the application of these techniques. Similarly, many of these entities have systemic effects impacting donor site selection (e.g., peroneal atherosclerosis in fibula free flap).

Previous treatment history is of critical importance in preoperative planning with particular reference to recipient vessels. Vein grafts are usually avoidable through careful planning and flap choice. Irradiation not only affects the microcirculation but also major vessels in terms of accelerating atherosclerotic degeneration, intimal and media thickening, and endothelial friability and dehiscence. Knowledge of total dose and volume radiation source, port size, and direction and dates of treatment are critical to treatment planning. Previous surgery either independent of or in addition to radiation history adds an additional degree of difficulty in terms of recipient vessel dissection, quality, and choice.

POINTS OF TECHNIQUE

There is no substitute for a broad and varied experience in applied clinical microsurgery in order to ensure success. Such expertise is generally available in most major locations and must overcome prevailing political, subspecialty, and personal interests for the greater goal of optimal care of the surgical patient. Some aspects of resective surgery should be modified when a microsurgical transfer is anticipated. Routine sacrifice of the external jugular vein destroys a potential recipient vein or vein graft conduit and is usually not of oncologic significance. Major arterial and venous vessels that are to be transected should be handled with the utmost technical care and sacrificed somewhat away from their takeoff, to allow a satisfactory stump for end-to-end anastomosis. This includes the internal jugular vein stump in radical dissections. Flap ischemia times are generally to be minimized, but are rarely defining issues in contemporary flap survival. Most times are under 1 hour, with the exception of osseous transfers, which require insetting and osteosynthesis of skeletal components prior to revascularization. Enteric (jejunum), muscle, and osteocyte components of flaps are most sensitive to ischemia. Complete dissection of the flap in situ and microscopic positioning and recipient vessel preparation *prior to* pedicle transection maximize success and minimize overall ischemia time. Flap cooling with iced saline throughout the ischemic period significantly reduces the tissues' metabolic demand and extends available time (warm versus cold ischemia time) prior to the onset of critical and irreversible changes.

COMPLICATIONS

In the most expert of hands, flap failure should occur in about 5% or fewer of cases, including the most complex of reconstructions. Free flap loss, usually an all-or-none phenomenon, occurs most frequently within the first 72 hours of revascularization. Anastomotic failures may be successfully salvaged through timely recognition and revision.[16] Myriad philosophies of perioperative management and monitoring techniques exist, and specialized instrumentation for free flap monitoring may improve survival only through increasing the vigilance of the nursing staff caring for the patient rather than through some intrinsic superiority to clinical observation alone.[17]

RADIAL FOREARM FLAP

The radial forearm flap was one of the first free flaps commonly applied to intraoral head and neck reconstruction and represents one of the most common transfers in contemporary reconstruction. Fasciocutaneous vessels from the *radial* vessels are transmitted to the skin paddle via the lateral intermuscular (brachioradialis, flexor carpi radialis) septum. The flap may incorporate a segment of the radius bone by including a cuff of flexor pollicis longus muscle. Sensate capabilities are provided by the *lateral* and *medial antebrachial cutaneous nerves*. The phenomenon of "sensory upgrading" has been observed in sensate reconstruction of the oral cavity where the transferred forearm flap, anastomosed to the recipient lingual nerve, demonstrates greater fidelity in two-point discriminatory capability *after transfer* into the mouth than when in situ in the forearm *prior to* transfer.[5] This is believed to be due to a greater cortical representation devoted to orolingual structures subserved by the lingual nerve.

In addition to the capabilities above, the flap's most intrinsic advantage is its thin, pliable soft tissue component, which has made it outstanding for intraoral reconstruction. Fascia-only designs may facilitate tongue mobility and better allow reconstitution of contours, sulci and vestibules. Inclusion of the palmaris longus tendon with the flap offers some theoretic advantage in suspending the flap laterally in palatal and in total lower lip reconstruction. The flap is also well suited to complex full-thickness defects of the cheek.

Drawbacks to this flap center around its distal and obvious donor site deformity, with mandatory skin grafting in most applications. The bone stock provided by this transfer is far inferior to alternatives where osseointegrated implantation is anticipated for oromandibular rehabilitation.[14] The combination of reconstruction plate plus fasciocutaneous flap, although an apparently attractive alternative to composite bone-containing free flaps, is usually an inferior choice in mandible reconstruction, and is neither time- nor resource-conserving.

LATERAL ARM FLAP

Fasciocutaneous perforators from the *radial collateral* vessels are transmitted to the overlying skin through the lateral intermuscular (brachialis, brachioradialis triceps) septum. It may include the *posterior cutaneous nerve* of the arm for sensate capability and/or the posterior cutaneous nerve to the forearm for vascularized interposition grafting. Transfer of a portion of the humerus and fascia-only designs have been described. The skin and subcutaneous tissues of this region of the arm are somewhat thicker and less pliable than the forearm counterpart. Pedicle caliber is similar to the radial forearm vessels. Flap geometry involving pedicle entry in the midportion of the cutaneous paddle complicates application to certain defects. Flap pedicle dissection is more difficult and it is shorter than that of the radial forearm flap. The donor site may be closed primarily with the single linear scar positioned in a place more easily camouflaged by clothing, making this flap appropriate to female and younger patients. In the male patient, this area of the arm may bear less hair than the forearm.

LATISSIMUS DORSI FLAP

The latissimus dorsi flap is based on the *thoracodorsal* pedicle, which is part of the subscapular system of flaps. The branch to

the serratus anterior may be sacrificed, producing a very long pedicle of large caliber facilitating anastomosis in the neck. It is generally not capable of supporting sensate reconstruction and must be harvested in a lateral decubitus position, which may require intraoperative repositioning. Motor reconstruction with this flap has been described.

RECTUS ABDOMINIS FLAP

The rectus abdominis flap is based on the *deep inferior epigastric* vascular pedicle and is generally transferred as a myocutaneous flap or as a muscle-only flap. It does not support sensate needs and is usually not applied as a functional motor reconstruction. The flap may be designed in a multitude of orientations but is usually oriented vertically or horizontally (transverse rectus abdominis muscle [TRAM]). The flap is capable of supporting a large volume of overlying soft tissue and finds additional application in massive combined head and neck defects.

Simultaneous flap harvest and resection are conducted with ease. Unilateral transfers may result in measurable abdominal wall weakness, which is well compensated by retained obliques, contralateral rectus, and muscle-sparing harvest techniques. This weakness is not noticed in the vast majority of individuals. Hernia is infrequent.

FIBULA FLAP

This transfer has revolutionized functional and aesthetic oromandibular reconstruction and rehabilitation since its application to the mandible by Hidalgo as reported in 1985. Subsequent refinements in technique have extended its application and usefulness. The flap is based on the *peroneal* vessels of the tibial peroneal trunk and the cutaneous component is perfused primarily by septocutaneous vessels transmitted via the posterior crural septum. Skin and muscle (flexor hallucis longus) may be reliably transferred with the bone and may be critical components in intraoral and external resurfacing (skin) and in submandibular contouring (flexor). These soft tissue components may be differentially inset, adding to the flexibility in application of this flap. The osseous component may be utilized to reconstruct the entire mandible. Its dimensions are aesthetically ideal for mandibular reconstruction and functionally ideal for osseointegrated implant placement. Simultaneous and independent maxillary reconstruction has also been accomplished with this flap.[23] Recent refinements of this transfer have included the *lateral sural cutaneous nerve* adding sensate capability to the skin paddle.

Disadvantages of this flap are occasional difficulties in soft tissue wound healing characteristic of the lower extremity and the potential involvement of pedicle vessels with atherosclerotic vascular disease. Studies of postoperative function have demonstrated no significant long-term donor site morbidity and only short-term ankle stiffness. An STSG is required to resurface the donor site in larger reconstructions.

The potential for osseointegrated implantation of dental prostheses represents a significant technical advancement over tissue-borne prosthodontics with the direct transfer of masticatory force to the underlying bone. It is important to realize, however, that this is an expensive and multistaged series of procedures, out of the reach of many head and neck patients. In most larger series, fewer than one quarter of patients complete this rehabilitative sequence.

ILIAC CREST FLAP

The iliac crest flap is based on the *deep circumflex iliac system* and is capable of transferring large amounts of soft tissue and bone into massive defects. The composite flap may include skin, subcutaneous tissue, iliac crest, and internal oblique muscle. Disadvantages include the large volume of tissue and donor site morbidity, relegating it to a secondary role behind the fibula flap for most oromandibular defects. Simultaneous flap harvest and resection are conducted with ease. This flap does not support motor or sensate reconstructions.

JEJUNUM

The attractiveness of transferring a secretory mucosal surface to the oral and pharyngeal axis is real, particularly in the context of radiation. In such instances, the flap may be divided along its antimesenteric border and inset as a patch graft. Potential disadvantages are those of laparotomy and enteric anastomosis. A feeding jejunostomy is usually performed. Laparoscopic harvest promises to minimize donor site morbidity. Mesenteric vessels must be respected for their friability and tendency toward rosetting and intimal separation.

ALLOPLASTIC IMPLANTATION, GRAFTING, AND TISSUE ENGINEERING

Major oromandibular reconstruction involves primarily implant systems for osteosynthesis and reconstruction of bony discontinuity, and biomaterials aimed at decreasing donor site morbidity (e.g., bone extenders such as hydroxyapatite cement). Titanium and Vitallium form the basis of rigid internal fixation systems and are eminently biocompatible as permanent implants. Absolute attention to detail in the proper application of these systems is essential and must resist an oft prevalent "hardware store" mentality.[11]

Continuity defects of the mandible spanning 4 to 6 cm in relatively favorable recipient beds (e.g., nonunion, comminution, no previous treatment or irradiation) may be grafted with particulate bone-cancellous marrow from the iliac crest. Longer defects require revascularized transfer techniques. The morbidity attendant to iliac crest bone graft harvest in cases requiring a large volume of material has provided the impetus to explore bone graft extenders such as hydroxyapatite cement, which has been recently released for craniomaxillofacial application.

POSTOPERATIVE MANAGEMENT

Perioperative antibiotics, effective against oral and pharyngeal flora, are continued for 24 to 48 hours with no proven benefit for more extended courses. Topical antibiotic mouth rinses are of benefit until intraoral wound healing is complete. Clindamycin 300 mg in 500 cc NS has been shown to decrease ambient oral flora tenfold and is used four times daily by mouth as a swish and spit/suction solution.

Tracheotomy is an essential part of many ablative procedures involving the oral cavity structures. Significant edema is made possible by loose mucosal covering of the floor of mouth, buccal spaces, and lips, as well as underlying loose adipose and areolar tissues. The floor of mouth spaces are continuous posteriorly with the submandibular space (behind the posterior border of the mylohyoid muscle) and the submental space (between the anterior bellies of the digastric muscles). Edema attendant to surgery and/or inflammatory processes (Ludwig's angina) may decompress/extend into these spaces, impinging on the airway through elevation and retrodisplacement of the tongue. In addition to providing the potential for purely mechanical airway obstruction, tracheotomy facilitates pulmonary toilet and respiratory mechanics because clearance of mucous secretions is often not possible via physiologic means (expectoration, swallowing).

In general, with the resolution of orolingual edema, bedside trials of manual occlusion of the tracheotomy tube should allow the patient nearing decannulation to "breathe around the tube" and to phonate with relative ease. The return of functional voice at this time is a significant psychologic boost to all such patients. Decannulation may follow, with the patient instructed to manually occlude the tracheotomy site for coughing and for speech in order to facilitate secondary intent closure of the tracheotomy site. In general, this process might begin on or about the third postoperative day, with decannulation complete by postoperative day 5 to 7. Suture or local flap closure of these sites is unnecessary and closure is complete within 1 to 2 weeks. Most patients, including those with free flap reconstructions, should be decannulated prior to discharge. The morbidity and potential for fatality, with inadequate care (through complete airway obstruction), of this relatively minor surgical procedure is ever-present and is not to be discounted.

Decannulation will also facilitate swallowing function inasmuch as a patent tracheotomy tube dampens the effectiveness of attempts to swallow, limits the effectiveness of the cough and pulmonary toilet, and, as any tube here will do, limits the physiologic excursion of the larynx during this effort. Vertical incision design may allow the tube to rise and fall with physiologic swallowing efforts, minimizing its tethering effect while in place. Not all procedures require tracheotomy (e.g., partial peroral glossectomy with or without supraomohyoid neck dissection, purely lateral composite resection with minimal soft tissue component).

An oral full liquid diet might begin within days, depending on edema and complexity of reconstruction. When protracted nutritional support is anticipated, nasogastric or percutaneous endoscopic feeding gastrostomy tube placement is required. It is important to remember that about a liter of saliva is created and swallowed each day, and the event of fistula formation is determined by multifactorial aspects of care.

Mandibular loading in cases involving skeletal surgery (osteotomy or replacement) may begin at about 2 months, consistent with the time course of secondary bone healing. The clinical assessment of stability is key as radiographic evidence of osseous healing will significantly lag behind adequate clinical osteosynthesis. Hardware removal procedures are typically required only to facilitate the placement of osseointegrated implants or in unusual cases of plate exposure, sensitivity, or failure of physiologic bone healing.

Although the primary placement of osseointegrated implants has been described in significant series of osseous free flap reconstructions, delayed placement at about 1 year after the completion of postoperative therapeutic radiation is more common. Removal of hardware and STSG vestibuloplasty or other flap modification and refinement procedures may be combined. Several months later, implant uncovering and transmucosal abutment placement follow. After soft tissue healing around these abutments (several additional months), implant-borne prosthodontics are fitted.

Adjuvant radiotherapy should generally begin within a 6-week postoperative period. Although it may be delayed in the presence of significant wound-healing problems, radiation may begin in the presence of minor ones (e.g., small fistula, STSG nontake) with continued conservative wound care through complete healing. Metallic mandibular reconstruction plate implant materials have been studied for their interaction with external beam therapeutic radiation fields. Amplification on the incident side of the beam (buccolabial aspect) to about 120% of the incident dose and attenuation to about 80% have been observed with falloff to normal dose characteristics within millimeters of such plates. A lesser effect may be expected for fracture or craniofacial type plates used for osteotomy synthesis. The radiophysiologic rationale justifying the primary placement of osseointegrated implants in the context of observed effects on osteocytes and bone regenerating capacity is that maximal radiotoxicity to bone is observed at about 6 to 8 weeks after initiating treatment. When added to the lag time from surgery to the initiation of treatment, adequate time has passed to allow complete osseointegration of such implants. The external hardware required for transport distraction osteogenesis, in addition to the internal defect-bridging reconstruction plate required to maintain occlusal relationships, confounds postoperative adjuvant RT planning and delivery, emphasizing the need for selective application of such techniques.

OUTCOMES

Overall survival for oral cavity malignancies is about 50%, a percentage that has remained essentially unchanged throughout the era of modern head and neck surgery despite advances in surgical and therapeutic technique. Cure is generally declared after a 5-year posttreatment surveillance period, with most local recurrences (80% to 90%) occurring within the first 2 years. Metastatic nodal involvement is the most powerful predictor of prognosis and outcome.

Locoregional recurrence is the most common cause of treatment failure and mortality, although improvements in local and regional disease control have increased the proportion of deaths due to distant metastasis (up to 20%). The appropriate addition of postoperative adjuvant external beam radiation therapy has contributed significantly to the control of disease above the clavicles, yet has unmasked this significant potential for systemic metastasis, with lung, liver, and bone the most common sites of distant involvement.

Second primary (metachronous) upper aerodigestive tract malignancies occur most frequently in people with oral cavity primaries (15% to 30%). The risk of this phenomenon is about 4% per year, cumulatively, to about 5 years where the risk levels off. This observation ties together concepts of "field cancerization," condemned mucosa, and the prevalent spectrum of premalignant dysplastic mucosal change. Ongoing risk factors (tobacco smoking, ethanol consumption) are not required for this phenomenon. Metachronous primaries most commonly involve the hypopharynx, lung, larynx, oropharynx, and esophagus and are the main cause of treatment failure and death in patients with controlled index disease. Continued posttreatment surveillance beyond the first 2 years (where emphasis is on the detection of primary disease recurrence) through at least 5 years posttreatment is indicated because of this potential.

RESULTS

A significant proportion of patients in this disease group present with advanced stage disease, despite the accessibility of this region to direct physical examination, underlining the continued need for public and professional awareness of this entity.

Overall 5-year survival for lip cancer is about 70%, with the presence of cervical metastasis lowering this figure below 50%. Stage I and II lesion curability should be about 90%, and stage 3 and 4 lesions about 60% and 40%, respectively. Lesions of the upper lip and commissure portend a survival rate about 10% to 20% lower than overall figures. About 5% to 15% of patients will present with clinically overt adenopathy and an additional 15% may manifest adenopathy over long-term follow-up.

Retromolar trigone lesions provide an approximate 80% (T1), 60% (T2), 45% (T3), and 25% (T4) 5-year survival. Floor of mouth primaries reveal a 5-year survival of about 60% to 88% (T1 and T2), 60% to 70% (T3), and 10% to 40% (T4). Locoregional recurrence is the major cause of treatment failure for these sites. Buccal mucosal carcinomas present a formidable challenge to local control, with recurrence in up to 45% of cases depending on stage. Five-year survival approximates 75% and 60% for stages I and II disease, and 40% and

25% for stages III and IV disease. Tumor thickness of greater than 6 mm, regardless of stage, has been correlated with poorer survival for this subsite.

The oral tongue subsite demonstrates a propensity for locoregional failure. Survival figures of 80%, 60%, 40%, and 20% are typical for stages I to IV, respectively. Whether or not tumors of the oral tongue and lip behave more aggressively in persons under 40 remains controversial, although recent matched-pair analyses (gender, stage) have shown a similar prognosis overall and a significant incidence of second primary malignancies.[13]

Nonsquamous Carcinomas

Survival for extranodal lymphomas is dependent on histologic pattern and clinical stage. Overall 5-year survival is about 50%. Mucosal melanomas are far more lethal than their cutaneous counterparts, with about 25% to 35% 5-year overall survival and a 5% to 6% 5-year survival for those with cervical metastasis. Late recurrence (to 10 years), with local failure associated with distant metastasis, underlines the unpredictability of this tumor and the need for effective systemic therapeutics and for long-term follow-up of apparent survivors. Adenoid cystic carcinoma is legendary for its long apparent disease-free interval, which should be measured in multiples of the typical 5-year period and which mandates long-term follow-up. The 5-, 10-, and 15-year survivals have been reported at approximately 45%, 30%, and 20%, respectively.

COMPLICATIONS

Complications are to be distinguished from expected sequelae of procedures directed at the ablation of oral cavity malignancies. In general, the sequelae are predictable and the anticipated impact may be addressed through thoughtful decision making in planning reconstructive maneuvers (e.g., provision of sensate lining through microvascular free flaps). Complications may occur at the skeletal or soft tissue level and may be major or minor. Skeletal complications might include malocclusion and nonunion, which are increasingly rare with contemporary rigid internal fixation systems. Preoperative planning utilizing lateral and transverse templates for mandibular and maxillary reconstruction has added significantly to the accuracy of maxillofacial free flap reconstruction. Failure of implant hardware is usually due to improper technique and/or poor judgment. Nonunion requires hardware removal, aggressive debridement, bone grafting, and revision osteosynthesis. Pathologic fracture in cases of conservation mandibulectomy may be minimized through the concurrent use of reconstruction plates across these sites of structural weakness—this is especially common in previously treated (irradiated) and elderly patients.

Soft tissue complications include dehiscence, partial flap loss, and orocutaneous fistulization, most of which are initially managed conservatively through debridement and dressing changes. The latter is more common in previously treated patients and rarely requires additional surgery for resolution.

Significant time (weeks, months) may be required for complete closure, and this adds significant morbidity to an otherwise nominal postoperative course. Despite the provision of reliable soft tissue components, most mandibular reconstructive flaps will require subsequent STSG vestibuloplasty at the time of secondary implant placement in order to recreate adequate sulcus anatomy and lip posture.

CHEMOTHERAPY

Head and neck oncologists await the development and discovery of curative therapeutic drugs for this class of malignancies. Current regimens are characterized by significant response rates, but limited duration of response and short time to recurrence/progression on discontinuation of therapy. Current treatment strategies are aimed at predicting and increasing radioresponsiveness in neoadjuvant and concurrent settings, respectively. Current therapeutics remain an important tool in palliative-intent and salvage-intent modes.

CHEMOPREVENTION

The effects of carotenoids and vitamins C and E in chemoprevention of oral cavity carcinogenesis have been demonstrated in epidemiologic and laboratory studies. Retinoic acid derivatives are currently most intensively studied and are observed to exert a cytodifferentiating effect on premalignant tissues. The oral cavity provides an ideal clinical model for the study of chemoprevention with its accessibility to evaluation, spectrum of premalignant pathology, and propensity to second primary disease. Clinical trials have heretofore been limited by drug toxicity but have demonstrated effectiveness in reducing second primary malignancy (although not in decreasing the recurrence of index primary lesions). Less toxic drugs are being evaluated in clinical trials.

FUNCTIONAL OUTCOMES ANALYSIS

Articulation

The complex interplay of the tongue, buccal vestibules, lips, and anterior dentition largely determines success in the articulation of speech. Disturbances in speech are most commonly the result of multifactorial impact of treatment on several of these structures, the most critical of which is tongue mobility. Reconstructive methods must avoid tethering tongue, augment and restore sulcus anatomy, and prevent excess bulk in the oral cavity.

Deglutition

The oral cavity initiates the swallowing mechanism by forming the bolus and moving it back to the pharynx. The provision of sensate linings where possible, tongue mobility, oral competence, and near-normal sulci, will maximize posttreatment functional rehabilitation. The addition of postoperative adjuvant external beam radiotherapy, with its field effect on mucosal linings, delicate musculature, and major and minor salivary glands, also impairs the process of swallowing in the oral phase and also at points distal to the surgical field.

The efficiency of eating is significantly and adversely impacted. What was previously a subconscious process often assumes a high level of frustrating and conscious effort, as compensatory mechanisms attempt to facilitate swallowing and to avoid social embarrassment. This can be a significant source of long-term morbidity and may turn patients into social recluses.[15] The resumption of a completely normal premorbid varied diet is a luxury known only to those presenting with early-stage disease. An additional minority of patients will require percutaneous enteral gastrostomy feeding tube placement for supplemental or long-term complete nutritional support.

Mastication

The provision of a stable bony base for the support of tissue-borne or implant-retained dental prosthesis is essential to the complete functional rehabilitation of the oral cancer patient after composite resection. The challenge of anterior mandibular reconstruction has been successfully addressed through the reliable transfer of both osseous and soft tissue components for replacement of similar tissues removed in resection. Similarly, advanced full-thickness defects resected for palliative intent can be reliably and confidently confronted. The major portion of masticatory function, however, resides posteriorly, in the molar regions. Here osseous reconstruction may be achieved via nonvascularized bone graft techniques (up to about 4 to 6 cm of continuity defect) or by vascularized osseous free flaps in larger defects. The maintenance of bicondylar architecture is of significant functional importance for comfort, resistance of unbalanced muscular forces, and cicatricial deformation, particularly in the dentate patient.

Despite the capability of accepting osseointegrated implants, a variety of fiscal, ethical, and delivery issues restrict these techniques to a minority of patients (about 25% or fewer) in large series of osseous free tissue transfer mandible reconstructions. Despite obvious intrinsic benefit, these restorations still fall short of allowing the full restoration of oromandibular function, and are often of greater impact aesthetically, reestablishing appropriate lower lip posture, facilitating oral competence and articulated speech, and normalizing lower third facial profile.

Salivation

Xerostomia attendant to oral cavity ablative procedures is most commonly due to the postoperative adjuvant use of external beam radiotherapy. The removal of the submandibular gland does not result in a perceptible diminution of function for most individuals, even when performed on a bilateral basis. Although the parotid gland is usually avoided surgically in addressing most oral cavity malignancies in this country, there is a growing awareness of the need to consider this gland surgically in buccal mucosal malignancies.

There is compelling evidence for a cytoprotective effect in the pretreatment institution of parasympathomimetic sialogogue agents (pilocarpine, Salagen) in minimizing the impact of radiation-induced damage. Therapeutic saliva substitutes are poor and expensive replacements for physiologic function. Many patients are relegated to carrying along a personal water supply to facilitate comfort, speech, swallowing, and eating functions. The variability in individual response to similar treatments is impressive. These treatment-related morbidities are significant, and are constant reminders of disease history.

Maxillary Reconstruction

Prosthodontic rehabilitation of maxillary defects has evolved from simple obturation to more complex techniques including osseointegration. Problems include the need to remove and replace prosthetic devices for maintenance and cleaning as well as the often difficult aspects of retention of larger, bulkier prostheses. Autogenous tissues via microvascular transfer offer the potential to avoid many of these issues, and in addition, make possible bony reconstruction and even sensate coverage of these formidable defects. Local pedicled flaps have been inadequate as viable alternatives to standard prosthodontics. It is expected that, as in mandibular reconstruction, the functional rehabilitation of these defects may be revolutionized by these free tissue transfer techniques.

Historical impediments to such applications have included the concept that open cavity inspection allowed earlier detection and treatment of recurrent disease and that flap techniques might potentially "bury" recurrences. Advances in diagnostic imaging and familiarity with the imaging characteristics of such flaps have largely invalidated such dogma. Furthermore, much recurrent disease in this region occurs at the skull base or deep infratemporal fossa where aggressive attempts at salvage are rarely advisable.

OSSEOINTEGRATED MANDIBULAR IMPLANTS—PRIMARY VERSUS DELAYED PLACEMENT

Despite the fact that osseointegrated implants are not covered by most third party payers, external pressure may influence the current predominant practice of secondary placement. Prolongation of an already extended operative time, theoretic potential for increased flap complications, and perceived difficulties in planning implant placement must be balanced against the need for a second general anesthetic and operating theater costs, STSG vestibuloplasty, hardware removal procedures, and additional morbidity and expense related to this potentially optional step in the otherwise necessarily staged reconstructive procedure. The integration process is, furthermore, well along the way to completion by the time postoperative adjuvant radiotherapy is instituted (4 to 6 weeks postoperation) and the peak of acute radiation toxicity is reached at the bone level. Implant uncovering and abutment placement are generally office procedures and are of little comparative fiscal impact.

SECONDARY PROCEDURES

The requirement for secondary procedures in patients undergoing major ablative and reconstructive surgery of the oral cavity, other than those mentioned for osseointegrated dental rehabilitation, is remarkably rare. The most common procedures might include flap revision/reduction/release, tracheotomy scar revision, soft tissue symmetry procedures, and the like. Generally, such secondary procedures are comparatively trivial and are performed on an outpatient same-day basis.

AREAS FOR FUTURE INVESTIGATION

Supraomohyoid Neck Dissection as Therapeutic
Supraomohyoid neck dissection was conceived as a staging procedure that would remove all first echelon lymph nodes draining oral cavity primary sites (level II) as well as one echelon proximal and distal to this region (levels I and III). This provided a rational approach to the staging of primaries with a high risk of clinically occult metastasis and to the selection of postoperative adjuvant radiotherapy or complete neck dissection (levels IV and V) for those with pathologically involved lymph nodes. A measure of its effectiveness could be found in the percentage of patients who later failed in those levels where no other treatment was selected.[24] As the technique has gained acceptance, its application has been extended to that of a therapeutic procedure for selected patients with pathologic N1 disease where there is no evidence of extracapsular extension. The academic and scientific merit of this approach is only now beginning to be studied.

Sentinel Lymph Node Biopsy
Despite the leadership of head and neck surgeons in modified radical and selective lymphadenectomy procedures, additional refinement in terms of more minimally invasive procedures is of interest. Although clearly established for cutaneous malignancies (malignant melanoma, Merkel cell carcinoma), the role of intraoperative lymphoscintigraphy remains unclear at present for mucosal disease. The potential for selecting only those patients with clinically N0 necks who actually harbor occult metastases (P+ about 30%) would allow potentially significant fiscal savings and limitation of treatment-related morbidity over currently necessary selective lymphadenectomy procedures. The avoidance of otherwise unnecessary surgery through such superselective sampling techniques offers obvious advantage and resource savings to the 70% of patients who are actually pathologically N0 as well. Initial experience with chromatic identification of sentinel lymph nodes utilizing mucosal injection of isosulfan blue has been disappointing.[21]

Mandibular Distraction Osteogenesis versus Free Flap
Although a potentially attractive technical alternative to microsurgical free tissue transfer techniques for the restoration of mandibular continuity defects, bifocal or trifocal transport distraction osteogenesis carries its own significant costs.

External appliance requirement, internal and external fixation and distraction hardware, and surveillance radiographic imaging result in costs approximating the surgical fees for free flap procedures. The appropriate application of this exciting technique and other forms to the arena of oncologic reconstruction awaits further definition.

Resorbable Plate Technology
The advent of resorbable plating systems offers the theoretic advantage of creating a more favorable environment for the progressive transfer of stress to bone grafts and osteotomies, a favorable biomechanical phenomenon in the course of bone healing. Furthermore, the avoidance of amplification and attenuation of external beam therapeutic radiation doses, presently a consideration with metallic plating systems, is eliminated.

REFERENCES

1. Anain SA, Yetman RJ: The fate of intraoral free muscle flaps: is skin necessary? *Plast Reconstr Surg* 91(6):1027-1031, 1993.
2. Ariyan S: The pectoralis major myocutaneous flap: a versatile flap for reconstruction in the head and neck, *Plast Reconstr Surg* 63:73, 1979.
3. Bakamjian VY: A two-stage method of pharyngoesophageal reconstruction with a primary skin flap, *Plast Reconstr Surg* 48:8, 1941.
4. Boyd TB, Morris S, Rosen IB, et al: The through-and-through oromandibular defect: rationale for aggressive reconstruction, *Plast Reconstr Surg* 93:44-53, 1994.
5. Boyd B, Mulholland S, Gullane P, et al: Reinnervated lateral antebrachial cutaneous neurosome flaps in oral reconstruction: are we making sense? *Plast Reconstr Surg* 93(7):1350-1359, 1996.
6. Byers RM, Weber RS, Andrew T, et al: Frequency and therapeutic implication of "skip metastases" in the neck from squamous carcinoma of tongue, *Head Neck* 19(1):14-19, 1997.
7. Conley J, Baker DC: Hypoglossal-facial nerve anastomosis for reinnervation of paralyzed face, *Plast Reconstr Surg* 63(1):63-72, 1979.
8. Cordiero PG, Santamaria E, Kraus DH, et al: Reconstruction of total maxillectomy defects with preservation of the orbital contents, *Plast Reconstr Surg* 102:1874, 1998.
9. Davidson BJ, Kulkarny V, DeLacure MD, et al: Posterior triangle metastases in squamous cell carcinoma of the upper aerodigestive tract, *Am J Surg* 166:395-398, 1993.
10. DeLacure MD: Special considerations in the management of mandible for cancer of the oral cavity: current opinion, *Otolaryngol Head Neck Surg* 4(2):98-105, 1996.
11. DeLacure MD, Friedman CD: Metal plate and screw technology, *Otolaryngol Clin North Am* 27(5):983-1000, 1994.
12. Edgerton MT Jr: One-stage reconstruction of the cervical esophagus or trachea, *Surgery* 31:239-250, 1952.
13. Friedlander PL, Schantz SP, Shaha AR, et al: Squamous cell carcinoma of the tongue in young patients: a matched-pair analysis, *Head Neck* 20(5):363-368, 1998.

14. Frodel JL Jr, Funk GF, Capper DT, et al: Osteointegrated implants: a comparative study of bone thickness in four vascularized bone flaps, *Plast Reconstr Surg* 92(3):449-455, 1996.

15. Harrison LB, Lee HJ, Pfister DG, et al: Long-term results of primary radiotherapy with/without neck dissection for squamous cell cancer of the base of tongue, *Head Neck* 20(8):668-673, 1998.

16. Hidalgo DA, Jones CS: The role of emergent exploration in free-tissue transfer: a review of 150 consecutive cases, *Plast Reconstr Surg* 86(3):492-498, 1996.

17. Jones NF, Monstrey S, Gambier BA: Reliability of the fibular osteocutaneous flap for mandibular reconstruction: anatomical and surgical confirmation, *Plast Reconstr Surg* 97(4):707-716; discussion 717-718, 1996.

18. Kirchner J, Edberg SC, Sasaki CT: The use of topical antibiotics in head and neck prophylaxis: is it justified? *Laryngoscope* 98(1):26-29, 1988.

19. Loree TR, Stong EW: Significance of positive margins in oral cavity squamous carcinoma, *Am J Surg* 160:410, 1990.

20. Netterville JL, Wood DE: The lower trapezius flap: vascular anatomy and surgical technique, *Arch Otolaryngol Head Neck Surg* 117(1):73-76, 1991.

21. Pitman KT, Johnson JT, Edington H: Lymphatic mapping with isosulfan blue dye in squamous cell carcinoma of the head and neck, *Arch Otolaryngol Head Neck Surg* 124:790-793, 1998.

22. Rassekh CH, Janeka IP, Calhoun KH: Lower lip splitting incisions: anatomic considerations, *Laryngoscope* 105(8):880-883, 1995.

23. Sadove RC, Powell LA: Simultaneous maxillary and mandibular reconstruction with one free osteocutaneous flap, *Plast Reconstr Surg* 92(1):141-146, 1993.

24. Spiro RH, Huvos AG, Wong GY, et al: Predictive value of tumor thickness in squamous cell carcinoma confined to the tongue and floor of the mouth, *Am J Surg* 152:345-350, 1986.

25. Stuzin JM, Wagstrom L, Kawamoto HK, et al: Anatomy of frontal branch of facial nerve: the significance of temporal fat pad, *Plast Reconstr Surg* 83(2):265-271, 1989.

26. Taylor GI, Palmer JH: The vascular territories (angiosomes) of the body: experimental study and clinical applications, *Br J Plast Surg* 40(2):113-141, 1987.

27. Urken ML, Weinberg H, Vickery C, et al: Oromandibular reconstruction using microvascular composite free flaps: report of 71 cases and a new classification scheme for bony, soft-tissue, and neurologic defects, *Arch Otolaryngol Head Neck Surg* 117(7):733-744, 1991.

28. Wei F-C, Demirkan F, Chen HC, et al: Double free flaps in reconstruction of extensive composite mandibular defects in head and neck cancer, *Plast Reconstr Surg* 103(1):39-47, 1999.

The Mandible

J. Brian Boyd*

INTRODUCTION

Diseases of the mandible may involve tongue, oral lining, floor of mouth, and lower lip. Reconstruction follows trauma, infection, the resection of congenital anomalies and the extirpation of tumors and cysts.

Benign cysts of the mandible are effectively treated by curettage. Small tumors, localized areas of infection, and osteoradionecrosis may occasionally be handled with a localized resection including a margin of healthy bone, leaving the mandibular arch intact. If the tumor originates in adjacent mucosa, larger locally invasive and malignant tumors require segmental resection as part of a composite resection, with neck dissection when there are metastases in the neck. Large areas of osteomyelitis and osteoradionecrosis may also require segmental resection for their complete elimination. Smaller areas are treated more conservatively.

The functional outcomes of dental rehabilitation, maintenance of tongue mobility, and restoration of intraoral sensation are now considered essential adjuncts to restoring the mandibular arch. Thus quality of dental rehabilitation, articulation of speech, ease of swallowing, and maintenance of normal intraoral sensation have come to reflect our abilities as reconstructive surgeons as much as anastomotic patency rates, bony union, absence of complications, cosmetic appearance, and decreased hospital stay.

INDICATIONS

MANDIBULAR DEFECT CLASSIFICATION

The HCL classification of Boyd et al[13] allows the surgeon to define segmental defects of the mandible in order to allocate treatment options (Figure 77-1). Major difficulties in

*The section on *Mandibular Pathology* is by Chris Assad.

mandibular reconstruction arise when a condyle requires replacement, when the defect has a mucosal and/or skin component, and when the area to be reconstructed involves the anterior arch. These difficulties form the basis of the HCL system.[13]

The classification uses the characters H, C, L, and o, m, s. H defects are lateral, of any length including the condyle, and do not significantly cross the midline. L defects are the same but without the condyle. C defects consist of the entire central segment containing the four incisors and the two canines. For C to be included in the description, the major part of it must be resected. Combinations of these letters are possible: an angle-to-angle defect, for example, is represented as LCL. Thus H and L defects may reach or even extend slightly beyond the midline, but are not referred to as LC or HC unless they contain the entire central segment. The letters o (neither a skin nor a mucosal component), s (skin), m (mucosa), and sm (skin plus mucosa) denote the epithelial requirement.

OCCLUSAL TILT AND MANDIBULAR SWING

It was once common to leave L and H defects unreconstructed and concentrate on soft tissue closure. This simplified reconstruction, maintained oral continence, and allowed the patient to subsist on a soft diet. Moreover, it avoided the risks of mandibular reconstruction, which were considerable before microvascular surgery. Unopposed muscle pull acting on the mandibular remnant causes a swing to the resected side, leading to a significant crossbite in dentulous patients but serving to decrease the size of the defect. This produces abnormal dental wear, caries, and loss of function. In addition, the patient's face has a flattened or even concave appearance on the affected side. Malocclusion is exacerbated by an occlusal tilt caused by unilateral shortening of mandibular height. Excessive dental wear occurs when the lower dentition presents its side enamel to the cusps of the upper teeth during chewing.

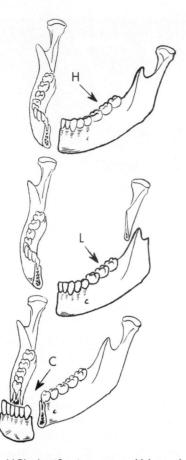

Figure 77-1. HCL classification system. *H,* Lateral segment, any length, containing condyle, not significantly crossing midline; *L,* lateral segment, any length, no condyle, not significantly crossing midline; *C,* central segment of mandible containing both canines and all four incisors. Whole segment must be present to use C designation; *o,* bone only; *m,* mucosa; *s,* skin; *m, s,* mucosa and skin. (Redrawn from Boyd JB et al: *Plast Reconstr Surg* 92:1266, 1993.)

LIP AND CHIN PTOSIS

Anterior arch defects present the greatest functional and cosmetic problems and the most difficult surgical challenge. According to the HCL classification (see Figure 77-1), the anterior arch or central segment is defined as that portion of the mandible containing the incisors and canines, and is represented by the letter C. Reconstruction of this C segment presents unique problems, frequently resulting in *lip and chin ptosis* (Figure 77-2), in which the soft tissues slide off the reconstructed arch, producing eversion of the lower lip and salivary incontinence. If edentulous, the mandibular arch tends to *overclose* rotating upward and carrying the intraoral flap with it. The anterior oral floor thereby becomes visible above a ptotic lower lip. Several factors contribute:

1. The C segment has four powerful mouth-opening muscles, two geniohyoid and two digastric, attached to its inner inferior border. When the bone is resected, these are necessarily detached. They may even be excised as part of the ablative procedure. As a result, the mandible, free of its anterior muscular tethering and pulled by the pterygoids and masseter, rides upward. In edentulous patients, this is not limited by occlusion. The detached muscles, now only attached to soft tissues, retract inferiorly, pulling the same soft tissues with them (see Figure 77-2). Even with massive bony resections, good oral function may be maintained by the preservation of the C segment and its muscular attachments. When this is not possible, it is occasionally feasible to reattach either the submental musculature or the soft tissues of the chin to the reconstructed symphysis (Figure 77-3).

2. The detached soft tissues may become ptotic, rather like the "witch's chin" seen occasionally in orthognathic and cosmetic surgery after overzealous degloving of the mentum.

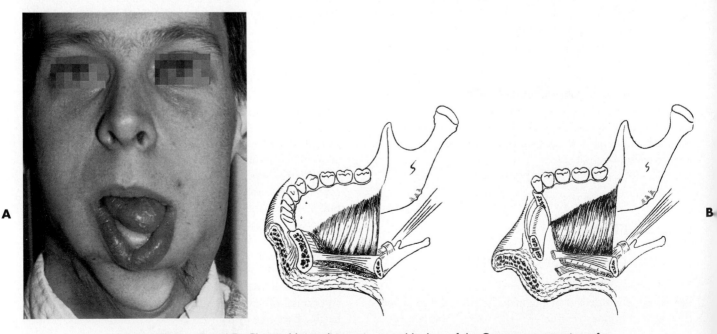

Figure 77-2. **A** and **B,** Chin and lower lip ptosis caused by loss of the C segment, resection of submental musculature, degloving of the chin, lower lip paralysis, and gravity. (**B,** Redrawn from Boyd JB et al: *Plast Reconstr Surg* 92:1266, 1993.)

(The mentum is automatically degloved in C-containing resections.) Here gravity plays a major role. Soft tissues of the chin should be reattached to the reconstructed mentum whenever possible.

3. Bilateral neck dissections and extensive anterior ablative surgery can result in destruction of the lower branches of the facial nerve on both sides. Lack of good oral sphincter tone contributes to a patulous and ptotic lower lip, exacerbating lip and chin ptosis.

4. If during reconstruction a large, anterior, floor-of-mouth "dead space" is not adequately filled with soft tissue, the resulting contracture tends to either distort the new bony arch or, alternatively, draw the soft tissues inferiorly, contributing to the same inferior displacement described above.

MANDIBULAR PATHOLOGY*

Mandibular pathology may present with swelling (fibrous dysplasia, cherubism, cysts, and cancer), pain (osteoradionecrosis, osteomyelitis, and invasive squamous cell carcinoma), numbness (neoplastic invasion of the inferior alveolar nerves), loosening of teeth (weakening of socket by many disease processes), or oral mucosal involvement (mandibular sarcomas breaking out, mucosal carcinomas breaking in, osteoradionecrosis causing inflammation, breakdown, and bone exposure). Rarely, mandibular conditions present with skin involvement (oral tumors, unusual cysts, and infections). Commonly, the patient's dentist is the first to identify the problem.

Diagnosis is made on the basis of a thorough history, physical examination, and appropriate tests. These include panorex, computed axial tomography (CAT) scan, chest x-ray, and quadroscopy with biopsy of the lesion. Magnetic resonance imaging (MRI) may be useful to define the soft tissue component of the process, but CAT with bone windows is more definitive for the bone involvement. A tissue biopsy is essential for planning appropriate therapy. Treatment may involve dental extraction, curettage, curettage with cancellous bone grafting, marginal resection, segmental resection, or "commando resection." The last mentioned refers to a composite excision of oral cancer (squamous cell carcinoma) together with an ipsilateral neck dissection; the intervening mandibular segment is removed en bloc with the specimen. The mandible was sacrificed on the historical observation, subsequently discredited, that lymphatics passing directly through the bone may contain cancer cells. However, today the mandible is spared unless clinically or radiologically invaded, with reliance on adjunctive radiotherapy to take care of any microscopic in-transit metastases.

Mandibular surgery is also required for infective processes. Osteomyelitis of the mandible is a rare condition usually associated with a dental abscess, or with a fracture with oral contamination, occurring most frequently in individuals with poor oral hygiene, in debilitated individuals, and in poorly fixed or inadequately immobilized fractures. It responds well to 6 weeks of intravenous antibiotics, dietary diversion if oral contamination is present, and sequestrectomy when indicated. In extensive cases and in those with significant bone loss, wide excision and reconstruction using a free vascularized bone graft is appropriate.

Osteoradionecrosis is a more difficult problem. Following large doses of radiotherapy, often years later, it may be precipitated by dental caries. Osteoradionecrosis is characterized by primary bone necrosis, which becomes secondarily infected, and its x-ray has an irregular moth-eaten appearance. Early cases may respond to local sequestrectomy, antibiotics,

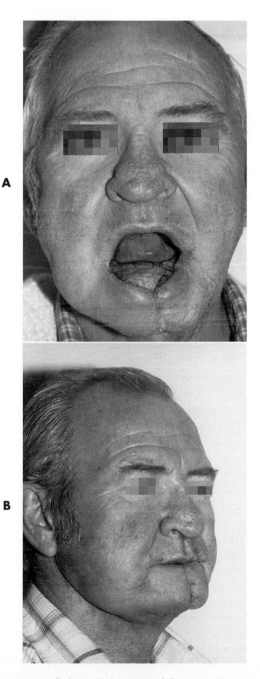

Figure 77-3. **A,** Lip and chin ptosis following anterior mandibular reconstruction. **B,** Correction at a second procedure by suturing soft tissues of the chin to drill-holes in the bone graft.

*By Chris Assad.

dietary diversion, and hyperbaric oxygen; however, the reconstructive surgeon is more likely to encounter those with persistent infection despite prolonged therapy. Extensive osteoradionecrosis induces breakdown of the overlying gingival mucosa, bone exposure, and secondary infection, leading to severe pain and trismus. En bloc excision with composite reconstruction using free tissue transfer offers the best hope of relief.

It is important to have a simple classification of mandibular cysts and tumors on which to base a working differential diagnosis. Unfortunately, no single unifying classification exists; most combine a mixture of odontogenesis and embryology, the propensity for inductive changes on surrounding tissues, histologic appearance, and clinical behavior.[39] The system shown in Table 77-1 borrows heavily from Kramer et al[39] and Reichart and Ries[54] and is designed to include the entities most likely to be encountered by a reconstructive surgeon. It omits many rare conditions and includes only the briefest comments on the less common pathologies listed.

Common conditions are illustrated in Figure 77-4. Please refer to Table 77-1 for information on these and other mandibular cysts and tumors.

MANDIBULAR PATHOPHYSIOLOGY

Many mandibular reconstructions are carried out unnecessarily. Fixation of the tumor to the inner cortex of the mandible (even without radiologic evidence of bony invasion) has commonly led to a T4 classification and resulted in segmental bone removal as part of a composite resection. Complex reconstruction ensues, with the associated risk, morbidity, and expense. Many published series on microvascular reconstruction contain individuals who may have been better served by a marginal mandibulectomy with a simple cutaneous flap for oral lining.

Earlier concepts of lymphatic spread from floor of mouth and tongue directly through the mandible have been discredited. McGregor and MacDonald[46] have shown that invasion of the dentate mandible occurs primarily through its apex along the alveolar ridge (Figure 77-4, D). This soft cancellous bone is the path of least resistance to tumor spread. The dense medial cortex presents a more effective barrier. It follows that the last portion of the mandible to be invaded is the lower border. In some cases where the intraoral tumor appears "attached" to the mandible, the inner cortex has not been breached and the apical invasion has not even started. By leaving a lower rim of mandible (marginal mandibulectomy), the "attached" portion is removed, as well as the most likely point of invasion, the apex. McGregor and MacDonald have presented convincing histopathologic data supporting this approach. Notwithstanding advances in free tissue transfer, an intact mandibular arch—even a rim—greatly simplifies reconstruction and improves the functional and cosmetic outcome. It also significantly shortens the surgery and minimizes the donor defect.

Exceptions are made where the tumor extends under the mandible and is fixed to the lower border and in those cases where radiologic invasion of the medial cortex is documented. To minimize the risk of pathologic fracture, the height of the rim should be at least 11 mm.[3] This applies to edentulous patients as well.[46] Careful preoperative and intraoperative assessment using panorex, CAT scan, and physical examination will allow selection of the appropriate patients for marginal mandibular resection.

PRIMARY VERSUS SECONDARY VERSUS NO RECONSTRUCTION

Noncutaneous squamous cell carcinoma of the head and neck has an annual incidence of 17/100,000, or 5% of all new cancers. Some 55% will involve the oral cavity or orohypopharynx. The more advanced (T4) lesions invading the mandible will require resection of bone as well as mucosa. In the past, many surgeons have left major mandibular defects unreconstructed due to the daunting extent of bony and soft tissue requirements and the hostile irradiated recipient bed; however, their patients were condemned to exist as oral cripples, suffering from a varying inability to chew, swallow, articulate, or maintain oral competence. These poor functional and aesthetic outcomes were most dramatic in anterior defects[48] where *Andy Gump*—a chinless comic character of the 1930s—lent his name to the condition. With lateral defects, a flattening of the affected side of the face and a lower facial asymmetry must be added to the problems of mandibular swing and occlusal tilt mentioned previously.

Primary reconstruction is presently the standard of care, since it immediately restores function and appearance, avoids further hospitalizations, and maximizes the quality of life for those patients with little remaining. Furthermore, it is simpler. Secondary reconstructions are still performed in patients who, for some reason, were denied immediate mandibular reconstruction, and in those patients in whom primary reconstruction failed. Secondary reconstruction is generally more difficult because:

1. Estimation of the length of the missing bone segment is difficult.
2. The mucosal requirement is difficult to predict.
3. Dissection of the posterior mandibular fragment puts the facial nerve at risk. If there has been a hemimandibular resection, it extends all the way up to the condylar fossa. Identification of the nerve is laborious and dangerous due to scarring and altered anatomy.
4. Contracture and fibrosis make it a challenge to position the mandibular fragments in their original spatial relationship.
5. The posterior mandibular fragment rotates upward due to unopposed muscle pull. It is often necessary to detach the coronoid process and strip off the medial pterygoid muscle in order to bring it down.
6. With previous neck dissections, there are fewer recipient vessels.

Text continued on p. 1251.

Table 77-1.
Summary of Mandibular Cysts and Tumors

MANDIBULAR CYSTS
Epithelial Odontogenic

SUBTYPE	FEATURES INCIDENCE	LOCATION	CLINICAL PRESENTATION	ETIOLOGY	RADIOGRAPHIC FEATURES	TREATMENT AND PROGNOSIS
Dentigerous cyst	24% of odontogenic cysts; peak incidence in childhood and early adolescence; AKA follicular cyst	Surrounds crown of unerupted second and third molars	Asymptomatic unless secondarily infected; slow growing; may cause displacement of teeth and facial asymmetry; can be locally destructive	Reduced enamel epithelium after crown formation, with fluid accumulating between the epithelium and crown	Well-defined (usually unilocular) radiolucency with sharp margins; larger lesions may have scalloped borders	Enucleation or marsupialization; approximately 6% recur; questionable ameloblastic transformation
Keratocyst	~5% of all jaw cysts; all ages peaking in second and third decades; male predilection	~50% around third molar and ascending ramus	Often slow growing, painful swelling with discharge; possible paresthesias; mean size 3 cm; aggressive with increased mitotic activity and cellularity	Dental lamina (also disputed origin from primordial cyst)	Often multiloculated with scalloped borders; marked cortical thinning and root resorption; may be confused with ameloblastoma	Enucleation with curettage for small cysts; resection, including soft tissue margin, if bony perforation; recurrence up to 60% with incomplete excision

Continued

Table 77-1.
Summary of Mandibular Cysts and Tumors—cont'd

SUBTYPE	FEATURES INCIDENCE	LOCATION	CLINICAL PRESENTATION	ETIOLOGY	RADIOGRAPHIC FEATURES	TREATMENT AND PROGNOSIS
MANDIBULAR CYSTS—cont'd						
Epithelial Odontogenic—cont'd						
Nevoid basal cell carcinoma (Gorlin's) syndrome	Incidence ~1 in 200; autosomal dominant; presents in early childhood	As for keratocyst	Multiple often bilateral keratocysts; multiple cutaneous basal cell carcinomas; calcified pineal; mental retardation; skeletal anomalies and dyskeratotic pitting of palms and soles; lifelong development of keratocysts and basal cell carcinomas	Cystic origin as above; autosomal dominant transmission	As for keratocysts	As for keratocyst; lifelong surveillance; difficult to distinguish recurrence from new cyst formation
Lateral periodontal cyst	Less than 2% of cysts; male:female ratio = 2:1	Develops on lateral aspect of root of tooth; usually between canine and premolar	Asymptomatic, small, and slow growing between vital (living) teeth	Growth of epithelial rests within periodontal ligament; often associated with supernumerary teeth	Well or poorly circumscribed radiolucency with sclerotic margins	Enucleation with preservation of vital teeth; does not tend to recur

Calcifying odontogenic (Gorlin's) cyst	Oral analogue of calcifying epithelioma of Malherbe; ~2% of jaw cysts; occurs in all ages	75% are located anterior to the first molar; 2/3 intraosseous and 1/3 extraosseous	May be cystic or solid; slow growing; asymptomatic swelling; average size 3 cm	From dental epithelium of unerupted developing teeth	Well-demarcated unilocular radiolucencies; can cause cortical expansion with resorption of tooth roots; seen with intraluminal opacifications	Complete excision; low recurrence rate
Residual cyst	Any odontogenic cysts that persist in bone after a tooth is removed; ~20% of odontogenic cysts	Any location in relation to teeth	Static or slowly enlarges; asymptomatic or painful with inflammation	From epithelial remnants in periapical granuloma ("root abscess")	Well circumscribed in edentulous area	Enucleation; low recurrence rate
Radicular cyst	Apical periodontal cyst; ~55% of odontogenic cysts; any age (greatest in third, fourth, and fifth decades)	Posterior mandible most common	Asymptomatic; pain and swelling with inflammatory sequence; may have sinus tract to oral mucosa or even skin	From rests of Malassez in periodontal ligament	Pear or ovoid radiolucency with sharp sclerotic borders; in continuity with apex of tooth root	Extraction of tooth with enucleation; low recurrence rate
Epithelial Nonodontogenic						
Fissural: median mandibular cyst	Rare; nonaggressive	Midline symphyseal	Asymptomatic with adjacent teeth remaining vital; pain if secondarily infected	Controversial: from trapped epithelial remnants of mandibular arch fusion vs. periodontal cyst	Well-circumscribed unilocular radiolucency with divergent tooth roots; can extend to alveolar crest	Enucleation; uncertain of prognosis due to rarity of lesion

Continued

Table 77-1.
Summary of Mandibular Cysts and Tumors—cont'd

MANDIBULAR CYSTS—cont'd

Nonepithelial (Pseudocysts)

SUBTYPE	FEATURES INCIDENCE	LOCATION	CLINICAL PRESENTATION	ETIOLOGY	RADIOGRAPHIC FEATURES	TREATMENT AND PROGNOSIS
Traumatic bone cyst	Known as a simple "unicameral bone cyst"; rare, solitary, osteolytic lesion	Mostly anterior mandible but also molar area	Size extremely variable; asymptomatic and found on routine examination; associated with labial or buccal expansion; teeth remain vital	Trauma with intramedullary hematoma	Smooth radiolucency with scalloped borders extending beyond tooth roots	May resolve spontaneously; curettage with possible bone grafting of large lesions; low recurrence rate
Aneurysmal bone cyst	Rare in mandible; benign expansile lytic lesion	Body of mandible	Pain and swelling; growth rate variable	Possibly traumatic origin with localized alterations in hemodynamics, or persistent connection between the damaged vessel and hematoma; possibly an AV fistula	Expansile eccentric cyst with thin cortices; soap bubble or honeycombed appearance	Curettage; excision bloody; recurrence rate not determined for mandibular lesions

MANDIBULAR TUMORS
Epithelial Odontogenic Benign

Ameloblastoma	Locally invasive; 1% of jaw tumors and cysts; commonest odontogenic tumor (11% of all); peak incidence in third and fourth decades; male:female ratio = 1:1; propensity for dangerous, disfiguring growth and late recurrence	80% occur in mandible, 20% in maxilla; most commonly molar area of mandible; often associated with unerupted third molar	Slow growing painless swelling with or without a soft tissue mass; size ranges from 1-16 cm; large lesions can cause facial asymmetry, loose or displaced teeth, and malocclusion; can expand bone, erode through it, or produce pathologic fractures	May arise from remnants of enamel organ, dental lamina, or previous keratocysts (origins from dentigerous cysts controversial)	Great variability: *Unilocular* Round or ovoid appearance with no calcified or radiopaque components; distinct border with slight marginal sclerosis, may have scalloped margins; no periosteal reaction *Multilocular* Honeycombed or soap bubble appearance; marked expansion with cortical thinning and bony destruction	Curettage or enucleation **condemned** due to up to 90% recurrence; partial mandibulectomy or segmental resection with margins of normal bone recommended (recurrence rate ~4-5%); radiation therapy palliative for unresectable tumors (usually maxillary); metastases rare; reported deaths from recurrent *mandibular* tumors extremely rare
Calcifying epithelial odontogenic tumor (Pindborg tumor)	Rare, locally aggressive tumor; ~2% of odontogenic tumors; bimodal incidence occurring in third and fourth decades	Usually in premolar and molar area (in contrast to ameloblastoma); many associated with unerupted teeth	Painless slow-growing mass; produces a mineralized substance	Tissue of origin debated but probably from the enamel organ	Well-circumscribed loculated radiolucency with varying amounts of centralized mineralization	Treatment similar to ameloblastoma; up to 14% recurrence reported

Continued

Table 77-1.
Summary of Mandibular Cysts and Tumors—cont'd

SUBTYPE	FEATURES INCIDENCE	LOCATION	CLINICAL PRESENTATION	ETIOLOGY	RADIOGRAPHIC FEATURES	TREATMENT AND PROGNOSIS
MANDIBULAR TUMORS—cont'd						
Epithelial Odontogenic Benign—cont'd						
Adenomatoid odontogenic tumor	Rare nonaggressive tumor; 2:1 female:male predilection; most patients present before 20 years of age	Usually anterior to canines and frequently associated with impacted or unerupted teeth	Slow growing; asymptomatic mandibular swelling; small, ~1.5-3 cm, painless anterior tumor	From the enamel organ	Well-demarcated unilocular radiolucency often associated with crown of unerupted tooth; rare resorption of tooth roots	Conservative excision; low recurrence rate
Mesenchymal Odontogenic Benign						
Myxoma	Locally aggressive; ~3% of odontogenic tumors; peak incidence second and third decades	Most commonly posterior mandible but rarely in condyle	Slow or rapidly growing; progressive swelling with bony expansion; can cause malpositioning of teeth	Odontogenic mesenchyme, most likely dental papilla	Multiple radiolucent areas of varying sizes separated by bony trabeculae; margins variably demarcated; can extend through bone and into soft tissues	En bloc excision; recurrence rate ~25%
Benign cementoblastoma	Common slow growing neoplasm containing cementum; most commonly in mid 20's	Premolar or molar teeth; usually 2-3 cm and attached to a tooth root	Swelling, pain, and hypoesthesia common; may cause severe facial asymmetry	Mesenchyme of periodontal ligament	Well-defined radiopaque lesion with radiolucent periphery; fused to a partially resorbed tooth root	Complete excision including involved tooth; low recurrence rate

Odontogenic fibroma	A rare, poorly defined, and controversial entity; may occur at any age; nonaggressive	Central, intraosseous, body of mandible	Slow persistent growth with asymptomatic cortical expansion	Speculative; arises from either dental papilla or dental sac	Multiloculated and well-circumscribed radiolucency; can be associated with unerupted or displaced teeth	Conservative excision or enucleation; low recurrence rate
Mixed Epithelial Mesenchymal Odontogenic Benign						
Ameloblastic fibroma	Rare tumor that may be confused with ameloblastoma or fibrosarcoma; rarely aggressive; occurs in younger ages with tooth formation and eruption	Premolar or molar area of mandible	Asymptomatic expansile swelling of mandible	Arises from ameloblasts and dental papilla	Well-defined unilocular or multilocular radiolucency associated with an unerupted tooth	Curettage; ~18% recurrence rate
Ameloblastic fibroodontoma	Nonaggressive; features of ameloblastic fibroma but also contains elements of dentin and enamel; also younger age group	Premolar or molar area of mandible; varying size from a few millimeters to half of mandible	Asymptomatic expansile swelling of mandible	Arises from ameloblasts and odontoblasts	Well-circumscribed with solitary or multiple radiopacities	Enucleation with curettage; low recurrence rate
Odontoma	Common; likely a hamartoma; all ages but mostly second decade	Posterior mandible; usually <1 cm but can grow to 6 cm	Most are asymptomatic but swelling may interfere with tooth eruption	From odontogenic apparatus (i.e., enamel, dentin, and cementum)	Well-circumscribed, unilocular or multilocular, with irregular radiodensities and often a surrounding halo	Early enucleation to prevent interference with tooth eruption; low recurrence rate

Continued

Table 77-1.
Summary of Mandibular Cysts and Tumors—cont'd

SUBTYPE	FEATURES INCIDENCE	LOCATION	CLINICAL PRESENTATION	ETIOLOGY	RADIOGRAPHIC FEATURES	TREATMENT AND PROGNOSIS
MANDIBULAR TUMORS—cont'd						
Epithelial Odontogenic Malignant						
Malignant ameloblastoma	Rare; classified as an odontogenic carcinoma; occurs any age after first decade but most commonly in men >50 years	Generally the same as ameloblastoma	History of multiple unsuccessful treatments of benign but persistent odontogenic epithelial lesions; pain, swelling, ulceration, and paresthesias; regional lymphadenopathy with metastases to lung, liver, vertebrae	Arises from residual odontogenic apparatus or from transformation of an odontogenic cyst or ameloblastoma	Poorly defined radiolucencies with gross expansion and thinned cortices	Full oncologic screening; radical resection; too few tumors reported to state ideal treatment but radiotherapy and chemotherapy are used; poor prognosis
Mesenchymal Odontogenic Malignant						
Ameloblastic fibrosarcoma	Rare; average age 15-18 years	Posterior mandible	Swelling preceding pain, paresthesias, ulceration	Rare reports of developing in preexisting ameloblastic fibromas or fibroodontomas	Like malignant ameloblastoma; may resemble ameloblastoma except peripheral margins are indistinct	Radical resection; chemotherapy for intractable cases; radiotherapy ineffective; fatal cases associated with uncontrolled infiltration

Nonodontogenic Benign

Fibrous dysplasia	Uncommon but not rare; usually first and second decades; fibroosseous lesion; developmental derangement due to undifferentiated mesenchymal bone-forming cells replacing normal lamellar by woven bone; monostotic and polyostotic variants; latter associated with **Albright's syndrome**	Commoner in maxilla; most often involves area of mandibular angle	Small lesions may be static and asymptomatic; usually progressive, unilateral swelling; variable facial asymmetry; pain and decreased function with progressive deformity; dentition can be shifted but teeth remain vital; burns out after puberty	Various theories: a. Trauma-induced b. Congenital anomaly of development c. Abnormal activity of mesenchymal cells d. Endocrine disturbance	Ground glass or orange peel appearance; poorly circumscribed with diffuse borders; pagetoid or cystlike appearance	If required, definitive reconstruction done when disease has burned out; earlier intervention with partial resection, curettage, or bony contouring indicated for pain and functional loss; rare malignant change postradiotherapy; prognosis generally good
Giant cell granuloma	Uncommon; ~3.5% of benign jaw tumors; locally aggressive; children and young adults	Typically symphyseal and bicuspid regions	Growth intermittent and variable; pain may be dominant symptom	Debated; reactive process vs. osteoclastic or odontogenic apparatus origin	Uniloculated or multiloculated; well circumscribed	Curettage or excision; recurrence rare with complete excision

Continued

Table 77-1.
Summary of Mandibular Cysts and Tumors—cont'd

SUBTYPE	FEATURES INCIDENCE	LOCATION	CLINICAL PRESENTATION	ETIOLOGY	RADIOGRAPHIC FEATURES	TREATMENT AND PROGNOSIS
MANDIBULAR TUMORS—cont'd						
Nonodontogenic Benign—cont'd						
Osteoma	Osteogenic tumor; 15-40 years of age; peripheral variants commoner than central	Commonly lingual surface of mandibular body; attached to cortical bone by a stalk	Asymptomatic lingual mass	Unknown	Well-circumscribed radiopaque mass; resembles exostosis	Usually not required, but if symptomatic, local excision is sufficient with no risk of recurrence
	Gardner's syndrome: Autosomal dominant with multiple osteomas, epidermal cysts, colon polyposis, and pigmented lip macules					
Cherubism	An uncommon bilateral condition; early childhood between 2 and 6 years of age; destructive fibrous swelling of the maxilla and mandible; sporadic or autosomal dominant inheritance with 100% penetrance in males	Entire body and ramus with sparing of condyles; extends into alveolar process	Painless rapid early growth; alveolar involvement causes shedding of deciduous teeth, delayed eruption, and malocclusion (**Maxillary** fullness produces retraction of lower eyelids, increased scleral show causing "cherubic" appearance)	Unknown	Bilateral, well-defined multilocular radiolucencies; cortical thinning or absence	Postpone treatment unless decreased function; treatment individualized depending on amount of regression or deformity; good prognosis if mandible solely involved

Nonodontogenic Malignant (Primary)

Osteosarcoma	Although most common primary bone malignancy, rarely encountered in the mandible (~6% of osteosarcomas); occurs in second and third decades, male:female ratio = 2:1	Most commonly in body of mandible	Rapidly progressive painful swelling; loose teeth; paresthesias	Radiation; radiotherapy of Paget's disease or fibrous dysplasia; disturbance of growth and maturity of bone during osteoblastic activity	Early: widening of periodontal space. Late: variable appearance; either poorly demarcated, radiolucent, unicentric areas or dense radiopaque lesions with "sunburst" appearance	Radical resection with radiotherapy; lymph node dissection if palpable nodes; metastases to lungs; 5-year survival rate up to 71%
Chondrosarcoma	Rare overall but approximately 10% of chondrosarcomas occur in the jaws; average age 32 years	Posterior mandible	Painless, slow- or fast-growing with loose teeth; invasive and destructive, becoming painful; metastases to lungs	Possible causes include: a. Radiation b. Malignant transformation of cartilaginous remnants of Meckel's cartilage	Variable; central radiolucency with thick walls and "cotton-wool" calcifications; late cortical erosion in soft tissues	Radical excision with wide margins followed by chemotherapy; radioresistant; poor prognosis
Central mucoepidermoid carcinoma	Uncommon; primary intraosseous salivary gland tumor; all ages, with average age in mid-50's	Posterior mandible associated with impacted third molar (resembles odontogenic cyst or osteoclastic odontogenic tumor)	Rapid onset of painless swelling; slow growth and pain also reported; metastases reported to regional lymph nodes	Debated: ectopic salivary gland tissue vs. follicular cyst origin	Multiloculated cystic appearance	No standardized treatment; en bloc resection with or without radiotherapy; 5-year survival excellent

Continued

Table 77-1.
Summary of Mandibular Cysts and Tumors—cont'd

SUBTYPE	FEATURES INCIDENCE	LOCATION	CLINICAL PRESENTATION	ETIOLOGY	RADIOGRAPHIC FEATURES	TREATMENT AND PROGNOSIS
MANDIBULAR TUMORS—cont'd						
Nonodontogenic Malignant (Primary)—cont'd						
Burkitt's lymphoma	Poorly differentiated B-cell lymphoma; most common childhood malignancy in East Africa, with mean age 7-9 years; rare in North America, with mean age 11-12 years; fastest growing neoplasm	80% of tumors; found in all four jaw quadrants; jaw less commonly involved in North American cases	Enlarges very rapidly; shifting and exfoliation of teeth; associated with adrenal, kidney, and gonadal masses; lymphadenopathy rare	Obscure relationship to Epstein-Barr virus; genetic association; environmental link to malaria	Early break in lamina dura distinctive; scalloped lytic lesions that coalesce; cortical expansion with "floating teeth"	Chemotherapy; 50% relapse rate; poorer prognosis if gonadal involvement
Nonodontogenic Malignant (Secondary)						
Metastatic carcinoma	~1% of malignant bony metastases involve the jaw	Body and angle most common	Usually elderly; pain, paresthesias, swelling, loose teeth, pathologic fractures	Commonest primaries are breast, kidney, lung, colon, prostate, and thyroid—in that order	Generally irregular "moth eaten" expansile radiolucencies, but breast and prostate may be osteoblastic, thus appearing sclerotic	Palliative procedures; poor prognosis

| Squamous cell carcinoma | 90% of oral cancers, 30% of head and neck cancers, 6% of all cancers; male:female ratio = 2:1, but increasing female incidence due to smoking **Morphology:** a. Exophytic (least bad) b. Ulcerative c. Mixed **Histologic variants:** a. Basaloid (worst variant) b. Verrucous—5% of oral SCC (better prognosis) | Commonly arises in mucosa of posterior alveolar ridge, but can spread from any part of the oral cavity, including lips; 35-50% have bone invasion histologically and radiographically at time of diagnosis; spread is thought to be via occlusal surface (gingiva, tooth socket), since periosteum is considered an effective barrier to tumor spread; may extend along inferior alveolar nerve; 10% of oral SCCs arise at alveolar ridge | **Risk factors:** a. Smoking, 6× risk b. Snuff, 4× risk c. Betal chewing—increased risk when combined with tobacco d. Alcohol, 6× risk e. Alcohol plus tobacco, 15× risk f. Malnutrition: iron, vitamins A and C deficiencies g. Solar exposure (lip) h. Viral i. Poor dentition j. Genetic | Can present as an incidental finding or as advanced disease; presents with a nonhealing sore, pain, loose teeth, poorly fitting dentures, difficulty with mastication, or numbness and pain if the inferior alveolar nerve is involved; weight loss is common | Invasive, poorly circumscribed lytic areas of bone that may be associated with a soft tissue mass | *Initial screening:* History and physical, biopsy with toluidine blue staining, chest X-ray, and liver function tests; CT to assess infiltrative nodal disease and distant metastases; MRI useful for soft tissue and perineural involvement; bone scan if bone pain; panendoscopy *Consultations:* H&N team, oncologist, nutritionist; treatment varies with TNM staging and patient factors *Modalities:* Surgery, radiotherapy, chemotherapy 50% reduction in cure rate with nodal involvement; prognosis generally poor |

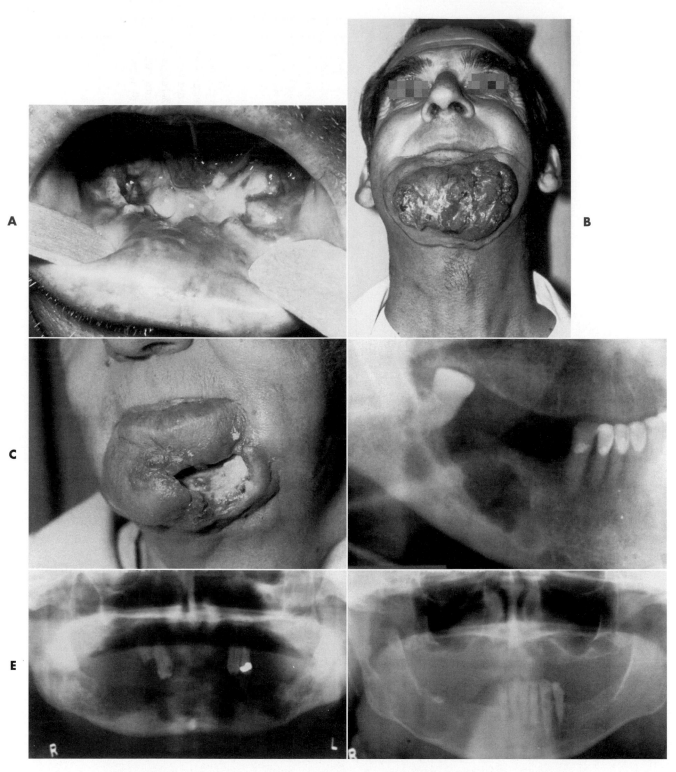

Figure 77-4. Common mandibular conditions. **A,** Anterior floor of mouth squamous cell carcinoma invading mandible. **B,** Exophytic oral squamous cell carcinoma invading mandible and overlying skin. Resection produces a through-and-through defect. **C,** Ulcerative, basaloid squamous cell carcinoma. This type is more aggressive and has a much poorer prognosis than **B. D,** X-ray of an advanced squamous cell carcinoma invading the mandible via its apex (the alveolar process)—the path of least resistance. Note the poorly circumscribed lytic areas. **E,** Extensive osteoradionecrosis of the mandible with trismus, chronic pain, and narcotic addiction. Friable oral mucosa has broken down, exposing bone in the floor of mouth. The radiographic appearance is described as moth-eaten. This case is too extensive for local measures and requires wide excision with composite reconstruction. **F,** Ameloblastoma in the mandibular body with soap bubble appearance, marginal sclerosis, cortical thinning, and bony expansion. *Continued*

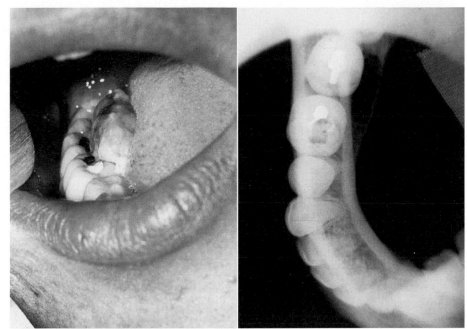

Figure 77-4, cont'd. **G** and **H,** Theoretically, any bony tumor may occur in the mandible. However, 10% of chondrosarcomas occur in the jaw. This one arises, as is usual, in the posterior mandible. A radiolucent lesion is seen breaching the medial cortex and extending into the oral cavity.

OPERATIONS

MANDIBULAR RECONSTRUCTION

Although the rib, metatarsal, humerus, and clavicle have all been used in composite oromandibular reconstruction, they have been largely abandoned due to the inadequacy of the bone, the morbidity of the donor site, or both. The four free flap donor sites in common use are the iliac crest,[70,71] fibula,[34,35] radius,[66] and scapula.[61,72] The option of using alloplastic reconstruction in conjunction with a cutaneous flap also exists.[15] For small defects in nonirradiated and noncontaminated beds, a nonvascularized graft may be satisfactory with this method.

The majority of mandibular resections in patients suffering from oral cancer involve mucosa. Composite tissue transfer is therefore required; however, in the younger patient, resections are most commonly performed for primary tumors of the mandible. In this group bone-only reconstructions are more common.[9]

Resections for locally invasive or malignant mandibular cysts are much rarer, but the defects are reconstructed using exactly the same principles. The same may be said for osteomyelitis and osteoradionecrosis, although the latter is more likely to require oral lining replacement in addition to the bony reconstruction.

Patient Assessment and Preparation

The extent of the disease must be assessed prior to proceeding with surgery. The assessment usually includes a full head and neck examination, biopsy of the lesion, chest x-ray, quadroscopy, liver function tests, and CT scan. Other tests may beindicated as a result of these investigations and as a result of a complete physical examination. Patients with disseminated disease are not generally considered for surgery unless it is to be performed as a "toilet procedure" to alleviate suffering from a necrotizing, fungating, foul-smelling, and painful intraoral lesion.

Since many of the individuals requiring mandibular resection are debilitated, they should also be assessed with regard to anesthetic risk and ability to heal. Preliminary (and ongoing) nutritional supplement (by the peroral or nasoenteral route) and respiratory therapy may be necessary.

With segmental mandibular resection it is advisable to perform a tracheotomy either before or during the procedure. This secures the airway from accidental extubation in the immediate postoperative phase and facilitates operation. When the continuity of the mandible is not breached or where there is minimal involvement of the tongue, this is usually unnecessary. In all but the simplest excisions it is necessary to have ample crossmatched blood on hand.

The reconstructive surgeon should be part of a team that includes a head and neck surgeon, a pathologist, a radiation oncologist, a pulmonologist, an anesthesiologist, and a radiologist familiar with the region and with modern techniques of imaging. Responsibility for difficult decisions is then shared, and combined protocols may be followed for the patients' benefit. Decisions on the best approach, the extent of resection, the place of radiotherapy, and the form of reconstruction are made at an indications conference. During surgery, a two-team approach is employed whenever possible. The duration of surgery is predictive of the incidence of systemic complications, the length of intensive care unit (ICU) stay, the total hospitalization, and the cost to the health care system. It should be minimized.

Iliac Crest

The deep circumflex iliac artery (DCIA) originates from the external iliac artery and passes laterally on the deep surface of the inguinal ligament (Figure 77-5). It continues along the inside of the iliac crest, sending some perforators into the bone and others over the crest into the muscle attached to it. The skin paddle receives a blood supply from the latter. Thus the flap consists of bone, an obligatory muscle cuff[37] (Figure 77-6) through which the perforators are transmitted, the overlying skin, and a vascular pedicle.

SURGICAL ANATOMY. The flap is based on the DCIA and the deep circumflex iliac vein (DCIV). The DCIA joins its vein a short distance lateral to the iliac vessels, forming the vascular pedicle. Passing medially from this point, the DCIV diverges superiorly from the DCIA, lying either in front of or behind the external iliac artery, before entering the external iliac vein. The DCIV receives one or two tributaries in this region and, as a result, has a fairly large diameter at its termination. The artery's diameter is approximately 2 mm, while the vein can measure between 2 and 4 mm. In the lateral part of the pedicle, the DCIV is represented by paired venae comitantes. These usually unite lateral to the convergence of artery and vein, but may remain paired for all or part of their terminal course.

The pedicle travels laterally, a few millimeters from the lower free edge of the inguinal ligament, occupying a fibrous tunnel composed of transversalis fascia. An ascending branch arises a couple of centimeters medial to the anterior superior iliac spine (ASIS), passing superior and lateral into the abdominal musculature and occupying the neurovascular plane between transversus abdominis and internal oblique. It supplies the muscle and skin of the abdominal wall above the iliac crest. Its significance is threefold: it can be used as a pedicle for a different free flap[75]; it is subject to anatomic variations; and, most important, it can be mistaken for the DCIA itself.

The ascending branch can have an early or late take-off, can be represented by multiple branches, and can even originate separately from the external iliac artery.[70,71] This last variation is uncommon (~5%), but important: it signifies a dominance of the ascending branch in the blood supply of the muscle and skin overlying the iliac crest. In this rare instance, the DCIA's main trunk plays a lesser part in supplying the skin, although it continues to supply bone from the medial side of the iliac crest. When this variation occurs, the skin component of the osteocutaneous flap based on the DCIA is at risk, unless a double pedicle is used. Further problems may ensue should the two be confused during dissection and the DCIA accidentally ligated.

The vascular pedicle passes onto the iliacus muscle just medial to the ASIS (see Figure 77-5). Continuing its linear course on this muscle, it passes behind the ASIS a couple of centimeters below the crest where it lies in the groove between the attachments of the iliacus and transversus abdominis. Sometimes there is a low attachment of transversus where some of the fibers actually arise from the iliacus fascia and "bury" the pedicle within its insertion.

The DCIA passes along the inside of the iliac bone 2 to 3 cm below the crest. However, as the iliac crest curves inferiorly

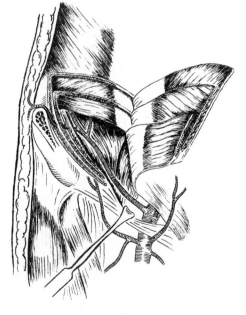

Figure 77-5. The deep circumflex iliac artery passes laterally on the deep surface of the inguinal ligament, reaching the inside of the pelvis just below the anterior superior iliac spine. It comes to lie in a groove between the iliacus and the transversus abdominis, sending perforators into the bone and through the abdominal musculature into the overlying skin. (Redrawn from Baker S, editor: *Microsurgical reconstruction in the head and neck,* New York, 1986, Churchill Livingstone.)

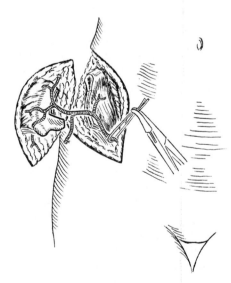

Figure 77-6. The osteomusculocutaneous deep circumflex iliac groin flap severed from the body showing the obligatory muscle cuff retained to protect the perforators passing to the overlying skin. (Redrawn from Baker S, editor: *Microsurgical reconstruction in the head and neck,* New York, 1986, Churchill Livingstone.)

toward the sacrum, the vessels, continuing in a straight line, pass superior to it, entering the neurovascular plane of the abdominal wall (see Figure 77-5). This occurs 6 to 8 cm posterior to the ASIS. The major perforators to the overlying skin arise in this region. Other perforators originate more proximally, entering the abdominal musculature via the transversus abdominis and passing over the crest to supply muscle and skin. Multiple branches of the pedicle enter the iliac crest directly. Others pass downward and inward on the iliacus muscle supplying both it and other parts of the iliac bone.

SURGICAL LANDMARKS AND PREOPERATIVE PLANNING. An estimate of the mucosal, skin, and bony deficit is obtained by a careful examination of the patient, reference to x-rays, CT scans, and discussion with the ablative surgeon. With secondary reconstruction, an estimate is made based on x-rays of the normal side (if present) and on experience. It is now possible to create mirror image models of the contralateral (normal) side from three-dimensional CT scans. This computer assisted design/computer assisted manufacture (CAD/CAM) technology[57] is expensive and in its infancy but may become a routine part of mandibular reconstruction.

The iliac crest, the pubic tubercle, the inguinal ligament, the external iliac artery, and the course of the DCIA are all marked on the patient's skin. The surface marking of the DCIA is almost a straight line between its origin 1 cm above the inguinal ligament and the scapula tip. It passes deep to the ASIS and emerges from the pelvis 6 to 8 cm behind. Its ascending branch is variable but usually passes laterally a few centimeters above the ASIS.

Usually, the crest forms the lower border of the mandible; the ASIS, the angle; and the anterior inferior iliac spine (AIIS), the condyle (Figures 77-7 and 77-8). The ipsilateral crest is therefore preferred.

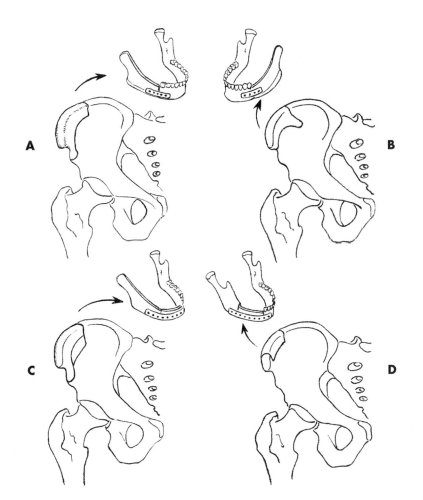

Figure 77-7. **A,** Usual orientation of bone graft for reconstruction of hemimandibular and most other bony defects. The ipsilateral iliac crest is harvested, and the pedicle emerges from under the newly reconstructed angle. This facilitates access to the vessels of the ipsilateral neck. **B,** Orientation of bone graft for reconstructing the contralateral mandible. The pedicle emerges anteriorly to access recipient vessels on the contralateral side. This is used when the ipsilateral crest is unavailable or when vessels are unavailable on the same side. **C,** Subtotal mandibular reconstruction is accomplished using ipsilateral iliac crest. An osteotomy is necessary. **D,** Short segments of mandible are essentially straight, and the orientation of bone grafts can be varied to fit the circumstances. (Redrawn from Baker S, editor: *Microsurgical reconstruction in the head and neck,* New York, 1986, Churchill Livingstone.)

A, B

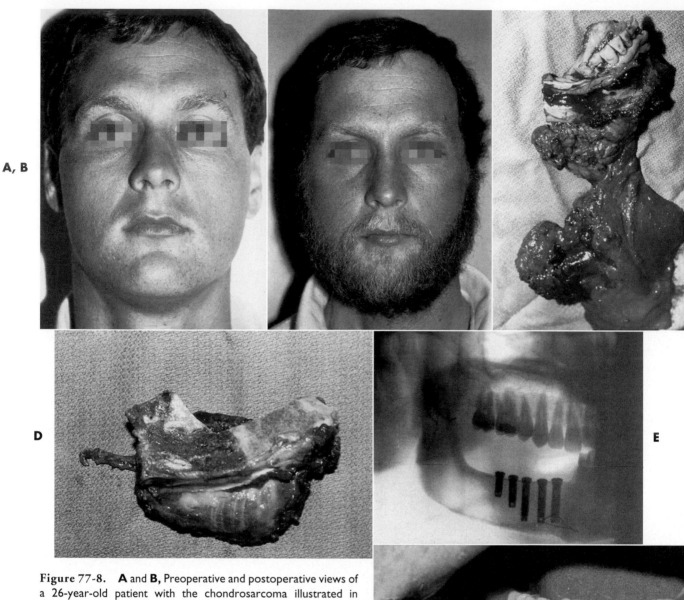

C

D

E

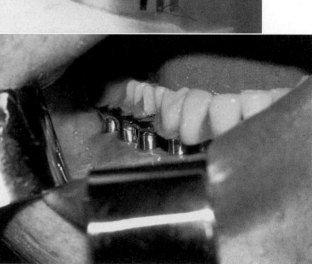

F

Figure 77-8. **A** and **B,** Preoperative and postoperative views of a 26-year-old patient with the chondrosarcoma illustrated in Figure 77-4, *G* and *H*. **C,** Resected specimen included hemimandible and neck dissection and a little oral mucosa. **D,** The iliac graft was harvested as in Figure 77-7, A. No osteotomies were required. The outer cortex was contoured to match the shape of the resected mandible. **E,** Osseointegrated implants were inserted later. The iliac bone accommodates them easily. **F,** Dental prosthesis in place.

The orientation of any skin paddle must correspond to the anticipated defect; for most purely oral lesions, this takes the form of an ellipse parallel to the crest. Only the flap's lower edge should overlie the perforators. Thus the skin paddle, when elevated, has a "mesentery" of subcutaneous tissue and muscle, which allows it some independence in positioning with regard to the bone.

For combined intraoral and extraoral use, the skin paddle should assume a more vertical orientation lying at right angles to the crest.

SURGICAL TECHNIQUE. The patient lies supine with a sandbag under the hip. The sandbag is removed for wound closure.

The paddle is elevated from the external oblique fascia toward the obligatory muscle cuff. This resembles a fringe, starting just lateral to the ASIS, where it measures 2 to 3 cm in vertical height, and extends posteriorly for 6 to 8 cm.

The incision passes medially to the pubic tubercle just above the inguinal ligament. Medially it is deepened through the external oblique aponeurosis and the inguinal canal. The fibers of the internal oblique and transversus abdominis muscles are then divided, allowing the external iliac artery to be palpated beneath the transversalis fascia. Extraperitoneal fat makes visualization difficult, so the great vessels are approached on their (safer) medial side.

The DCIA and the DCIV are located within fatty extraperitoneal tissues just above the femoral canal, and their junctions with their parent vessels are surgically defined. They are followed laterally on the deep surface of the inguinal ligament where they can be palpated and protected, allowing safe division of the residual abdominal musculature as far as the ASIS. The pedicle lies within a fibrous tunnel roofed posteriorly by transversalis fascia. The tunnel is unroofed from behind, dividing small branches and identifying the ascending branch of the DCIA, which may be confused with the DCIA itself. Although usually arising a couple of centimeters medial to the ASIS, it may originate anywhere along the course of the DCIA. Generally, the ascending branch passes superior to the ASIS while the DCIA passes inferior to it.

After the superior margin of the skin paddle has been elevated downward to within 3 cm of the crest, the inferior margin is elevated upward to its outer lip. The muscle cuff is defined by dissection in the following way. A finger is introduced into the full thickness groin incision just medial to the ASIS. It is then directed laterally and used to sweep away extraperitoneal fat from the transversalis and iliacus fascia. The peritoneum is simultaneously cleared from the underside of the abdominal wall in the region of the flap. The DCIA can easily be palpated and protected as it runs in the groove between the iliacus and transversus abdominis muscles. Using the finger as a guide, the abdominal wall muscles are divided in unison, leaving a 2- to 3-cm cuff attached to the crest.

Posteriorly, an incision is made down through this cuff to the crest 8 to 10 cm behind the ASIS. (In pure osseous reconstructions no obligatory muscle cuff is required.)

Laterally, the origin of the tensor fascia lata is divided and the muscle attachments removed from the outer surface of the ilium. The periosteum is preserved to avoid bone exposure at the recipient site.

The lateral femoral cutaneous nerve passes under the lateral portion of the inguinal ligament. It is preserved. This ligament and the originating fibers of the sartorius muscle are then sharply divided from the ASIS, and the bone is cleared of attachments right down to the AIIS.

Inside the ilium, the iliacus fascia, muscle, and periosteum are divided 1 cm below the DCIA. The incision is parallel to the iliac crest and therefore curves downward posteriorly. In making the incision, there is a tendency to drift upward in relation to the crest and, in so doing, leave very little muscle on the most posterior part of the graft. The muscle and periosteum are essential to maintain perfusion to the distal segment should an osteotomy be required. Some major branches from the DCIA feed the iliacus and these are ligated when the muscle is divided. The pelvic portion of the iliacus muscle is then swept inferiorly to clear a space for the saw.

Harvesting the bone graft requires a thin-bladed reciprocating saw, which can be guided to shape the graft and remove it in one continuous cut. The curve of the crest is paralleled posteriorly lest the saw run out of bone prematurely. The blade is introduced below the ASIS and its tip observed on the inside of the pelvis by an assistant who retracts the medial structures out of its way. Posteriorly, the osteotomy is completed with a vertical cut down through the crest. To maintain hip contour, and when the mandibular defect is relatively small, the inner table may be split off the ilium as a unicortical graft by an osteotomy passing downward from the superior border of the crest external to the muscle cuff. The outer cortex maintains normal contour, but the graft is thinner and has less capacity to accept osseointegrated implants.

Finally, after observing the blood flow in both skin and bone, the DCIA and DCIV are individually cross clamped at their junction with the external iliac artery and vein. After division, the stumps are suture-ligated and the flap is transferred to a separate table for shaping.

In primary reconstruction, the resected specimen is analyzed. The mandibular angle, the external length(s) of the mandibular body or bodies, and the splay (shortest distance between their ends) are measured along the lateral cortices. In secondary cases, estimations must be made after the remaining fragments have been freed and positioned in a normal plane. Old radiographs, previously removed reconstruction plates, and computer-generated models[57] can be helpful.

During shaping, the vertical height of the bone graft is reduced to approximately 2 cm and the external cortex may be partly or completely removed, particularly in the region of the iliac tubercle, to improve jaw contour and limit bulk (see Figure 77-8, D).

For central defects an opening osteotomy is employed. The periosteum on the medial surface is raised along the line of the proposed osteotomy and preserved to provide continuity of the blood supply to the distal segment. The lateral periosteum is incised to allow division of the bone, but the soft tissue bridging the two fragments along the superior margin of the crest is carefully elevated and preserved, not only to maintain perfusion, but also to stabilize the bones during fixation. During osteotomy, the soft tissues are protected by a narrow malleable retractor. A piece of corticocancellous bone is shaped to precisely fill the gap produced when the osteotomy is opened.

Fixation is achieved with 26-gauge wires passed through drill holes in each fragment of the graft and either around or through the bone block, filling the osteotomy. Additional fixation can be obtained by transfixion of all three pieces with a threaded K-wire. Most screws hold poorly in the cancellous iliac bone. The most rigid method of bony fixation does not rely on the stability of the junction between graft and adjacent bone. Before the graft is inserted, the mandibular fragments may be brought into their correct anatomic positions and fixed there with a sturdy reconstruction plate. If possible, the plate is bent and the holes drilled prior to mandibular resection. With the plate back in position, the crest is osteotomized and tailored to fit the defect, bringing it precisely end to end with the mandibular remnants. Simple interosseous wiring of the osteotomy allows some final adjustment of splay as the bone is lag-screwed to the inside of the plate. The graft should be positioned so that the screws penetrate the upper outer lip of the iliac crest, which contains the highest density of cortical bone.

It is unnecessary to carry out more than one osteotomy on an iliac crest, and postoperative intermaxillary or external fixation is redundant. With the iliac crest, fusion rates exceed 90% with all methods except miniplates and dynamic compression plates.[12]

For through-and-through defects, the iliac crest is usually not first choice. Nevertheless, there are two possibilities for soft tissue replacement using this flap. A strip of skin across the center of the paddle can be deepithelialized to receive the lip or cheek. Thus the same skin paddle acts as both lining and cover. This is best suited for central defects (Figure 77-9). The alternative is to use an accessory flap such as the pectoralis major or radial forearm flap for one surface and the iliac crest paddle for the other.[14]

The microvascular anastomoses are usually performed to the ipsilateral superior thyroid vessels or another branch of the external carotid artery. Prior irradiation is not a contraindication to their use.[51] If no ipsilateral vessels are present, then the flap can be designed with its pedicle emerging anteriorly to access contralateral recipients (see Figure 77-7). Vein grafts may be necessary.

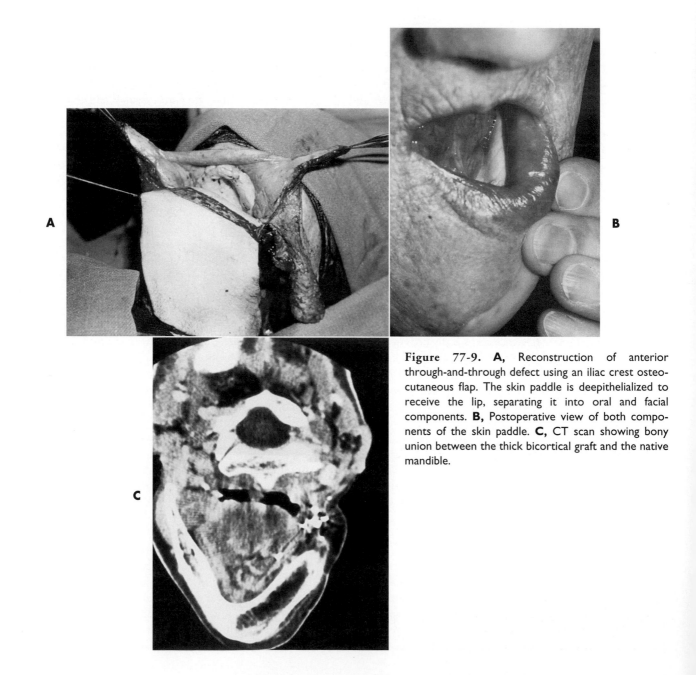

Figure 77-9. A, Reconstruction of anterior through-and-through defect using an iliac crest osteocutaneous flap. The skin paddle is deepithelialized to receive the lip, separating it into oral and facial components. **B,** Postoperative view of both components of the skin paddle. **C,** CT scan showing bony union between the thick bicortical graft and the native mandible.

MANAGEMENT OF DONOR SITE AND COMPLICATIONS. The wound is closed in layers. The transversalis fascia and the transversus abdominis are sutured to the iliacus fascia, and the internal and external oblique to the tensor fascia lata using heavy synthetic absorbable sutures. The inguinal region is repaired as for a herniorrhaphy. Suction drains are placed under both skin and muscle. The patient is mobilized on the third postoperative day.

Even with the best surgical technique, donor site complications may occur (Tables 77-2 and 77-3), but the morbidity is generally well tolerated. Early postoperative pain and long-term sensory changes are the most frequent problems encountered. Postoperative pain usually resolves in a few weeks but occasionally becomes chronic, leading to an antalgic gait, particularly in the elderly patient.

Femoral neuropathy has been described,[27] emphasizing the importance of careful dissection and gentle retraction during flap elevation.

Sensory changes are present in about 38% of cases,[45] occurring after transection or traction injuries involving the lateral cutaneous branch of the subcostal nerve (T12), the lateral cutaneous branch of the iliohypogastric nerve (L1), and the lateral femoral cutaneous nerve of the thigh (L2, L3). Attempts are made to preserve these structures, although inclusion of a cutaneous paddle necessitates transecting the lateral cutaneous branches of the subcostal and iliohypogastric nerves.

Taking the obligatory muscle cuff (see Figure 77-6) appears to increase the chance of hernia formation, as shown by a 12% (7/59) incidence following osteocutaneous flaps compared to 4% (1/23) with pure osseous flaps.[27] Meticulous technique supplemented, if required, by synthetic mesh should minimize the incidence. Secondary repair usually requires mesh.

Injury to the tensor fascia lata resulting from reflection, retraction, and incomplete reattachment leads to both pain on ambulation and gait disturbance because of its function as a leg stabilizer and hip flexor. Reflection of the gluteus medius and minimus, although not primary muscles of ambulation, may also contribute to pain and gait abnormalities (even to a degree of Trendelenburg's symptom). For these reasons, gait disturbances are relatively common following harvesting of iliac bone, either as vascularized (10.9%) or nonvascularized (16%) bone grafts. Although usually self-limiting, they may be minimized by meticulous wound closure and muscle reattachment.[27]

ADVANTAGES AND DISADVANTAGES. The iliac crest supplies abundant callus to ensure primary bony union. It accommodates osseointegrated implants with ease[28] and allows three-dimensional carving into the shape of a hemimandible without the need for osteotomy (see Figure 77-8). Although it may be osteotomized, the iliac crest is not the ideal solution for angle-to-angle defects because the curvature makes shaping difficult, and the associated intraoral soft tissue defect is not handled easily by the bulky skin paddle.

The skin paddle is reliable and may be 10 × 20 cm or greater. It is well placed to reconstruct facial skin but is less suitable for oral lining. Since the skin is attached to the outside of the crest, it has to be rotated either over or under the graft to reach the mouth. Rotation beneath the mandible is difficult due to lack of space. Rotation over the mandible produces an external bulge, which can compromise (or be compromised by) wound closure. Either way there is a shearing and compressive effect on the perforating vessels supplying the skin paddle, leading to

Table 77-2.
Early Complications in 82 Cases of Free Iliac Crest Tissue Transfer[27]

		NUMBER OF CASES	
	TOTAL (%)	BONE AND SKIN FLAP*	BONE FLAP†
Pain	27.0	18	4
Delayed healing	4.8	2	2
Femoral nerve palsy	4.8	2	2
Vascular	3.6	2	1
Infection	3.6	1	2
Operative	2.4	2	—
Hematoma and seroma	—	—	—
GI/GU	—	—	—

*Used in 59 of the 82 cases.
†Used in 23 of the 82 cases.

Table 77-3.
Late Complications in 82 Cases of Free Iliac Crest Tissue Transfer[27]

		NUMBER OF CASES	
	TOTAL (%)	BONE AND SKIN FLAP*	BONE FLAP†
Sensory changes	27.0	14	9
Contour irregularity	20.0	14	2
Poor scar	12.0	7	3
Gait	10.9	6	3
Hernia	9.7	7	1
Pain (>1 year)	8.4	5	2
Tightness	6.1	4	1
Meralgia paresthetica	4.8	2	2
Clothing difficulties	3.6	3	—
Cold sensitivity	2.4	—	2
Revisionary surgery	2.4	—	2
Impotence	1.2	1	—
Barometer effect	1.2	—	1

*Used in 59 of the 82 cases.
†Used in 23 of the 82 cases.

partial or complete skin necrosis in over 20% of cases.[37] Alternatively, the skin paddle may be discarded and an internal oblique muscle flap, based on the ascending branch of the deep circumflex artery,[75] used instead. This has more independence of movement and sustains reepithelialization from the surrounding oral mucosa. Harvesting the muscle flap increases the donor defect, increasing the risk of a denervation bulge or frank hernia.

Cosmetically, the donor site is excellent and easily hidden by underwear. Contour irregularities may be minimized by a linear tapering osteotomy or by taking the inner cortex alone.[23] The color match of the skin with that of the face is poor in Caucasian patients.

Indications for the iliac crest have become more specific with the advent of newer flaps. Ideally, defects should exclude soft tissue and occupy lateral (L, H) segments—up to a complete hemimandible (see Figure 77-8). The composite flap is capable of reconstructing facial skin with ease, but—as with other free flaps—the color match is poor. Although mucosal defects are generally handled badly, the flap can replace soft tissue bulk and mandibular height following anterior full-thickness excisions (see Figure 77-9). Where donor site cosmesis is of paramount importance, the iliac crest is one of the best flaps available.

Fibula

See Chapter 78.

Radius

The radial forearm flap[65,66] is based on the radial artery, its venae comitantes, and the subcutaneous venous system. Perforators pass from the radial artery to the overlying forearm skin via a soft tissue "mesentery" between the brachioradialis and the flexor carpi radialis muscles (Figure 77-10). They are distributed along the course of the radial artery and permit two separate paddles of skin to be taken together with a strip of radial bone (Figure 77-11). The bone comprises the dorsolateral third of the radius between the insertions of flexor carpi radialis and brachioradialis (see Figure 77-10, B). It is nourished by the radial artery via perforators passing through the flexor pollicis longus, which clothes the distal radius and upon which the vessel resides. A segmental blood supply allows the radial bone to be osteotomized for shaping, but it is best bridging lateral defects as if it were a biocompatible reconstruction plate (Figures 77-11 and 77-12).

Sensation to forearm skin is supplied by the medial and lateral antebrachial cutaneous nerves, the watershed between them lying down the midline of the forearm (see Figure 77-10, C). To enhance oral continence and improve speech,

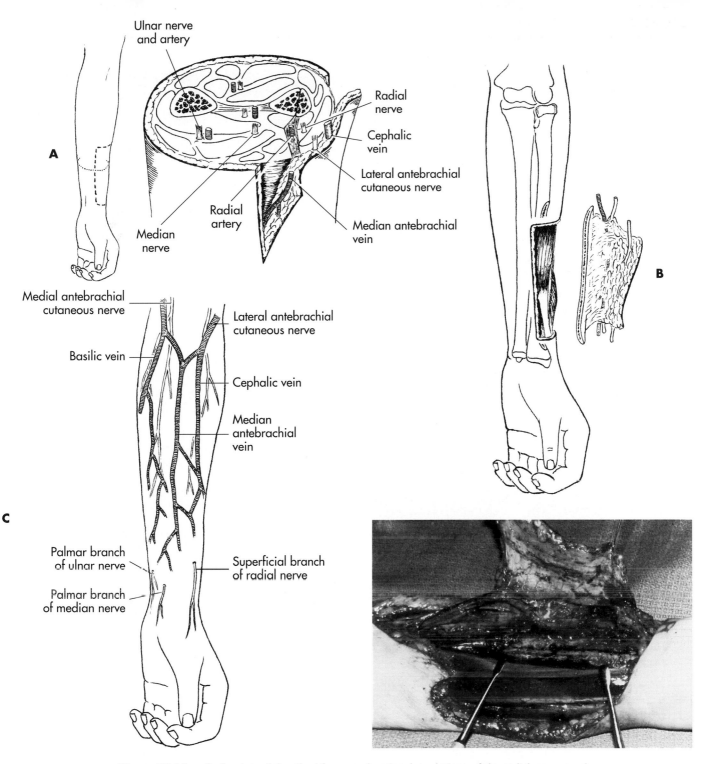

Figure 77-10. **A,** Section of the distal forearm showing the relations of the radial artery to the lateral intermuscular septum, the flexor pollicis longus, and the osteotomy. One third of the radial cross-section is taken with an osteotomy passing posterolaterally from the middle of its anterior surface. The skin paddle lies over the dorsoradial aspect of the wrist to include the cephalic vein. This vein facilitates venous access in the neck but the resulting dorsoradial wrist scar is detrimental to donor site cosmesis. **B,** Muscular attachments to the left anterior radius and ulna. The bone graft extends between the insertions of pronator teres and brachioradialis (some of which are included for extra length). The osteotomy is boat-shaped to avoid cross-cutting at the corners and excessive weakening. **C,** The lateral antebrachial cutaneous (LABC) neurosome flap is centered along a line running between the radial artery and the cephalic vein. This is the area of maximal cutaneous innervation (neurosome) of the LABC nerve. The watershed between the LABC and medial antebrachial cutaneous nerve (MABC) neurosomes lies down the midline of the anterior forearm. The main trunks of the LABC and MABC are located internal to their associated veins in the proximal forearm. **D,** Anterior aspect of left forearm, hand to the right. The flap is elevated in preparation for osteotomy. The origin of the flexor pollicis longus has been incised longitudinally and the exposed radius marked for the osteotomy. The radial artery sends perforators to the skin as well as to the flexor pollicis longus. It is from the latter that the bone derives its blood supply. (Redrawn from *Oper Tech Plast Reconstr Surg* 3(4):241, 1996.)

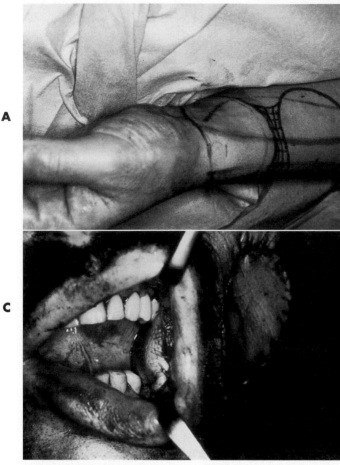

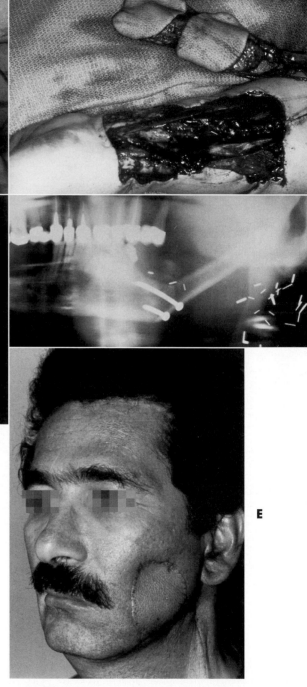

Figure 77-11. A, Double paddle forearm flap for lateral full-thickness defect. **B,** Osteocutaneous flap elevated. **C,** Flap sutured into position. **D,** Bony fixation using lag-screw technique (see text). **E,** Final result.

mastication, and swallowing, the paddle may be reinnervated,[76] providing sensation like that of the normal mouth.[16]

SURGICAL ANATOMY. The septocutaneous perforators from the radial artery are plentiful in the distal third of the forearm, but proximally—where tendons give way to muscle bellies—they become rather sparse. Nevertheless, it is safe to raise a skin flap anywhere along the lateral intermuscular septum (see Figure 77-10, *A*). Thus two skin islands may be raised—one proximal and one distal—facilitating reconstruction of the through-and-through defect (see Figure 77-11).

After emerging from the septum, the vessels branch laterally and medially, piercing the deep fascia and quickly passing to the subdermal plexus. As a result, very little of the deep fascia needs to be harvested with the flap.

The brachial artery bifurcates into radial and ulnar arteries a few centimeters distal to the antecubital fossa. The radial artery and its venae comitantes are invested by the fascia of the lateral intermuscular septum. They pass distally along the radial side of the pronator teres, initially lying between the biceps tendon and the bicipital aponeurosis, and then cross anterior to the pronator teres just proximal to that muscle's insertion into its

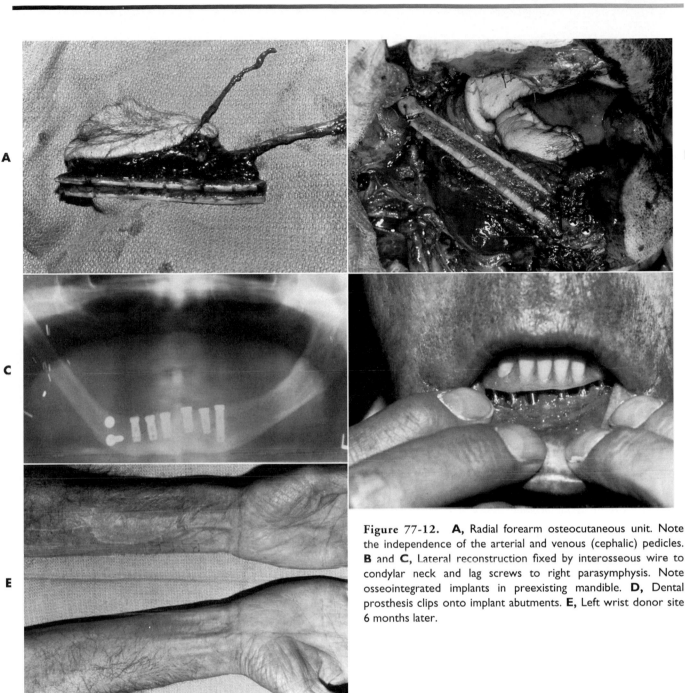

Figure 77-12. A, Radial forearm osteocutaneous unit. Note the independence of the arterial and venous (cephalic) pedicles. **B** and **C,** Lateral reconstruction fixed by interosseous wire to condylar neck and lag screws to right parasymphysis. Note osseointegrated implants in preexisting mandible. **D,** Dental prosthesis clips onto implant abutments. **E,** Left wrist donor site 6 months later.

tubercle on the lateral surface of the radius. On entering the distal third of the forearm, the vessels first overlie the flexor pollicis longus and finally the pronator quadratus. These two muscles intimately clothe the flat anterior surface of the distal radius (see Figure 77-10, *B*). Muscular branches from the radial artery give periosteal twigs to the underlying bone and are the basis for the osseous portion of the flap (see Figure 77-10, *D*).

The venae comitantes of the radial artery are constant but of variable diameter. They are often inconveniently small for microvascular anastomosis. In the region of the bifurcation of the brachial artery there is a confluence of veins. Here the venae comitantes of both ulnar and radial arteries communicate with each other, as well as with one or more of the large

subcutaneous veins of the forearm (see Figure 77-10, *C*). Classically, there are three major subcutaneous veins in the anterior forearm: the cephalic, the median, and the basilic. In the distal forearm the cephalic vein lies on the dorsoradial, and the basilic on the dorsoulnar, aspect of the wrist. They pass around their respective borders at the midforearm level, and then proceed proximally on the radial and ulnar sides of the anterior forearm. The median vein lies in the midline of the anterior forearm. Just distal to the antecubital fossa it bifurcates into two: the median cephalic and the median basilic. The former angles radially to join the cephalic and the latter ulnarly to join the basilic. The cephalic and basilic veins then pass up the arm on either side of the biceps muscle. There are significant variations on this basic pattern. Perforating veins connect the superficial veins to the deep system at various points. Of most interest here is the communication at the level of the brachial artery bifurcation. This may be single or multiple and may be from any of the superficial veins (commonly the median).

Either the venae comitantes or the large subcutaneous veins of the forearm are capable of draining the osteocutaneous forearm flap. The superficial veins are often preferred because of their greater diameter and their independence from the arterial pedicle. However, care should be taken to ensure that the superficial veins have not previously been canalized and undergone partial or complete thrombosis. When a radial forearm flap is first contemplated, the nondominant arm should be marked with indelible ink warning phlebotomists and anesthetists to refrain from venepuncture.

The medial antebrachial cutaneous nerve (C8, T1) enters the forearm in the company of the basilic vein (see Figure 77-10, C). It soon gives off a number of large anterior branches, which pass down the radial side of the basilic vein and supply the ulnar half of the anterior forearm as far as the wrist. An ulnar branch supplies the ulnar border of the forearm. The lateral antebrachial cutaneous nerve (C5, C6) is the forearm continuation of the musculocutaneous nerve. It enters the forearm on the ulnar side of the cephalic vein and, via multiple branches, supplies the radial half of the forearm as far as the wrist as well as the dorsoradial aspect of the forearm.

SURGICAL LANDMARKS AND PREOPERATIVE PLAN-NING.
The radial artery's course is a straight line from the brachial pulse in the antecubital fossa to the radial pulse at the wrist. The cephalic and basilic veins may be identified on the lateral and medial aspects of the anterior forearm, respectively. Proximally these vessels are accompanied by the lateral and medial antebrachial cutaneous nerves, which in the midforearm divide into numerous small filaments. The watershed between the neurosomes of these two nerves lies down the midline of the anterior forearm.

An Allen test helps predict potential postoperative ischemia. However, the surgeon should be prepared to reconstruct the artery. The vessels are marked on the skin surface. The paddle overlies the artery and is best positioned over the anterior or anterolateral aspect of the wrist where the subcutaneous tissue is thinnest, the pedicle length is maximal, and the cephalic vein facilitates venous drainage. The bone graft occupies the dorsolateral aspect of the radius between the insertions of pronator teres and brachioradialis. The longitudinal positioning of skin flap in relation to bone is designed according to the expected recipient defect.

The skin flap may be extremely large as long as a significant portion of it overlies the vascular septum. It may be a longitudinal ellipse overlying the radial artery or a rectangular flag flap with the short edge in contact with the septum. That portion overlying the vascular septum represents the "base" of the flap. Length/width ratios of greater than 2:1 should be avoided.

With small skin islands, it is possible to primarily close the donor site.[26] Such islands are positioned transversely, with one edge overlying the radial artery. Closure is by means of a long,

ulnar-based rotation-advancement of the forearm skin. The proximal defect thus created is closed as a V to Y. Wrist flexion facilitates closure.

Since the watershed between the neurosomes of the lateral and medial antebrachial cutaneous nerves lies down the midline of the anterior forearm, flaps positioned over the cephalic vein and extending to the midline need only the lateral antebrachial cutaneous nerve for full reinnervation. Those positioned centrally—straddling two neurosomes—require both superficial nerves.[16]

SURGICAL TECHNIQUE.
Under tourniquet control the skin paddle is incised around its periphery and dissection is carried down to the deep fascia. At the proximal margin of the flap superficial veins are preserved. The incision is extended to the antecubital fossa and the selected venous system traced proximally. For innervated flaps, the subcutaneous nerves entering the flap should be preserved in a sheath of fascia. They lie immediately superficial to the deep fascia, but in the distal forearm are branched, fine, and difficult to identify. Localization of their main trunks in the proximal forearm is simple—they run with the cephalic and basilic veins (see Figure 77-10, C). These nerves and their branches are traced distally into the proximal margin of the flap.

The ulnar side of the flap is then elevated just superficial to the deep fascia, working toward the intermuscular septum between the brachioradialis and the flexor carpi radialis. Approximately 1 cm to the ulnar side of this septum, the deep fascia is incised, allowing dissection to proceed under it. Preservation of the deep fascia in this way facilitates skin grafting of the donor site.

Dissection passes superficial to the paratenon of the flexor carpi radialis, extending around the radial border of the tendon into the space beneath. Fibers of the flexor digitorum superficialis are now visible. They are retracted ulnarward, exposing the flexor pollicis longus arising from the anterior surface of the distal radius and the adjacent interosseous membrane (see Figure 77-10, B and D).

The radial dissection passes immediately superficial to the deep fascia until a point is reached 1 cm lateral to the intermuscular septum where the deep fascia is divided, and dissection then proceeds at this deeper level. The brachioradialis tendon is seen, and the dissection hugs it in the same way that the ulnar dissection hugged the flexor carpi radialis tendon. Paratenon is preserved. Once around the ulnar border of the tendon, the plane of dissection passes laterally and a space filled with loose adventitial tissue is entered. Blunt dissection exposes the dorsoradial "bare area" of the radius.

Distally, the radial artery is identified, ligated, and divided. The insertion of the brachioradialis defines the distal limit of the bone graft, but it may be stripped distally allowing a little more radius to be taken. The superficial branch of the radial nerve passing through the deep portion of the flap is preserved.

The proximal portion of the lateral intermuscular septum is then entered and communicated with the distal dissection. The radial artery and its venae comitantes are isolated proximally, clipping or coagulating small muscular branches. The communication between superficial and deep venous systems may be preserved as part of a combined venous pedicle.[29]

The osteotomy is the most critical part of the operation (see Figure 77-10, B). Perforators to the radius from the radial artery pass through the flexor pollicis longus, which obscures the bone by clothing its anterior surface (see Figure 77-10, D). Unlike the lateral border, the medial border is not easily palpated due to the tightness of the interosseous membrane. Passing a fine hemostat through the flexor pollicis longus muscle is a way of establishing where bone ends and where interosseous membrane begins. A line is then drawn longitudinally down the anterior surface of the flexor pollicis longus muscle at a point corresponding to the midline of the flat anterior face of the radius. The osteotomy will pass from here, dorsally and laterally, toward the bare area (Figure 77-10, A). A cuff of muscle is thus taken to safeguard the perforators to the bone. If the osteotomy were to pass perpendicularly through the radius, half of the cortex would be harvested. However, by angling the osteotomy in this way, only one third is taken.

The muscle is incised down to bone from the distal radius proximally for about 12 to 14 cm. The periosteum is elevated a few millimeters on either side to expose the bone along the line of osteotomy. The insertion of the pronator teres marks the proximal extent of the graft; however, the tendon may be detached from the radius and a little more bone taken if required (see Figure 77-10, B).

In preparation for the osteotomy, it only remains to communicate the flexor pollicis longus–splitting incision distally with the bare area of the radius immediately proximal to the remaining insertion of the brachioradialis. The osteotomy is best performed using a reciprocating saw with a blade narrow enough to be guided through bone. With assistants retracting the vital structures and providing irrigation, the reciprocating saw enters the distal radius under the tendon of the brachioradialis at approximately 45 degrees to the bone surface and angled proximally. The axis of the saw cut is dorsal and radial, passing from the midline of the radius anteriorly to the bare area of the radius dorsolaterally (see Figure 77-10, A). As the saw enters the bone, the saw is turned to follow the predetermined line along the anterior surface of the radius. The saw blade is observed emerging at the bare area. The osteotomy extends to the pronator teres insertion, angling out through the lateral cortex to follow the predetermined cut in the soft tissues. With this continuous osteotomy the graft is boat- or keel-shaped and there is no cross cutting (see Figure 77-10, B).

Blood flow to the flap is ensured, the pedicle is divided, and the flap removed. At the recipient site, the bone is trimmed, osteotomized (if necessary), and fitted into the defect. (Closing wedge osteotomies are performed. Fixation is best achieved by a five-hole miniplate applied to the cut surface of the bone.) Fixation of the graft to the recipient mandible may be performed using miniplates, lag-screws (see Figures 77-11, D, and 77-12, B and C), or a reconstruction plate. Miniplates require precise end-to-end abutment. The lag screw method involves an external decortication of the mandibular fragments. The reconstruction plate method was described earlier. All methods give excellent fusion rates.

The skin paddle is sutured to the intraoral defect. Microvascular anastomosis is performed to the ipsilateral facial artery and external jugular vein, if available. The lateral antebrachial cutaneous nerve is trimmed and sutured to the stump of the ipsilateral lingual nerve. If this is unavailable, the inferior alveolar nerve is equally effective. Exposure may require drilling out the mandibular canal. Alternatively, an end-to-side anastomosis with an intact lingual nerve may be accompanied by some expectation of success.[78]

MANAGEMENT OF DONOR SITE AND COMPLICATIONS. The surgeon must reconstruct the radial artery in the face of arterial insufficiency, but this is rare unless an aberrant superficial ulnar artery is accidentally ligated.

To facilitate wound closure, the palmaris longus tendon is removed. The proximal wound is sutured directly. Although the paratenons of the flexor carpi radialis and the brachioradialis accept a skin graft, it is safer to bury the tendons among the fibers of the flexor digitorum superficialis. Muscle fibers are sutured over them, producing a well-vascularized bed for a skin graft (see Figure 77-12, E).

The immediate result of harvesting a radial bone graft is a weakening of its breaking strength by 76%.[68] The risk of fracture following relatively minor trauma mandates cautious rehabilitation. Accordingly, an above-elbow cast is worn for 2 months and a below-elbow cast for a further month. The risk of radial fracture is inversely related to the experience of the surgeon but in most series is less than 10%.[67] The condition should be treated with rigid internal fixation and bone grafting to prevent a debilitating nonunion.

Loss of the radial artery has been postulated as a cause of cold intolerance; however, there is little evidence for this in the studies that are available.[64]

More common is delayed healing of the skin graft, often with tendon exposure.[67] This complication, which occurs more often in heavy smokers and diabetics, may be the result of infection, hematoma, seroma, excessive mobility, or desiccation of the bed prior to graft application. It is minimized by meticulous surgical technique and use of unmeshed skin graft and treated with wet-to-dry dressings, immobilization, and debridement.

Despite intimate dissection of the superficial branch of the radial nerve, and harvesting of the lateral antebrachial cutaneous nerve, surprisingly few patients develop chronic radial neuroma pain.

SUMMARY. The small bulk of the radial forearm flap and limited bone length reduce its usefulness. However, in those cases where it is indicated, it is second to none. When good appearance requires minimal bulk; when tongue mobility relies on thin, supple lining; and when speech, mastication, and oral continence are enhanced by oral sensibility, it is an excellent method. Finally, when early postoperative mobility is considered crucial, the radial forearm flap imposes no ambulatory restrictions.

Small osseointegrated implants may be inserted in the radial bone graft, but this is seldom required since there is usually

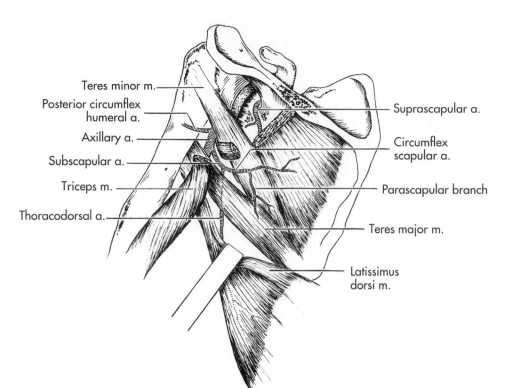

Figure 77-13. The circumflex scapular artery sends branches to the lateral border of the scapula, then emerges from the triangular space and bifurcates into transverse (scapula flap) and descending (parascapula flap) branches. The space is usually palpable 2 cm superior to the posterior axillary crease. (Redrawn from Baker S, editor: *Microsurgical reconstruction in the head and neck,* New York, 1986, Churchill Livingstone.)

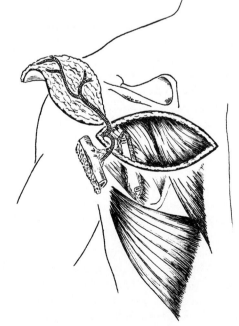

Figure 77-14. The skin flap is elevated toward the triangular space. The branches of the circumflex scapular artery are located emerging from this space. As the pedicle is dissected inward, branches to the lateral border are carefully preserved. The bone graft is selected anywhere between the glenoid fossa and the scapular tip. (Redrawn from Serafin D, editor: *Atlas of microsurgical composite tissue transplantation,* Philadelphia, 1996, WB Saunders.)

enough native mandible remaining (see Figures 77-12, *C* and *D*) in the short defects handled best by this technique.[50]

Even though functional impairment is minimal at the donor site, the radius is significantly weakened.[68] This is a problem in manual workers and those with osteoporosis. Radial fracture is an uncommon complication in those centers that routinely use the flap and take the appropriate steps to minimize the risk (see above). Cold sensitivity is uncommon.[64] However, the skin graft constitutes a significant cosmetic deformity and is often subject to delayed healing.

Scapula

The circumflex scapular artery forms the arterial pedicle of a versatile free flap capable of carrying large areas of back skin together with bone from either the lateral[61,72] or medial[73] border of the scapula. After supplying the lateral border, the vessel emerges from the triangular space formed by the teres major below, the teres minor above, and the long head of the triceps laterally (Figure 77-13). It then bifurcates into a transverse branch and a descending branch, each capable of sustaining an independent skin paddle.

Although the lateral is more commonly utilized (Figure 77-14), use of the medial border produces a very long artery-bone pedicle (Figure 77-15). This may be elongated further by incorporating the subscapular artery. By using this vessel, the latissimus dorsi and the serratus anterior may be included in a truly massive free tissue transfer.

SURGICAL ANATOMY. The subscapular artery originates from the third portion of the axillary artery and, after a short course of 3 to 4 cm, bifurcates into the thoracodorsal and the circumflex scapular arteries. The former descends on the deep surface of the latissimus dorsi muscle while the latter travels posteriorly around the lateral border of the scapula to emerge from the triangular space between teres major, teres minor, and long head of triceps (see Figure 77-13). The arterial "crotch" between the circumflex scapular artery and the thoracodorsal artery bestrides the teres major muscle, which must be divided if the territories of both are to be carried on one pedicle.

The lateral border is a thickened termination of the thin dorsal blade, and its usable length—extending from the subglenoid region to the tip—measures 10 to 14 cm. Its thickness varies between 1 and 2.5 cm, and a width of 3 or 4 cm is possible. As the circumflex scapular artery passes through the triangular space, it sends numerous twigs into the bone.

The length of the vascular pedicle from the axillary artery to the scapular border is approximately 6 cm and from there to the overlying skin flap 2 to 3 cm. The diameters of the subscapular and circumflex scapular arteries are approximately 3 to 3.5 mm. The accompanying veins are of similar dimensions.

Two large independent skin paddles are commonly designed to overlie the major cutaneous branches of the circumflex scapular artery. One skin paddle is parallel to and 2 cm below the scapular spine and based on the transverse branch of the circumflex scapular artery; the other is parallel and 2 cm medial to the lateral border and based on the descending branch. Allowing for primary closure, dimensions of about 15 × 30 cm are possible. More skin may be taken if the donor site is grafted, and longer parascapular flaps are feasible if the skin paddle is designed to pass laterally through the axilla, ending in the inframammary sulcus.[62] This may be used for cosmetic advantage. Because the blood supply to the skin is independent of that supplying bone, three-dimensional positioning of the different components is facilitated. This is ideal for complex full-thickness defects.

The medial border of the scapula (see Figure 77-15) is 10 to 12 cm long, 7 to 15 cm thick, and 3 to 4 cm wide. Its posterior surface is clothed with the infraspinatus muscle through which perforating vessels connect bone to the overlying skin. (A cuff of infraspinatus muscle is therefore taken to preserve blood supply to the bone graft.) Use of the medial border of the scapula effectively doubles the length of the vascular pedicle as measured from anastomosis to bone edge, allowing vessel access in the contralateral neck. On the negative side, the bone is more remote from its blood supply and may receive inadequate perfusion. Furthermore, it is thinner, shorter, and weaker than that of the lateral border.

SURGICAL LANDMARKS AND PREOPERATIVE PLANNING.

Positioning the patient laterally with the arm free-draped and resting on a padded Mayo stand, the scapula is palpated and its boundaries surface-marked on the skin. The triangular space can often be seen, or at least felt, in thin individuals, and here the surgeon is aided by the emaciation of the typical oral cancer patient (Figure 77-16). Obesity remains the bane of the reconstructive surgeon and can render ungainly results no matter how great the artistry. When the triangular space is not palpable, its approximate location may be established by drawing a line from the midpoint of the spine down the lateral border to the inferior angle. It is located two fifths of

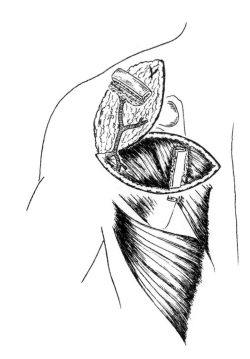

Figure 77-15. Harvesting the medial border of the scapula. The scapula flap is left attached to the soft tissues directly overlying the desired bone graft. Dissection is performed lateral to this in order to elevate the skin paddle. A tunnel is thus formed between the vascular pedicle and the medial attachment between skin and bone. Elevation is completed by osteotomizing the bone and detaching its medial and anterior muscle attachments. (Redrawn from Serafin D, editor: *Atlas of microsurgical composite tissue transplantation,* Philadelphia, 1996, WB Saunders.)

the way down this line. If the medial scapular osteocutaneous flap is being elevated, the medial border is easily palpated and marked.

The cutaneous vessels are located with a Doppler probe and traced back into the triangular space. It is usual to design single skin islands along the course of the descending branch, since an excellent cosmetic result is obtained if the inferior portion is curved into the axilla.[62] Double paddles are obtained by adding a transverse ellipse along the presumed course of the transverse branch (Figure 77-17).

SURGICAL TECHNIQUE. The skin islands are elevated in a centripetal direction beneath the deep fascia of the underlying muscles. On reaching the triangular space, it is from within the emerging tissue that the cutaneous vessels will be isolated. Incising the dense axillary fascia and retraction of the posterior fibers of the deltoid muscle expose the space fully. Under loupe magnification the vessels are traced to their common stem, which is then dissected deeply. Movement of the free-draped arm opens up the space and facilitates exposure. One or more major branches are encountered passing to the lateral border of the scapula. They are carefully preserved as the dissection proceeds inward. The vascular pedicle is dissected as far as is necessary to gain sufficient length. It can include the subscapular artery, but this requires division of the thoracodorsal vessels. To facilitate dissection of the subscapular artery, it helps to make a separate incision in the midaxilla. In 4% of cases the

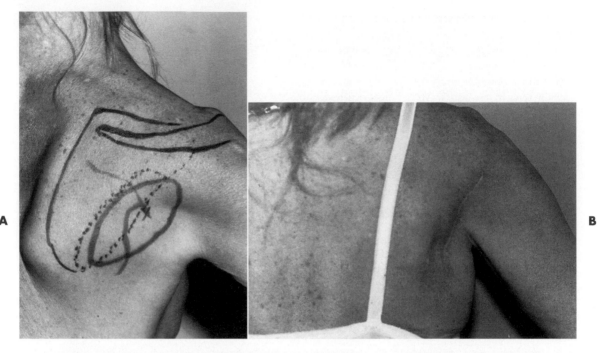

Figure 77-16. A, Preoperative markings for a unipedicled osteocutaneous flap. The triangular space may be palpated and the presence of the circumflex scapular artery confirmed by Doppler. **B,** Donor scar from the same patient. Cosmesis is improved by orienting the flap toward the axilla.

circumflex scapular artery originates not from the subscapular, but directly from the axillary artery.

Once the vessels have been isolated, an incision is made through the posterior musculature of the scapula vertically down to bone along the transition between the thick lateral border and the blade. The incision exits the bone inferiorly at the tip of the scapula, and a lateral cross-cut immediately below the glenoid fossa completes the exposure for osteotomy. Division of the bone is achieved using an oscillating saw. Isolation of the composite flap on its vascular pedicle is completed with division of the remaining subscapular muscle attachments, leaving a muscle cuff on the undersurface of the lateral border to preserve its blood supply.

The scapula may be osteotomized for mandibular reconstruction (see Figure 77-17). The preferred method of fixation is by reconstruction plate, although the bone has a high cortical component allowing fairly rigid direct interosseous fixation using miniplates or even K-wires combined with interosseous wire loops. As with other vascularized bone grafts used in mandibular reconstruction, the union rate is high no matter which of these techniques is employed.[12]

Elevation of the medial scapula flap is also begun in a distal to proximal direction. From the outset, the skin paddle is designed to overlie the medial border of the scapula (see Figure 77-15). It is necessary to elevate the bone and define its attachments to the skin paddle right at the beginning so that pedicle dissection may be aided by full mobility of the osteocutaneous unit. The skin flap is incised around its periphery and elevated from medial to lateral until the medial border of the scapula is encountered. The rhomboid muscles are then divided and the medial border elevated sufficiently for the serratus anterior muscle attachments to be severed from its anterior surface. A

vertical tunnel is made 3 to 4 cm lateral to the medial border of the scapula deep to the deep fascia of the infraspinatus (see Figure 77-15). Medial to this tunnel, the skin flap is left attached to the infraspinatus, which clothes the posterior surface of the scapula. The flap is retracted outward and the infraspinatus divided down to bone, again 3 to 4 cm lateral to the medial scapular border. Osteotomies are then performed and the osseous unit elevated out of the wound attached to the medial tail of the skin flap.

MANAGEMENT OF DONOR SITE AND COMPLICATIONS. The wound is closed in layers. Drill-holes in the new lateral or medial borders facilitate reattachment of the divided musculature. With large skin paddles, undermining may be required to permit skin closure.

Considerable amounts of serum may be drained for several days. Retention of the drains beyond a week is probably counterproductive, since they provide a pathway for infection. Further collections may be removed by weekly aspiration with a large bore needle.

Postoperatively, the shoulder should be immobilized in a sling for approximately 5 days. Physiotherapy is commenced after that time and continued on an outpatient basis. It involves both elbow and shoulder, and starts with range of motion exercises. These are active and active-assisted and their repetitions are tailored to the patient's progress and abilities. After a few weeks the patient commences a strengthening program, which is continued until recovery is complete. By 6 months most patients will be back to normal. A neck dissection performed on the same side may compromise shoulder rehabilitation by weakening or paralyzing the trapezius muscle.

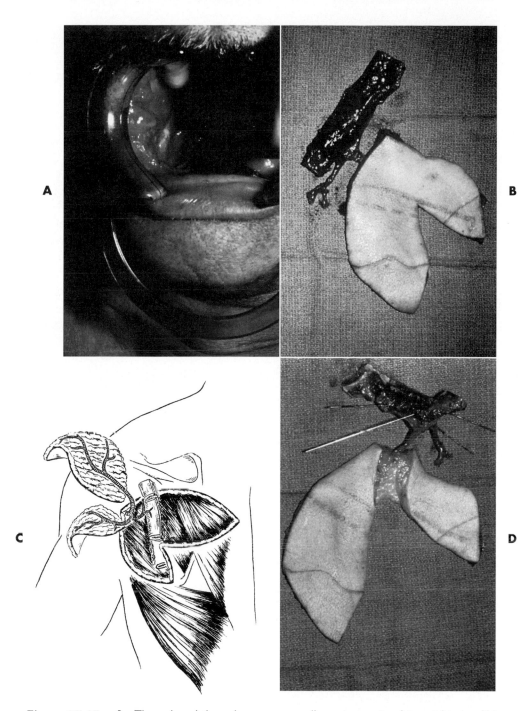

Figure 77-17. A, Through-and-through squamous cell carcinoma involving right mandible. **B,** Double paddle scapula flap elevated. **C,** Spatial relationship of skin paddles planned using the reverse template technique. **D,** Bone osteotomized using two closing wedges. The scapula and parascapula skin paddles are formally separated. This gives them greater independence of placement in relation to each other as well as the bone. *Continued*

ADVANTAGES AND DISADVANTAGES. The scapula flap is not difficult to elevate and the donor defect is only moderate. For complex compound oromandibular reconstructions, the scapula flap has no peer because two large skin paddles can be moved independently of each other and of the attached bone (see Figure 77-17). The main limitation is the bone graft, which is limited to 14 cm.

Equivalent or even greater flexibility with full-thickness reconstructions may be obtained by the use of two simulta-

neous free flaps (e.g., a fibula osteocutaneous flap together with a radial forearm neurocutaneous flap[59]), but this raises the complexity to a higher level and should be reserved for situations beyond the scope of single-flap alternatives. Indications include through-and-through oromandibular defects with a bone requirement of greater than 14 cm.

Apart from concerns with intraoperative turning, the skin paddles can be a little bulky for intraoral use and the bone is insufficient for extensive mandibular reconstruction. After all,

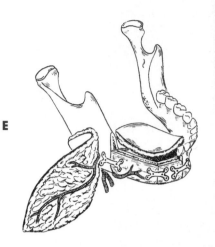

E

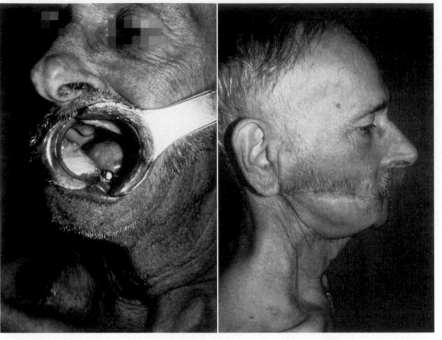

F, G

Figure 77-17, cont'd. **E,** Diagram of final bone position and direction of osteotomies. **F** and **G,** Postoperative result.

cases with massive through-and-through defects—the main indication for the scapula flap—often have large bone defects too. Color match with facial skin is poor in the average Caucasian patient but better than the alternatives.

Excessive bulkiness of the skin paddle is only an issue when the recipient skin or mucosal defect is small (a contraindication for this flap) or when the patient is obese (a problem with any flap). Bone defects greater than angle-to-angle, which are associated with massive skin and mucosal loss, constitute the main and rare indication for double free flap reconstruction.[11] The scapula works extremely well in lateral defects (L, LC) with large soft tissue loss, but osteotomies permit its use in only moderate LCL defects. Fortunately, the surgeon is unlikely to find himself or herself committed to the scapula without knowing the extent of the bony defect because the resection will be complete before the patient is turned to elevate the scapula.

Both medial and lateral borders of the scapula are thick enough to accommodate osseointegrated implants.[28] There are now a great variety of implants available for use in almost any size of graft. Since even the unicortical radius can accommodate implants,[50] suitability for osseointegration is no longer a major issue in the choice of flap.

SUMMARY. The scapula flap is available both as a cutaneous and as an osteocutaneous unit. The donor site is tolerated well, both functionally and aesthetically. For those not subscribing to the "magic bullet" notion of mandibular reconstruction, the scapula flap holds a unique place: it is invaluable for large full-thickness composite defects with a bone gap of less than 14 cm. The major objection remains the need for intraoperative turning.

The Plate-Flap Option

The combination of a reconstruction plate for mandibular replacement and a radial forearm flap for oral lining has been advocated by a number of authors[15,17,24] because it allows use of the best flap for intraoral replacement, avoids the risk of radial fracture, and minimizes postoperative elbow and wrist immobilization (Figure 77-18). In those patients with only a few months to live, prolonged hospitalization and immobilization because of a donor defect are avoided. If, prior to bony resection, the plate is bent and the existing mandible drilled, precise realignment of the mandibular fragments is ensured and oral function maximized. The flap may be reinnervated to improve oral function. The elimination of bone harvesting and shaping minimizes operating time, and complex soft tissue defects are handled more easily when skin flap positioning is not constrained by attached bone. Gullane[30] has shown that the presence of the metallic plate does not compromise postoperative radiotherapy. The method is ideal for low volume defects but unsuitable when the requirement is for bulk.

Most patients with large T4, N+ tumors will die before fatigue fracture of the plate occurs. Nevertheless, the longer the plate remains in place, the more likely a fracture becomes. Those few survivors with plate fracture may be rescued by a bone-only vascularized bone graft or, if their prognosis is still believed to be poor, a second plate.[15,17,24]

Poor long-term durability of the plates makes the plate-flap option unsuitable in young patients with a reasonable prognosis. Furthermore, osseointegration into adjacent bone is difficult due to the encroachment of the necessary hardware. Functional results are occasionally compromised by this method

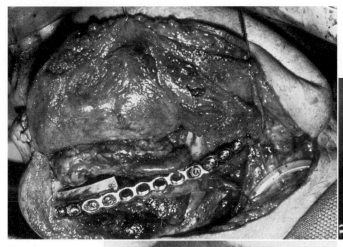

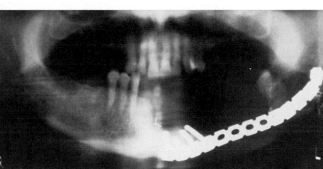

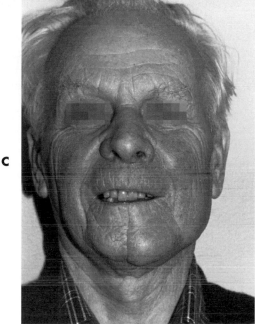

Figure 77-18. **A** to **C,** Lateral defect reconstructed using a stainless steel reconstruction plate and a radial forearm flap. Mandibular alignment remains anatomic because the plate was bent and its holes drilled prior to excision. Five screws were used in each bony fragment. With a similar titanium system, only three screws are required, since they are able to osseointegrate. A factor mitigating against a good result is the retention of the patient's own teeth and the possibility of heavy chewing causing plate failure.

because dentures worn directly over the plate can lead to intraoral exposure. Defects requiring bulk replacement are not adequately handled by the plate-flap option. Use in this situation leads to soft tissue contraction and plate exposure. Finally, it has been shown that use of the plate for anterior (C-containing) defects has a failure rate (plate removal) of 35% or above compared with only 5% for lateral defects.[17]

Indications for the plate-flap option are advanced tumors with an abysmal prognosis, elderly or frail patients, and patients with lateral or posterior bony defects.

Rigid mandibular fixation using a reconstruction plate permits nonvascularized bone grafting under ideal circumstances. These include small defects (<6 cm), minimal or no oral contamination, no scarring of the recipient bed, and well-vascularized cover. However, studies have shown that conventional reconstruction in the primary setting is generally unreliable even when reconstruction plates are used.[38,42] Due to the high success rate of vascularized bone grafting, many centers would use vascularized bone grafts even under these conditions.

Choice of Flap

These five methods represent a spectrum of options covering most reconstructive challenges. At one end is the radial forearm flap with its reliable, thin, supple skin, capable of lining most of the mouth or being split into two components for small full-thickness defects. At the other end, the skin of the iliac crest is poorly positioned for intraoral use, it is very thick, and its blood supply is compromised by the unavoidable tight inserting. The bone, however, is ideal for mandibular replacement: its curvature matches that of the jaw, its size allows the modeling of an entire hemimandible as a single piece, and it has plenty of stock for osseointegrated implants.[28,55] By contrast the radial bone is thin, short, and straight—unsuitable for extensive defects and more difficult to osseointegrate.[10] The fibula and the scapula fit in between.

Although iliac crest bone is generally superior to the fibula for hemimandibular reconstruction, the fibula handles large angle-to-angle defects better because of its greater length. Its skin is not as versatile as the scapula flap nor as supple as the radial forearm flap but it is less bulky than the iliac crest and well positioned for intraoral use. These factors make the fibula the most versatile flap and the most commonly indicated. The scapula's advantage lies in its large independent skin paddles, which facilitate the reconstruction of massive through-and-through defects. It should be noted, however, that these paddles cannot be innervated and that they are somewhat bulky.

The following considerations determine the choice of free flap:

1. Extent of the defect. The HCL classification (see Figure 77-1) gives the functional extent and the epithelial requirements of the area to be reconstructed. For example, a Ho defect would best be handled by an iliac crest bone-only flap, while a fibula osteocutaneous flap would be most appropriate for a LCLm defect. The absolute length of the bony gap should also be considered. For example, only a fibula would be suitable to reconstruct a 20-cm defect.

2. Height of the native mandible. In dentulous patients, the vertical height of the anterior arch is significantly greater than that provided by either a fibula, a radius, or a reconstruction plate. Loss of anterior mandibular height, although not a major functional problem, can constitute a significant cosmetic deformity, leading to the choice of iliac crest or scapula over these alternatives.

3. The bulk of the proposed excision in relation to that of the reconstructive options. Clearly a massive floor of mouth resection including tongue, mandible, and some overlying skin would not be adequately reconstructed using a radial forearm flap even if the bony gap were small.

4. The donor site. Some sites may not be available as a result of previous harvesting, scars, arteriopathy, vascular anomaly, or injury. Often for functional or cosmetic reasons one donor site is selected over another. The iliac donor site is best when appearance is the overriding issue.

5. Rehabilitation. All four bone grafts described here accept osseointegrated implants. However, the iliac crest closely followed by the fibula are the most favored sites for their placement.

6. The desirability for simultaneous dissection. All except the scapula permit simultaneous dissection. Here it is necessary to turn and redrape the patient twice during the procedure.

7. Recipient vessels. Size and availability of the recipient vessels should not be a prime consideration in flap selection for head and neck reconstruction. Neither should their previous radiation status.[51] Nevertheless, the iliac crest, with its short pedicle, can present technical difficulties unless vein grafting is used. The best recipient artery for the iliac crest in terms of size-match and positioning is the superior thyroid, whereas the larger facial or external carotid vessels are more commonly employed for the other osseous transfers. Ideally, venous drainage is provided by the external jugular vein. Alternatives are the internal jugular used end to side, the superior thyroid used in retrograde fashion, or, if all else fails, the cephalic vein brought up as a Corlett loop.[51] Frequently vessels are sought in the opposite neck. The radial forearm flap has a great advantage in this scenario.

8. Age, prognosis, and complexity of the reconstruction. The plate-flap option is an expedient means of treating older patients and those with a poor prognosis. If the soft tissue defect is complex, there is some advantage in not having to worry about the spatial relationship between bone graft and two attached skin paddles. The donor defect is minimized, and where life expectation is short the plate will probably outlive the patient. This method is not recommended in C-containing defects, however. For short segments, where there has not been any intraoral contamination (rare), there is still a place for a nonvascularized bone graft used in conjunction with a reconstruction plate. The properties and applications of the four vascularized bone grafts are summarized in Tables 77-4 and 77-5.

Special Considerations

DENTAL REHABILITATION. Many patients undergoing mandibular reconstruction are edentulous prior to their surgery and have been subsisting on a soft (liquid) diet for years. They often have poor motivation and insufficient means to provide for the upkeep of any dental rehabilitation given. Other patients have resections of their ascending rami and posterior mandibular bodies and do not require dental reconstruction at all. Individuals with small segmental defects and good surrounding dentition may be left unreconstructed or may receive a conventional dental plate. This is particularly true for bone-only reconstructions. An expensive alternative is to place osseointegrated titanium implants in the graft to support a dental prosthesis. Although optional for small gaps, patients with hemimandibular, anterior arch, or larger reconstructions nearly always require these implants[19,55,58] for optimal dental function (see Figures 77-8 and 77-12). A minimum of three may be placed at the time of the primary reconstruction[74] to shorten the process as much as possible. Secondary insertion would have to await wound healing, radiation, and possibly chemotherapy. Primary insertion maximizes the quality of life for those with limited survival prospects and may be a way of "burying" the cost of the implants in the surgical fee. However, the disadvantages include the likelihood of malalignment (and therefore wastage of implants), the extra operative time, and the fact that many patients will not survive long enough to complete their reconstructions. A more prudent approach would be to wait 6 months and only reconstruct those individuals who appear to be survivors. Unfortunately few insurance policies cover the cost of dental rehabilitation regardless of method used.

Osseointegrated implants may be placed either in the vascularized bone graft or in the adjacent edentulous mandible. The advantage of preoperative over postoperative radiotherapy is that the bone graft avoids radiation damage and remains a hospitable host. The failure rate of implants in radiated bone is significantly higher.

Finally, the oral lining is very important for the underlying implants to succeed. Fat, wobbly flaps do not provide a stable seal for the emerging posts, resulting in infection and loosening. It is better to remove the skin flap at a second stage and replace it with a skin graft, which, by becoming adherent to the bone, more closely mimics normal oral mucosa and provides excellent cover for the implant.

Table 77-4.
Comparison of the Qualities Provided by the Four Major Osteocutaneous Free Flaps Used in Mandibular Reconstruction*

	CREST	FIBULA	SCAPULA	RADIUS
Bone length	+++	++++	++	+
Bone quality	++++	+++	++	+
Bone shape	++++	++	++	++
Skin versatility	+	++	++++	++++
Skin quality	+	+++	++	++++
Lack of bulk	+	+++	++	++++
Innervation potential	–	++	–	++++
Donor site cosmesis	+++	++	++	+
Donor site recovery	++	+++	+++	+

*++++ is the best, + the worst.

Table 77-5.
Flap Option According to Defect*

DEFECT	o	m	s	ms
H	Iliac crest Fibula	Iliac crest Fibula	Iliac crest Fibula	Iliac crest+* Fibula+ Scapula
L	Iliac crest Fibula	Iliac crest Radius Fibula	Iliac crest Radius Fibula	Iliac crest+ Radius Scapula
C	Iliac crest Fibula	Iliac crest Radius Fibula	Iliac crest Radius Fibula	Iliac crest Scapula Fibula
LC	Fibula Iliac crest	Fibula Iliac crest	Fibula Iliac crest	Iliac crest+ Scapula Fibula+
HC	Fibula Iliac crest	Fibula Iliac crest	Fibula Iliac crest	Iliac crest+ Fibula+ Scapula
LCL	Fibula Iliac crest	Fibula Iliac crest	Fibula Iliac crest	Iliac crest+ Fibula+ Scapula
HCL	Fibula Iliac crest	Fibula Iliac crest	Fibula Iliac crest	Fibula+ Iliac crest+
HCH	Fibula	Fibula	Fibula	Fibula+

*For key to symbols "HCL" and "oms" see text and Figure 77-1.
+, Indicates an *accessory* flap, for example a radial forearm skin-only flap or a pectoralis major flap.

TEMPOROMANDIBULAR JOINT. Rarely, a temporomandibular joint requires reconstruction following ablative surgery. The native condyle should be preserved whenever oncologically permissible, even if—as Hidalgo[36] has shown—this means rescuing it from the excised specimen and fixing it to the graft. The choice of methods is not bone-dependent. Condylar head prostheses (Figure 77-19), soft tissue interposition, and precise shaping of the graft have all been successfully employed. However, fitting vascularized bone into the condylar fossa when the meniscus is absent risks ankylosis. The meniscus should always be preserved if possible.

For condylar reconstruction, the portion of the graft constituting the ascending ramus is tapered and abutted against the meniscus. If the meniscus has been removed, soft tissue, either attached to the graft itself or in the region of the mandibular fossa, is interposed between the end of the bone graft and the fossa. Temporary support for the graft is achieved using a heavy nonabsorbable suture passed over the zygomatic arch (using an awl) and through a drill hole in the tapered end of the new ascending ramus. Alternatively, a reconstruction plate with an attached prosthetic condyle can be used to span the gap between mandibular remnant and condylar fossa, the bone graft tailored to the defect and lag-screwed to the inside of the plate (see Figure 77-19).

ORAL LINING. Oral lining should be soft, moist, supple, and sensate.[16] A stable alveolar ridge is needed to support a dental prosthesis and a mobile sensate tongue is required for speech and swallowing.

The ability of oral mucosa to secrete mucus facilitates the lubrication of ingested food and aids swallowing. Oral cancer patients frequently suffer from dry mouth due to the effects of radiotherapy on their salivary and mucosal glands. The use of a revascularized jejunal patch may be considered for mucosal replacement, since it has the capacity to secrete mucus and relieve the patient's discomfort, as well as provide an excellent substitute for oral lining.[33] Nevertheless, due to the versatility of the radial forearm flap and a natural reluctance to avoid an intraabdominal donor site, this technique is not in common use in the primary setting.

Reconstruction of the alveolar ridge is important for the patient's rehabilitation with either dentures or osseointegrated implants. The mucosal replacement should be thin and adherent. The flaps described here, including jejunum, are less than ideal due to either their relative thickness or excessive mobility. Unfortunately, the gingiva is usually reconstructed in conjunction with underlying bone, and so a cutaneous flap is commonly used. As mentioned earlier, it is possible to resurface the floor of mouth with vascularized muscle such as the internal oblique.[75] This shrinks down and becomes somewhat adherent to the underlying iliac crest. Yousif et al[80] have used the fascial component of a radial forearm flap covered by a skin graft to achieve the same purpose. Peritoneal tissue has even been employed.[49] However, there may be some concern as to the reliability of the intraoral seal achieved in these ways, particularly for larger defects. An alternative is to remove the cutaneous paddle at a later stage and replace it with a skin graft. At the same time, sulci can be deepened (or created) and lined by the same means. Postoperative splinting with dental compound is essential to prevent contracture.

Sensory restoration is believed to be important in soft tissue reconstruction insofar as it allows the presence of food to be detected within the mouth. This prevents the pooling of saliva and may initiate the afferent arc of the swallow reflex. Minimizing abnormal accumulations of food may have a beneficial effect on oral hygiene as well as oral continence. Both the radial forearm flap and the fibula are capable of bearing sensory paddles and their reinnervation should be attempted whenever possible.

After total glossectomy no active tongue function remains. Haughey[32] used a free latissimus skin-muscle flap, with the muscle sutured transversely to the residual muscles of mastication at the level of the mandibular angles. A sagittally oriented skin component provided additional bulk, as well as lining for the neotongue. He was able to demonstrate tongue elevation during swallowing and most of his 11 patients were able to tolerate a soft diet. Obviously sensory, in addition to motor,

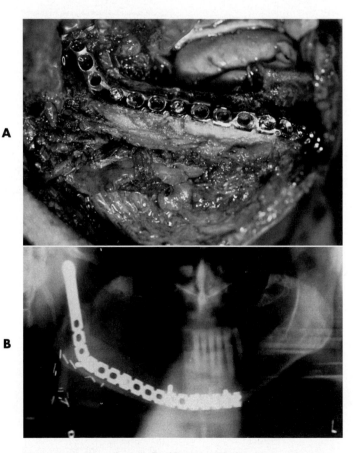

A

B

Figure 77-19. **A** and **B,** Hemimandibular bone-only reconstruction for ameloblastoma using an iliac crest fixed with a reconstruction plate. Since the condyle was resected, a condyle bearing–plate was employed. It is probably unnecessary to reconstruct the ascending ramus with bone in such a case. It is important to retain the meniscus whenever possible to avoid upward displacement of the head. Immediate downward displacement is avoided by suture suspension from the zygomatic arch.

reinnervation would have improved function even more. Sensation in the region of the posterior tongue is essential to protect the airway following total glossectomy.

OUTCOMES

CONVENTIONAL BONE GRAFTING

By the beginning of the twentieth century, surgeons were using a variety of nonvascularized autogenous bones, including the iliac crest, tibia, and calvarium, to reconstruct the mandible.[6,8,21,63] The multitude of reconstructive options described suggests the suboptimal outcome of any given technique. Bone grafts have taken the form of small or large corticocancellous blocks[18,21,44,47] or cancellous grafts housed in a metallic mesh.[1,2] When employed in irradiated beds, extrusion, infection, or resorption occurred in up to 50%, with an overall complication rate near 80%.[1]

To eliminate donor site morbidity, surgeons have used allograft bone in mandibular reconstruction, again with unacceptably high failure rates in radiated beds.[2,25,43] They have also subjected excised (autogenous) mandibles to various "purging" treatments, including the use of soldering irons, diathermy, caustic materials, and cryotherapy, in an attempt to kill neoplastic cells. The purified, lifeless bone was then recycled to act as a framework for creeping substitution. Investigators reported failure rates of 50% with this technique.[7,79]

Even with advances in excision, reconstruction, chemotherapy, and radiotherapy, oral cancer patients now have an overall 5-year survival of only 40%.[56] With such limited life expectancy, reconstructive techniques with failure rates of 50% severely affect the quality of life remaining. The late 1960s and the 1970s were a golden age of discovery for regional flaps suitable for head and neck reconstruction. These flaps enlisted undamaged, well-vascularized tissue for poorly healing radiated wounds, thus facilitating mandibular reconstruction. However, donor morbidity, the uncertainty of "random" cutaneous components, bulky soft tissue, limited arc of rotation, and poor bone vascularity prevented these regional skin,[5] skin-muscle,[4] and skin-muscle-bone[20,22] flaps from fulfilling their early potential. Even with rigid fixation, conventional bone grafts covered by regional flaps had an unacceptably high failure rate in the primary setting.[38,42]

The success of "conventional" or nonvascularized bone grafting is dependent on the size of the defect, the vascularity of the bed, the absence of bacterial contamination, and the rigidity of the fixation. The failure rate becomes unacceptably high when the defect exceeds 6 cm; when the bed is irradiated, contaminated, or fibrotic; when there is communication with the oral cavity; and when there is motion at the synostosis. In other words, "conventional" bone grafting is risky in most of the situations encountered in modern head and neck surgery.[1,31,52]

Although some surgeons have advocated the combination of repeated hyperbaric oxygen dives with "mesh and mush,"

corticocancellous blocks, or medullary-packed cadaveric shells, the results have not proven reproducible, and the expense in terms of cost, quality of life, and time lost has not justified their labored application. Conventional bone grafting is reasonable for the short lateral defect when approached via an extraoral incision without breaching the oral mucosa. Fixation should be rigid (reconstruction plate preferred) and bone contact should be exact and generous.

ALLOPLASTIC RECONSTRUCTION

To be successful, alloplastic reconstruction must include rigid and durable mandibular fixation, must prove resistant to the massive stresses and strains produced by normal chewing, and must not interfere with the healing of the overlying soft tissue. Alloplastic materials must be covered with well-vascularized mucosal replacement, usually a regional or free flap.

The history of alloplastic mandibular reconstruction is littered with failures in these areas. Nevertheless, progress has been made, particularly in the concept of rigid fixation and with the phenomenon of osseointegration. Rigid fixation may be produced by six or more stainless steel bicortical screws in each fragment. Alternatively, three titanium screws osseointegrated with the native mandibular bone can provide equal stability.[53]

The weakness lies in the metal plate itself—stainless or titanium—which, although strong enough to bear the weight of a man, will inevitably submit to the repeated stresses and strains of normally loaded mastication. Patients with alloplastic mandibular reconstruction who continue to enjoy a normal diet and who do not succumb to their disease will often fracture their plates 2 to 3 years postoperatively.[15,17,24,30]

The interaction of metal and mucosa can prove equally noxious. The remedy lies in placing the plate far from skin or mucosa. Laborious attempts have been made to secure the plate low on the medial cortex but this is difficult and needs complex instrumentation. To avoid contact with the oral mucosa and to gain purchase on the densest bone, the plate is generally placed laterally along the lower border of the mandibular remnants.

Use of reconstruction plates has proven effective in elderly patients and in those with poor prognosis. However, a long-term study has shown that the outcome is suboptimal when the plate is used to reconstruct the anterior arch (C segment).[17] In the series in question, there was a 35% removal rate when the plate was used anteriorly and only a 5% failure rate when the flap was used laterally. In addition to this, the aesthetically debilitating condition of "lip and chin ptosis" often accompanied a technical "success" with anterior reconstructions (see Figures 77-2 and 77-3). This technique is therefore only recommended for lateral defects.

The complications related to the various methods of mandibular reconstruction are dealt with under the appropriate headings and will not be discussed in this section.

Use of complex free tissue transfers for composite oromandibular defects previously repaired by soft tissue pedicled flaps alone has raised issues of cost-effectiveness, morbidity, and suitability, particularly in those with poor prognosis.

The most objective outcome is the survival of the free tissue transfer, which, in centers publishing their work, stands at 93% to 100%. These figures are consistent with the survival of free flaps used in other parts of the body and are superior to the survival rate for replanted digits. Problems of vessel spasm encountered in replants and in lower leg free flaps are not seen in the head and neck. However, positional problems, kinking, and oral contamination can lead to vessel thrombosis in this area.

Flap survival, however, tells us nothing about its effectiveness, either from a cost or a functional/aesthetic standpoint. Many seminal articles have reviewed the outcome of free flap mandibular reconstruction in terms of oral continence, masticatory function, speech, swallowing, and appearance; however, only a few have compared the alternatives. Urken et al[77] compared 10 reconstructed and 10 unreconstructed patients with lateral defects using a battery of tests to assess their overall well-being, appearance, deglutition, oral competence, speech, length of hospitalization, and dental rehabilitation. They also measured masticatory function in terms of interincisal opening, bite force, chewing performance, and chewing stroke. The results showed a clear advantage for the reconstructed patients in almost all categories, but the issue of cost was not tackled. This was left to Talesnik et al[69] who compared the cost and outcome of osteocutaneous free tissue transfer (iliac crest excluded) with pedicled soft tissue reconstruction for composite defects. Operating times were greatest for osteocutaneous free flaps, least for pedicled soft tissue flaps, and intermediate for soft tissue free flaps used in conjunction with a plate. (Scapula flaps took longest because simultaneous dissection could not be performed.) Surprisingly, blood loss was greatest in the pedicled group. Hospital stay was similar for all, but time spent in the ICU was longest for osteocutaneous free flaps, the scapula being the worst. ICU stay appeared proportional to operating time. The pedicled flaps had a greater incidence of flap complications including partial necrosis and fistulas, but pulmonary complications were commoner in the free flap group (another factor of longer operating time).

Aesthetically, the appearance of the patients receiving a plate and a free tissue transfer was rated highest by patient and surgeon alike. Next came composite free flap patients, while the pectoralis patients were rated poorest. Many of these had severe mandibular deviation to the affected side and flattening of mandibular contour. Several patients requested further surgery to remedy their iatrogenic deformities.

Social function mirrored aesthetic outcome, with the plate group being most comfortable in public. Speech quality was not related to the extent or location of the osseous defect or the form of reconstruction, but more to the degree of scarring and mobility of the remaining tongue. Ease of swallowing and oral continence were similar in all groups, but the plate and the free tissue transfer patients had greater diet tolerance than the pectoralis major patients.

Readmissions for complications and cancer recurrence were more frequent in the pectoralis musculocutaneous flap group, but the total cost of free osteocutaneous transfer was still higher. The total costs for the plate-flap group were on par with the pectoralis patients. Looking at individual flaps, radial bone was only a little more expensive than pectoralis reconstructions, while the scapula was the costliest. The fibula was intermediate. Clearly, costs relate to the duration of surgery, which impacts on intensive care recovery time and the length of hospital stay.

The authors argue that the superior aesthetic and functional results of the osteocutaneous transfers justify the additional costs, although they advocate reducing those costs by simultaneous dissection whenever possible, the use of intermediate care units, and early discharge with home care. The results with pectoralis flap alone were considered unpredictable, while the plate-flap option was found to be highly cost-effective.

Kroll et al[40] looked at three different groups of patients receiving oromandibular resection: 20 patients underwent vascularized bone reconstruction, 15 received a metallic plate (plus either a pectoralis major or a radial forearm flap), and 15 were reconstructed with soft tissue alone. They found that with bone, immediate reconstruction was more cost-effective than delayed and had a lower complication rate. However, soft tissue reconstructions were less expensive than those involving vascularized bone—notwithstanding their inferior functional and cosmetic results, particularly with anterior defects. They also had fewer complications. Plate reconstructions had an unacceptably high failure rate when used to reconstruct the anterior arch.

Some of these findings are supported and amplified by another outcome study from the same center in which free flaps used for intraoral reconstruction are compared with pectoralis flaps used for the same purpose.[41] In this study, defects involving the mandible were regrettably excluded. The mean costs of surgery were higher for free flaps but more than offset by shorter hospital stays. Failure rates in the two groups were similar. However, it would be incorrect to extrapolate these findings to osteocutaneous free flaps, since the addition of the osseous component increases donor site morbidity, magnifies the complexity of the surgery, and lengthens operating time, ICU recovery, and, presumably, hospital stay. These factors, as we have seen, serve to drive up costs. Rather, the findings are supportive of the plate-flap option in which the osseous defect is addressed simply and accurately, adding little to a simple flap transfer.

Clinical nonunion with a vascularized bone graft results in extra hospitalization, further surgery, suffering, and an increase in "days life lost" for a patient whose days are already numbered. There is an increase in costs associated with this course of events. Fortunately, primary union occurs in over 90% of synostoses, whether so-called rigid or nonrigid methods of fixation are employed.[12] The only form of fixation shown to be ineffective is the use of miniplates with the iliac crest. Although they hold well in the fibula, the screws cannot gain purchase on the crest's soft cancellous bone.

There have been no large-scale outcome studies on the efficacy of reinnervated flaps in the mouth. One series compared 15 patients receiving reinnervated radial forearm flaps with 15 receiving noninnervated ones and 15 receiving pectoralis major flaps.[16] The reinnervated flaps achieved a level of sensation comparable to the contralateral normal side of the mouth and significantly superior to forearm skin in its native site. The noninnervated flaps regained little or no measurable sensation. Exactly how this translates into improved speech, oral continence, mastication, and swallowing is a matter for detailed outcome review. It seems logical, however, that reinnervation must confer some beneficial effect.

Finally, what patient factors mitigate against a good outcome in free osteocutaneous reconstruction of oromandibular defects? The use of irradiated vessels has been thought to increase the risks of thrombosis and flap failure. The evidence is based on gut feeling and animal experiments whose clinical applicability is questionable. Two large clinical series (226 and 308 patients)[51,60] could not relate failure to previous irradiation. One included a case control study that related flap failure with only two factors: postoperative wound infection, and time interval between radiation and surgery. In a multifactorial analysis of delayed reconstruction, tobacco use, alcohol consumption, and previous irradiation, flap loss only related to previous surgery and the use of vein grafts. The use of vein grafts to bypass radiated vessels is therefore illogical.

SUMMARY

Primary mandibular reconstruction has not been well served by conventional methods of bone grafting or by pedicled musculocutaneous flaps with bone attachments. The outcomes of vascularized bone grafting are superior. The costs are more than leaving the mandible unreconstructed, but doing nothing is always cheaper than doing something; by taking the appropriate measures, the expense may be significantly reduced. We still do not know the postdischarge costs of the various types of reconstruction, but it is likely that patients with an intact autogenous mandibular arch will incur less secondary surgical or dental treatment than those with other forms of reconstruction.

Survival rates, fusion rates, and complications are similar in the four vascular bone grafts described here. A knowledge of all four methods is important so that the most appropriate flap may be selected in a particular situation; also, when the first choice is unavailable, a backup may be employed.

In patients with poor prognosis, the plate-flap option is a viable alternative, provided the defect is lateral or posterior. The true incidence of long-term plate fracture is unknown, since many patients succumb to their disease before this occurs.

REFERENCES

1. Adamo A, Szal RL: Timing, results and complications of mandibular reconstructive surgery: report of 32 cases, *J Oral Surg* 37:755, 1979.

2. Alonso MR: Reconstruction of the mandible, *Otolaryngol Clin North Am* 53:501, 1972.

3. Ariyan S, Abrahams JJ, Brattlebort SW, et al: Tomographic studies of human jaws to assess potentials for preserving the blood supply in rim mandibulectomies, *Plast Reconstr Surg* 96:816, 1995.

4. Baek S, Lawson W, Biller HF: An analysis of 133 pectoralis major musculocutaneous flaps, *Plast Reconstr Surg* 69:460, 1982.

5. Bakamjian VY: A two-stage method for pharyngo-esophageal reconstruction with primary pectoral skin flap, *Plast Reconstr Surg* 36:173, 1965.

6. Bardenheuer D: Ueber unterkiefer und oberkiefer Resection, *Arch Klin Chir* 4:604, 1892.

7. Blair VP: *Surgery and diseases of the mouth and jaws,* St Louis, 1918, Mosby.

8. Blocker TG, Stout RA: Mandibular reconstruction in World War II, *Plast Reconstr Surg* 4:153, 1949.

9. Boyd JB: Mandibular reconstruction in the young adult using free vascularized iliac crest, *Microsurgery* 9:141, 1988.

10. Boyd JB, Rosen IB, Freeman J, et al: The iliac crest and the radial forearm flap in vascularized oromandibular reconstruction, *Am J Surg* 159:301, 1990.

11. Boyd JB: Osteocutaneous free flap options in oral cavity reconstruction, *Op Tech Otol Head Neck Surg* 4:104, 1993.

12. Boyd JB, Mulholland S: Fixation of the vascularized bone graft, *Plast Reconstr Surg* 91:274, 1993.

13. Boyd JB, Gullane PJ, Rotstein LE, et al: Classification of the mandibular defect, *Plast Reconstr Surg* 92:1266, 1993.

14. Boyd JB, Morris SF, Rosen IB, et al: The 'through-and-through' oro-mandibular defect, *Plast Reconstr Surg* 93:44, 1994.

15. Boyd JB: Use of reconstruction plates in conjunction with soft tissue free flaps for oromandibular reconstruction, *Clin Plast Surg* 21:69, 1994.

16. Boyd JB, Mulholland S, Gullane P, et al: Lateral antebrachial cutaneous neurosome flaps in oral reconstruction: are we making sense? *Plast Reconstr Surg* 93:1350, 1994.

17. Boyd B, Mulholland S, Davidson J, et al: The free flap and plate in oromandibular reconstruction: long-term review and indications, *Plast Reconstr Surg* 95:1018, 1994.

18. Boyn PJ, Zaren H: Osseous reconstruction of the resected mandible, *Am J Surg* 132:49, 1976.

19. Branemark P-I, Lindstrom J, Hallen O, et al: Reconstruction of the defective mandible, *Scand J Plast Surg* 9:116, 1975.

20. Conley T: Use of composite flaps containing bone for major repairs in the head and neck, *Plast Reconstr Surg* 49:522, 1972.

21. Converse JM, Campbell RM: Bone grafting on surgery of the face, *Surg Clin North Am* 34:375, 1954.

22. Cuono CB, Ariyan S: Immediate reconstruction of a composite mandibular defect with a regional osteo-musculo-cutaneous flap, *Plast Reconstr Surg* 65:477, 1980.

23. David JD, Tan E, Katsaros J, et al: Mandibular reconstruction with vascularized iliac crest, *Plast Reconstr Surg* 82:792, 1988.

24. Davidson J, Boyd JB, Gullane PJ, et al: A comparison of the results following oromandibular reconstruction using a radial forearm flap with radial bone versus a radial forearm flap with a metallic reconstruction plate, *Plast Reconstr Surg* 88:201, 1991.

25. Defries HO, Marble HB, Snell KW: Reconstruction of the mandible: use of a homograft combined with autogenous bone and marrow, *Arch Otolaryngol* 93:426, 1971.

26. Elliot D, Bardsley AF, Batchelor AG, et al: Direct closure of the radial forearm flap donor defect, *Br J Plast Surg* 41:358, 1988.

27. Forrest C, Boyd JB, Manktelow RT, et al: The free vascularized iliac crest tissue transfer: donor site complications associated with eighty-two cases, *Br J Plast Surg* 45:89, 1992.

28. Frodel JL, Funk GF, Capper DT, et al: Osseointegrated implants: a comparative study of bone thickness in four vascularized bone flaps, *Plast Reconstr Surg* 92:449, 1993.

29. Gottlieb LJ, Tachmes L, Pielet RW: Improved venous drainage of the radial artery forearm flap: use of the profundus cubitalis vein, *Ann Plast Surg* 9:281, 1993.

30. Gullane PJ: Primary mandibular reconstruction: analysis of 64 cases and evaluation of interface radiation dosiometry on bridging plates, *Laryngoscope* 101(6 pt 2):1, 1991.

31. Harrison DNF: Problems of reconstruction following preoperative radiotherapy, *Proc R Soc Med* 67:601, 1974.

32. Haughey BH: Tongue reconstruction: concepts and practice, *Laryngoscope* 103:1132, 1993.

33. Hester TR, McConnel FMS, Nahai F, et al: Reconstruction of the cervical esophagus hypopharynx and oral cavity using free jejunal transfer, *Am J Surg* 140:487, 1980.

34. Hidalgo DA: Fibula free flap: a new method of mandible reconstruction, *Plast Reconstr Surg* 84:71, 1989.

35. Hidalgo DA: Aesthetic improvements in free flap mandibular reconstruction, *Plast Reconstr Surg* 88:574, 1991.

36. Hidalgo DA: Condyle transplantation in free flap mandibular reconstruction, *Plast Reconstr Surg* 93:770, 1994.

37. Jewer DD, Boyd JB, Manktelow RT, et al: Orofacial and mandibular reconstruction with the iliac crest free flap: a review of 60 cases and a new method of classification, *Plast Reconstr Surg* 84:391, 1989.

38. Komisar A, Warman S, Danziger E: A critical analysis of immediate and delayed mandibular reconstruction using A-O plates, *Arch Otolaryngol Head Neck Surg* 115:830, 1989.

39. Kramer IRH, Pinborg JJ, Shear M: Histological typing of odontogenic tumors. In: *WHO international histological classification of tumors,* ed 2, New York, 1992, Springer-Verlag.

40. Kroll SS, Schusterman MA, Reece GP: Costs and complications in mandibular reconstruction, *Ann Plast Surg* 29:341, 1992.

41. Kroll S, Evans GRD, Goldberg D, et al: A comparison of resource costs for head and neck reconstruction with free and pectoralis major flaps, *Plast Reconstr Surg* 99:1282, 1997.

42. Lawson W, Loscalzo L, Baek S, et al: Experience with immediate and delayed mandibular reconstruction, *Laryngoscope* 92:5, 1982.

43. Mainous EG: Restoration of resected mandible by grafting with combination of mandible homograft and autogenous iliac marrow and post-operative treatment with hyperbaric oxygenation, *Oral Surg* 35:13, 1973.

44. Manchester WM: Immediate reconstruction of the mandible and temporomandibular joint, *Br J Plast Surg* 18:291, 1965.

45. Marx RE, Morales MJ: Morbidity from bone harvest in major jaw reconstruction: a randomized trial comparing the lateral, anterior and posterior approaches to the ileum, *J Oral Maxillofac Surg* 48:196, 1988.

46. McGregor IA, MacDonald DG: Spread of squamous cell carcinoma to the non-irradiated edentulous mandible: a preliminary report, *Head Neck Surg* 9:157, 1987.

47. Millard DR: Immediate reconstruction of the resected mandibular arch, *Am J Surg* 114:685, 1957.

48. Millard DR, Maisels DO, Batotone J: Immediate repair of radical resection of the anterior arch of the lower jaw, *Plast Reconstr Surg* 39:153, 1967.

49. Mixter RC, Mayfield K, Dibbell DG, et al: Intraoral reconstruction with a microvascular peritoneal flap, *Plast Reconstr Surg* 88:452, 1991.

50. Mounsey RA, Boyd JB: Mandibular reconstruction with osseointegrated implants into the free vascularized radius, *Plast Reconstr Surg* 94:457, 1994.

51. Mulholland S, Boyd JB, McCabe S, et al: Recipient vessels in head and neck microsurgery: radiation effect and vessel access, *Plast Reconstr Surg* 92:628, 1993.

52. Parel S, Drane J, Williams E: Mandibular replacement: a review of the literature, *JADA* 94:120, 1977.

53. Raveh J, Stich H, Sutter F, et al: Use of titanium-coated hollow screw and reconstruction system in bridging of lower jaw defects, *J Oral Maxillofac Surg* 42:281, 1984.

54. Reichart PA, Ries P: Considerations on the classification of odontogenic tumors, *Int J Oral Surg* 12:323, 1983.

55. Reidiger D: Restoration of masticatory function by microsurgically revascularized iliac crest bone grafts using enosseous implants, *Plast Reconstr Surg* 81:861, 1988.

56. Rice DH, Spiro RH: In: *Current concepts in head and neck cancer,* New York, 1989, American Cancer Society, pp 2-3.

57. Rose EH, Norris MS, Rosen JM: Application of high tech three-dimensional imaging and computer generated models in complex facial reconstructions with vascularized bone grafts, *Plast Reconstr Surg* 91:252, 1993.

58. Sanger JR, Head MD, Matloub HS, et al: Enhancement of rehabilitation by the use of implantable adjuncts with vascularized bone grafts for mandibular reconstruction, *Am J Surg* 15:243, 1988.

59. Sanger JR, Matloub HS, Yousif NJ: Sequential connection of flaps: a logical approach to customized mandibular reconstruction, *Am J Surg* 160:402, 1990.

60. Schusterman MA, Miller MJ, Reece GP, et al: A single center's experience with 308 free flaps for repair of head and neck cancer defects, *Plast Reconstr Surg* 93:472, 1994.

61. Schwarz WM, Banis JC, Newton ED, et al: The osteocutaneous scapular flap for mandibular and maxillary reconstruction, *Plast Reconstr Surg* 77:530, 1986.

62. Siebert JW, Longaker MT, Angrigiani C: The inframammary extended circumflex scapular flap: an aesthetic improvement of the parascapular flap, *Plast Reconstr Surg* 99:70, 1997.

63. Skyloff W: Zur Fragder-Knochen-Plastik am Unterkiefer, *Centralbl Chir* 27:881, 1900.

64. Smith A, Bowen VA, Boyd JB: Donor site deficit of the osteocutaneous radial forearm flap, *Ann Plast Surg* 32:372, 1994.

65. Song R, Gao Y, Yu Y, et al: The forearm flap, *Clin Plast Surg* 9:21, 1982.

66. Soutar DS, Scheker LR, Tanner NSB, et al: The radial forearm flap: a versatile method for intraoral reconstruction, *Br J Plast Surg* 36:1, 1983.

67. Swanson E, Boyd JB, Manktelow RT: The radial forearm flap: reconstructive applications and donor site complications in 35 consecutive patients, *Plast Reconstr Surg* 85:258, 1990.

68. Swanson E, Boyd JB, Mulholland RS: The radial forearm flap: a biomechanical study of the osteotomized radius, *Plast Reconstr Surg* 85:267, 1990.

69. Talesnik A, Markowitz B, Calcaterra T, et al: Cost and outcome of osteocutaneous free tissue transfer versus pedicled soft tissue reconstruction for composite mandibular defects, *Plast Reconstr Surg* 97:1167, 1996.

70. Taylor GI, Townsend P, Corlett R: Superiority of the deep circumflex iliac vessels as supply for free groin flaps: experimental work, *Plast Reconstr Surg* 64:595, 1979.

71. Taylor GI, Townsend P, Corlett R: Superiority of the deep circumflex iliac vessels as a supply for free groin flaps: clinical work, *Plast Reconstr Surg* 64:745, 1979.

72. Teot L, Bosse JP, Moufarrege R, et al: The scapular crest pedicled bone graft, *Int J Microsurg* 3:257, 1981.

73. Thoma A, Young JEM, Archibald SD: *The medial scapula osteofasciocutaneous free flap for head and neck reconstruction.* Presented at the fourth annual meeting of the American Society for Reconstructive Microsurgery, Baltimore, MD, September 17-19, 1988, p. 80.

74. Urken ML, Buchbinder D, Weinberg H, et al: Primary placement of osseointegrated implants in microvascular mandibular reconstruction, *Otolaryngol Head Neck Surg* 101:56, 1989.

75. Urken ML, Vickery C, Buchbinder D, et al: The internal oblique—iliac crest osseomyocutaneous free flap in oromandibular reconstruction, *Arch Otolaryngol Head Neck Surg* 115:339, 1989.

76. Urken ML, Weinberg H, Vickery C, et al: The neurofasciocutaneous radial forearm flap in head and neck reconstruction: a preliminary report, *Laryngoscope* 100:161, 1990.

77. Urken ML, Buchbinder D, Weinberg H, et al: Functional evaluation following microvascular oromandibular reconstruction of the oral cancer patient: a comparative study of reconstructed and non-reconstructed patients, *Laryngoscope* 101:935, 1991.

78. Viterbo F, Trindade JC, Hoshino K, et al: End to side neurorrhaphy with removal of the epineural sheath: an experimental study in rats, *Plast Reconstr Surg* 94:1038, 1994.

79. Weaver AW, Smith DB: Frozen autogenous mandibular stent-graft for immediate reconstruction in oral cancer surgery, *Am J Surg* 126:505, 1972.

80. Yousif NJ, Matloub HS, Sanger JR, et al: Soft tissue reconstruction of the oral cavity, *Clin Plast Surg* 21:15, 1994.

Mandible Reconstruction with the Fibula Free Flap

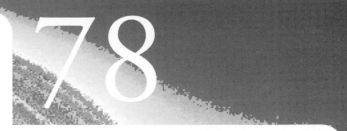

Gregory A. Mantooth
Jeffrey D. Wagner

INTRODUCTION

Free vascularized fibula transfer was first described by Taylor et al in 1975.[24] In 1989, Hidalgo was the first to report a significant series of vascularized fibula grafts for mandibular reconstruction.[12] The fibula free flap has since become one of the most important resources in head and neck reconstructive surgery, with a number of significant advantages over other commonly used osteocutaneous donor sites.

Perhaps the greatest utility of the fibula is that it can provide up to 24 cm of straight, dense cortical vascularized bone, which can be shaped using multiple osteotomies to accommodate a mandibular defect. The fibula may be harvested with an associated fasciocutaneous segment, allowing transfer of soft tissue for intraoral or facial reconstruction. The skin paddle may be up to 15×25 cm, is thin and pliable, and may be harvested with the sural nerve to provide sensation.[1] The vascular pedicle length is adequate for most reconstructive needs, and the peroneal vessels are well suited for microvascular anastomosis. The location of the fibula allows a two-team surgical approach such that tumor extirpation and fibula free flap harvest may be performed simultaneously.

Mandibular reconstruction with a fibula free flap permits prosthodontic dental rehabilitation using osseointegrated implants to be performed.[21] Donor site morbidity is low, with nearly all patients ambulating within a few weeks of surgery. This chapter will address preoperative assessment of patients who are candidates for fibula free flaps, the technical details of graft harvest, and the limitations of the free fibula transfer for mandibular reconstruction.

ANATOMY OF THE FIBULA FREE FLAP

The fibula is located at the junction of the four fascial compartments of the leg. It articulates proximally with the tibia and distally with the tibia and talus. The distal fibula is important to ankle stability and normal motion. The bone is triangular in cross-sectional shape, approximately 1.5 to 2 cm in diameter, and 40 cm in length. It is comprised primarily of dense cortical bone with a relatively small amount of cancellous bone.

The fibula has a type V blood supply consisting of a dominant nutrient pedicle and several secondary segmental pedicles to the periosteum that originate from the lateral aspect of the peroneal artery.[18] The dominant pedicle enters posterior to the interosseous membrane at the junction of the upper and middle thirds of the fibula. For the purpose of fibula transfer, the segmental periosteal blood supply from the peroneal artery is the most clinically important because it permits multiple osteotomies to shape the vascularized bone graft. Depending on the length of bone harvested, the peroneal vascular pedicle provides a pedicle length ranging from 5 to 10 cm, with an average diameter of 1.8 to 2.5 mm. Venous drainage of the fibula is via paired venae comitantes, each with a diameter of 2 to 4 mm.

The skin territory of the peroneal artery is located over most of the lateral leg. The blood flow to this skin is supplied by 4 to 8 septocutaneous and musculocutaneous perforators derived from the peroneal artery.[14,23,26] Septocutaneous perforators reach the skin by traveling posterior to the fibula through the posterior crural septum. A variable number of peroneal artery–derived musculocutaneous perforators lie within the flexor hallucis longus and soleus muscles. The

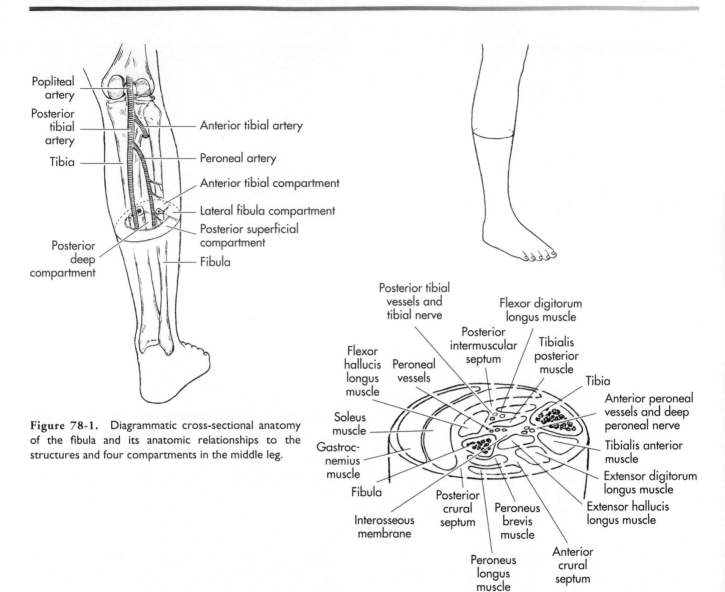

Figure 78-1. Diagrammatic cross-sectional anatomy of the fibula and its anatomic relationships to the structures and four compartments in the middle leg.

fasciocutaneous paddle, which may be transferred with the fibula free flap, can be up to 25 cm in length and 15 cm wide. Diagrammatic anatomy of the fibula and surrounding structures is illustrated in Figure 78-1.

Motor innervation to the muscles of the lateral compartment, the peroneus longus and brevis, is supplied by the superficial peroneal nerve. Sensory innervation to the corresponding lateral calf skin territory is largely supplied by the sural nerve, which is of adequate size to allow microscopic anastomosis, potentially providing sensation to the fasciocutaneous portion of the fibula free flap.

PREOPERATIVE ASSESSMENT

Preoperative assessment to determine whether a patient is a suitable candidate for a vascularized fibula transfer begins with a careful medical history to identify any conditions that could indicate unreliability of the peroneal artery as a pedicle for tissue transfer. These conditions include peripheral vascular disease, arteritis, deep vein thrombosis, or trauma to the lower extremities. Any history of lower extremity surgery, particularly revascularizations or reconstructive procedures, should also be elucidated.

Detailed physical examination is performed. The knee and ankle joints should be assessed for range of motion, which can suggest the need for extended postoperative rehabilitation. Joints should also be examined for hyperlaxity, which can be an indicator of possible ankle or knee instability after fibula harvest.[9] Physical examination should include assessment for signs of peripheral vascular disease such as hair loss, decreased capillary refill, dependent rubor, venous insufficiency, or skin lesions. One of the most important components of preoperative assessment is evaluation of the arterial supply to the lower extremity. A modified foot Allen's test is performed. Both the dorsalis pedis and posterior tibial arteries should be easily palpable with occlusion of the other vessel. If they are not, further evaluation is indicated.

When use of the fibula free flap was first described, contrast angiography was routinely performed prior to surgery to assess patency of the peroneal artery and ensure there would be no significant vascular compromise to the foot after the flap harvest. Some authors still feel preoperative arteriography should be performed on all patients, since it can result in a change in the operative plan in a significant number of cases.[4] Others contend arteriography should be reserved for patients with abnormal findings on physical examination, particularly absent or diminished pedal pulses.[6,17]

Duplex ultrasonography provides a potential compromise for preoperative evaluation. Without the invasiveness, potential risk, and expense associated with arteriography, duplex scanning provides reliable information about the vascular anatomy of the leg.[20] Color flow Doppler can also provide the number and location of septocutaneous and musculocutaneous perforating vessels from the peroneal artery to the skin paddle overlying the fibula.[8] Although not as sensitive for segmental vascular detail as an arteriogram, the combination of careful physical examination and duplex ultrasonography provides an adequate preoperative assessment of the pertinent lower extremity vasculature prior to vascularized fibula harvest in the majority of patients. Angiography may then be reserved for patients with equivocal findings on physical examination or noninvasive studies.[17]

Whether angiography is performed routinely or selectively, there are radiographic indications that the fibula cannot be safely transferred as a free flap. Peripheral vascular disease or trauma may result in decreased or absent flow in the peroneal artery, rendering it unreliable as a vascular pedicle for the flap. Vascular disease or injury can also result in diminished or absent flow in the anterior tibial or posterior tibial arteries. In severe cases of peripheral vascular occlusion, harvest of the peroneal artery could result in a limb-threatening situation. Rare congenital vascular anomalies restricting the use of fibula free flaps exist. Peroneal arteria magna, which occurs in 0.2% to 5% of the population, is associated with hypoplasia or absence of both the anterior tibial and posterior tibial arteries, with the peroneal artery as the sole arterial supply for the foot.[15] In this situation, vascularized fibula transfer is contraindicated.

Other imaging modalities may occasionally be useful in preoperative assessment. Magnetic resonance angiography evaluation of the lower extremity can provide a reliable map of the major arterial anatomy of the leg without the potential risks associated with arteriogram. The cost, however, currently argues against routine use of this modality.[5,19]

VASCULARIZED FIBULA HARVEST

OSSEOUS FLAP

The entire leg should be prepared circumferentially to include the calf for fibula harvest, the course of the saphenous vein (in case a vein graft is required), and the upper thigh for a skin

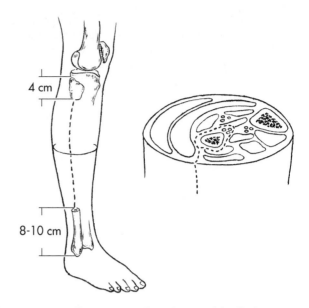

Figure 78-2. Diagrammatic lateral view of the fibula osteocutaneous free flap after division of the proximal and distal bone and ligation of distal peroneal vessels. Lateral retraction on the distal end of the fibula facilitates exposure.

graft donor site. Some surgeons prefer to perform fibula graft harvest under tourniquet control. The use of a tourniquet facilitates the four-compartment muscular dissection that must be performed.

When harvesting only the fibula bone for transfer as a vascularized bone graft, the procedure begins with an incision along the lateral aspect of the leg from the fibula head to approximately 4 cm proximal to the lateral malleolus. The lateral compartment is opened first, exposing the peroneus longus and brevis muscles. These muscles are retracted anteriorly and dissected from the lateral fibula, leaving a 1-to 2-mm cuff of muscle on the bone to preserve periosteal blood supply. The muscles are dissected for the entire length of the fibula to facilitate exposure of the vessels. Careful dissection should be performed at the fibula head, identifying the superficial peroneal nerve, which must be preserved. Once this nerve is identified, proximal and distal osteotomies may be performed using either an oscillating or reciprocating saw. Early fibula division greatly facilitates subsequent exposure and speeds the dissection of the pedicle. Care should be taken to preserve at least 4 cm of fibula proximally to protect the superficial peroneal nerve and 5 to 10 cm distally to ensure ankle joint stability. After the osteotomies have been completed, the fibula may be gently retracted laterally for better visualization of the peroneal vessels (Figure 78-2). The distal peroneal artery and venae comitantes are identified just medial to the site of distal fibular osteotomy and are ligated, allowing further lateral retraction of the fibular segment.

Dissection then proceeds from distal to proximal, anterior to posterior. Dissection is layer by layer, along the entire length of the graft for each compartment. The anterior compartment is first opened by incising the anterior crural septum. The extensor hallucis longus and the extensor digitorum longus are dissected for the entire length of the graft, revealing the dense interosseous membrane, which connects the fibula to the tibia. This is incised, leaving a 1-to 2-mm cuff of muscle on the fibula to preserve the periosteal blood supply. At this point, the anterior tibial vessels are often seen just anterolateral to the fibula and must be preserved.

The posterior crural septum is then divided, exposing the superficial compartment musculature. The lateral gastrocnemius and soleus muscles are dissected from the length of the fibula graft. The deep posterior compartment may be entered from either a posterior or anterior approach, with the anterior approach affording better exposure of the peroneal vessels.[18] The peroneal artery and paired venae comitantes are identified, usually found lying anterior to the flexor hallucis longus and tibialis posterior muscles. The muscles are transected lateral to the peroneal vessels, taking a narrow cuff of muscular tissue. The posterior tibial vessels and the tibial nerve are visualized posterior to the tibia, about 1 to 1.5 cm medial and parallel to the peroneal vessels in the midcalf, and must be preserved. Care must be exercised in dissecting the midportion of the fibula because the dominant nutrient pedicle from the peroneal artery enters the fibula at the junction of the upper and middle thirds of the bone.

After dissection of the deep posterior compartment, the peroneal vessels should be the only remaining attachment between the fibula flap and the leg. The pedicle is then dissected proximally to the junction of the peroneal and posterior tibial vessels. Perforating vessels at this level from the peroneal artery and veins to the soleus muscle should be identified and ligated to avoid bleeding. Once dissected to the

tibioperoneal trunk, the vascular pedicle is usually 5 to 7 cm long. Pedicle length can be increased an additional 1 to 2 cm by ligation of the lateral posterior tibial vein. More commonly, subperiosteal dissection and resection of a proximal portion of the fibula graft is performed to add functional length to the vascular pedicle. Depending on the bone requirement, up to 7 to 10 cm of additional pedicle length can be obtained in this manner. The nutrient branch of the peroneal artery may be safely sacrificed during this maneuver, provided the distal periosteal blood supply to the fibula has been preserved.

OSTEOCUTANEOUS FLAP

The skin and soft tissue overlying the fibula are routinely transferred as a fasciocutaneous component of the fibula free flap for oromandibular reconstruction. Although the reliability of the fibula skin paddle has been questioned, skin flap transfer is successful in over 90% of cases.[12] Typically, larger skin paddles are more reliably transferred than very small ones.

The fasciocutaneous paddle is designed over the lateral aspect of the leg, and may be up to 15×25 cm in size (Figure 78-3). The skin flap was originally described as centered over the midportion of the fibula.[11,12,23] Recent anatomic studies suggest improved fasciocutaneous paddle survival can be achieved if the skin paddle is located more distally, with the flap centered over the junction of the middle and distal thirds of the fibula.[14] The blood supply to paddles overlying the proximal fibula is less consistent, relying mainly on musculocutaneous perforators. The distal skin and subcutaneous tissues are predominantly supplied by septocutaneous perforators, allowing for more reliable tissue transfer.

To facilitate skin paddle design, cutaneous perforators should be localized with a Doppler (Figure 78-4). The anterior

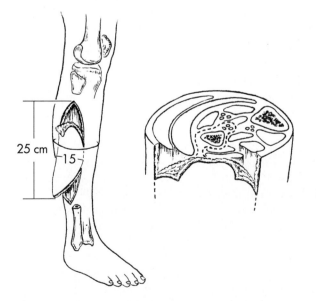

Figure 78-3. The fasciocutaneous paddle, which may be reliably transferred with the fibula free flap, can be up to 25 cm in length and 15 cm in width, depending on the body habitus of the patient.

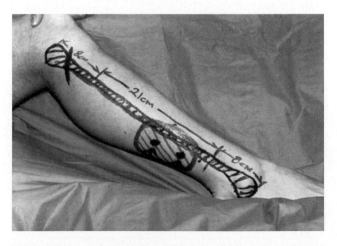

Figure 78-4. Preoperative markings for fibula osteocutaneous free flap harvest. Note distally located skin paddle with Doppler localized septocutaneous perforators.

portion of the skin paddle is dissected first with an incision through the skin, subcutaneous tissues, and deep muscular fascia. The flap is elevated in a posterior direction in the subfascial plane, over the peroneus longus and brevis muscles to the posterior crural septum, which carries the cutaneous perforators. The perforating septocutaneous branches previously identified by Doppler on the skin surface are visualized coursing perpendicular to the fibula along the anterior surface of the posterior crural septum and should be carefully preserved. This septum and the septocutaneous perforators must be gently handled to ensure perfusion to the skin paddle. The posterior portion of the flap is similarly incised along its length to the level of the deep fascia. It is also dissected in the subfascial plane from the lateral gastrocnemius and soleus muscles toward the posterior crural septum. The sural nerve should be identified and preserved. Alternatively, it can be harvested with the fasciocutaneous flap to provide a sensate flap.

There is controversy with regard to the inclusion of muscle with the osteocutaneous flap to ensure adequate blood flow to the skin paddle. To ensure a sufficient blood supply, a 1-cm cuff of soleus and flexor hallucis longus muscles should be included with the fibula graft, particularly if the skin paddle is large (15×25 cm) or centered over the midportion of the fibula. There will be improved flap survival with inclusion of musculocutaneous perforators, particularly for skin overlying the proximal portion of the fibula.[23] Somewhat less reliably, a fasciocutaneous flap may be elevated without a muscular cuff, based only on septocutaneous perforators. If this technique is used, the skin flap should be based over the distal portion of the leg to provide a greater possibility of graft survival.[14] The remainder of the dissection is similar to standard osseous flap elevation.

The fibula is shaped while still attached to its vascular pedicle (Figure 78-5). Using a template of the excised mandible as a guide, the necessary osteotomies are performed with an oscillating or reciprocating saw. Limited subperiosteal dissection allows access to the fibula cortex while preserving maximal periosteal attachments to the bone. Closing wedge osteotomies are performed as needed and individual segments are rigidly affixed using any of a variety of plating systems. The fibula free graft is transferred after modeling of the fibula has been completed and the recipient site prepared for microvascular anastomosis. A clinical case of oromandibular reconstruction using a free fibula osteocutaneous flap is illustrated in Figure 78-6.

Prior to closure, closed suction drains are placed and the peroneal muscles are reapproximated to the soleus muscle. When an osteocutaneous flap is harvested, primary closure of the defect is generally not possible because it will result in undue tension on the skin, potentially severe enough to result in a compartment syndrome.[22] It is best to primarily close only the proximal and distal ends of the incision that approximate easily, covering the remainder of the defect with a split-thickness skin graft. The postoperative dressing should include a well-padded posterior splint to keep the ankle in 90 degrees of flexion.

Postoperative care, in addition to routine wound care, should include lower extremity physical therapy. Ambulation with protected weight bearing can generally begin at postoperative day two to seven. Therapy should include passive and active range of motion exercises for the knee, ankle, and foot once the patient has started ambulating. Unrestricted weight bearing is usually possible within several weeks after surgery.

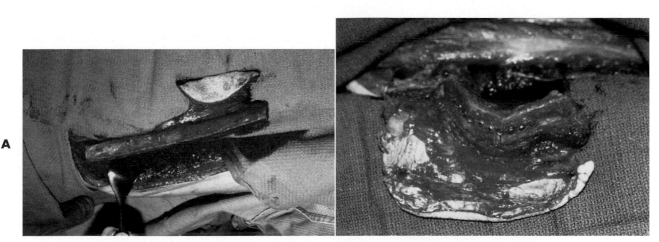

Figure 78-5. **A,** Fibula osteocutaneous flap harvest. The flap is perfusing at the leg after completion of vascular pedicle dissection, prior to osteotomies. **B,** Bone modeling at leg donor site while the flap perfuses. Two closing wedge osteotomies performed to simulate a resected anterior segment of mandible. Osteotomies fixed with miniplates.

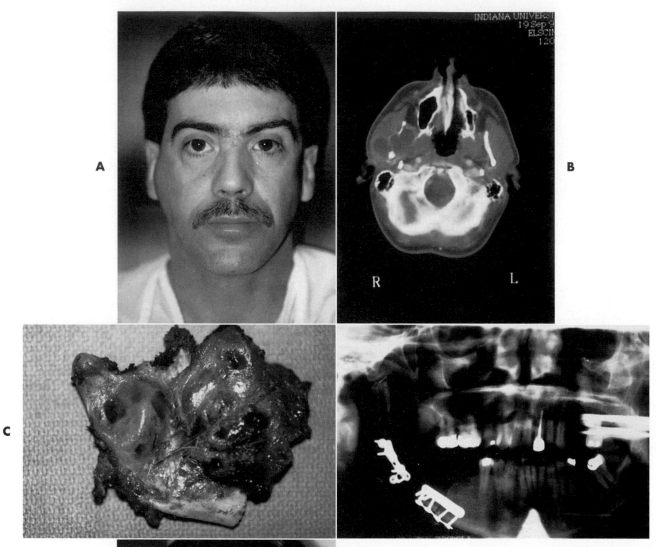

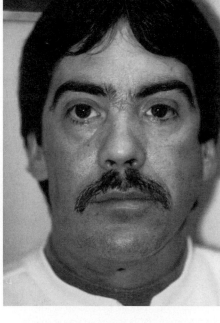

Figure 78-6. **A,** Preoperative frontal view of a patient with a massive posterior right mandibular keratocyst with malignant degeneration. **B,** CT scan demonstrating mandibular destruction. **C,** Surgical specimen after resection of the posterior body, ramus, and condyle to remove keratocyst. **D,** Radiograph of right posterior neomandible reconstructed using a fibula osteocutaneous free flap. **E,** Postoperative frontal view.

DONOR SITE MORBIDITY

Several studies have examined the potential morbidity associated with harvest of the fibula flap. Major wound complications associated with fibula free flap harvest are relatively rare, with a reported incidence of 3% to 7%.[2] Skin grafts to fibula donor sites consistently heal well, usually with a satisfactory cosmetic result.[14] Occasionally, some skin graft loss is seen, particularly over the peroneal tendons. Secondary healing in these cases may be prolonged but is usually successful. Pain with ambulation is reported in the immediate postoperative period in approximately 17% of patients. Almost all patients can expect to have minimal or no discomfort with walking by an average of 5 weeks after surgery.[10]

Postoperative weakness of ankle or great toe dorsiflexion is seen in approximately 15% to 30% of patients. Similarly, joint stiffness about the ankle and great toe is seen in 10% to 40% of patients.[2] These limitations are typically mild and of short duration. Ankle instability has been reported following fibula free flap harvest. To minimize this problem, at least 4 cm of fibula proximally and 6 to 8 cm distally should be preserved.[3] Clinical series have consistently shown that with routine physical therapy, virtually all patients can expect to resume normal ambulation and their preoperative level of activity.

Other rare complications include heterotopic bone formation in the donor site (Figure 78-7) and nerve injury. Neuropraxia of the superficial peroneal nerve, the most common nerve injury seen with fibula harvest, is probably related to retraction compression; however, most cases are self-limited with no associated long-term sequelae.[16]

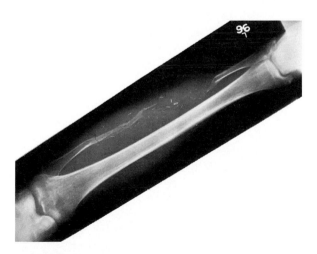

Figure 78-7. Postoperative radiograph of a fibula harvest site 2 years after oral cavity reconstruction with an osteocutaneous fibula free flap. Note heterotopic bone formation in the proximal fibula bed. The patient suffered a symptomatic fracture of this area.

LIMITATIONS OF THE FIBULA FREE FLAP

There are some limitations to the use of the fibula free flap. The presence of vascular disease or congenital vascular anomalies of the lower extremity can preclude use of the fibula as a vascularized tissue transfer.

Although the fibula free flap can be transferred with a fasciocutaneous component, the skin paddle may not satisfy large soft tissue requirements due to its limited bulk. With large floor of mouth or glossectomy defects requiring mandibular reconstruction, a free fibula graft can be supplemented with a pectoralis myocutaneous flap. In instances involving extensive oral cavity and lip resection, two free flaps may be required. Alternatively, a single composite flap with a larger amount of skin and muscle, such as a subscapular system flap, may be better suited to this type of reconstruction.

Bone height in neomandibles reconstructed with fibula flaps generally ranges from 10 to 15 mm, which may be significantly shorter than the remaining mandible, particularly in a dentate patient.[21] Because of this difference in bone height, there have been concerns about the use of osseointegrated implants. Animal studies have shown some bone resorption around implants secondary to excessive load forces.[13] However, several patient studies indicate reliable incorporation of osseointegrated implants into a fibular graft, with limited bone loss around implants seen only in those patients receiving radiation therapy.[21] In dentate patients having 3 to 4 cm bone height, particularly with short, straight lateral segment, bone-only mandible defects, the iliac crest may be a better bone source than the fibula.

Another concern not necessarily unique to the fibula free flap is the number of osteotomies that can be safely performed in shaping the bone. It is possible to perform multiple osteotomies along the length of the fibula, taking care to maintain maximal periosteal attachments to the segments.[11] Others recommend caution, describing possible bone loss or nonunion when more than two osteotomies are performed.[7]

ALTERNATIVE OSTEOCUTANEOUS FLAPS

The fibula is the single most versatile bone flap for mandible reconstruction and satisfies most oromandibular reconstructive needs. There are alternatives to the fibula free flap that have particular characteristics that may make them more applicable in certain cases of mandibular reconstruction[25] (Table 78-1).

Table 78-1.
Characteristics of Major Osteocutaneous Free Flap Donor Sites

DONOR SITE	BONE LENGTH	SOFT TISSUE CHARACTERISTICS	PEDICLE	MORBIDITY
Fibula	20-24 cm	Skin and muscle; potential sensation	Peroneal artery; up to 10-12 cm	Low
Iliac crest	15 cm	Skin and muscle (often bulky); no potential sensation	Deep circumflex iliac artery; 5-6 cm	Moderate to high
Radius	10 cm (unicortical)	Skin only; sensate	Radial artery; up to 15 cm	Moderate to high
Scapula	14 cm	Skin and muscle; no potential sensation	Subscapular artery; 10 cm	Moderate

Adapted from Wagner JD: Preoperative assessment and preparation for mandible reconstruction, *Oper Tech Plast Reconstr Surg* 3:220, 1996.

SUMMARY

The development of the fibula free flap has been one of the most important advances in head and neck reconstructive surgery, particularly for the composite oromandibular defect. The fibula osteocutaneous flap provides ample, easily shaped bone for mandibular replacement, as well as skin and soft tissue for facial and intraoral reconstruction. The fibula is readily harvested with minimal donor site morbidity. Despite some limitations, the free fibula graft remains the best option for most patients who require composite tissue oromandibular reconstruction.

REFERENCES

1. Anthony JP, Foster RD: Mandibular reconstruction with the fibula osteocutaneous flap, *Oper Technique Plast Reconstr Surg* 3:233, 1996.
2. Anthony TP, Rawnsley JD, Benhaim P, et al: Donor leg morbidity and function after fibula free flap mandible reconstruction, *Plast Reconstr Surg* 96:146, 1995.
3. Babhulkar SS, Pande KC, Babhulkar S: Ankle instability after fibula resection, *J Bone Joint Surg* 77B:258, 1995.
4. Blackwell KE: Donor site evaluation for fibula free flap transfer, *Am J Otolaryngol* 19:89, 1998.
5. Cambria RP, Yucel K, Brewster DC, et al: The potential for lower extremity revascularization without contrast angiography: experience with magnetic resonance angiography, *J Vasc Surg* 17:1050, 1993.
6. Disa JJ, Cordeiro PG: The current role of preoperative arteriography in free fibula flaps, *Plast Reconstr Surg* 102:1083, 1998.
7. Ferri J, Piot B, Ruhin B, et al: Advantages and limitations of the fibula free flap in mandibular reconstruction, *J Oral Maxillofacial Surg* 55:440, 1997.
8. Futran ND, Stack BC: Preoperative color Doppler assessment of the lower extremity in fibula free flap reconstruction, *Conjoint Symposium on Contemporary Head and Neck Reconstruction,* 1995.
9. Ganel A, Yaffe B: Ankle instability of the donor site following removal of vascularized bone graft, *Ann Plast Surg* 24:7, 1990.
10. Goodacre TEE, Walker CJ, Iawad AS, et al: Donor site morbidity following osteocutaneous free fibula transfer, *Br J Plast Surg* 43:410, 1990.
11. Hidalgo DA: Discussion of the osteocutaneous free fibula flap: is the skin paddle reliable? *Plast Reconstr Surg* 90:797, 1992.
12. Hidalgo DA: Fibula free flap: a new method of mandible reconstruction, *Plast Reconstr Surg* 84:71, 1989.
13. Hoshaw SJ, Brunski JB, Cochran GV: Mechanical loading of Branemark implants affects interfacial bone modeling and remodeling, *Int J Oral Maxillofacial Implant* 9:345, 1994.
14. Jones NF, Monstrey S, Gambier BA: Reliability of the osteocutaneous flap for mandibular reconstruction: anatomical and surgical confirmation, *Plast Reconstr Surg* 97:707, 1996.
15. Kim D, Orron DE, Skillman JJ: Surgical significance of popliteal artery variants: a unified angiographic classification, *Ann Surg* 210:776, 1989.
16. Lee EH, Goh JCH, Helm R, et al: Donor site morbidity following resection of the fibula, *J Bone Joint Surg* (Br) 72B:129, 1990.
17. Lutz BS, Wei F, Chang SCN, et al: Routine donor leg angiography before vascularized free fibula transplantation is not necessary: a prospective study in 120 clinical cases, *Plast Reconstr Surg* 103:121, 1999.
18. Mathes S, Nahai F: *Reconstructive surgery principles, anatomy, and techniques,* New York, 1997, Churchill Livingstone, pp 1353-1370.
19. McDermott VG, Meakem TJ, Carpenter JP, et al: Magnetic resonance angiography of the distal lower extremity, *Clin Rad* 50:741, 1995.

20. Moneta GL, Yeager RA, Antonovic R, et al: Accuracy of lower extremity arterial duplex mapping, *J Vasc Surg* 15:275, 1992.

21. Roumanas ED, Markowitz BL, Lorant JA, et al: Reconstructed mandibular defects: fibula free flaps and osseointegrated implants, *Plast Reconstr Surg* 99:356, 1996.

22. Saleem M, Hashim F, Manohar MB: Compartment syndrome in a free fibula osteocutaneous flap donor site, *Br J Plast Surg* 51:405, 1998.

23. Schusterman MA, Reece GP, Miller MJ, et al: The osteocutaneous fibula free flap: is the skin paddle reliable? *Plast Reconstr Surg* 90:787, 1992.

24. Taylor GI, Miller GDH, Ham FJ: The free vascularized bone graft: a clinical extension of microvascular techniques, *Plast Reconstr Surg* 55:533, 1975.

25. Wagner JD: Preoperative assessment and preparation for mandible reconstruction, *Oper Tech Plast Reconstr Surg* 3:217, 1996.

26. Wei F, Chen H, Chuang C, et al: Fibular osteoseptocutaneous flap: anatomic study and clinical application, *Plast Reconstr Surg* 78:191, 1986.

The Pharynx

John J. Coleman III

INDICATIONS

The pharynx connects the oral cavity to the cervical esophagus and creates a passageway for food from the mouth to the stomach. This muscle-lined tubular continuation of the oral cavity is functionally complex: it not only regulates food entry to the esophagus, but also, because of its location immediately above and behind the larynx, acts as the aditus to the respiratory tree and modulator of voice and speech. Coordinated function of the intact or reconstructed pharynx and larynx is necessary to continue the vegetative functions of alimentation and respiration. Impairment of this synergy may result in dysphagia, leading to starvation, airway obstruction, or aspiration.

Although the pharynx is comprised of similar tissue throughout, each of its three parts has a somewhat specialized task to ensure continued progress of the food bolus. The *nasopharynx* is a rigid mucosa-lined, box-shaped structure that is bounded by the base of the skull cephalad, the nasal side of the soft palate caudad, the vertebral bodies and prevertebral fascia posterior, and the posterior openings of the nasal cavity (the choanae) anterior. Within the nasopharynx are the orifices of the eustachian tubes, the adenoids, and numerous other nests of lymphatic tissue. The *oropharynx* includes the tonsils and tonsillar pillars, the base of the tongue, and the cephalad portion of the middle constrictor, which lies subjacent to the posterior mucosa of the pharyngeal wall. The *hypopharynx* lies lateral and posterior to the larynx and lateral to the pyriform sinuses; the postcricoid hypopharynx is surrounded by the cricopharyngeus muscle (Figure 79-1).

Although the synergy of structures that allow speech and swallowing is incredibly complex, a simple outline can be described to facilitate subsequent reconstruction. The oral cavity serves as the acceptance and capacitance unit for swallowing. The food bolus is prepared here, being liquefied with saliva, immunoglobulins, and enzymes, and reduced in size by mastication. The bolus is kept inside the oral cavity by the anterior sphincter action of the lips; the superior elevation of the velum, which obturates the nasopharynx; and the anterior movement of the middle constrictor, which approximates the base of the tongue. When the bolus is ready to be swallowed, the tongue pushes it up and back, the velum remains elevated, the middle constrictor relaxes, the larynx elevates and moves anteriorly to close beneath the epiglottis, and the food moves into the oropharynx and hypopharynx. The pharyngeal constrictors now strip the bolus caudad. The cricopharynx relaxes and allows movement down into the esophagus, where the bolus progresses toward the stomach by means of peristalsis. As the bolus passes, the larynx descends, the velum descends, the tongue moves forward, and the airway is reopened so that exhalation or inhalation of air, or its corollary function of speech, can proceed.[18,20] Sensory supply to the pharynx and larynx is primarily by the internal laryngeal branch of the superior laryngeal nerve; a branch of the vagus, which descends from high in the neck; and, more cephalad, by the glossopharyngeal nerve. Motor supply to the upper pharynx is derived from the external laryngeal branch of the vagus nerve; the lower pharynx and larynx receive their motor supply from the nerve's recurrent laryngeal branch. The combined motor and sensory loss that comes from a lesion of the vagus nerve above the carotid bifurcation results in severe functional disruptions in the pharynx and larynx, with cord paralysis and pharyngeal dyskinesia that usually result in disabling aspiration and pneumonitis, requiring gastrostomy feedings. Injury to the vagus nerve lower in the neck or to the recurrent laryngeal nerve above is usually compensated for with or without surgical intervention since this is primarily a motor palsy (Figures 79-1 and 79-2).

The coordinated activity of swallowing and respiration relies on both voluntary and involuntary neuromuscular activity and is subject to significant disruption by extirpative or reconstructive surgery. Although each anatomic region is essential, as is each part of the process, most studies demonstrate direct relationship between dysphagia or swallowing dysfunction and the amount of tongue resected. Interference with elevation and depression of the larynx and its protective relationship with the base of the tongue and epiglottis is also a major cause of morbidity from aspiration and subsequent pneumonitis.

Congenital defects of the oral cavity and the head and neck, such as cleft palate, can result in pharyngeal dysfunction, most particularly the obturation of the nasal cavity by the soft palate. Velopharyngeal insufficiency may require surgical intervention, and pharyngeal myomucosal flaps or dynamic muscle slings are effective methods of restoring such lost function.

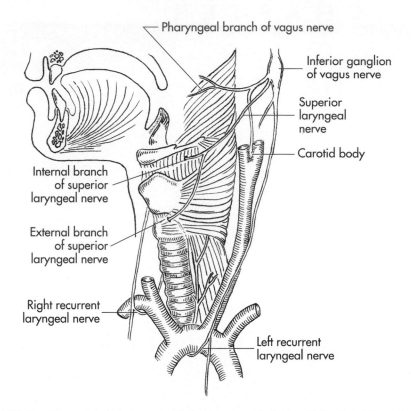

Figure 79-1. Neurovascular anatomy of the larynx and pharynx. Mixed motor and sensory innervation is carried by the superior laryngeal and recurrent laryngeal nerve branches of the vagus. The cephalad pharynx also receives sensory innervation from the glossopharyngeal nerve.

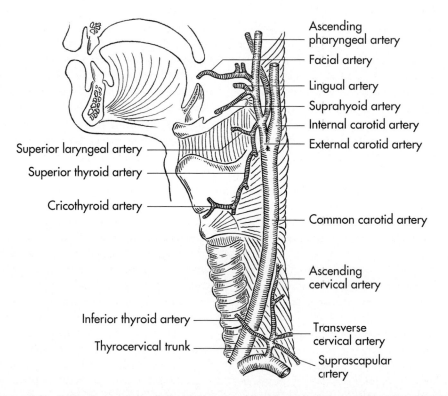

Figure 79-2. Vascular anatomy of the pharynx. A rich collateral system of blood flow from the external carotid branches, superior laryngeal and thyroid, ascending pharyngeal, facial, and lingual, and from the thyrocervical trunk branches, inferior thyroid, ascending pharyngeal, and transverse cervical.

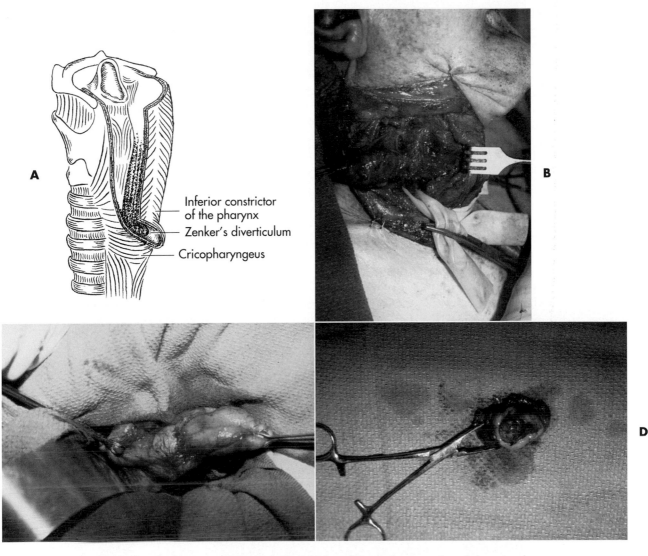

Figure 79-3. **A,** Anatomy of Zenker's diverticulum. Chronic hypertension of the cricopharyngeus muscle results in outpouching of the mucosa through a weak point laterally just above the muscle. This results in postprandial regurgitation of undigested food, dysphagia, aspiration pneumonitis, and sometimes obstruction. Therapy requires cricopharyngeus myotomy with or without resection of the diverticulum. **B** and **C,** Approach to Zenker's diverticulum through lateral cervical approach. **D,** Squamous cell carcinoma in the apex of Zenker's diverticulum.

Occasionally in the presence of a very wide cleft, the introduction of soft tissue from a distance may be necessary to adequately separate the oropharynx and nasal cavity. Microvascular transfer of the radial forearm or scapula flap is an excellent choice in these cases. Congenital neurologic disorders or injuries frequently manifest as dyskinesias of the pharyngeal musculature and difficulty with speech or swallowing. Surgical intervention is sometimes useful after careful analysis of residual function and anatomy by direct endoscopy, videofluoroscopy, or manofluorography.

Tracheoesophageal fistula is a rare cause of pharyngeal problems, but may require cervical esophageal or total esophageal reconstruction. Various diverticula of the pharynx and esophagus have been described, the most common being Zenker's diverticulum at the cephalad margin of the cricopharyngeus muscle. Usually seen in the seventh to eighth decade and characterized by delayed regurgitation of undigested food, this mucosal outpouching was once originally thought to be secondary to weakness in the wall of the hypopharynx; however, manometric studies have shown continuous hypertension of the cricopharyngeus muscle, and therapy consists of a cricopharyngeus myotomy with or without resection of the diverticulum (Figure 79-3).

Trauma to the pharynx and esophagus is relatively uncommon. Penetrating trauma, gunshot, knife wounds, and perforations from ingested objects (e.g., pins, fish bones) rarely cause significant deformity and can usually be repaired primarily or allowed to fistulize and heal. Larger wounds are likely to be fatal because of the proximity of the carotid artery and jugular vein laterally and the spinal cord posteriorly.

Ingestion of caustic substances such as alkali (e.g., lye, cleaning fluid) and acids may cause extensive damage to the pharynx; the majority of such patients are toddlers, although there is a second peak of incidence when suicidal or psychotic individuals in their twenties present. Depending on concentration and volume of the substances ingested, there may be damage to the oral cavity structures, the pharynx, the larynx, the cervical and thoracic esophagus, and the stomach. Coagulation of mucosal proteins may result in a full-thickness burn and perforation at any site. Contracture and epithelialization of the surface injury results in stenosis of the pharyngeal tube and synechiae of the walls of the pharynx and esophagus or portions of the larynx, pharynx, and tongue. Endoscopic and manometric studies of the esophagus and careful inspection of computed axial tomography (CAT) or magnetic resonance imaging (MRI) of the oral cavity and pharynx will help delineate the extent of injury. Because of extensive scarring, lysis of the adhesive surfaces and replacement of contracted tissues with epithelium-lined, supple vascularized tissues are usually necessary. Major caustic ingestion can result in immobility of the oral tongue, caused by scarring to the floor of the mouth; velopharyngeal insufficiency, caused by shortening of the soft palate and uvula and fixation to the lateral pharyngeal wall; supraglottic stenosis, caused by synechiae of the epiglottis and the lateral and posterior pharyngeal walls; and esophageal stricture of varying length.

Iatrogenic injuries to the cervical esophagus or hypopharynx may result in fistula, stenosis, or complete obstruction. Injury or transection of the pharynx during thyroidectomy for goiter or other problems may not be recognized and can result in postoperative abscesses, with stricture of the pharynx. Such injuries are frequently compounded by damage to the recurrent laryngeal nerve or superior laryngeal nerve, creating further disruption of the laryngopharyngeal synergistic function by loss of motor and sensory capacities (Figure 79-4).

The great majority of defects in the pharynx are created by the treatment of malignancy. Pediatric tumors such as rhabdomyosarcoma may be treated with chemotherapy and

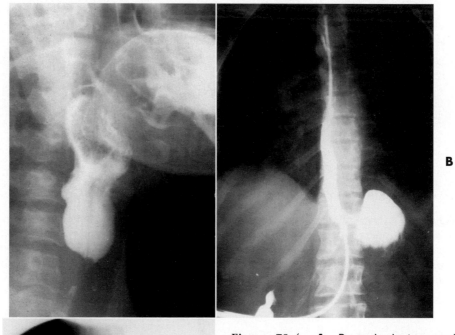

Figure 79-4. **A,** Prograde barium swallow demonstrating complete obstruction of the postcricoid hypopharynx after inadvertent injury to the esophagus and transection of the left recurrent laryngeal nerve during thyroidectomy. Postoperative infection and fistula resulted in stenosis and obstruction. **B,** Retrograde injection through the gastrostomy tube demonstrates a short segment of complete obstruction. **C,** Because the lesion was below the larynx, a jejunal free autograft was chosen to reestablish alimentary continuity. Normal swallowing function was reestablished despite the injury to the recurrent laryngeal nerve.

radiotherapy without surgery, but subsequent retardation of growth or stricture at the site of tumor necrosis may require reconstruction early in life. Squamous cell carcinoma of the larynx is relatively common in the United States, and the various sites of pharyngeal epidermoid carcinoma also frequently require reconstruction. Although larynx preservation has been achieved in some patients with combined chemotherapy and radiotherapy, the standard treatment for advanced-stage squamous cell carcinoma of the larynx and pharynx is resection with a margin of normal tissue, with or without neck dissection, followed by postoperative adjuvant radiotherapy. Carcinoma arising in the oropharynx and hypopharynx (base of tongue), posterior pharyngeal walls, tonsils and tonsillar pillars, and pyriform sinuses has a great predilection for cephalad spread into the nasopharynx and lateral spread into the lymph nodes of the ipsilateral or bilateral neck, as does carcinoma of the supraglottic larynx (epiglottis, arytenoids, false cords). Carcinoma of the intrinsic larynx (vocal cords) is less likely to demonstrate early neck metastasis and may remain confined to the larynx for a significant period of time (Figure 79-5). Carcinoma of the cervical esophagus is characterized by extensive submucosal spread into the thoracic esophagus, perhaps even perineural invasion or "skip metastases," and nodal spread to the mediastinum rather than the neck. Thus, although segmental resection of the pharynx with neck dissection is usually adequate therapy for laryngeal and pharyngeal tumors, cervical esophageal carcinoma may require laryngectomy and total esophagectomy with mediastinal dissection. Because it tends to remain within the larynx for a longer portion of its natural history, intrinsic laryngeal carcinoma, even T2 and T3 lesions, is frequently treated with definitive radiotherapy, saving surgery for salvage of persistent disease or subsequent recurrence. Pharyngeal tumors greater than T1 are usually treated by resection and postoperative adjuvant radiotherapy. Definitive radiotherapy for laryngeal tumors is usually 5500 to 6500 cGy to the central neck without lateral neck fields. For postoperative adjuvant radiotherapy, 5000 to 6000 cGy are administered to the primary site and one or both necks.

Despite its functional complexity, the pharynx is a compact area where numerous structures are in close juxtaposition. The surgical oncologic tenet of removing the tumor with a margin of 2-cm normal tissue around it frequently results in complete removal of the larynx and pharynx, creating a circumferential defect extending from the base of the tongue anterior around to the posterior pharynx. The distal extent of the defect is usually near the thoracic inlet, which allows reconstruction to proceed within the neck. By surgical maneuvers such as release of the sternocleidomastoid muscle from the sternum and medial clavicle or by resection of the manubrium, the esophagus can be visualized to the arch of the aorta. After resection of some lesions of the larynx, pyriform sinus, or posterior pharyngeal wall, a strip of mucosa may be left along the prevertebral fascia. Because of the unopposed action of the longitudinally transected constriction muscles immediately beneath the mucosa, this tissue bunches up on the prevertebral fascia and may seem very thin and small. Careful stretching to both sides and repositioning it on the prevertebral fascia with resorbable

stitches will demonstrate muscle and mucosa's true extent and determine whether it should be preserved for use in reconstruction or discarded. Preservation of the larynx after resection of pharyngeal cancer is occasionally possible, particularly when the tumor presents in the base of the tongue, tonsillar pillars, or posterior pharynx. In such cases, reconstruction must aim to facilitate normal function of the larynx, not impairing its motion, and to provide sensation to the area surrounding the larynx so that the airway will not be presented with such substances as saliva or food without sensory warning. Naturally, similar mucosal tissue is best in such cases, but innervated distant tissue such as the radial forearm, lateral arm, or other neurotized free flaps may be acceptable.

The pharynx is a complex structure comprised of rather tenuous musculomucosal walls and containing a number of mobile structures. The motor activity of the tongue and the pharyngeal constrictors creates an intraluminal pressure wave that may exceed 130 mm of mercury. Maintenance of a watertight closure in such circumstances may be difficult, and whether because of high pressures, mobility, tissue ischemia, postoperative radiotherapy, or surgical misadventure, fistula is common in pharyngeal resection and reconstruction, ranging from 15% to 40% in various series.[4,16,32] Anastomotic leakage beneath the skin flaps may result in abscess and invasive infection affecting the remaining pharynx or the great vessels. Open drainage will usually allow the wound to stabilize, and depending on the local milieu, secondary healing may occur. Because of the high incidence of pharyngocutaneous fistula in head and neck reconstruction, the concept of surgically created controlled fistula had been advocated until recently. At a site where saliva would be diverted from the great vessels usually laterally on the neck, the skin is sewn to the mucosa, creating a permanent opening through which the fluids will flow, thus improving the likelihood of primary healing of the remainder of the repair. This planned diversion could be permanent, and dealt with by bagging, or temporary, and closed at a later date by an elective procedure.

Stenosis or stricture of the pharynx is another common cause for reconstruction of the pharynx. The approach of primary closure of the postlaryngopharyngectomy mucosa results in a 15% to 45% fistula rate. In those patients developing fistulas that may go on to heal by secondary intention (i.e., contraction and epithelialization), the subsequent stenosis rate may reach 80%.[19] Since the ability to take adequate alimentation by mouth is an important quality-of-life consideration in these patients, who often present with late-stage disease and are at high risk for recurrent disease and death, avoidance of fistula and subsequent stenosis is paramount. Technical problems, particularly with the distal esophageal suture line, may also result in stenosis at the distal aspect of the pharyngeal reconstruction. Extrinsic compression by the trachea or thyroid may impede the intraluminal passage of food. Stenosis of a pharyngeal reconstruction either early or late must be carefully investigated to rule out recurrent tumor.[11]

Major tumor resections in the laryngopharyngeal area and their complications may result in total failure of the operation in 3% to 20% of cases.[28] The nature of the wound and the

LARYNX (ICD-O 161)

Data Form for Cancer Staging

Patient identification

Name _____

Address _____

Hospital or clinic number _____

Age _____ Sex _____ Race _____

Institutional identification

Hospital or clinic _____

Address _____

Oncology Record

Anatomic site of cancer _____

Chronology of classification* [ ] Clinical-diagnostic (cTNM)
                                [ ] Surgical-evaluative (sTNM)

Date of classification _____

Histologic type† _____ Grade _____

[ ] Postsurgical resection–pathologic (pTNM)

[ ] Retreatment (rTNM) [ ] Autopsy (aTNM)

Definitions: TNM Classification

Primary Tumor (T)

[ ] TX Minimum requirements to assess the primary tumor cannot be met.

[ ] T0 No evidence of primary tumor

Supraglottis

[ ] Tis Carcinoma *in situ*

[ ] T1 Tumor confined to site of origin with normal mobility

[ ] T2 Tumor involves adjacent supraglottic site(s) or glottis without fixation

[ ] T3 Tumor limited to larynx with fixation or extension to involve postcricoid area, medial wall of piriform sinus, or preepiglottic space

[ ] T4 Massive tumor extending beyond the larynx to involve oropharynx, soft tissues of neck, or destruction of thyroid cartilage

A

Glottis

[ ] Tis Carcinoma *in situ*

[ ] T1 Tumor confined to vocal cord(s) with normal mobility (including involvement of anterior or posterior commissures)

[ ] T2 Supraglottic or subglottic extension of tumor with normal or impaired cord mobility

[ ] T3 Tumor confined to the larynx with cord fixation

[ ] T4 Massive tumor with thyroid cartilage destruction or extension beyond the confines of the larynx, or both

Subglottis

[ ] Tis Carcinoma *in situ*

[ ] T1 Tumor confined to the subglottic region

[ ] T2 Tumor extension to vocal cords with normal or impaired cord mobility

[ ] T3 Tumor confined to larynx with cord fixation

[ ] T4 Massive tumor with cartilage destruction or extension beyond the confines of the larynx, or both

Nodal Involvement (N)

[ ] NX Minimum requirements to assess the regional nodes cannot be met.

[ ] N0 No clinically positive nodes

[ ] N1 Single clinically positive homolateral node 3 cm or less in diameter

[ ] N2 Single clinically positive homolateral node more than 3 but not more than 6 cm in diameter or multiple clinically positive homolateral nodes, none more than 6 cm in diameter

[ ] N2a Single clinically positive homolateral node more than 3 cm but not more than 6 cm in diameter

[ ] N2b Multiple clinically positive homolateral nodes, none more than 6 cm in diameter

[ ] N3 Massive homolateral node(s), bilateral nodes, or contralateral node(s)

[ ] N3a Clinically positive homolateral node(s), one more than 6 cm in diameter

[ ] N3b Bilateral clinically positive nodes (in this situation, each side of the neck should be staged separately; *i.e.*, N3b: right, N2a: left, N1)

[ ] N3c Contralateral clinically positive node(s) only

Distant Metastasis (M)

[ ] MX Minimum requirements to assess the presence of distant metastasis cannot be met

[ ] M0 No (known) distant metastasis

[ ] M1 Distant metastasis present
Specify _____

Location of Tumor

Supraglottis

[ ] Ventricular band

[ ] Arytenoid

[ ] Suprahyoid epiglottis

[ ] Infrahyoid epiglottis

[ ] Arytenoepiglottic fold

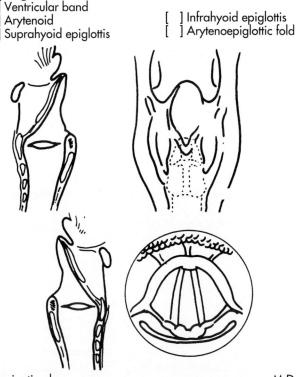

Examination by _____ M.D.

Date

* Use a separate form each time a case is staged.
† See reverse side for additional information.

American Joint Committee on Cancer

Figure 79-5. **A** to **C,** American Joint Council on Cancer staging forms for cancers of the pharynx and larynx. (From *Manual for staging of cancer,* ed 2, 1983, JB Lippincott.)   *Continued*

Glottis
[ ] Vocal cords (including commissures)

Subglottis

Characteristics of Tumor
[ ] Superficial
[ ] Exophytic
[ ] Moderate infiltration
[ ] Deep infiltration
[ ] Impaired cord mobility
[ ] Cord fixation
[ ] Cartilage destruction
[ ] Tumor confined to larynx

[ ] Tumor extension to the following:
[ ] Base of tongue
[ ] Piriform sinus
[ ] Postcricoid region
[ ] Preepiglottic space
[ ] Trachea
[ ] Soft tissue or skin of neck

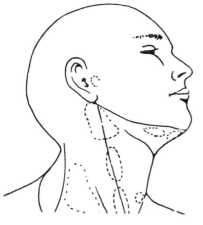

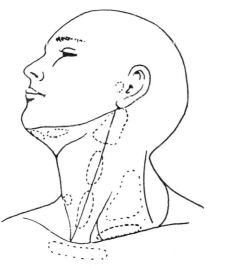

Indicate on diagram primary tumor and regional nodes involved.

Stage Grouping
[ ] Stage I   T1, N0, M0
[ ] Stage II   T2, N0, M0
[ ] Stage III T3, N0, M0
              T1, T2, T3; N1, M0
[ ] Stage IV T4, N0, N1; M0
              Any T, N2, N3; M0
              Any T, any N, M1

Staging Procedures

A variety of procedures and special studies may be employed in the process of staging a given tumor. Both the clinical usefulness and cost efficiency must be considered. The following suggestions are made for staging a cancer of the larynx:

Essential for staging

1. Complete physical examination of the head and neck including indirect laryngoscopy and nasopharyngoscopy
2. Biopsy of primary tumor
3. Chest roentgenogram
4. Roentgenograms of skull (nasopharynx)
5. Direct examination of hypopharynx

May be useful for staging or patient management

1. Multichemistry screen
2. Soft-tissue roentgenograms of neck, CT scans
3. Barium swallow
4. Performance status (Karnofsky or ECOG scale)

May be useful for future staging systems or research studies

1. Panendoscopy (direct laryngoscopy, bronchoscopy, esophagoscopy)
2. Studies of immune competence
3. Assay of antibodies to Epstein–Barr viral capsid antigen (nasopharynx)

Histologic Type of Cancer

The predominant cancer is squamous cell carcinoma.

Histologic Grade
[ ] G1   Well differentiated
[ ] G2   Moderately well differentiated
[ ] G3–G4   Poorly to very poorly differentiated

Postsurgical Resection–Pathologic Residual Tumor (R)

Does not enter into the staging but may be a factor in deciding further treatment

[ ] R0   No residual tumor
[ ] R1   Microscopic residual tumor
[ ] R2   Macroscopic residual tumor
         Specify _____

Performance Status of Host (H)

Several systems for recording a patient's activity and symptoms are in use and are more or less equivalent as follows:

AJCC	Performance	ECOG Scale	Karnofsky Scale (%)
[ ] H0	Normal activity	0	90–100
[ ] H1	Symptomatic but ambulatory; cares for self	1	70–80
[ ] H2	Ambulatory more than 50% of time; occasionally needs assistance	2	50–60
[ ] H3	Ambulatory 50% or less of time; nursing care needed	3	30–40
[ ] H4	Bedridden; may need hospitalization	4	10–20

B

Figure 79-5, cont'd.   For legend see p. 1294.

PHARYNX (ICD-O 146–148)

Data Form for Cancer Staging

Patient identification

Name _____

Address _____

Hospital or clinic number _____

Age _____ Sex _____ Race _____

Institutional identification

Hospital or clinic _____

Address _____

Oncology Record

Anatomic site of cancer _____

Chronology of classification* [ ] Clinical-diagnostic (cTNM)

                                 [ ] Surgical-evaluative (sTNM)

Date of classification _____

Histologic type† _____ Grade (G) _____

[ ] Postsurgical resection–pathologic (pTNM)

[ ] Retreatment (rTNM) [ ] Autopsy (aTNM)

Definitions: TNM Classification

Primary Tumor (T)

[ ] TX Minimum requirements to assess the primary tumor cannot be met.

[ ] T0 No evidence of primary tumor

Oropharynx

[ ] Tis Carcinoma *in situ*

[ ] T1 Tumor 2 cm or less in greatest diameter

[ ] T2 Tumor more than 2 cm but not more than 4 cm in greatest diameter

[ ] T3 Tumor more than 4 cm in greatest diameter

[ ] T4 Massive tumor more than 4 cm in diameter with invasion of bone, soft tissues of neck, or root (deep musculature) of tongue

Nasopharynx

C

[ ] Tis Carcinoma *in situ*

[ ] T1 Tumor confined to one side of nasopharynx or no tumor visible (positive biopsy only)

[ ] T2 Tumor involving two sites (both posterosuperior and lateral walls)

[ ] T3 Extension of tumor into nasal cavity or oropharynx

[ ] T4 Tumor invasion of skull, cranial nerve involvement, or both

Hypopharynx

[ ] Tis Carcinoma *in situ*

[ ] T1 Tumor confined to one site

[ ] T2 Extension of tumor to adjacent region or site without fixation of hemilarynx

[ ] T3 Extension of tumor to adjacent region or site with fixation of hemilarynx

[ ] T4 Massive tumor invading bone or soft tissues of neck

Nodal Involvement (N)

[ ] NX Minimum requirements to assess regional nodes cannot be met.

[ ] N0 No clinically positive nodes

[ ] N1 Single clinically positive homolateral node 3 cm or less in diameter

[ ] N2 Single clinically positive homolateral node more than 3 but not more than 6 cm in diameter or multiple clinically positive homolateral nodes, none more than 6 cm in diameter

[ ] N2a Single clinically positive homolateral node more than 3 cm but not more than 6 cm in diameter

[ ] N2b Multiple clinically positive homolateral nodes, none more than 6 cm in diameter

[ ] N3 Massive homolateral node(s), bilateral nodes, or contralateral node(s)

[ ] N3a Clinically positive homolateral node(s), one more than 6 cm in diameter

[ ] N3b Bilateral clinically positive nodes (in this situation, each side of the neck should be staged separately; *i.e.*, N3b: right, N2a: left, N1)

[ ] N3c Contralateral clinically positive node(s) only

Distant Metastasis (M)

[ ] MX Minimum requirements to assess the presence of distant metastasis cannot be met

[ ] M0 No (known) distant metastasis

[ ] M1 Distant metastasis present

      Specify _____

Location of Tumor

Oropharynx

[ ] Faucial arch

[ ] Tonsillar fossa, tonsil

[ ] Base of tongue

[ ] Pharyngeal wall

Nasopharynx

[ ] Posterosuperior wall

[ ] Lateral wall

Hypopharynx

[ ] Piriform fossa

[ ] Postcricoid area

[ ] Posterior wall

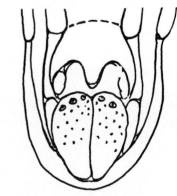

Size of primary tumor: _____ cm

Examination by _____ M.D.

Date _____

* Use a separate form each time a case is staged.

† See reverse side for additional information.

American Joint Committee on Cancer

Figure 79-5, cont'd. For legend see p. 1294.

general condition of the patient are the key parameters for determining whether immediate secondary reconstruction is appropriate or whether temporizing procedures and later definitive closure are necessary. Careful analysis of the wound including consideration of previous radiotherapy or surgery or the need for subsequent radiotherapy, the presence of infection or bacterial colonization, and the condition of the great vessels will all impact on not only the choice of operation but also its timing.[9]

OPERATIONS

Total esophagectomy with or without laryngectomy is performed for malignancy stricture or occasionally motility disorders. Visceral interposition has become the most commonly used method of reconstruction, with stomach used most frequently for malignancy because of its relative ease and single-stage nature as either a total transposition or reversed gastric tube from the greater curvature of the stomach. There is some evidence that the injured esophagus from pediatric caustic ingestion is at increased risk of development of malignancy, a situation comparable to Marjolin's ulcer. Because of this concern and the severe structural damage caused by the caustic ingestion, total esophagectomy may be necessary. Reconstruction with the right, left, or transverse colon based on its respective mesocolon as a pharyngogastric conduit either in the subcutaneous or substernal position is appropriate. Although this can usually be performed in a single stage, the body habitus of the patient and the history of previous surgery may limit its efficacy. Pedicled jejunum transposition has also been advocated as a total esophageal replacement, although at present it is the least commonly used of these methods. Further length to accommodate a pharyngoenteric anastomosis without ischemia has been obtained by performing a vascular anastomosis of the mesenteric vessels in the most distal arcade to vessels in the neck in such a pedicled flap.[28] Visceral interpositions are subject to higher mortality rates because of the necessity for transgression of both the abdominal and thoracic cavities. Fistula at the pharyngoenteric anastomosis is usually an indication of distal ischemia and is thus unlikely to resolve without subsequent therapy.[25,31] Combined vascular transposition and free tissue transfer may be used to obtain adequate length for total esophageal reconstruction. Although skin tubes fashioned on the anterior chest wall and joined to the pharynx proximally and the stomach distally are primarily of historic interest, recent description of long skin flaps tubed and transferred by microvascular anastomosis, such as the posterior thigh flap, may resolve the occasional unusual problem. A more common problem presenting for reconstruction is the segmental total or partial defect of the pharynx in the neck or upper mediastinum, usually a consequence of laryngopharyngectomy or some complication of that procedure. When laryngectomy for intrinsic laryngeal carcinoma alone is the cause of the defect, there may

be enough mucosa from the pyriform sinuses to close the defect primarily in two layers. This results in a T-shaped closure, the horizontal limb along the base of the tongue and the vertical limb extending down into the neck toward the cervical or thoracic esophagus (Figure 79-6). Although this narrow channel may distend with subsequent swallowing allowing an adequate passage for food, previous or subsequent radiotherapy or fistula may limit the elasticity of this myomucosal tube, causing stenosis and dysphagia. When tumors of the pyriform sinuses or extensive tumors of the larynx are the cause of laryngopharyngectomy, the amount of mucosa left after resection is considerably less and primary closure has much higher risk of fistula (30%) and stenosis (80%).[19]

The use of local tissue to reconstruct small pharyngeal defects has been successfully attempted. Lateral defects of the oropharynx, particularly above the level of the larynx, may be closed with a tongue flap, with its rotation point at the base of the tongue and carried up into the oral tongue (Figure 79-7). This can be transferred inferiorly or laterally and, if designed correctly, should not tether the tongue. Island flaps of palatal or buccal mucosa and muscle may be transposed on the palatine or facial vessels to close small defects in the lateral pharynx, with the donor site closed either primarily by split-thickness skin grafting or by contraction and epithelialization. The small amounts of tissue available, the limited arcs of rotation, the shared morbidity with the created defect, and the scarring at the donor site all limit the usefulness of such methods of reconstruction.

Previously, the most widely accepted surgical oncologic tenet was extirpation as a primary procedure, with 2- to 5-year follow-up to ensure cure from the cancer and then attempts at secondary closure; this created a population of patients with pharyngocutaneous fistula of various sizes. Depending on the size of the defect and the condition of the adjacent neck, a combination of cervical skin flaps could be designed to provide both internal lining or replacement of the mucosal defect and external coverage. Smaller turnover flaps based on the margin of the defect could be covered by axial pattern skin flaps to create a two-layer closure. Various attempts at reconstruction of the pharynx relied on skin grafting over a tube of tantalum or other material to create an inner lining. The horizontal neck flap designed by Wookey in 1942 was laterally based and provided access for the laryngopharyngectomy.[33] At the first stage of the procedure, this was laid into the defect and its cephalad and caudad margins sutured to the posterior portion of the pharyngeal defect at the oropharyngeal and esophageal margin. At a second procedure after neovascularization of the skin flap from the underlying bed, the lateral base of the flap is transected and the two free margins sutured to themselves and to the base of the tongue and anterior margin of the cervical esophagus to complete the tube. The external coverage was by advancement flaps from the lateral neck or split-thickness skin grafting. Although conceptually attractive, this method depended on excellent blood supply in the neck. Furthermore, the length of the defect was sometimes greater than the available neck skin, resulting in a smaller but persistent fistula. Most important, the likelihood of having healthy, hairless, well-

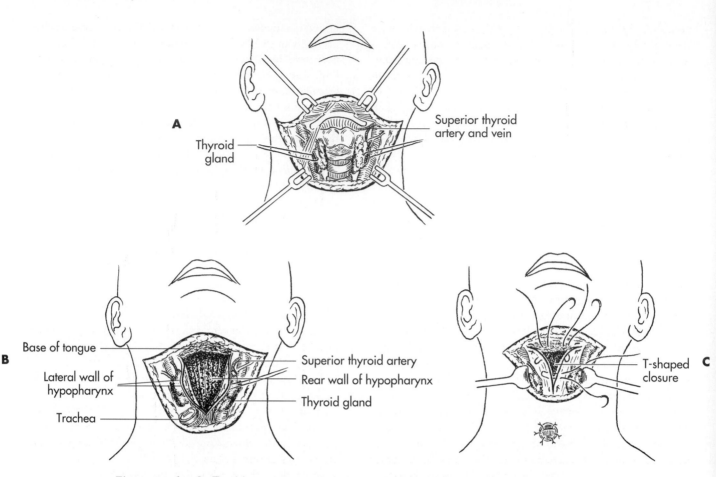

A

Thyroid gland

Superior thyroid artery and vein

B

Base of tongue

Lateral wall of hypopharynx

Trachea

Superior thyroid artery

Rear wall of hypopharynx

Thyroid gland

T-shaped closure

C

Figure 79-6. **A,** Total laryngectomy removes the cartilaginous framework and mucosa of the larynx with or without posterolateral mucosa of the adjacent pyriform sinus. **B,** The defect after laryngectomy usually extends from just below the cricoid to the base of the tongue. If enough lateral mucosa is available, the defect can be closed primarily over a nasogastric tube. **C,** The T-shaped closure in two layers, with the horizontal limb along the base of the tongue and the vertical limb running down the pharynx. The end tracheostomy is brought out through a separate distal site above the manubrium.

Figure 79-7. Small defects of the lateral pharynx can be closed with a posterior tongue flap. Depending on flap design, this can be an axial pattern or random pattern flap.

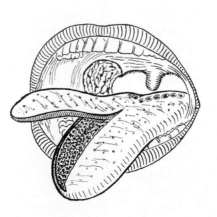
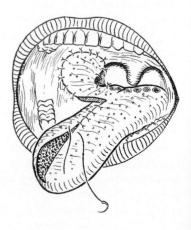

vascularized skin in the neck was small in patients who were often treated initially by definitive radiotherapy. The donor site including the great vessels of the neck often required skin grafting for closure. In addition to laterally based flaps, apron flaps of cervical skin based on the facial vessels and bipedicle bucket handle flaps were also described for oral and pharyngeal reconstruction. These flaps shared the same limitations as other axial pattern neck skin flaps in attempting major reconstructions.[51]

Although cervical flaps had the advantage of proximity to the defect, their disadvantages made them less popular than the subsequently developed thoracic skin flaps. These flaps were initially prepared by one or more delay procedures wherein an attempt was made to direct the blood supply in an axial pattern followed by division of the most distal point of attachment and rotation of the flap into the defect. After 10 to 21 days, the proximal attachment of the flap to the donor site is divided and the tissue used to close the remaining defect. These flaps suffered the usual limitations of random pattern flaps, unreliable blood supply at the most operant distal end, limitation of the amount of tissue that could be transferred, and their use in an environment that was not conducive to either immediate or delayed reconstruction.

The deltopectoral skin or fasciocutaneous flap, described by Bakamjian in 1965, demonstrated some distinct advantages over other thoracic flaps in reconstruction of the pharynx.[3] With an axial blood supply from a transverse branch of the perforating branch of the internal mammary artery, the deltopectoral flap could be designed to extend to the anterolateral margin of the shoulder. Further extension down the arm or onto the posterior shoulder is possible if surgical delay is performed. The deltopectoral flap has a distal blood supply that is considerably more reliable than that of the thoracic random pattern flaps and provides enough length and width of skin to create a tube to be inset to the base of the tongue and proximal pharynx, then sutured to itself and left as a controlled fistula. At a second-stage operation after 14 to 21 days, the base of the flap is divided and inset into the distal esophageal segment for completion of the alimentary tube.[3] The donor site on the shoulder and chest is decreased in area by advancement of adjacent mobile tissues and split-thickness skin grafts, avoiding exposure of the carotid and jugular veins. Although greatly superior to previous methods with respect to the amount of tissue available and the blood supply, the deltopectoral flap suffers the limitations of being at least a two-stage procedure and of requiring revascularization from the compromised local milieu. Most series had high complication rates.

The recognition that the large, flat thoracic muscles, the pectoralis major, trapezius, and latissimus dorsi, and the smaller cervical muscles, the platysma and sternocleidomastoid, could carry a paddle of overlying skin provided a number of new approaches to reconstruction of the pharynx. Although all of the thoracic musculocutaneous flaps have been used for reconstruction of the pharynx, by far the most commonly described is the pectoralis major musculocutaneous flap.[2,24] Its proximity to the pharynx, the abundant amount of soft tissue available for transfer, the presence of muscle that can be used to cover the

carotid[10] and other structures of the neck, and the possibility of its combined use with the deltopectoral flap all added to its popularity as an oral or oropharyngeal reconstructive technique (Figure 79-8). Because a total skin island can be developed on the muscle, the complete inset of the flap and thus reconstruction of pharynx can be carried out at a single stage. Although somewhat cumbersome in females, because of the overlying breast, and in patients with thick thoracic wall skin (like most Americans, even those with head and neck cancer), the flap may be constructed as a tube to reconstruct a circumferential defect of the pharynx. Similarly, less than complete defects of the pharynx may be addressed by using the skin island as an onlay patch sutured to the base of the tongue and the remaining lateral pharyngeal mucosa and muscle. The thickness and bulk of the pectoralis flap, the gravitational pull back down to the chest, and the somewhat random blood supply of its skin paddle make the likelihood of fistula formation or other unsat-

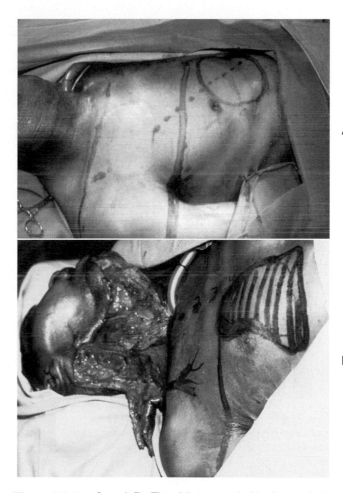

A

B

Figure 79-8. **A** and **B,** The deltopectoral skin flap and the pectoralis major musculocutaneous flap can be raised together by designing the skin paddle of the pectoralis flap so it does not include the perforating branches of the internal mammary vessel branches through the second, third, and fourth intercostal spaces. Even when the deltopectoral flap is not necessary in the primary reconstruction, it is useful to design the pectoralis flap in such a way that it remains available as a secondary procedure in the event of complication or recurrence.

isfactory result fairly high (Figure 79-9). A technique to decrease the likelihood of separation of the pectoralis flap from the cephalad or lateral margin is to use the pectoralis flap skin only as a 270-degree reconstruction of the circumferential defect, suturing its cephalad margin to the base of the tongue and its lateral margins to the prevertebral fascia immediately medial to the carotid vessels. The rigid prevertebral fascia

provides a more secure anchor point for the heavy flap, decreasing the likelihood of separation. The posterior 90-degree portion of the repair, that covering the prevertebral fascia, is covered with a split-thickness skin graft or allowed to epithelialize from the margins[13] (Figure 79-10).

The sternocleidomastoid musculocutaneous flap may be useful for closure of relatively small pharyngeal defects in the

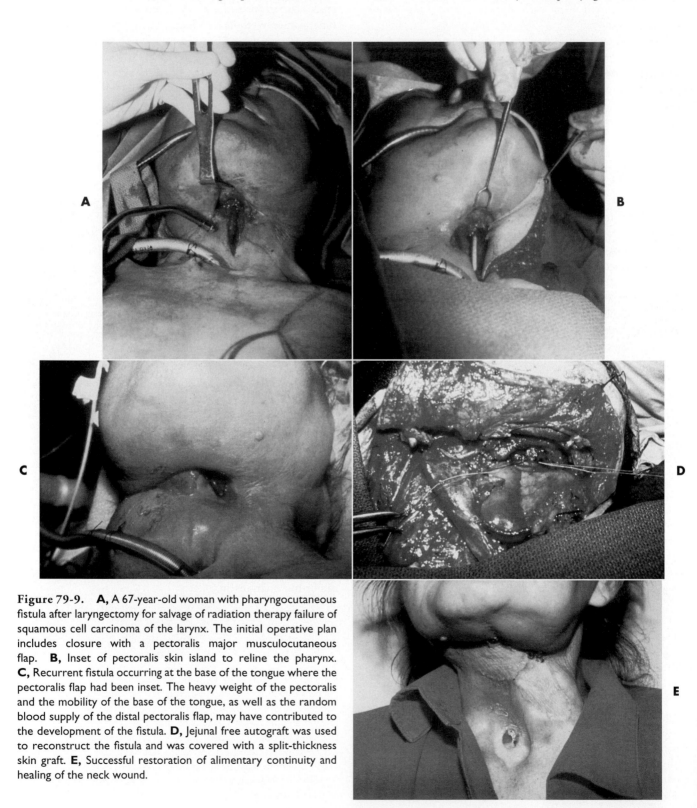

Figure 79-9. **A,** A 67-year-old woman with pharyngocutaneous fistula after laryngectomy for salvage of radiation therapy failure of squamous cell carcinoma of the larynx. The initial operative plan includes closure with a pectoralis major musculocutaneous flap. **B,** Inset of pectoralis skin island to reline the pharynx. **C,** Recurrent fistula occurring at the base of the tongue where the pectoralis flap had been inset. The heavy weight of the pectoralis and the mobility of the base of the tongue, as well as the random blood supply of the distal pectoralis flap, may have contributed to the development of the fistula. **D,** Jejunal free autograft was used to reconstruct the fistula and was covered with a split-thickness skin graft. **E,** Successful restoration of alimentary continuity and healing of the neck wound.

neck, particularly pharyngocutaneous fistulas. Although the island skin paddle is not particularly reliable, a peninsula design of the flap and careful attention to leaving as much of the cephalad blood supply to the muscle from the occipital and superior thyroid vessels as is possible will allow a segment of well-vascularized muscle to be introduced into the defect. The

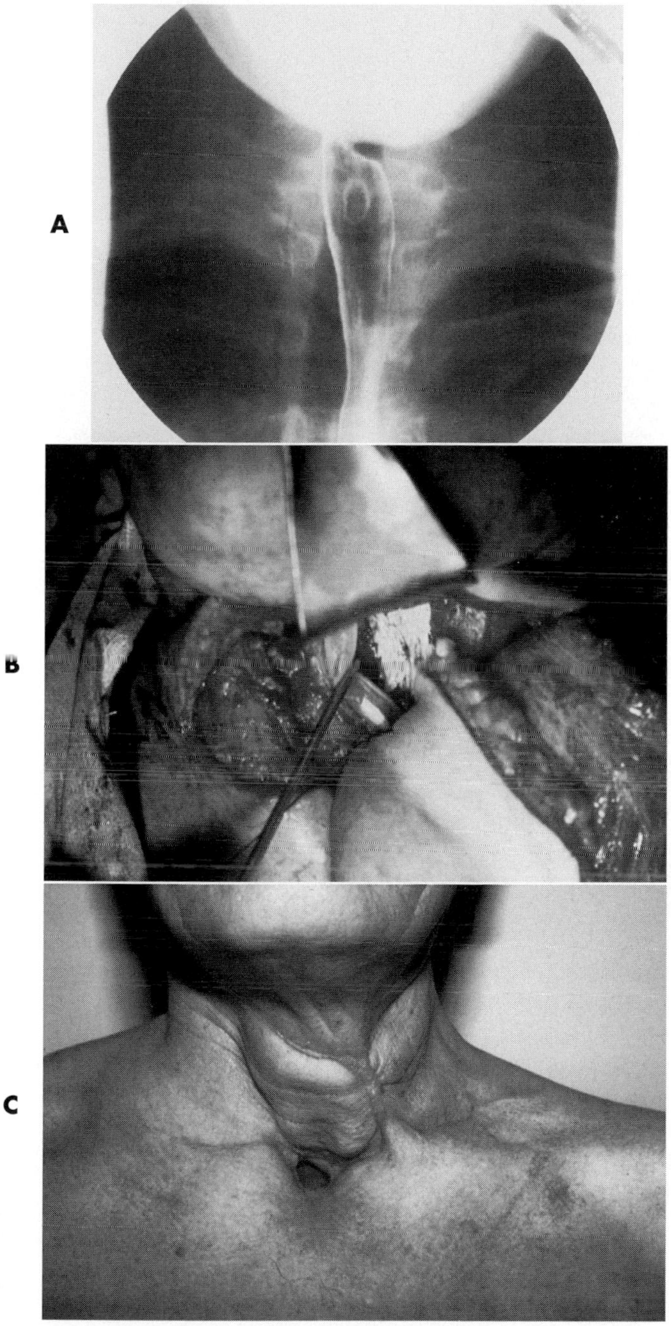

Figure 79-10. **A,** Obstruction of the pharynx secondary to recurrent carcinoma of the pharynx. **B,** Reconstruction of the total laryngopharyngectomy defect with split-thickness skin graft to prevertebral fascia and inset of the edges of the pectoralis major skin paddle to the edge of the prevertebral fascia and skin graft. This fixation to the more rigid prevertebral fascia prevents pulling away of the flap and fistula. **C,** Successful restoration of alimentary continuity and closure of the wound.

internal lining of the repair can be provided by turnover flaps from the margin of the wound or a split-thickness skin graft on the deep layer of the sternocleidomastoid muscle. Closure is performed in two to three layers, mucosa to deep surface or turnover flaps, soft tissue to soft tissue, and skin to skin (Figure 79-11).

The transfer of segments of the intraabdominal viscera with revascularization in the neck has been sporadically practiced since the early 1960s,[15,26] but became more widely accepted in the late 1970s and early 1980s. Although colon, gastric antrum, and small bowel have all been used, the greatest experience has been with the jejunal free autograft. Carried by the jejunal branches of the superior mesenteric artery and vein, segments of bowel from 10 to 30 cm in length can be transferred by a single arterial and venous anastomosis in the neck. Because of its mucosal lining with considerable secretory capacity, the diameter of the lumen (which is similar to that of the pharynx or esophagus), the relative abundance and expendability of bowel, and the reasonable size of the jejunal vessels, the jejunal free autograft has become an extremely popular mechanism for reconstruction of large pharyngeal defects. Either after or during the resection of the tumor, a second operative team can explore the abdomen, selecting a segment of jejunum far enough from the ligament of Treitz to allow easy resection and reanastomosis with a tube jejunostomy just distal to it. An appropriate length of jejunum is identified and its blood supply traced down to the superior mesenteric vessels, ensuring its pattern of arborization supplies the selected bowel. The proximal jejunum is a better choice than more distal small bowel because the smaller vasa recta and the larger jejunal vessels have a more direct relationship, passing through only one arcade, whereas there may be several vascular arcades separating the distal bowel from the jejunal branch of the superior mesenteric artery.[7] When the mesentery has been divided and the vessel isolated, the bowel is divided and the segment left attached to its blood vessels. The proximal and distal margins of the segment to be transferred, as well as the remaining jejunum, are observed for 5 to 10 minutes to ensure adequate perfusion. Then, a jejunojejunostomy is performed between the remaining intraabdominal bowel segments and a tube jejunostomy placed distal to the suture line and brought through the abdominal wall. The reconstructive segment of jejunum is left attached to its blood supply until the tumor has been resected, tumor-free margins have been confirmed, and the recipient vessels in the neck have been prepared for microvascular anastomosis. The jejunal vessels are divided and the segment transferred to the neck. The abdomen is closed. Although branches of the external carotid artery are frequently used for microvascular anastomosis, the transverse cervical vessels are an excellent choice because of their lateral position and relative protection from previous surgery and radiotherapy (Figure 79-12). To minimize the likelihood of fistula, the most difficult pharyngoenteric anastomosis should be performed prior to microvascular anastomosis while the bowel can be freely manipulated. Two-layer closure with absorbable or nonabsorbable suture (3-0 Vicryl) is preferable. Because it is important to minimize ischemic time (preferably less than 1½ to 2 hours), the micro-

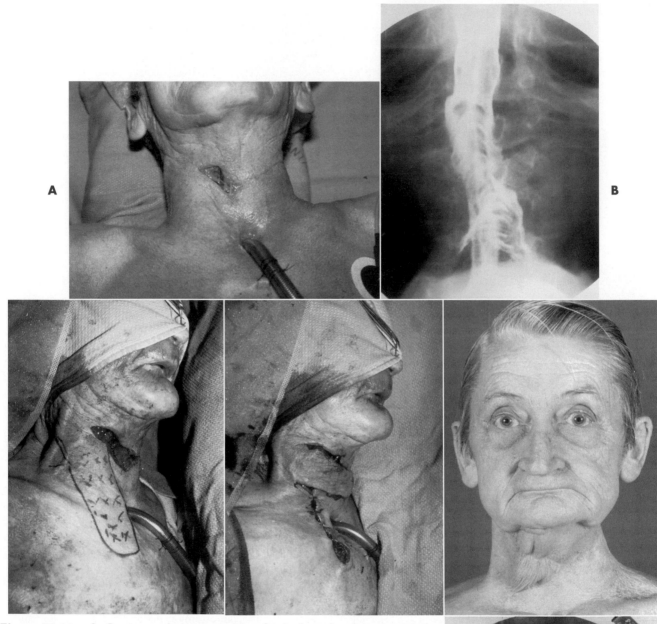

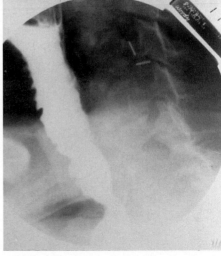

Figure 79-11. **A,** Persistent pharyngocutaneous fistula 6 weeks after pharyngeal reconstruction with jejunal free autograft after laryngopharyngectomy for squamous cell carcinoma of the pyriform sinus. **B,** Barium swallow demonstrating fistula at distal anastomosis of autograft. **C,** Sternocleidomastoid musculocutaneous flap design as a peninsula rather than an island flap to ensure better blood supply to skin. **D,** Transposition of the flap based on its cephalad blood supply (occipital and superior thyroid vessels). A split-thickness skin graft was applied to the deep surface of the flap to provide lining. **E,** Postoperative appearance. **F,** Barium swallow demonstrating closure of fistula and reestablishment of continuity of the alimentary tract.

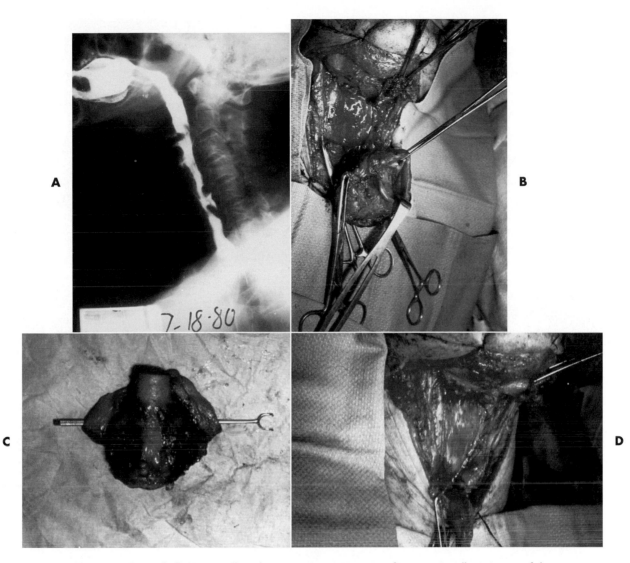

7-18-80

Figure 79-12. **A,** Barium swallow demonstrating recurrence of squamous cell carcinoma of the posterior pharynx. **B** and **C,** Operative approach required total laryngopharyngectomy. **D,** Defect from base of tongue to cervical esophagus at the thoracic inlet. Prevertebral fascia is visible as deep margin of resection. *Continued*

vascular anastomosis is performed next and, after demonstration of good revascularization, the other pharyngoenteric anastomosis completed. Usually the proximal enteric anastomosis is done first, followed by the microvascular anastomosis, followed by the esophageal anastomosis. In cases where a mediastinal enteric anastomosis is necessary, the distal suture line should be placed first. Access to the site of enteric anastomosis to ensure accurate suture placement is crucial to avoid fistula and possible abscess with subsequent invasive infection and pedicle thrombosis. Mandibulotomy to visualize the proximal suture line or sternotomy or resection of the manubrium to expose the esophageal suture lines is occasionally necessary. A circumferential reconstruction of the pharynx can be accomplished by an end-to-end or end-to-side anastomosis of the bowel to the base of the tongue and pharynx. By splitting the jejunum along its antimesenteric

border, a wide enough area can be obtained to accommodate either partial or total reconstruction of the floor of the mouth as well as the pharynx as a combined tube filled when partial or total glossectomy accompanies laryngopharyngectomy (Figure 79-13). For less than circumferential defects, the jejunum can be opened and used as a patch. Its homogeneous blood supply and light weight make it an excellent choice for pharyngeal defects or pharyngocutaneous fistula after primary closure of another type of reconstruction.[30]

Although the jejunum has been widely used for pharyngeal reconstruction, there is growing enthusiasm for other free tissue autografts such as the radial forearm, lateral arm, lateral thigh, and scapula flaps. When designed correctly, these flaps share the beneficial characteristics of homogeneous luxuriant blood supply and light weight (Figure 79-14). Further advances are avoidance of laparotomy, potential for sensory

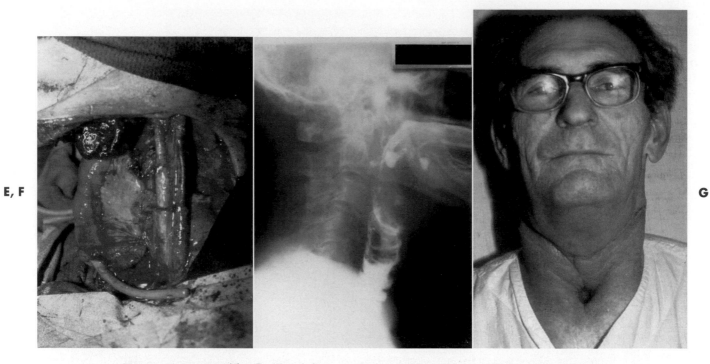

E, F

G

Figure 79-12, cont'd. **E,** Jejunal free autograft revascularized in neck by anastomosis to superior thyroid artery and internal jugular vein. **F,** Barium swallow at 10 days demonstrates restoration of continuity of alimentary tract. **G,** Postoperative appearance.

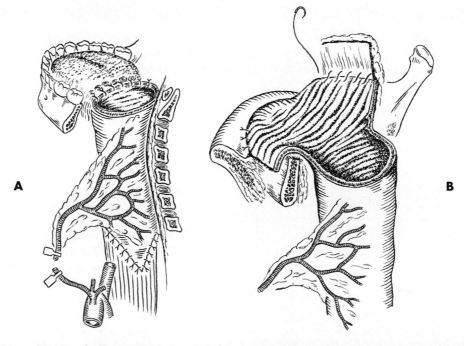

A

B

Figure 79-13. **A,** The jejunal free autograft as a tube graft. **B,** When the defect includes both planar and circumferential elements, one end of the tubular segment can be split along the antimesenteric border to create a tube fillet. This is particularly useful for total or subtotal glossectomy with laryngectomy.

reinnervation, and relatively ample supply. A number of authors have demonstrated sensation in the pharynx and oral cavity reconstruction that approximates that of normal oropharyngeal tissue and that is superior with regard to two-point discrimination to that of the donor area on the arm after performing end-to-end or end-to-side neuroanastomosis to the lingual, alveolar, or cervical plexus sensory nerves. Whether this improved sensation will translate into improved swallowing function is yet unclear.

The gastroomental free flap is particularly useful when a long vascular pedicle is necessary to bring the microvascular anastomosis out of an inflamed or ischemic neck.[20] The gastroepiploic vessels that supply the greater curvature of the stomach can reach the axillary vessels carrying gastric tissue to

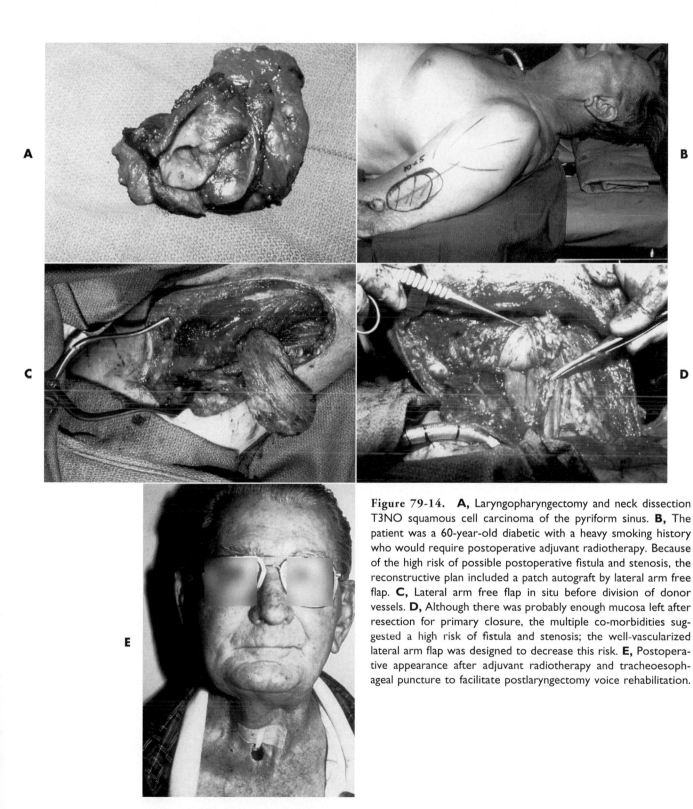

Figure 79-14. **A,** Laryngopharyngectomy and neck dissection T3N0 squamous cell carcinoma of the pyriform sinus. **B,** The patient was a 60-year-old diabetic with a heavy smoking history who would require postoperative adjuvant radiotherapy. Because of the high risk of possible postoperative fistula and stenosis, the reconstructive plan included a patch autograft by lateral arm free flap. **C,** Lateral arm free flap in situ before division of donor vessels. **D,** Although there was probably enough mucosa left after resection for primary closure, the multiple co-morbidities suggested a high risk of fistula and stenosis; the well-vascularized lateral arm flap was designed to decrease this risk. **E,** Postoperative appearance after adjuvant radiotherapy and tracheoesophageal puncture to facilitate postlaryngectomy voice rehabilitation.

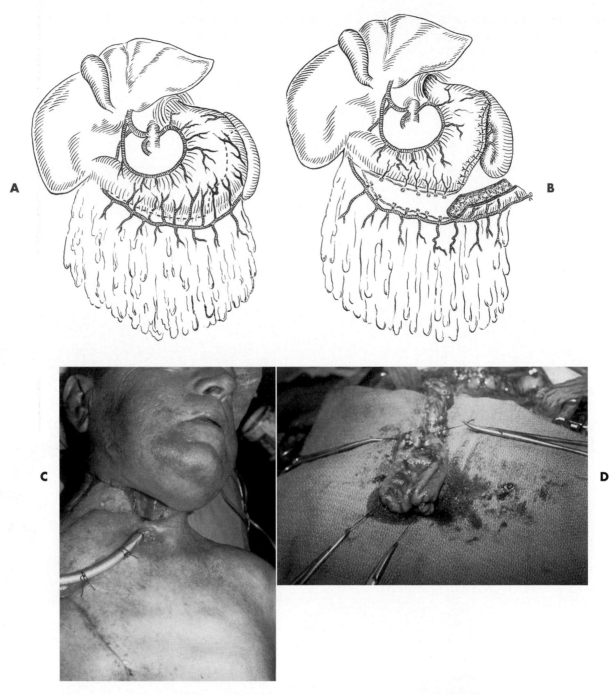

Figure 79-15. **A,** The gastroomental or greater epiploic free flap consists of a segment of the greater curvature of the stomach based on the greater epiploic vessels. **B,** A long vascular pedicle can be created to carry enough tissue to create a tubular or patch graft for mucosal replacement. If soft tissue coverage of the neck or face is needed, the omentum can be included in this flap. **C,** A 63-year-old patient with large pharyngocutaneous fistula after laryngopharyngectomy and bilateral radical neck dissection for surgical salvage of radiotherapy treatment failure of squamous cell carcinoma of the larynx. A pectoralis major musculocutaneous flap was unsuccessful in closing this wound, but did cover the exposed right common carotid artery. **D,** Patch autograft of gastric fundus based on the greater epiploic vessels. *Continued*

replace the gullet and omentum to cover exposed vessels or neck structures (Figure 79-15).

An important consideration in pharyngeal reconstruction is not only closure of the wound and reestablishment of the alimentary conduit, but also facilitation of voice rehabilitation. Alaryngeal speech depends on the passage of a column of air through the oral cavity for its modification by the tongue, palate, buccal musculature, and lips. Whether this air comes from the stomach, having been previously swallowed, or from the trachea through a tracheoesophageal puncture, it must pass in reasonable volume unobstructed into the oral cavity.[27] The best pharyngeal reconstructions will provide enough diameter

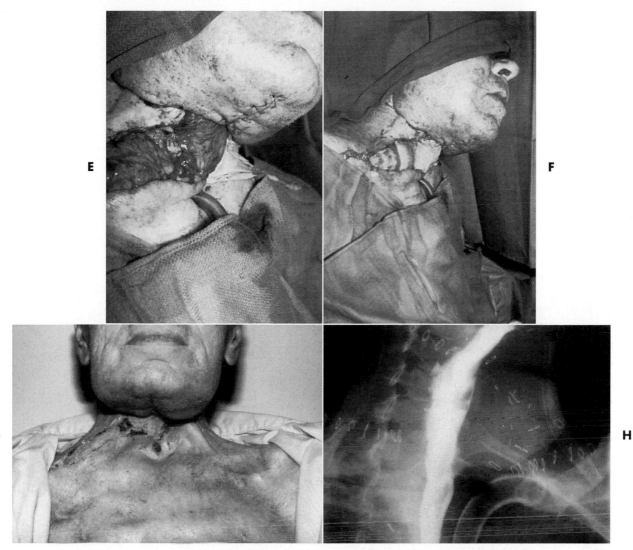

Figure 79-15, cont'd. **E** and **F,** Because of the previous surgery and radiotherapy to the neck and the pectoralis major flap, the axillary vessels were chosen as the recipient blood supply. The omentum was used to cover the neck and a split-thickness skin graft was applied for external cover. **G** and **H,** Postoperative appearance and barium swallow demonstrating a healed wound and restoration of alimentary continuity.

to the pharyngoesophagus to allow such free passage of air to create fluent speech. Provision of ample well-vascularized tissue will minimize the likelihood of scarring and secondary obstruction and allow manipulation of excess tissue to beneficially modify air flow as in shunts or neolarynx construction. Although reasonable function using such fistulas has been reported with the jejunal free flap, there is some evidence that its contractibility and highly secretory nature may impede speech production and that skin or fasciocutaneous flaps such as the radial forearm, lateral arm, or scapula flap may provide superior speech rehabilitation.[1]

There are a number of reasons for the high rate of fistula and stenosis in primary closure of the larynx and the remarkable rate of complications when earlier techniques were employed. Primary healing of a functional reconstruction will occur most readily when well-vascularized tissue is approximated without tension with a minimum amount of foreign material present. Although there is excellent collateral circulation in the head and neck, the effects of radiotherapy, previous surgery, and neck dissection may combine to render the tissues relatively ischemic and subject to dehiscence or wound necrosis.[4] Primary reconstruction of a previously untreated neck provides a very different environment from reoperation after definitive radiotherapy or as a result of fistula. The need for subsequent radiation may later render tissues that are marginally perfused ischemic, resulting in scar contracture or fistula.[9] The mobility of the area and the pressures generated in the normal functions of the area must be considered.[21] The mobile base of tongue generates high pressures on distal suture lines, and when these pressures are added to the weight of the heavy thoracic musculocutaneous flaps, the combined force acts on the superior suture line. Pharyngocutaneous fistulas then are most likely to occur at the superolateral suture line of flap with base of the tongue, the very area where the most distal and thus poorly vascularized segment of the deltopectoral or pectoralis flap is placed (see Figures 79-9 and 79-15). The presence of inflammation, bacterial coloniza-

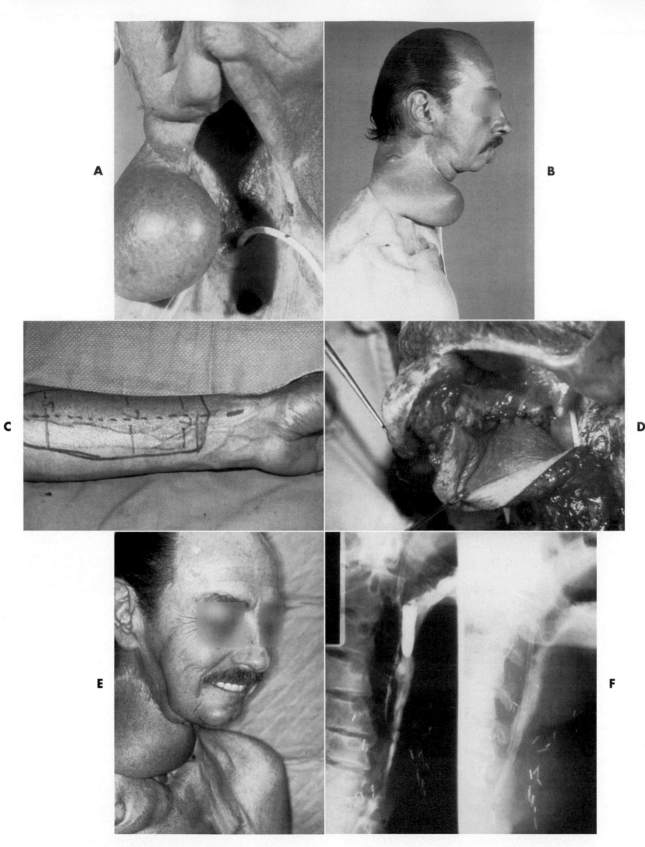

Figure 79-16. A and **B,** A 57-year-old man 3 years after hemimandibulectomy, total glossectomy, laryngopharyngectomy, and right neck dissection with adjuvant postoperative radiotherapy for squamous cell carcinoma of the tongue. Multiple previous attempts at reconstruction including bilateral pectoralis major, right latissimus dorsi, and trapezius musculocutaneous flaps and deltopectoral flap had all failed, leaving a large oropharyngocutaneous fistula. **C** and **D,** Analysis of the defect suggested that the lining of the alimentary tract required a lightweight, homogeneously well-vascularized segment of tissue, and the radial forearm free flap was chosen for internal lining. The previously attempted trapezius flap was unfurled and used for external coverage. **E** and **F,** Compartmentalization of the reconstruction resulted in a single-stage successful closure of the wound and restoration of alimentary continuity that allowed peroral feeding and subsequent esophageal speech.

tion, or invasive infection in the complicated pharyngeal wound requires vigorous debridement to decrease the infectious load and local or systemic antibiotic therapy. Actual inspection and analysis of the wound are the obvious necessities to ensure good wound healing, but anticipation of common problems and selection of lightweight tissues with luxuriant homogeneous blood supply are the remaining key components. Since there are a number of methods available for pharynx reconstruction, a combination may be most appropriate for particularly complex problems. Breaking the wound into its component parts, internal lining or mobile oral and pharyngeal tissue and external cover or relatively stationary thick protective tissue, is critical in achieving the healed wound (Figure 79-16).

The restoration of vascularized tissue to the environment, particularly vascularized tissue with a homogeneous blood supply such as provided by a free tissue transfer, improves the tolerance of the reconstruction to postoperative radiotherapy and increases the likelihood of spontaneous healing of the created wound or fistula and ultimate normal function.[22]

OUTCOMES

For the majority of cases of pharyngeal reconstruction, the desired outcome is a survival free of the initiating event, usually cancer, with a closed wound and normal function. Although more aggressive surgical extirpation and routine use of adjuvant radiotherapy have made a modest impact on survival, restoration of function (mainly swallowing) and achievement of a closed wound with alimentary continuity have been greatly improved by recent advances in reconstruction. Such improvements have stimulated more aggressive surgical approaches, thus restoring reasonable function to some patients who would previously never have been approached surgically.

Until recently, most reports of pharynx reconstruction emphasized techniques rather than results, either in terms of survival or function. Before the deltopectoral flap was widely used, it was impossible to assess the effectiveness of local cervical or random or waltzed thoracic flaps. Although the deltopectoral flap was a major improvement, several large series have shown unplanned fistula rates of from 40% to 78% and a high likelihood of subsequent revisional surgery and ultimate functional failure (40%).[6] Thoracic musculocutaneous flaps, mainly the pectoralis major, have an improved fistula rate (23% to 75%), but again with high requirement for secondary surgery (50%) and a disappointing rate of functional failure (40%).[6,8,13]

Visceral interposition such as right and left colon and stomach transposition have a high rate of perioperative mortality (8% to 30%), with even the most recent reports showing 10% to 15% mortality, usually secondary to respiratory complications. Ischemia of the distal pharyngovisceral anastomosis results in a high rate of fistula and need for secondary surgery.[28,29]

Free tissue transfer has become the predominant method in reconstruction of the major defect of the pharynx. Large series of jejunal free autografts have shown that the initial success rate in achieving alimentary continuity and a closed wound is high (87% to 97%) and that the ultimate success rate (94% to 100%) is even better.[11,23,29] Coleman demonstrated a series where the jejunum was statistically superior to the pectoralis major in ultimate success, spontaneous closure of fistula, and avoidance of a further operation, particularly in metachronous reconstruction.[8] The emphasis on restoration of function that has followed the ability to achieve a closed wound has increased the use of the radial forearm and lateral arm flaps for pharyngeal reconstruction, since it appears that the more flaccid skin and fasciocutaneous flaps allow better air passage and resonance, facilitating esophageal and tracheoesophageal speech.[1,17] Modification of the jejunum and the gastroomental flap have also proven beneficial in specialized cases in which the free tissue transfer would be useful, but local conditions are prohibitive.[14]

There are many methods of reconstruction that can be successfully employed in the patient who requires pharyngeal reconstruction. Careful analysis of the defect and knowledge of the natural history of the disease states that cause it will allow a choice of the optimal method and should allow successful wound closure and restoration of swallowing function in over 90% of cases. It has become obvious that single-stage procedures are most likely to decrease costs and time lost to normal life functions and should be planned with the extirpative portion of the surgery whenever possible and oncologically appropriate.

REFERENCES

1. Anthony JP, Singer MI, Deschler DG, et al: Long-term functional results after pharyngoesophageal reconstruction with the radial forearm free flap, *Am J Surg* 168:441-445, 1994.
2. Baek S, Lawson W, Biller HF: Reconstruction of the hypopharynx and cervical esophagus with pectoralis major island myocutaneous flap, *Ann Plast Surg* 7:18-24, 1981.
3. Bakamjian VY: A two stage method for pharyngoesophageal reconstruction with a primary pectoral skin flap, *Plast Reconstr Surg* 36:173, 1965.
4. Brown P, Coleman JJ: The role of radiotherapy and musculocutaneous flap in oropharyngocutaneous fistulas, *Am J Surg* 156:256-260, 1988.
5. Carlson GW, Coleman JJ, Jurkiewicz MJ: Reconstruction of the hypopharynx and cervical esophagus, *Curr Probl Surg* 30:425-480, 1993.
6. Carlson GW, Schustermann MA, Guillamondegui OM: Total reconstruction of the hypopharynx and cervical esophagus: a twenty year experience, *Ann Plast Surg* 29:408, 1992.
7. Coleman JJ: Reconstruction of the pharynx and cervical esophagus with jejunal free autograft, *Prob Gen Surg* 6:2:532-549, 1989.
8. Coleman JJ: Reconstruction of the pharynx after resection for cancer: a comparison of methods, *Ann Surg* 209:554-561, 1989.

9. Coleman JJ: Complications in head and neck surgery, *Surg Clin North Am* 66:149-167, 1986.

10. Coleman JJ: Treatment of the ruptured or exposed carotid artery, *South Med J* 78:262-267, 1985.

11. Coleman JJ, Searles JM, Hester TR, et al: Ten years experience with the free jejunal autograft, *Am J Surg* 154:394-398, 1987.

12. Reference deleted in pages.

13. Fabian RL: Pectoralis major myocutaneous flap reconstruction of the laryngopharynx and cervical esophagus, *Laryngoscope* 98:1227, 1988.

14. Guedon CE, Marmuse JP, Gehanno P, et al: Use of gastro-omental free flap in major neck defects, *Am J Surg* 168:491-493, 1994.

15. Jurkiewicz MJ: Vascularized intestinal graft for reconstruction of the cervical esophagus and pharynx, *Plast Reconstr Surg* 36:509, 1965.

16. Lavelle RJ, Maw RA: The etiology of post-laryngectomy pharyngocutaneous fistulae, *J Laryngol Otol* 86:785-793, 1972.

17. Martini DV, Har-El G, Lucente FE, et al: Swallowing and pharyngeal function in postoperative pharyngeal cancer patients, *ENT J* 450-456, 1997.

18. McConnel FMS, Cernko D, Jackson RT, et al: Timing of major events of pharyngeal swallowing, *Arch Otolaryngol Head Neck Surg* 114:1413-1418, 1988.

19. McConnel FMS, Duck S, Hester TR: Hypopharyngeal stenosis, *Laryngoscope* 94:1162-1165, 1984.

20. McConnel FMS, Mendelsohn MS, Logemann JA: Examination of swallowing after total laryngectomy using manofluorography, *Head Neck Surg* 8:3-12, 1986.

21. Moreno-Osset E, Thomas-Ridocci M, Paris F, et al: Motor activity of esophageal substitute (stomach, jejunal, and colon segments), *Ann Thorac Surg* 41:515, 1986.

22. Petruzzelli GJ, Johnson JT, Myers EN, et al: The effect of postoperative radiation therapy on pharyngoesophageal reconstruction with free jejunal interposition, *Arch Otolaryngol Head Neck Surg* 117:1265-1268, 1991.

23. Reece GP, Shusterman MA, Miller MJ, et al: Morbidity and functional outcome of free jejunal transfer reconstruction for circumferential defects of the pharynx and cervical esophagus, *Plast Reconstr Surg* 96(6): 1307-1316, 1995.

24. Rees R, Cary A, Shack RB, et al: Pharyngocutaneous fistulas in advanced cancer: closure with musculocutaneous or muscle flaps, *Am J Surg* 154:381-383, 1987.

25. Schusterman MA, Shestak K, deVries EJ, et al: Reconstruction of the cervical esophagus: free jejunal transfer versus gastric pull-up, *Plast Reconstr Surg* 85:16-21, 1990.

26. Seidenberg B, Rosenak SS, Hurwitt ES, et al: Immediate reconstruction of the cervical esophagus by a revascularized isolated jejunal segment, *Ann Surg* 149:162, 1959.

27. Singer M, Blom ED: An endoscopic technique for restoration of voice after laryngectomy, *Ann Otol Rhinol Laryngol* 89:529-533, 1980.

28. Surkin MI, Lawson W, Biller HF: Analysis of the methods of pharyngoesophageal reconstruction, *Head Neck Surg* 6:953-970, 1984.

29. Theile DR, Robinson DW, et al: Free jejunal interposition reconstruction after pharyngolaryngectomy: 201 consecutive cases, *Head Neck* 17(2):83-88, 1995.

30. Torres WE, Fibus TF, Coleman JJ, et al: The radiographic evaluation of the free jejunal graft, *Gastrointest Radiol* 12:226-230, 1987.

31. Wei WI, Lam KH, Choi S, et al: Late problems after pharyngolaryngoesophagectomy and pharyngogastric anastomosis for cancer of the larynx and hypopharynx, *Am J Surg* 148:509-513, 1984.

32. Weingrad DN, Spiro RH: Complications after laryngectomy, *Am J Surg* 146:517-520, 1983.

33. Wookey H: The surgical treatment of cancer of the pharynx and upper esophagus, *Surg Gynecol Obstet* 75:499, 1942.

CHAPTER

Trapezoidal Paddle Pectoralis Major Myocutaneous Flap for Esophageal Replacement

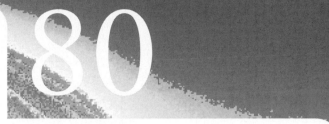

Berish Strauch
Carl Silver
Randall S. Feingold
Arthur Shektman

INTRODUCTION

Reconstruction of hypopharyngeal defects can be accomplished with pedicled myocutaneous flaps or with micro vascular free flaps. The authors contrast their results using the trapezoidal paddle pectoralis major myocutaneous (TPPMMC) flap with the reported results of two published series of free jejunal flaps. The severity of the defects, preprocedure irradiation, and mix of primary and secondary reconstruction were comparable between series. The benefits, complications, and functional results of either technique also appear to be comparable. However, the authors recommend the TPPMMC flap for its ease of performance, rapidity of surgery, and absence of intraperitoneal approach. With the current effort to achieve comparable results with shorter procedures, and greater conservation of patient, hospital, and public resources, this flap should be reconsidered.

INDICATIONS

Reconstruction of circumferential defects of the hypopharynx and cervical esophagus remains a challenge for the plastic surgeon. Various methods of reconstruction are available in our armamentarium, but two particular methods—the TPPMMC flap and free jejunal autografts—have proven to be consistently reliable and versatile. Yet, the debate as to which one of these procedures is best suited to reconstruct the hypopharynx and esophagus still continues.

Malignant disease in this area carries a poor prognosis; surgical intervention frequently plays only a palliative role. Therefore, a reconstructive procedure should have a low rate of major complications, allowing the patient to return to a normal or near-normal lifestyle as soon as possible after surgery. Ideally, reconstructive efforts should be easily executed, require little in the way of expensive equipment, and conserve hospital resources. The TPPMMC flap is a procedure with those characteristics.

Ten consecutive patients who underwent hypopharyngeal reconstruction with a TPPMMC flap were enrolled in the study; six were men and four were women. Their ages ranged from 45 to 89 years. All of the reconstructions were performed by the same surgeon from the Department of Plastic and Reconstructive Surgery at the Montefiore Medical Center between 1981 and 1988. Six patients had primary reconstruction, while the four remaining patients had secondary reconstruction after a previous laryngectomy. The defects were confined to the pharyngoesophageal region and were all above the clavicle. Six of the 10 patients had undergone preoperative radiotherapy. Among variables assessed were postoperative complications and return to normal or near-normal swallowing.

OPERATIONS

After the extirpative part of the procedure is completed, the resultant defect is measured; the vertical height of the defect will become the vertical height of the skin paddle. The skin paddle is outlined on the chest wall in a trapezoidal shape, with the longer edge of the paddle placed inferiorly and the short edge placed superiorly (Figure 80-1). These edges should be

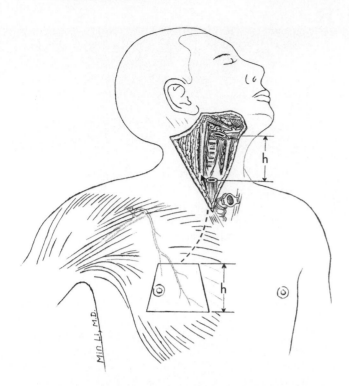

Figure 80-1. Measurement of defect; its vertical height will become the vertical length of the trapezoidal paddle. Skin paddle is outlined on the chest wall, with long width placed inferiorly and short edge placed superiorly. *h,* Height. (Redrawn from Shektman A, Silver C, Strauch B: *Plast Reconstr Surg* 100:1691-1696, 1997.)

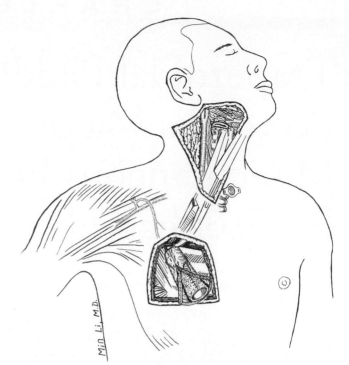

Figure 80-2. Tubing of the flap, with long suture line placed laterally, and muscle placed over the skin tube. (Redrawn from Shektman A, Silver C, Strauch B: *Plast Reconstr Surg* 100:1691-1696, 1997.)

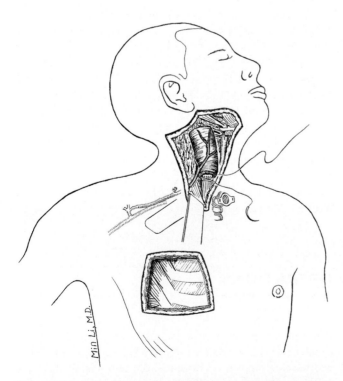

Figure 80-3. Muscle and skin paddle are passed subcutaneously into the neck wound, and the inferior anastomosis is begun. (Redrawn from Shektman A, Silver C, Strauch B: *Plast Reconstr Surg* 100:1691-1696, 1997.)

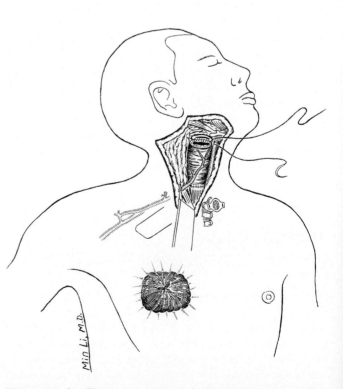

Figure 80-4. The superior repair (with the larger circumference) is now closed. The skin flap is closed. Any remaining area not covered with skin flap is skin grafted. (Redrawn from Shektman A, Silver C, Strauch B: *Plast Reconstr Surg* 100:1691-1696, 1997.)

equal in length to the circumference of the oropharyngeal and esophageal remnants, respectively. The skin paddle should lie entirely over the pectoralis major muscle, resulting in no "random" portion of the flap.

Once the skin is incised down to the pectoralis fascia, the muscle itself is freed from its sternal, costal, humoral, and clavicular attachments, and the entire musculocutaneous flap is rotated into the neck. Prior to performing the proximal and distal anastomoses, the flap is tubed, placing the long suture line lateral (Figures 80-2 to 80-4) and the muscle over the skin tube. The pectoralis major muscle is sutured to the prevertebral fascia and other surrounding tissues for support. A split-thickness skin graft is placed on any of the externally exposed muscle, and the chest wound is closed primarily.

OUTCOMES

No flap loss occurred in any of our patients. Normal or near-normal swallowing was attained by all patients. The time to deglutition was 1 to 3 weeks for nonirradiated patients and 3 to 13 weeks for irradiated patients. A fistula developed in four patients, all of whom had been previously irradiated. Two of the four fistulas healed with conservative management. One stenosis developed in this series and was successfully treated by a single dilation.

A previously published series of 10 cases of TPPMMC flaps from this institution[5,8] was compared to two other published series of free jejunal autografts[2,4,6] in terms of ease of execution and rates of complications. Coleman and colleagues[2,4] and Reece et al[6] published the results of their series of free jejunal transfers for correction of circumferential hypopharyngeal defects. The mix of patients, severity of defects, preprocedure irradiation, and number of primary and secondary reconstructions were similar (Table 80-1), as were the results (Table 80-2). There were major complications with both procedures; of these, fistulas, strictures, and flap losses are the most serious.

All series demonstrated nearly a 50% complication rate, with fistula appearing to be the most frequently encountered complication. The fistulization rate in our series was 40%; Coleman and colleagues[4] and Reece et al[6] reported 33% and 19%, respectively. Fistula formation may be expected to be between 20% and 40% of hypopharyngeal reconstructions,

Table 80-1.
Comparisons of the Three Reported Series

AUTHOR	NO. OF PATIENTS	METHOD	TYPE OF RECONSTRUCTION (%)	IRRADIATED PATIENTS (%)
Coleman et al[2,4]	$n = 101$ (111 flaps)	Free jejunal autograft	71 primary 29 secondary	50
Reece et al[6]	$n = 93$ (96 flaps)	Free jejunal autograft	97 primary 3 secondary	50
Cusumano et al[5] and Silver et al[8]	$n = 10$ (10 flaps)	TPPMMC flap	60 primary 40 secondary	60

From Shektman A, Silver C, Strauch B: A re-evaluation of hypopharyngeal reconstruction: pedicled flaps versus microvascular free flaps, *Plast Reconstr Surg* 100:1691-1696, 1997.

Table 80-2.
Comparison of Complications and Results of the Free Jejunal Autograft and the TPPMMC Flap for Pharyngoesophageal Reconstruction

AUTHOR	METHOD	FLAP LOSS (%)	FISTULA (%)	STENOSIS (%)	SWALLOW (%)
Coleman et al[2,4]	Free jejunal autograft	13.5	33	18	83
Reece et al[6]	Free jejunal autograft	3	19	15	80
Cusumano et al[5] and Silver et al[8]	TPPMMC flap	0	40	10	100

From Shektman A, Silver C, Strauch B: A re-evaluation of hypopharyngeal reconstruction: pedicled flaps versus microvascular free flaps, *Plast Reconstr Surg* 100:1691-1696, 1997.

regardless of the reconstructive method used. Half of these heal with expectant management, even in previously irradiated patients; half require surgical correction.

Stricture formation occurs in 10% to 25% of TPPMMC flaps, and in 15% to 20% of free jejunal transfers. Unless stricture is secondary to tumor recurrence, balloon dilation will usually alleviate the problem.

With both procedures, most patients can be expected to resume their preoperative diets within 3 weeks of surgery. Preoperative radiotherapy or history of previous radiotherapy appears to delay resumption of a peroral diet by several weeks.

Where TPPMMC flaps seem to have an appreciable advantage over free jejunal autografts is in the rate of flap loss. In a review of the Montefiore flap series, as well as eight others, Cusumano and colleagues[5] and Silver and colleagues[8] reported pectoralis flap loss to be 0% to 3%. The two series mentioned above, using free jejunal transfers, had flap losses of 13.5% and 3%, respectively. Another potential disadvantage of the jejunal flap is the large amount of mucus produced, which may increase aspiration if laryngectomy has not been done.[3]

The most significant advantage of the TPPMMC flap is its relative ease of execution, with an average operating time of 2.5 to 3 hours compared with an average of 6 to 6.5 hours for the free jejunal graft. Use of the flap also avoids the morbidity associated with opening the peritoneal cavity and avoids the need for bowel anastomosis.[7] Because of the large percentage of elderly patients in all series, the decrease in operating time and the elimination of an intraabdominal procedure favor the pectoralis flap. Moreover in the TPPMMC flap, the pectoralis muscle serves to cover the suture line closure and may cover adjacent irradiated carotid. This normal muscle cover is lacking in jejunal and in free radial forearm-flap reconstructions.[1]

In this era of limited health-care resources and managed-care plans, the TPPMMC flap, with its predictably good results, low complication rate, and relatively short time requirement for surgery, holds a particularly promising position in reconstruction of postextirpative defects of the hypopharynx and cervical esophagus.

REFERENCES

1. Boyd JB: Radial forearm cutaneous flap for hypopharyngeal reconstruction. In Strauch B, Vasconez L, Hall-Findlay E, editors: *Grabb's encyclopedia of flaps,* ed 2, New York, 1997, Thieme.
2. Coleman JJ III: Reconstruction of the pharynx after resection for cancer, *Ann Surg* 209:554, 1989.
3. Coleman JJ III: Jejunal free flap. In Strauch B, Vasconez L, Hall-Findlay E, editors: *Grabb's encyclopedia of flaps,* ed 2, New York, 1997, Thieme.
4. Coleman JJ III, Tan K-C, Searles JM, et al: Jejunal free autograft: analysis of complications and their resolution, *Plast Reconstr Surg* 84:589, 1989.
5. Cusumano RJ, Silver CE, Brauer RJ, et al: Pectoralis myocutaneous flap for replacement of cervical esophagus, *Head Neck* 11:450, 1989.
6. Reece GP, Schusterman MA, Miller MJ, et al: Morbidity and functional outcome of free jejunal transfer reconstruction for circumferential defects of the pharynx and cervical esophagus, *Plast Reconstr Surg* 96:1307, 1995.
7. Shah JP, Haribhakti V, Loree TR, et al: Complications of the pectoralis major myocutaneous flap in head and neck reconstruction, *Am J Surg* 160:352, 1990.
8. Silver CE, Cusumano RJ, Fell SC, et al: Replacement of upper esophagus: results with myocutaneous flap and with gastric transposition, *Laryngoscope* 99:819, 1990.

CHAPTER 81

Pharyngeal Reconstruction with the Gastric Pullup

Lorne E. Rotstein

INDICATIONS

Surgical reconstruction of the massive defect created by total laryngopharyngectomy remains a daunting task. The radical ablation and bilateral carotid vessel exposure, combined with the extensive mobilization of tissues required for the reconstruction, result in unfortunately high levels of perioperative morbidity and mortality.[5,7,18]

The earliest solutions to the problem of total pharyngeal replacement involved multistaged cervical skin flap manipulations, such as that designed by Wookey,[20] or staged tubed pedicle deltopectoral flaps. Both reconstructions are tedious, mutilating, and prone to failure.[20] Ong and Lee in 1960 first described the single-stage pharyngolaryngoesophagectomy with gastric transposition, a revolutionary concept at the time.[11] Tumors that involved the hypopharynx and/or upper cervical esophagus were removed en bloc with the entire esophagus. The mobilized stomach was transposed through the esophageal bed in the posterior mediastinum to the neck and anastomosed to the residual proximal pharynx. Several advantages were described. Among them, the procedure (1) involved a single-stage reconstruction; (2) required only a single gastrointestinal anastomosis; (3) avoided thoracotomy; (4) involved resection of potential "skip lesions" of the index tumor or synchronous occult primary malignancies in the esophagus; (5) provided predictability and plentitude of the gastric blood supply; (6) allowed adequate width for anastomosis to the patulous pharynx; and (7) decreased operating time by the simultaneous use of an extirpative and reconstructive operating team.

The initial report of Ong and Lee[11] was substantiated by Le Quesne and Ranger in 1966,[8] and "gastric pullup" rapidly became the operation of choice for reconstruction of the pharyngolaryngeal defect. High morbidity and mortality rates, attributed to poor patient preoperative nutritional status, prior radiation, and operator inexperience among other reasons,

were considered acceptable because of the lack of other feasible single-stage reconstructive techniques and the relentless natural history of the disease if left untreated.[7,17]

With the popularity of less morbid free visceral small intestine segmental transfer in the 1980s,[1,3,4,6,10] indications for gastric pullup have narrowed; however, the procedure remains important for reconstruction of the pharyngolaryngeal defect when the inferior end of the defect extends into the superior mediastinum, precluding the technical possibility of anastomosis of the lower end of a jejunal free flap to the intrathoracic esophagus through a cervical incision.[12,16]

There is obviously no effective way of restoring normal speech with laryngopharyngectomy, but the functional outcomes of any reconstructive procedure should include the potential for nonlaryngeal speech, as well as restoration of swallowing.

The indication therefore for a visceral reconstruction following laryngopharyngectomy is essentially that of a circumferential or near circumferential defect precluding primary or myocutaneous flap pharyngeal closure. The choice then falls between gastric transposition/pullup and jejunal segmental microvascular transfer. Numerous reports have shown that the morbidity and mortality of jejunal transfer are less than that for gastric pullup in the reconstruction of comparable defects.[2,16]

Furthermore, the length of the jejunal segment can always be "tailored" to fit the defect even when the resection margin extends proximally to the base of the tongue or nasopharynx, a potential problem with gastric pullup. Prior reports cite the requirement for a microvascular team as a disadvantage to jejunal transfer[7,18]; however, this has become a non-issue with the dramatic expansion and general availability of microsurgical expertise. Given the relative advantages of jejunal transfer over gastric transposition, the only remaining indications for the latter technique are: (1) the extension of the tumor to the superior mediastinum so that there is no disease-free cervical esophagus for jejunal anastomosis; or (2) a second primary squamous carcinoma of the thoracic esophagus necessitating total esophagectomy in addition to the circumferential laryngopharyngectomy.

Absolute technical contraindications to gastric transposition would include prior gastrectomy or gastroesophageal antireflux surgery and active peptic ulcer disease. Relative contraindications would include severe cardiopulmonary disease and prior peptic ulcer disease.

It is not the intent of this chapter to discuss indications for radical laryngopharyngectomy; however, given the significant morbidity and potential mortality of gastric transposition combined with laryngopharyngectomy, we believe this procedure should never be considered for palliative intent, but only when there is some reasonable potential for complete tumor ablation and cure.

OPERATIONS

The first step in gastric transposition is to assess the resectability of the disease in the neck prior to creating an abdominal incision. Since we do not advocate palliative gastric transposition, discovery of tumor involvement of the prevertebral fascia, carotid sheath, nasopharynx, or mediastinal soft tissues should result in a decision against proceeding with the ablative procedure.

Such procedures as laryngopharyngectomy, neck dissections, thyroidectomy, and parathyroid autotransplantations are done by the ablative team in the usual standard manner. In our experience, sternotomy or manubrial resection is not routinely required for esophageal mobilization and is only rarely performed for adequate tumor ablation if necessary (i.e., resectable stomal recurrence removal).

The abdominal team then mobilizes the stomach through a long upper midline abdominal incision with the aid of a Buchwalter or other similar multiblade self-retaining retractor. The lesser sac is entered through the gastrocolic omentum. The gastrocolic omentum is then divided below the gastroepiploic arcade all the way to the origin of the right gastric artery and to the left to the first short gastric artery (Figure 81-1, *B*). The viability of the mobilized stomach depends on preservation of both the right gastric and right gastroepiploic arteries, as well as preservation of the entire gastroepiploic arcade pedicled from the right gastroepiploic artery. The left gastroepiploic or short gastric arteries and veins are then generally divided close to the stomach, freeing up the greater curve proximally to the gastroesophageal junction (Figure 81-1, *C*). The spleen is left in situ. The lesser omentum is then entered, and the left gastric artery and its branches are generally divided along the lesser curve anterior and posterior to the lesser omental leaflet, as for a highly selective vagotomy (Figure 81-1, *A*). It is important that all of the blood vessels divided and ligated on the stomach are dealt with in small bites (i.e., one by one rather than "en masse") and that the division of vessels is immediately adjacent to the stomach serosa to avoid bunching or plication of the

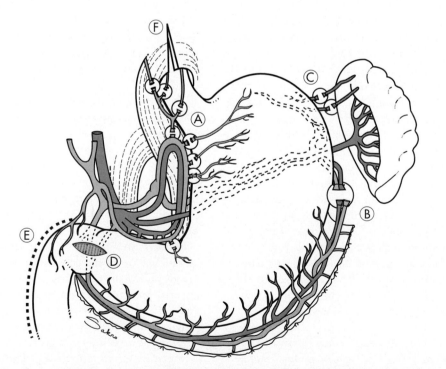

Figure 81-1. Surgical anatomy of abdominal portion of gastric interposition. **A,** Ligation and division of left gastric vasculature. **B,** Division of left gastroepiploic vessels. **C,** Division of short gastric vessels. **D,** Pyloromyotomy/pyloroplasty. **E,** Kocher maneuver. **F,** Vertical incision into diaphragmatic crura.

organ and subsequent shortening. The venous anatomy parallels that of the arterial except at the pylorus, where the right gastroepiploic artery and vein diverge with the artery heading posteriorly behind the proximal duodenum to its origin from the gastroduodenal artery. The vein, however, runs down inferiorly and medially toward the superior mesenteric vein into which it drains. Preservation of the right gastroepiploic vein is critical to prevent venous infarction of the transposed stomach.[8]

The hiatus is then mobilized or enlarged by manually stretching or by dividing the right crus of the diaphragm anteriorly from the esophagus toward the pericardium (Figure 81-1, F). The lower esophagus in the posterior mediastinum can then be mobilized under direct vision up to the level of the carina, with the feeding vessels clipped under direct vision.

A Kocher maneuver is next performed to allow for adequate proximal transposition of the mobilized stomach (Figure 81-1, E). A pyloromyotomy or pyloroplasty is essential for drainage of the stomach in view of the requirement for vagotomy in the neck or chest (Figure 81-1, D).

By this time the ablative surgery should be completed so that the team at the cranial end is free to mobilize the cervical esophagus downward into the mediastinum. The technique is essentially a downward stripping motion separating the esophagus from the prevertebral fascia posteriorly and off the membranous trachea anteriorly (Figure 81-2). To avoid injury to the membranous trachea, it is important to temporarily deflate the endotracheal tube balloon and to push the esophagus gently posteriorly off the trachea rather than pulling the trachea forward so as to avoid potential inadvertent laceration of the membranous portion of the trachea.

By this point the only remaining esophageal attachments are at the level of the carina and aortic arch. Throughout most of its thoracic course, the esophagus is surrounded by relatively loose areolar tissue, allowing for easy blunt dissection. The area between the carina and aortic arch, however, is more densely attached and unfortunately requires more vigorous blunt dissection. The abdominal operator must insert his or her entire hand through the hiatus and push the esophagus in a posterior vector off the carina and to the right off the aortic arch. The operator's other hand can be inserted through the neck incision simultaneously to assess the extent of mobilization; however, because of the tightness of the thoracic inlet, the majority of the dissection is performed by the abdominally placed hand. The operator must manipulate both hands in this dissection so that the palms and finger pulps are pointed posteriorly and so that the esophagus is pushed off the trachea from front to back, thereby avoiding inadvertent injury to the membranous trachea (Figure 81-2, B).

During the blunt intrathoracic portion of the procedure,

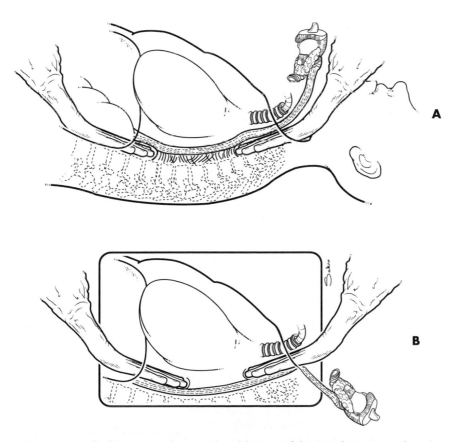

Figure 81-2. **A** and **B,** Blunt manipulation and mobilization of the intrathoracic esophagus.

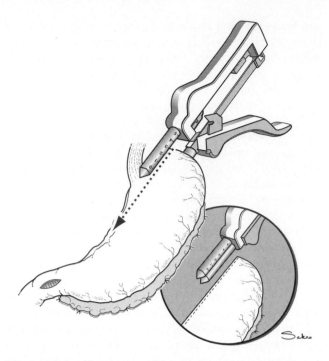

Figure 81-3. Transection of lesser curve of the stomach with stapling device.

pressure on the posterior aspect of the heart can initiate dysrhythmia or a sudden blood pressure drop, necessitating careful coordination between surgeon and anesthetist. Frequently, this portion of the procedure must be done in limited steps with intermittent removal of the operator's hands from the chest to allow for hemodynamic recovery.

There are two methods by which the stomach can then be transposed to the neck. The most common involves a combination of traction on the esophagus from above while the stomach is gently fed up through the hiatus. By a combination of gentle push and pull, the cardia and fundus are brought into the neck where the gastroesophageal (GE) junction is then transected with a stapling device (Figure 81-3). In the second method, the GE junction is transected by a stapler in the abdomen.[5] A sterile plastic bag is placed over the stomach and a small hole made in the bag at the level of the GE junction. A long, large rubber tube is placed through the hole and stitched to the GE junction. The other end of the tube is then brought through the esophageal bed into the neck and placed on suction (Figure 81-4). The bag with the stomach can then be gently pulled along the esophageal bed into the neck while manually guided through the hiatus from below simultaneously (Figure 81-5). The bag itself eases the

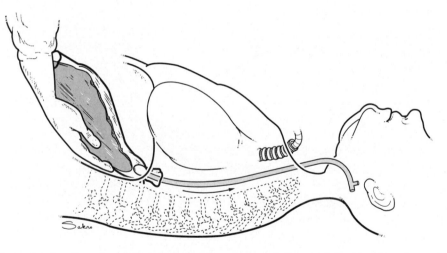

Figure 81-4. Transfer of the mobilized stomach through the esophageal bed into the neck.

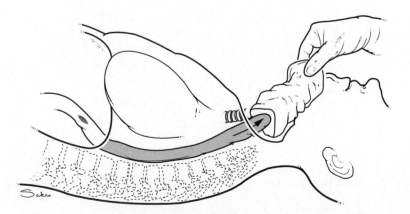

Figure 81-5. Completion of gastric transposition component of procedure.

sliding of the stomach to the neck and helps to avoid seromuscular traction injuries to the stomach.

The pharyngogastric anastomosis is then performed in two layers with interrupted monofilament absorbable 3-0 sutures. The fundus is used rather than the prior GE junction because it provides greater proximal length and easily is accommodated to the patulous oropharynx (Figure 81-6). This is a relative advantage compared with suturing discordantly sized jejunum to oropharynx in the procedure of free jejunal transfer.

If the transposed stomach does not reach far enough proximally, a number of maneuvers exist that may correct the problem.[13] Usually the difficulty is due to the ligation of the lesser curvature blood vessels being incorrectly performed in clumps rather than by single vessel division, resulting in plication or shortening of the stomach. Maximal length can be obtained in this situation by first reducing the stomach back into the abdomen and dividing it obliquely along the lesser curve from the GE junction to the incisura using a cutting stapler device as described by Shriver et al[15] (Figure 81-7, B). If length is still inadequate at this point (a rare event), other maneuvers can be employed (i.e., flexion of the head and/or the use of a "smile" incision in the anterior wall of the stomach as described by Schechter et al[13] (Figure 81-7, C and D). After completion of the pharyngogastric anastomosis, a nasogastric tube is placed and anchored firmly to the patient's nose because reinsertion postoperatively is associated with the potential risk of anastomotic disruption. My personal preference is to also place a feeding jejunostomy tube prior to abdominal closure so that if a persistent cervical anastomotic leak were to develop, percutaneous gastrostomy for feeding would obviously be precluded by the intrathoracic relocation of the stomach.

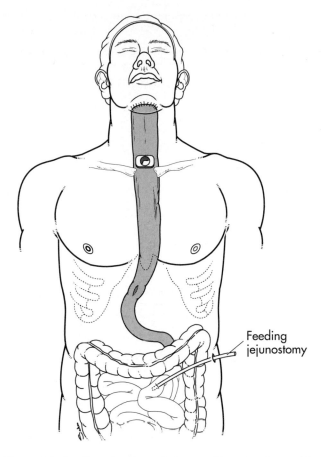

Feeding jejunostomy

Figure 81-6. Completed gastric interposition showing position of transposed stomach.

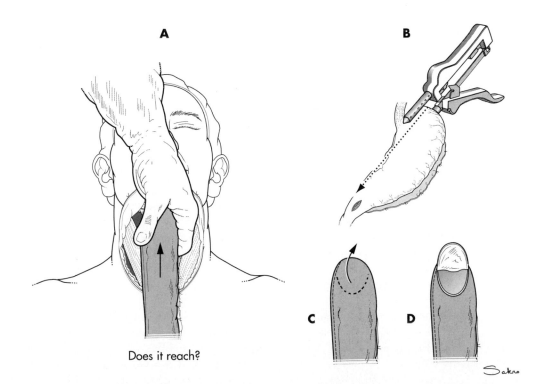

A

Does it reach?

B

C   D

Figure 81-7. Potential solutions for inadequate stomach length.

Table 81-1.
Morbidity and Mortality of Gastric Transposition

AUTHOR	NUMBER OF PATIENTS	MORTALITY (%)	FISTULA (%)	TOTAL COMPLICATIONS (%)
Wookey[20]	362	9	9	36
Biel and Maisel[1]	120	11	13	55
Silver et al[17]	317	9	9	49
Coleman et al[3]	41	19	20	54

Most technical descriptions of gastric transposition in this procedure vary little from that described above except for a recent preliminary presentation by Wei et al describing the use of transthoracic endoscopy for esophageal mobilization in a small number of patients.[19]

POSTOPERATIVE MANAGEMENT

Any operation that transgresses thorax, abdomen, and the neck, particularly in a relatively malnourished patient population, requires careful postoperative monitoring and care. These patients are generally nursed in an intensive care setting for 24 to 48 hours. The most immediate postoperative issues to be addressed are occult blood loss in the chest and/or pneumothorax. Portable chest x-rays are obtained immediately postoperatively and as frequently as necessary until the patient is stable. Hemodynamic and respiratory support and monitoring are likewise critical in the early postoperative period.

Assessment of the viability of the transposed stomach is a somewhat debatable issue but we generally use an esophagoscope to visualize the anastomosis and gastric mucosa once in the first 48 hours after operation.[5] Integrity of the anastomosis is assessed by a Gastrografin contrast swallow radiologic assessment at 7 to 9 days prior to initiating oral feeds.[5]

OUTCOMES

Early reports of high perioperative morbidity and mortality associated with gastric pullup for laryngopharyngeal reconstruction were attributed to lack of appreciation for potential problems,[5,7,18] inadequate postoperative support, or the "learning curve." Large series that compared outcomes at single institutions in earlier years with more recent outcomes, however, have clearly demonstrated that the high morbidity and mortality rates previously reported are still problematic and are intrinsic to the procedure rather than to lack of clinical experience or poor postoperative support.[2,16,18]

Perioperative mortality rates range widely, from 8% to 20%

in various reported series (Table 81-1); however, in most recent large series mortality approximates 10% overall. Similarly, major complication rates have varied from 25% to 55% and fistula rates from 2% to 22%.[2,16,18] A review from Memorial Sloan Kettering Cancer Center that reflects a large number of procedures performed in a single institution by a small group of experienced surgeons describes perioperative mortality of 11%, anastomotic fistula rate of 13%, and a total complication rate of 55%, indicating that significant problems can be anticipated with this procedure, even with refined surgical techniques and an excellent facility.[18]

In our institution the mean hospital stay is reported as 31.1 days.[5] Spiro et al have broken down duration of hospitalization at a median of 18 days in uncomplicated cases and 26 days in those with complications.[18]

FUNCTIONAL OUTCOME

Assessment of oral alimentation has been reported by a number of authors, and in general about 90% of those who survive this procedure regain the ability to maintain oral alimentation. Swallowing is generally reported as "good" or "easy," but early satiety and reflux are very common.[14]

Assessment of voice rehabilitation following gastric pullup is infrequent and anecdotal, but many of these patients develop intelligible esophageal speech.[18] Furthermore, for those who do not develop intelligible esophageal speech, the ability to use an electrolarynx device is not impaired. Schechter et al reported on speech quality after gastric pullup and found that when compared with patients who have had deltopectoral or pectoralis major myocutaneous reconstructions, these patients have poor quality speech limited to single words or short phrases, similar to the speech patterns attained with an electrolarynx.[17] There are scattered case reports of successful placement of tracheogastric voice prostheses; however, the potential risk of production of a tracheogastric fistula and its sequelae is daunting.

Wei et al have reviewed 136 patients after gastric transposition and found that only nine (6.6%) were able to produce an audible whisper and only six (4.4%) could communicate with an electrolarynx.[19] Mariglia and colleagues reported a series of five patients with tracheogastric puncture after gastric transposition and described their speech as low in pitch, slow, and wet sounding compared with those with tracheoesophageal puncture after primary closure. Three of the five patients subsequently voluntarily requested prosthesis removal.[9] Formal patient satisfaction surveys for gastric transposition have not been published.

ECONOMIC CONSIDERATIONS

Given that gastric pullup has high morbidity and mortality rates and a long duration of reported length of hospital stay, it is implicit that this is an expensive venture. No direct costing of this procedure has been published to date but any general comparisons that have been done with jejunal transposition demonstrate fewer complications and shorter mean and median length of stay for the latter.[16]

REFERENCES

1. Biel MH, Maisel RH: Free jejunal autograft reconstruction of the pharyngoesophagus: review of a ten year experience, *Otolaryngol Head Neck Surg* 96:369-375, 1987.

2. Carlson GW, Coleman JJ, Jurkiewicz MJ: Reconstruction of the hypopharynx and cervical esophagus, *Curr Probl Surg* 30(5):427-472, 1993.

3. Coleman JJ, Searles JM, Hester TR, et al: Ten years experience with the free jejunal autograft, *Am J Surg* 154:389-393, 1987.

4. Ferguson JL, DeSanto LW: Total pharyngolaryngectomy and cervical esophagectomy with jejunal autotransplant reconstruction, complications and results, *Laryngoscope* 98:911-914, 1988.

5. Goldberg M, Freeman J, Gullane PJ, et al: Transhiatal esophagectomy with gastric transposition for pharyngolaryngeal malignant disease, *J Thorac Cardiovasc Surg* 97:327-333, 1989.

6. Jurkiewicz MJ: Vascularized intestinal graft for reconstruction of the cervical esophagus and pharynx, *Plast Reconstr Surg* 361:509-517, 1965.

7. Lam KH, Ho CM, Lau WF, et al: Immediate reconstruction of the pharynx after resection for cancer, *Ann Surg* 209:554-561, 1989.

8. Le Quesne LP, Ranger D: Pharyngolaryngectomy with immediate pharyngogastric anastomosis, *Br J Surg* 53:101-109, 1966.

9. Mariglia AJ, Leder SB, Goodwin WJ, et al: Tracheogastric puncture for vocal rehabilitation following total pharyngolaryngoesophagectomy, *Head Neck* 11:524-527, 1989.

10. McConnel FMS, Hester TR, Nahai F, et al: Free jejunal grafts for reconstruction of pharynx and cervical esophagus, *Arch Otolaryngol Head Neck Surg* 107:476-481, 1981.

11. Ong GB, Lee TC: Pharyngogastric anastomosis after esophagopharyngectomy for carcinoma of the hypopharynx and cervical esophagus, *Br J Surg* 48:193-200, 1960.

12. Peracchia A, Bardini R: Total esophagectomy without thoracotomy: results of a European questionnaire (GEEMO), *Int Surg* 71:171-175, 1986.

13. Schechter GL, Baker JW, El-Mahd AM, et al: Combined treatment of advanced cancer of the laryngopharynx, *Laryngoscope* 92:11-15, 1982.

14. Schechter GL, Baker JW, Gilbert DA: Functional evaluation of pharyngoesophageal reconstructive techniques, *Arch Otolaryngol Head Neck Surg* 113:40-44, 1987.

15. Shriver CD, Spiro RH, Burt M: A new technique for gastric pull-through, *SGO* 177:519-520, 1993.

16. Shusterman MA, Shestek K, de Vries EJ, et al: Reconstruction of the cervical esophagus free jejunum vs. gastric pullup, *Plast Reconstr Surg* 85:16-21, 1990.

17. Silver CE, Cusumano RJ, Fell SC, et al: Replacement of upper esophagus: results with myocutaneous flap and with gastric transposition, *Laryngoscope* 99:819-821, 1989.

18. Spiro RH, Bains MS, et al: Gastric transposition for head and neck cancer: a critical update, *Am J Surg* 162:348-352, 1991.

19. Wei WI, Lam LK, Yuen PW, et al: Current status of pharyngolaryngoesophagectomy and pharyngogastric anastomosis, Presentation at 4th *International Conference on Head and Neck Cancer*, Toronto, Canada, July 1996.

20. Wookey H: The surgical treatment of carcinoma of the hypopharynx and the oesophagus, *Br J Surg* 35:249-266, 1948.

The Larynx

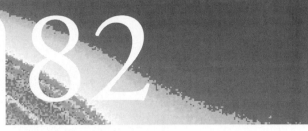

Daniel J. Kelley
Jatin P. Shah

INTRODUCTION

Surgical treatment of laryngeal disease is based on the embryology, anatomy, physiology, and pathology of the larynx. The surgical techniques available for the treatment of laryngeal disease can be divided into two general categories: open and closed (endoscopic) techniques. In general, endoscopic techniques are used more commonly in the management of benign laryngeal pathology. However, endoscopic excision of laryngeal cancer can be performed in select instances. The choice of procedure is determined by the extent to which a pathologic condition involves the larynx and the surgeon's ability to accurately diagnose and treat the particular disease entity. This chapter will discuss the indications, operations, and outcomes for the most common laryngeal surgical procedures.

Direct laryngoscopy is indicated as an essential part of the routine diagnostic evaluation of laryngeal pathology. It may be performed in the office utilizing flexible fiberoptic equipment or rigid telescopes under topical anesthesia for diagnostic purposes and in combination with stroboscopy and video recording (Figure 82-1). This procedure provides an adequate comprehensive view of the pharynx and larynx and also provides dynamic functional assessment. Vocal cord motion abnormalities and adequacy of airway can be easily evaluated. In a single field this examination provides a complete and thorough view of the larynx (Figure 82-2). In the operating room, rigid equipment under intravenous sedation or general anesthesia (Figure 82-3) can be used alone or in combination with either an operating microscope or fiberoptic telescopes to carefully assess laryngeal pathology (Figure 82-4). Although detailed surface evaluation of the larynx and subglottic region is feasible with the use of rigid telescopes (0, 30, 70, and 120 degrees), the disadvantage of microlaryngoscopy under general anesthesia is that it does not provide functional assessment of the larynx.

Computed tomography (CT) and magnetic resonance imaging (MRI) are the main modalities for radiologic examination of the larynx. Both techniques are comparable in delineating site and extent of pathology within soft tissue and characterizing cartilaginous tumors, laryngoceles, and cysts (Figure 82-5). CT scan is preferred in patients who may have rapid breathing or coughing, when assessing the integrity of the laryngeal skeleton for identification of occult or suspected fractures or injuries, or if MRI is contraindicated (e.g., patients with pacemakers, metallic implants). MRI is preferred in cooperative patients for evaluation of the larynx prior to partial laryngectomy or organ preservation protocol, and may be more sensitive than CT scan in detecting pathologic involvement of laryngeal cartilages.[18] MRI has an added advantage of providing coronal and sagittal images (Figure 82-6).

INDICATIONS

CONGENITAL

Congenital anomalies of the larynx are rare, presenting usually with stridor, airway distress, or failure to thrive in the newborn infant, and may be part of a syndrome of congenital anomalies.[20] Some of the more common congenital laryngeal anomalies include laryngeal cysts and webs, laryngomalacia, abnormalities of the epiglottis, hemangiomas, cystic hygromas, thyroid and cricoid cartilage anomalies such as subglottic stenosis, and laryngeal clefts.[11,116,119] The diagnosis of many congenital laryngeal anomalies can be reliably confirmed using flexible laryngoscopy in the office or direct laryngoscopy in the operating room. Flexible laryngoscopy in infants can be difficult, although safely done with topical anesthesia. Videolaryngoscopy can improve the diagnostic accuracy of office evaluation.[147]

Laryngomalacia, the most common congenital laryngeal anomaly, is more common in males[168] and presents with large, floppy arytenoid cartilages that prolapse into the glottis on inspiration, causing stridor.[93] Redundant mucosa over the lateral edges of the epiglottis, aryepiglottic folds, arytenoids, and corniculate cartilages and abnormal appearance of the epiglottis are also common in these patients. Although children with laryngomalacia may have height and weight deficits relative to the general population, mild symptoms of

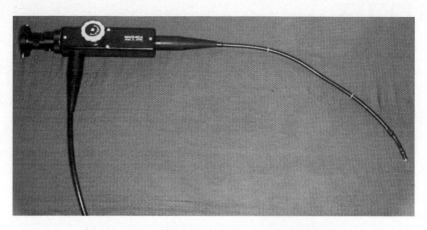

Figure 82-1. Fiberoptic flexible nasolaryngoscope.

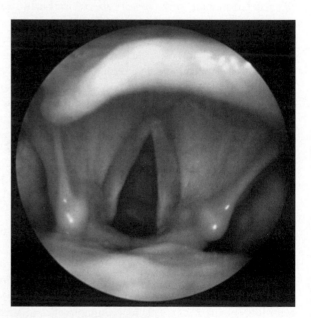

Figure 82-2. Comprehensive view of the larynx as seen with a flexible fiberoptic nasolaryngoscope or a rigid telescope.

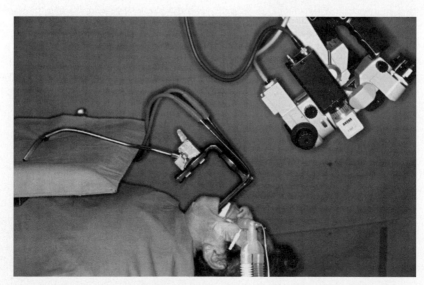

Figure 82-3. Suspension microlaryngoscopy under general anesthesia.

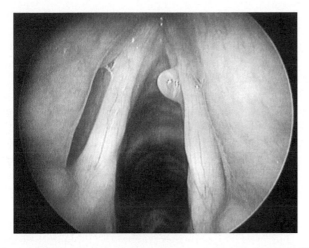

Figure 82-4. Microlaryngoscopic view of the endolarynx (×40), showing a mucosal polyp on the anterior one third of the right vocal cord.

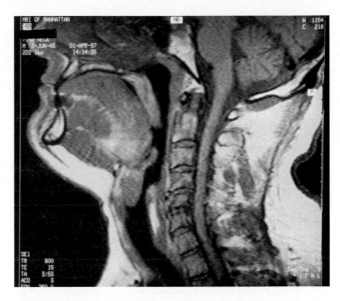

Figure 82-6. Sagittal view of the MRI scan of the larynx showing an adenoid cystic carcinoma of the infrahyoid portion of the epiglottis.

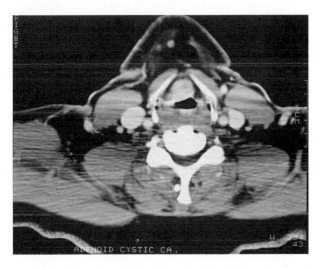

Figure 82-5. Axial view of a CT scan of a larynx showing an adenoid cystic carcinoma of the epiglottis extending into the preepiglottic space.

intermittent stridor improve over time, and surgical treatment is usually not indicated. In 10% of patients, laryngomalacia results in failure to thrive, apnea, or cardiopulmonary disease, warranting surgical intervention,[7] usually either epiglottoplasty or tracheostomy.[72]

Congenital cystic laryngeal anomalies include simple vallecular cysts, cystic hygromas, saccular cysts, and laryngoceles.[146] Laryngeal cysts are caused by retained mucus or dilation of the laryngeal saccule. External laryngoceles are distinguished by their presentation external to the larynx as a cystic, air-filled neck mass.[22] The annual incidence of simple congenital laryngeal cysts is reported as 1.82 cases per 100,000 live births.[147] Laryngeal involvement by cystic hygromas can be particularly difficult to manage due to extralaryngeal extensions.[139] Once diagnosed, treatment is indicated for these conditions because symptoms are progressive. Management options include needle aspiration, endoscopic marsupialization, and surgical removal via an external approach through the thyrohyoid membrane.[139] Tracheotomy can usually be avoided except in cases of large cystic hygromas.

Congenital laryngeal clefts result from failure of cephalad advancement of the tracheoesophageal septum and fusion of cricoid cartilage.[19] Most patients present with stridor and aspiration due to the presence of a communication between the larynx and esophagus.[42] Prognosis is related to the severity of other anomalies and the quality of respiratory and nutritional care in combination with surgical correction of the defect.[24] Surgical correction is indicated when the diagnosis is made and can be accomplished using endoscopic techniques, anterior laryngofissure, or lateral pharyngotomy approaches. The choice of technique is dictated by the severity of the cleft. Despite successful closure of the laryngeal cleft, abnormal swallowing with aspiration may persist. Any associated gastroesophageal reflux must be adequately treated by surgical antireflux procedures if necessary.

Congenital subglottic stenosis represents a spectrum of laryngeal anomalies that range from mild narrowing of the subglottis to complete atresia of the larynx.[61] A grading system has been developed to determine the severity of the stenosis and help guide treatment.[109] Treatment is indicated for patients with recurrent respiratory obstruction. Severe subglottic stenosis can be treated with a variety of surgical techniques, including endolaryngeal stents, endoscopic laser excision, cricoid split, cricoid cartilage augmentation, and partial or complete cricoid resection and primary tracheal anastomosis.[50] Many patients who are tracheotomy dependent at the time of surgery can eventually be decannulated following surgical treatment.[97] Children with high-grade subglottic stenosis and multiple prior surgeries are at high risk for poor voice outcome after reconstruction.[97]

Infantile hemangiomas are problematic laryngeal lesions and treatment options include observation, systemic steroids, interferon, electrocautery, CO_2 or neodymium:yttrium-aluminum-garnet (Nd:YAG) laser excision, and tracheostomy.[32,128] Small or moderate-sized lesions can be treated expectantly or with steroids. Tracheostomy and staged CO_2 laser excision are reserved for large lesions that are unresponsive to other therapies or that become symptomatic, causing dysphagia, recurrent bleeding, or airway obstruction.[128,158] The potential complication of electrocautery or laser treatment is the development of laryngeal stenosis.[128]

ACQUIRED

Traumatic

INTERNAL. Acquired lesions are more common indications for surgical treatment. Patients requiring both temporary and prolonged intubation are at risk for permanent injury to the larynx, such as web, granuloma, vocal cord paralysis, vocal cord nodules, arytenoid cartilage dislocation, or laryngeal stenosis.[138] At increased risk are patients with prolonged intubation, large endotracheal tube, or nasogastric tube, or patients having a seizure disorder or head injury[125] (Figure 82-7). In neonates, acquired subglottic stenosis is due to posttraumatic fibrosis following long-term endotracheal intubation.[62] Arytenoid subluxation and recurrent laryngeal nerve paralysis, both sequelae of intubation, may be difficult to distinguish.[65] Steroid therapy is not effective prophylaxis against intubation laryngeal injury and may increase the incidence of local or systemic sepsis.[138] Vocal cord nodules are caused by chronic vocal abuse, often in combination with mucosal irritants, such as cigarette smoking and gastroesophageal reflux disease (GERD).[84] Correction of GERD in some patients will often result in resolution of laryngeal inflammatory lesions.[36] Other patients, particularly those with

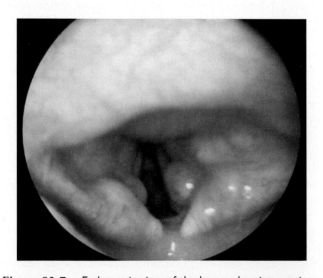

Figure 82-7. Endoscopic view of the larynx showing postintubation granulomas involving the posterior third of both vocal cords.

benign vocal cord nodules, respond to speech therapy or endoscopic microsurgical excision with or without the CO_2 laser.[85]

Strictures of the upper airway caused by burns have features distinct from other benign stenoses.[53] Caustic ingestion of household cleaning agents and lye-containing cosmetic products can result in injury to the face, oral cavity, larynx, pharynx, and esophagus, occurring most frequently in children. Chronic aspiration, dysphagia, and esophageal stenosis are common long-term problems in these patients.[126] More than half of the 150,000 burn patients hospitalized in the United States each year have head and neck involvement, with 3% to 7% sustaining concomitant inhalation injury.[115] Inflammation of the airway caused by exposure to hot gases and complicated by intubation results in a high incidence of laryngotracheal strictures in survivors.[57]

Treatment for internal laryngeal trauma depends on the site and extent of permanent injury.[156] Prolonged hoarseness or odynophagia after endotracheal intubation should alert the physician to the possibility of a cricoarytenoid joint injury. Endoscopic relocation of the displaced joint may bring resolution of the cricoarytenoid edema and return of vocal cord function. Persistent vocal fold dysfunction may occur secondary to joint arthritis, hemarthrosis, or nerve injury.[134] Permanent vocal cord paralysis can be treated by observation; reinnervation with either a motor nerve anastomosis to the recurrent laryngeal nerve or nerve-muscle pedicle; injection of fat, Gelfoam, Teflon, or silicon; or medialization laryngoplasty.[71,169] Subglottic stenosis can be treated by reintubation and subsequent extubation, tracheotomy, anterior cricoid split, laser vaporization, skin grafting, or laryngotracheal reconstruction.[64,113] Treatment options for the rare laryngeal burn injury include observation, steroids, and tracheostomy and stent placement with or without resection of the area of stricture. Early resection should be avoided and prolonged stenting is recommended to allow maturation of the contracture.[53]

EXTERNAL. Both blunt and penetrating trauma to the larynx can result in permanent injury and dysfunction. Motor vehicle injury, gunshot, and stab wounds can cause either isolated airway or combined airway/digestive tract injuries.[57] Since the introduction of seat belts, laryngotracheal trauma has become a rare injury, constituting less than 1% of blunt trauma cases seen at major trauma centers.[112] Although less common than penetrating injuries, blunt injuries are more often life-threatening because acute respiratory distress is more common and the potential for laryngotracheal disruption is higher.[48] Even seemingly minor events can result in life-threatening laryngeal injuries.[10] Seat belt syndrome, with skin abrasions of the neck, chest, and abdomen, is associated with injuries to the larynx and other neck structures.[59] Potential injuries include laryngeal fractures, mucosal lacerations, and arytenoid dislocation and subluxation.

Emergent airway management options include tracheostomy, endotracheal intubation, and cricothyrotomy.[164] MRI and CT studies are used to assess the degree of injury to the laryngeal framework.[34] Associated injuries, general health status of the patient, and length of time since the injury will dictate management.[118] Endoscopic evaluation followed by neck exploration and repair of laryngotracheal and esophageal injury with stent placement in severe cases should be performed once the patient is hemodynamically stable.[83] Cricoarytenoid subluxation is treated by endoscopic reduction of the dislocation.[134] Epiglottic laryngoplasty or tissue grafts can be used to repair mucosal defects and prevent the development of granulation tissue or stenosis.[169] Persistent vocal cord immobility may be due to arytenoid fixation or recurrent nerve injury.[86]

Recurrent laryngeal nerve injury occurs in 2% to 3% of patients following thyroid and parathyroid surgery, but may also be seen after central nervous system, intrathoracic, tracheoesophageal, or neck procedures.[63,164] Flexible laryngoscopy is the best method for evaluation of vocal cord paralysis, and laryngeal electromyography (EMG) is helpful in predicting return of function following injury.[10,83] Permanent vocal cord paralysis can be treated by observation; ansa cervicalis anastomosis to the adductor branch of the recurrent laryngeal nerve; injection of fat, Gelfoam, Teflon, or silicon; or medialization laryngoplasty.[51,71,169]

INFLAMMATORY

Systemic diseases involving the larynx, such as Wegener's granulomatosis, idiopathic pseudotumor, and sarcoidosis, are rare, are often misdiagnosed, and may be misinterpreted as infections or malignant neoplasms.[99,152] They manifest initially as upper airway obstruction, hoarseness, dysphonia, or rapidly progressive stridor.[89] Manifestations of systemic lupus erythematosus (SLE) can range from mild ulcerations, vocal cord paralysis, and edema to necrotizing vasculitis with airway obstruction.[137] Granulomas within the larynx may be caused by Crohn's disease, sarcoid, foreign body, or gout.[8,58,107,157] Laryngeal symptoms often improve with corticosteroid therapy and management consists of accurate assessment of the extent of disease and establishment of the diagnosis with a biopsy.[5] Local excision can be undertaken endoscopically or via a midline vertical thyrotomy. Laryngectomy is indicated only under rare circumstances.[94]

INFECTIOUS

Infections of the larynx vary from the common to the obscure, but few require surgical treatment. Scleroma may present with chronic ulceration. The identification of the infecting agent and exclusion of a malignant process, although difficult, are crucial.[105] Laryngeal tuberculosis may be indistinguishable both clinically and radiographically from carcinoma.[92] Immunocompromised patients are at risk for a variety of opportunistic infections, particularly cytomegalovirus and aspergillosis.[76,94] Infection by human papillomavirus can result in recurrent respiratory papillomatosis and chronic airway ob-

struction.[6] The histologic diagnosis must be established by biopsies, cultures, and special staining.

NEOPLASTIC

Benign

One of the most common benign laryngeal neoplasms is recurrent respiratory papilloma (RRP).[5] These lesions, caused by human papillomavirus and found throughout the larynx,[95] are often difficult to eradicate, requiring multiple attempts at laser ablation.[80] Secondary infection throughout the upper aerodigestive tract and malignant transformation to squamous cell carcinoma have been reported.[90,114] Laryngeal hemangiomas of the mixed or cavernous type may occur throughout the larynx. Dysphagia, recurrent bleeding, or airway obstruction may demand treatment with interferon, injection with sclerosing agents, laser photocoagulation, or excision via laryngotomy.[158]

A variety of other benign neoplasms of the larynx, including schwannomas, neurinomas, plexiform neurofibromas, hamartomas, adenomas, rhabdomyomas, oncocytic papillary cystadenomatosis, and junctional nevi, have been reported in the literature.* Unless symptoms of dysphagia, hoarseness, or airway obstruction occur, benign neoplasms are usually managed nonsurgically. Endoscopic microsurgical excision with or without the carbon dioxide laser or excision via laryngotomy or pharyngotomy may, however, be necessary.[131,153]

Malignant

Diagnosis and treatment of malignant tumors of the larynx require careful assessment of the primary site, histology, and extent of disease. For description and staging purposes, the larynx is divided into three parts: the supraglottis, glottis, and subglottis (Figure 82-8). The supraglottic larynx extends from the superior tip of the epiglottis to the apex of the laryngeal ventricle. The glottic larynx is bounded superiorly by the apex of the laryngeal ventricle. There are two commonly used boundaries for the inferior extent of the glottic larynx: 1 cm below the ventricle apex or 5 mm below the free edge of the true vocal cord. The subglottis extends from the inferior aspect of the glottis to the inferior aspect of the cricoid cartilage.

Certain anatomic structures play critical roles in determining the behavior of neoplastic conditions within the larynx and permit partial removal of intralaryngeal compartments in an oncologically sound manner.[77] The conus elasticus, a fibroelastic membrane, covers the surface of the vocalis muscle near the muscle's insertion at the thyroid cartilage. This structure helps create a barrier to invasion of adjacent structures by vocal cord cancers.[121] The hyoepiglottic ligament (HL) serves as the superior boundary of the paraglottic and the preepiglottic spaces separating the supraglottic larynx from the tongue base. It can be used as a surgical boundary in the resection of supraglottic cancer that is confined to the larynx and does not invade the suprahyoid epiglottis.[167]

---

*References 1, 44, 45, 100, 101, 106, 124, 127.

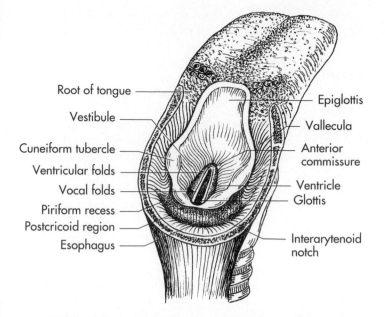

Root of tongue

Vestibule

Cuneiform tubercle

Ventricular folds

Vocal folds

Piriform recess

Postcricoid region

Esophagus

Epiglottis

Vallecula

Anterior commissure

Ventricle

Glottis

Interarytenoid notch

Figure 82-8. Anatomic sites within the larynx and pharynx.

Staging of the neck is critically important in the management of larynx cancer. Cervical metastases from laryngeal cancer are associated with decreased disease-free interval and overall survival, as well as increased risk of distant metastases. The incidence of metastasis to cervical lymph nodes varies with the tumor size and location of the primary site within the larynx,[108] with supraglottic lesions at highest risk, followed by subglottic and glottic. Occult neck metastases occur in as many as 30% of patients with T3/4 laryngeal cancer.[78] One of every six patients who present with clinically negative necks will develop regional lymph node metastases, most commonly in the deep jugular chain, and 10% of these patients will die of nodal disease. Lymph node metastases from vocal cord cancer are rare and the clinically negative neck in a patient with glottic cancer can be observed, reserving neck dissection or radiotherapy for salvage.

The choice of treatment of laryngeal cancer is based on careful consideration of multiple patient and tumor-specific factors. Advanced disease usually requires total removal of the larynx. Radiation therapy alone or in combination with chemotherapy, however, has been shown to be effective for both early and advanced disease, and patients should be informed of all therapeutic options before initiating treatment. Both CT scan and MRI provide reliable techniques to aid clinical staging.[74]

Although by far the most common malignant histology within the larynx is squamous cell carcinoma, adenocarcinoma of minor salivary gland origin, sarcoma, malignant fibrous histiocytoma, lymphoepithelioma, plasmocytoma, lymphoma, and melanoma have been reported.* Cutaneous melanoma and renal carcinoma are the most common secondary tumors; sporadic cases of solitary lung and

*References 2, 14, 38, 43, 106, 122, 155, 166.

colon metastasis have been described, although these are extremely rare.

GLOTTIC LARYNX

Early glottic cancer can be treated with comparable success with either radiation therapy or surgical removal. When resection is limited to the true vocal cord, laser vaporization, cord stripping, and cordectomy are all effective. In such instances, surgery offers a single procedure for both diagnosis and treatment at the potential expense of vocal quality. Radiation therapy may offer better vocal quality, but requires extended treatment over several weeks. Local recurrence following radiotherapy for early vocal cord cancer can be salvaged with partial or total laryngectomy.[12]

Glottic carcinoma with vocal cord fixation or extension into the hypopharynx or preepiglottic space may be treated by vertical partial pharyngolaryngectomy with tracheotomy or total laryngectomy as primary therapy and for surgical salvage following radiation therapy.[79,96,123] Clinical underestimation of the extent of the cartilage involvement occurs in half of patients with T3 lesions. Extensive cartilage ossification, glottic fixation, transglottic cancer, and extensive involvement of the anterior commissure all suggest microinvasion of the thyroid cartilage.[110] Involvement of the thyroid cartilage or soft tissues of the neck represents advanced disease (T4) and usually requires either total laryngectomy or combined chemotherapy and radiation therapy for organ preservation, with total laryngectomy reserved as surgical salvage.[17]

SUPRAGLOTTIC LARYNX

Tumors limited to one subsite within the supraglottis with normal vocal cord mobility (T1) are rare and can be treated with open or endoscopic excision or primary radiation therapy. Most supraglottic cancers, however, extend into the glottic larynx or pharynx at the time of presentation[150] (T2-4) and have a high incidence of occult, ipsilateral, or bilateral regional lymph node metastases, making treatment of both necks in addition to the primary site necessary. Treatment includes supraglottic or total laryngectomy and neck dissection, primary radiation therapy, or a combination of surgery, radiation, and/or chemotherapy.

SUBGLOTTIC LARYNX

Primary subglottic carcinoma is rare, accounting for less than 5% of all larynx cancers.[52] The most common histologies include squamous cell carcinoma and minor salivary gland malignancies.[40] Many patients are classified as having glottic cancers due to inappropriate staging.[9] Symptoms are identical to other laryngeal sites including hoarseness, respiratory difficulty, and hemoptysis.[130] Advanced stage due to invasion of

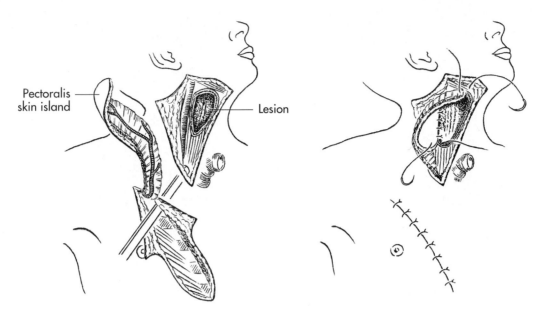

Figure 82-9. Pectoralis major myocutaneous flap reconstruction for partial pharyngeal defects.

cartilage and the thyroid gland is much more common. Primary radiation therapy with surgical salvage and a combination of surgery and postoperative radiotherapy[60] are treatment options.

TRANSGLOTTIC (ADVANCED)

In many cases, the tumor has invaded adjacent structures, and laryngopharyngectomy with resection of the base of tongue or cervical esophagus is necessary. In such cases, primary closure is rarely feasible, and regional pedicled flaps or free flaps including jejunum, radial forearm, rectus abdominis, and others are appropriate. The pectoralis major myocutaneous flap is useful for partial or circumferential defects either as a patch or tubed to create a lumen[30] (Figure 82-9). When there is extension into the cervical esophagus[98] and total esophagectomy is necessary, particularly when a cervical esophageal lesion extends into the upper thoracic esophagus, gastric pullup with pharyngogastrostomy is indicated (Figure 82-10). When a primary cancer involves the postcricoid region or is limited to the cervical esophagus, a circumferential pharyngolaryngectomy defect is best reconstructed with a free segment of jejunum with microvascular repair (Figure 82-11). Defects of the pharyngeal wall, after resection of pharyngeal cancer with preservation of the larynx, are suitable for reconstruction with a radial forearm free flap (Figure 82-12), since the secretory characteristics of the jejunum may result in unacceptable aspiration.

Although preservation of the larynx by either radiotherapy or surgery is desirable, life-threatening aspiration after treatment of malignancies of the tongue, hypopharynx, and cervical esophagus may dictate laryngectomy even in the absence of tumor. Although uncommon, full-thickness invasion of the larynx or trachea by well-differentiated thyroid carcinoma may require laryngectomy or tracheal resection.[39] Acute airway obstruction due to advanced carcinoma of the larynx may be managed by tracheotomy followed by elective definitive tumor surgery or laser debulking to maintain a patent airway in cases where only palliation is appropriate. Emergency laryngectomy, defined as total laryngectomy performed within 24 hours, for a previously untreated and undiagnosed malignancy does not appear to offer patients any survival advantage despite earlier reports of increased stomal recurrence in situations where staged laryngectomy after tracheostomy was performed.[111]

Tracheoesophageal puncture (TEP) is the most effective method of voice restoration following laryngectomy, either at the time of laryngectomy (primary) or as a secondary procedure.[87,141] A voice prosthesis is placed within the tracheostoma that communicates with the cervical esophagus, allowing continuous air flow and thus sound production (Figure 82-13). The successful production of voice with a TEP requires a compliant pharyngoesophageal segment, and failure may result from spasm of the pharyngoesophageal segment.[23] Because of this, some authors advocate incomplete approximation of the pharyngeal sphincters, cricopharyngeal myotomy, or pharyngeal neurectomy as an adjunct to total laryngectomy.[69,133] TEP can be performed following reconstruction with gastric pullup or microvascular free flap, although vocal quality may be inferior.[3,104,151] Patient motivation and compliance, manual dexterity, extent of initial surgery, history of irradiation, insufflation test results, the presence of pharyngeal stricture, as well as other medical comorbidities are important clinical factors that may impact on the success of TEP.[91] Potential complications include severe aspiration, pharyngocutaneous fistula, and poor voice outcome.[136]

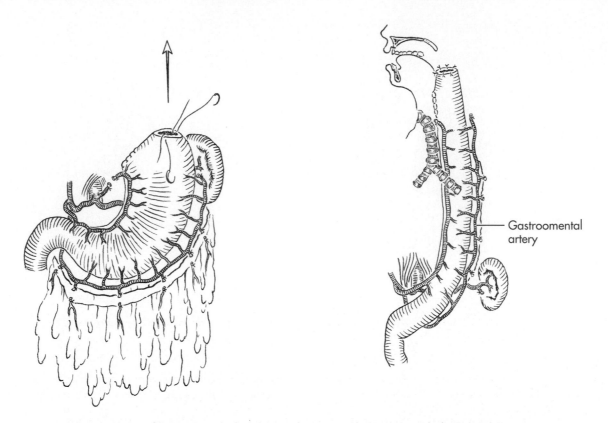

Figure 82-10. Operative steps for pharyngolaryngoesophagectomy and pharyngogastrostomy. Note that the blood supply of the transposed stomach is provided by the gastroepiploic and right gastric arteries.

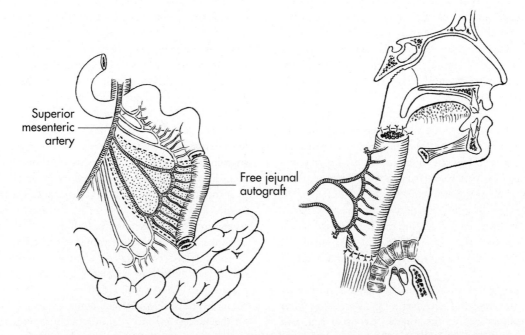

Figure 82-11. Reconstruction of total pharyngeal defect with a free segment of jejunum. The donor vessels are branches of the external carotid artery and tributaries of the internal jugular vein.

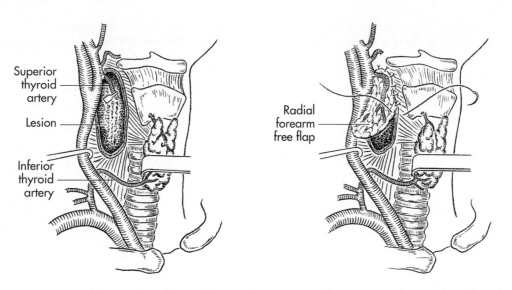

Figure 82-12. Lateral pharyngotomy and resection of posterior pharyngeal wall with preservation of the larynx. Reconstruction using a radial forearm free flap.

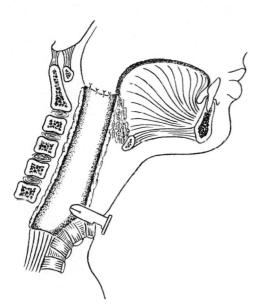

Figure 82-13. Tracheoesophageal puncture with insertion of a duckbill voice prosthesis.

OPERATIONS

CO₂ LASER EXCISION OF LARYNGEAL PAPILLOMA

Prior to the development of the laser for medical applications, recurrent papillomas of the larynx were removed with forceps via the transoral route. Laser vaporization with minimal risk of damage to normal laryngeal structures is currently the procedure of choice. Endotracheal intubation or intermittent jet ventilation allows exposure for laryngoscopy with suspension. Papillomas are vaporized under low energy to limit the possibility of damage to adjacent normal mucosa or underlying

structures within the larynx. Careful observation following the procedure is necessary to detect possible airway obstruction secondary to bleeding or edema.

EPIGLOTTOPLASTY

Hyomandibulopexy and tracheotomy were in the past the accepted treatments for infants with severe laryngomalacia. In 1987, Cotton described endoscopic epiglottoplasty, in which excision of redundant mucosa over the lateral edges of the epiglottis, aryepiglottic folds, arytenoids, and corniculate cartilages is performed via the transoral route.[163] Postoperative observation in the intensive care unit and intravenous steroids to minimize laryngeal edema may obviate the need for tracheostomy.

EXCISION OF LARYNGOCELE

Surgical excision of laryngoceles includes the lateral approach to the thyrohyoid membrane and laryngofissure in which the thyroid cartilage is divided in the midline to gain adequate exposure of the endolarynx.[91] Unless the laryngocele is massive or infected, patients can be managed without a tracheostomy. The surgical specimen should be carefully examined for the presence of occult carcinoma.

CRICOID SPLIT

Infants requiring prolonged endotracheal intubation are at high risk to develop subglottic stenosis. Microlaryngoscopy and bronchoscopy performed at the time of surgical repair identify the site of subglottic stenosis. A single midline vertical incision through the anterior cartilaginous ring of the cricoid cartilage and the upper two tracheal rings may release the stenosis.[27] Postoperative management consists of 7 to 10 days of endotracheal intubation, mechanical ventilation, neuromuscular blockade, sedation, and total parenteral nutrition followed by extubation and careful observation for stridor or obstructive apnea. Carbon dioxide laser can be used to vaporize residual granulation tissue at the level of the cricoid cartilage if necessary. Periodic postoperative micro-laryngoscopy and bronchoscopy are helpful in follow-up evaluation.[49]

LARYNGOTRACHEAL RECONSTRUCTION

A variety of techniques have been described to correct congenital or acquired subglottic stenosis, including hyoid interposition grafts, anterior and posterior costal cartilage grafts, and laser excision with long-term stenting. Our preferred method uses costal cartilage grafts to the anterior and posterior subglottis and short-term stenting as a single-stage procedure. Patients are maintained in an intensive care setting with sedation until removal of the stent. Repeated endoscopy assesses patency of the airway and the presence of granulation tissue.[25,26]

LARYNGOFISSURE

Laryngofissure is sometimes necessary to gain access and increased exposure of the larynx when the transoral route is limited. Its original use was to allow cordectomy for the management of laryngeal cancer limited to the true vocal cord[31] (Figure 82-14). The success of radiation therapy in the treatment of early vocal cord cancer has virtually eliminated laryngofissure for this purpose. It is, however, extremely useful in approach to the larynx for laryngotracheal reconstruction, exploration following laryngeal trauma, and keel placement for webs of the anterior commissure. A low collar incision is used and subplatysmal skin flaps elevated. The thyroid cartilage is exposed and divided in the midline

for access to the endolarynx (Figure 82-15). The extent of endolaryngeal resection depends on the pathology. For early vocal cord cancers confined to the true vocal cord, a cordectomy with adequate mucosal margins is satisfactory (Figure 82-16). Meticulous reapproximation of the anterior commissure is critical following laryngofissure. A nonsuction

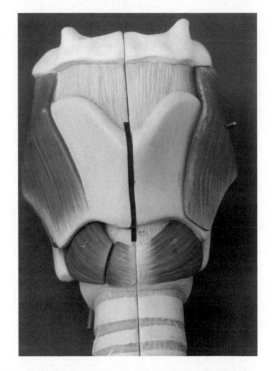

Figure 82-15. Midline thyrotomy for laryngofissure.

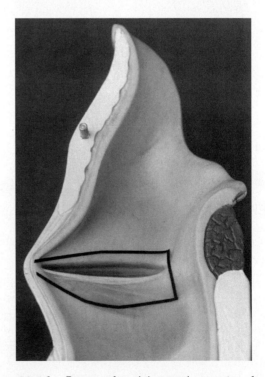

Figure 82-16. Extent of endolaryngeal resection for cordectomy.

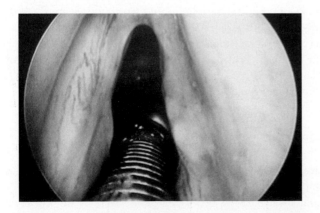

Figure 82-14. Microlaryngoscopic view of the larynx showing a localized superficial carcinoma involving the middle third of the right vocal cord.

drain is used to avoid trauma in the immediate post-operative period.[29]

LARYNGECTOMY

Total laryngectomy was first described in 1880, and subsequent modifications of supraglottic partial, vertical partial, subtotal, supracricoid with cricohyoidopexy, near-total, total laryngopharyngectomy, and laryngopharyngoesophagectomy have been described.[142,148]

VERTICAL PARTIAL LARYNGECTOMY

Early staged glottic cancers (T1, T2) with extension beyond the vocal cord or recurrent tumors of the glottic larynx, following radiotherapy, that are still confined to the hemilarynx are suitable for vertical partial laryngectomy (Figure 82-17). The extent of surgical resection in a vertical partial laryngectomy (hemilaryngectomy) is shown in Figure 82-18. The surgical specimen of hemilaryngectomy shows vocal cord cancer with subglottic extension (Figure 82-19).

SUPRACRICOID SUBTOTAL LARYNGECTOMY WITH CRICOHYOIDOEPIGLOTTOPEXY

Glottic cancers with bilateral vocal cord involvement can be resected by a supracricoid subtotal laryngectomy preserving the cricoid cartilage and at least one arytenoid. This operation can be performed as initial definitive treatment or for salvage after failure of radiotherapy (Figure 82-20). The entire thyroid cartilage is resected bilaterally to encompass the glottic larynx on both sides (Figure 82-21). The surgical specimen shows total excision of both vocal cords in a monobloc fashion with paraglottic space and thyroid cartilage intact (Figure 82-22). Reconstruction of the resultant defect requires reapproxima-

tion of the hyoid to the cricoid cartilage to achieve suspension of the laryngeal remnant. Postoperative appearance of the reconstructed larynx is shown in Figure 82-23. Most patients are able to swallow by mouth and have a reasonable airway and quality of voice.

SUPRAGLOTTIC LARYNGECTOMY

Supraglottic laryngectomy involves removal of all laryngeal structures superior to the vocal cords and below the base of

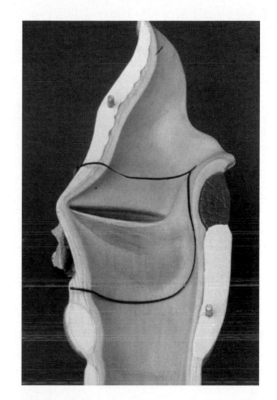

Figure 82-18. Extent of laryngeal resection for vertical partial laryngectomy (hemilaryngectomy).

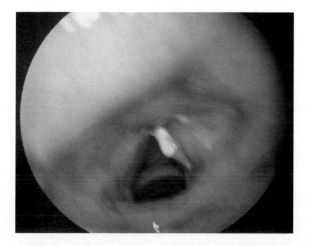

Figure 82-17. Endoscopic view of the larynx showing recurrent carcinoma of the anterior half of the right vocal cord following previous radiotherapy.

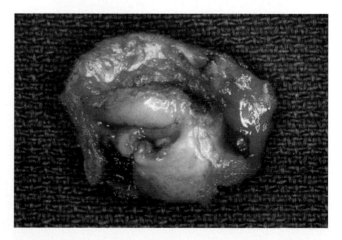

Figure 82-19. Surgical specimen of hemilaryngectomy for the tumor shown in Figure 82-17. Note subglottic extension from the vocal cord cancer.

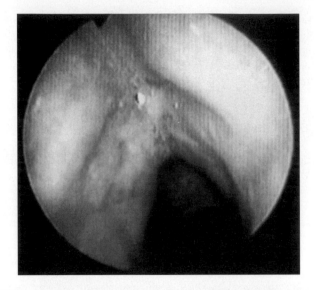

Figure 82-20. Endoscopic view of the larynx showing recurrent carcinoma involving the anterior half of both vocal cords following previous radiotherapy.

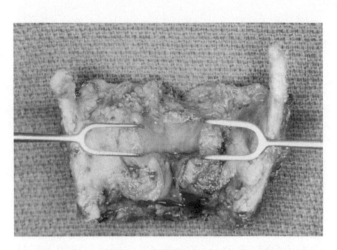

Figure 82-22. Surgical specimen of supracricoid subtotal laryngectomy showing the glottic larynx bilaterally with intact paraglottic space and thyroid cartilage.

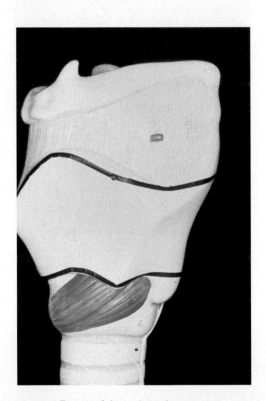

Figure 82-21. Extent of thyroid cartilage resection required for supracricoid subtotal laryngectomy.

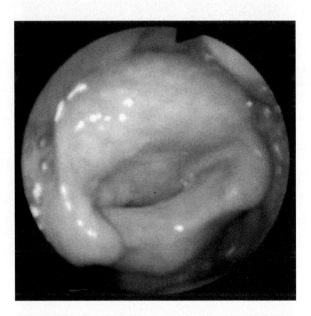

Figure 82-23. Postoperative endoscopic view of the reconstructed larynx after cricohyoidoepiglottopexy.

tongue (Figure 82-24). Endoscopic view of the larynx of a patient with squamous cell carcinoma of the laryngeal surface of the epiglottis is shown in Figure 82-25. The surgical specimen shows monobloc resection of the tumor with the preepiglottic space (Figure 82-26). Reconstruction is accomplished by approximation of the thyroid cartilage stump to the base of the tongue. This maneuver resuspends the larynx to the tongue and minimizes aspiration during swallowing. Decan-nulation can be achieved in most well-selected cases, but extension into the base of tongue and age older than 65 years predispose to significant aspiration and may necessitate total laryngectomy.[135]

Tumors that involve the infrahyoid epiglottis with preepiglottic space invasion are not amenable to supraglottic laryngectomy but may be treated with supracricoid partial laryngectomy and cricohyoidopexy.[81] This procedure is similar to the one described above and consists of resection of the thyroid cartilage, the paraglottic space, the epiglottis, and the entire preepiglottic space. The cricoid cartilage, the hyoid bone, and at least one arytenoid cartilage are spared.[21] Near-total laryngectomy with epiglottic reconstruction permits removal of

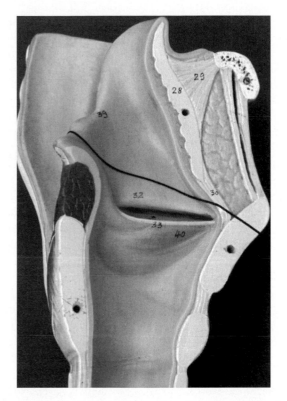

Figure 82-24. Extent of surgical resection required for supraglottic partial laryngectomy.

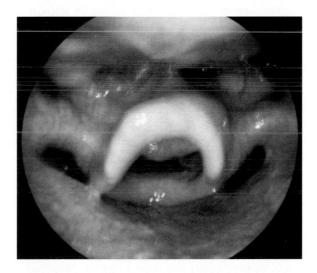

Figure 82-25. Endoscopic view of the larynx of a patient with carcinoma of the laryngeal surface of the epiglottis.

most of both vocal folds, with immediate reconstruction using the epiglottis without the need for stenting or multistage procedures.[143] This procedure usually requires permanent tracheostomy. The rationale for these subtotal laryngectomies is to preserve structures that might produce superior speech to TEP despite the fact that permanent tracheostomy is necessary.

Total laryngectomy involves the resection of the entire larynx with preservation of adequate pharyngeal mucosa for reconstruction of the pharynx. The larynx is separated from the base of tongue above the hyoid bone, from the trachea between

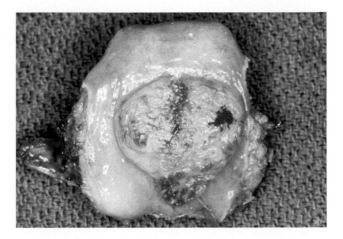

Figure 82-26. Surgical specimen of supraglottic partial laryngectomy for the tumor shown in Figure 82-25. Note adequate mucosal margins and monobloc resection of the preepiglottic space with the primary tumor.

the second and third tracheal ring, and from the pharynx at the posterior aspect of the thyroid cartilage alae. The pharyngeal defect is repaired by primary closure if sufficient pharyngeal mucosa is available.[68] Single-or multiple-layer closure of the pharyngeal remnant is acceptable.[23] A tracheostome is created in the anterior neck.

Some authors recommend cricopharyngeal myotomy in combination with laryngectomy to enhance the free flow of saliva and secretions past the pharyngeal repair into the upper esophagus and improve voice restoration by creating a more patulous conduit for airflow.[66] Hemithyroidectomy is performed when there is extension of tumor into the thyroid cartilage, soft tissues of the neck, pharynx, cervical esophagus, or subglottic region. The thyroid gland should be preserved when the laryngeal tumor is confined to the supraglottic and glottic regions without clinical evidence of thyroid gland involvement. Similarly, careful attention to parathyroid anatomy and their preservation is crucial in all laryngeal surgery.[161]

Resection of the pharynx and/or cervical esophagus in combination with total laryngectomy requires regional or free flap reconstruction to maintain the upper aerodigestive tract continuity. Preoperative care consists of appropriate counseling about the nature of the surgery, subsequent deformity, and alteration in the ability to communicate. Broad-spectrum antibiotics in the perioperative period have been shown to decrease the incidence of wound infection. Suction drainage is maintained until wound drainage is minimal, and patients receive nutrition via a small-diameter, soft nasogastric tube or percutaneous endoscopic gastrostomy, until oral feeding is initiated usually at 10 to 14 days.

THYROPLASTY

Thyroplasty, a technique of vocal cord medialization, was described in 1974 by Isshiki[70] for improvement in the quality of voice and to reduce aspiration in patients with a paralyzed vocal cord. It can be performed under local anesthesia, with fiberoptic laryngoscopy used to guide implant placement. The addition of arytenoid adduction improves vocal quality in patients with gaps in the posterior glottis. An incision is made over the thyroid cartilage and a small window placed in the thyroid lamina. The inner perichondrium is elevated and a Silastic implant positioned within the window to push the paralyzed vocal cord medially.

OUTCOMES

Unilateral carbon dioxide laser removal of redundant supraglottic tissue (supraglottoplasty) is effective in nearly all children with obstructive apnea, failure to thrive, cyanosis, and/or cor pulmonale secondary to severe laryngomalacia, and has a minimal risk of complications. A small percentage of patients will require a contralateral procedure.[75] Both aryepiglottoplasty and epiglottoplasty are effective as well, but bilateral supraglottoplasty increases the risk of complications.[72] Hemangiomas of the larynx often undergo involution over time or following steroid therapy but if resistant may require systemic interferon or laser photocoagulation. Results following repair of laryngeal clefts are more unpredictable and there is a paucity of outcome data in the literature for this rare entity. An initially successful surgical result can be compromised by postoperative aspiration, due to gastroesophageal reflux and impaired swallowing as a result of the cleft repair or preexistent abnormalities of the swallowing reflex.[61] Other congenital anomalies, such as laryngeal cysts, respond well to laser vaporization or marsupialization.[4]

Laser excision of mild subglottic stenosis as the treatment for stridor is effective in the majority of patients.[154] Laryngotracheal reconstruction with costal cartilage grafts in the anterior and posterior subglottis and stent placement for tracheotomy-dependent patients with moderate and severe laryngotracheal stenosis (Cotton grades III and IV) results in a better than 90% decannulation rate.[162] Partial cricoid resection with or without resection of trachea and primary tracheal anastomosis achieves a similar rate of decannulation. Vocal quality and exercise tolerance following cricoid resection are reported as normal in the majority of cases.[50] The complications of this procedure include pneumothorax, granulation tissue formation, and restenosis.[162] Strictures of the upper airway caused by burns are best managed with prolonged T-tube placement followed by resection after maturation of the scar. Of those patients who undergo resection, approximately 50% to 75% can be permanently decannulated, with a functional airway and adequate voice in most patients.[53]

Most laryngeal infections are adequately treated with antimicrobial agents and surgery is rarely indicated. Surgical intervention may, however, be necessary for patients with symptomatic subglottic stenosis secondary to Wegener's granulomatosis. Cartilage graft augmentation or primary thyrotracheal anastomosis during clinical remission is frequently successful despite concurrent use of prednisone and cyclophosphamide. Several small series report no evidence of local recurrence of granulomas following resection and reconstruction. The prognosis for recurrent laryngeal papillomas is determined in part by the extent of disease. Solitary lesions respond well to laser vaporization, but extensive disease requires repeated laser treatments with frequent recurrence and occasional malignant transformation.[16]

The results of treatment of benign laryngeal neoplasms is essentially anecdotal in the medical literature due to the rarity of these entities.

Outcome data for the treatment of malignant neoplasms of the larynx have focused on the effects of various clinical variables and treatments on patient survival and function. Factors associated with treatment failure above the clavicles include advanced tumor stage and the presence of nodal disease,[103] lymph node metastasis in the laryngectomy specimen (Delphian, pretracheal, tracheoesophageal, parathyroid), primary tumor more than 1.5 cm in greatest diameter, and subglottic extension.[46] Distant metastasis is associated with the presence of extracapsular spread of cancer within regional lymph nodes.[73] Recurrence at the tracheostoma is more common after salvage laryngectomy and is associated with advanced stage, bulky nodal disease, subglottic involvement, and possibly preoperative tracheostomy in patients treated with primary laryngectomy.[165] Elective neck dissection may offer some survival benefit in patients with T4 larynx cancer when compared with patients treated with total laryngectomy alone. In addition to the above parameters, long-term survival in patients with cancer of the larynx as with other upper aerodigestive sites is impacted by presentation of second primary cancers.[28] Five-year disease-free survival rates vary based on treatment technique and the use of adjuvant therapy, but for early vocal cord cancer (T1), they approach 95% regardless of therapy (endoscopic excision or external radiation therapy).[117] Survival at 5 years decreases to 80% to 90% in patients with T2 vocal cord cancer and 60% to 80% for T3 tumors.[21] Survival following total laryngectomy for all stages ranges from 35% to 50% at 5 years following treatment.[55] Organ preservation protocols offer cure rates comparable to surgical treatment but do not appear to improve local/regional tumor control or survival despite careful patient selection criteria.[41] Approximately one third of patients enrolled have successful preservation of the larynx, although voice quality is not uniformly excellent.[132]

Bilateral modified neck dissection performed in conjunction with supraglottic laryngectomy and postoperative radiation therapy does not appear to increase postoperative surgical morbidity.[149] Supraglottic laryngectomy with neck dissection offers improved locoregional control when compared with primary radiation therapy in patients who present with regional lymph node metastases.[56] Resection of the arytenoid cartilage is frequently associated with prolonged swallowing difficulty and aspiration is common.[54] Although subglottic cancer has a reputation for a dismal prognosis, the 5-year survival rates approach 70% in several small series.[52,60]

Surgical salvage for nonlaryngeal primaries (i.e., pharynx) who fail organ preservation is poor, although some patients can be effectively palliated.

Functional swallowing is usually achieved within 1 to 3 months of surgery for patients treated with vertical partial laryngectomy or total laryngectomy. Supraglottic laryngectomy, particularly with tongue base resection, is more problematic and significant swallowing impairment frequently persists up to 9 months. Early radiographic assessments of swallowing function are sometimes useful in predicting the time to swallow recovery. Prolonged swallowing dysfunction is common in patients who have not achieved oral intake prior to initiation of radiotherapy.[120] Intelligible fluent speech is obtained in 60% to 70% of patients within 1 to 6 months following near-total or total laryngectomy and immediate TEP.[55] Successful long-term prosthesis use is most common in patients who achieve good voice quality early and do not have a pharyngeal stricture.[87] Psychologic and socioeconomic factors play a significant role in patients unable to manage a tracheoesophageal prosthesis.[88]

Complications of surgical treatment of advanced laryngeal cancer include pharyngocutaneous fistulas, tracheostomal stenosis, and pharyngeal stenosis or spasm.[28,30,82] Pharyngocutaneous fistulas occur in 15% to 30% of laryngectomies for glottic and supraglottic cancer and are related to advanced disease, preoperative radiotherapy, wound sepsis, surgical technique, and patient nutritional status.[15,145] Fistulas in previously radiated patients are more likely to require surgical repair.[102] The timing of oral feeding after surgery or postoperative vomiting does not appear to contribute to fistula development.[140] Gastroesophageal reflux may predispose to fistula formation after laryngectomy, and mechanical and pharmacologic prophylaxis including antibiotics may decrease postoperative morbidity and length of hospital stay.[129,144] Pharyngocutaneous fistulas usually respond to conservative treatment consisting of local wound care and antibiotics, but occasionally regional or microvascular flaps are required for closure.

The incidence of tracheostomal stenosis ranges from 4% to 42%. The most important factors in prevention of stomal stenosis after laryngectomy are meticulous surgical technique and careful attention to tissue blood supply during stoma creation. Stomaplasty by various techniques is usually successful.[148] Pharyngeal stenosis frequently responds to serial dilation but may require surgery.[30] Management of patients with pharyngeal constrictor spasm following laryngectomy includes bougienage, pharyngeal myotomy, and/or pharyngeal neurectomy.[13] Pharyngeal myotomy as an adjunct to TEP is effective in selected patients.[69] Transcutaneous injection of botulinum toxin may improve voice and swallowing function.[28]

The most common sites for recurrence following total laryngectomy for advanced laryngeal carcinoma are the pharynx, regional lymph nodes, stoma, and lungs.[160] Treatment failure can occur within the undissected ipsilateral or contralateral neck despite previous adjuvant radiotherapy. Subglottic extension and nodal metastases are associated with failure above the clavicles and delayed metastasis within an undissected neck.[47] Peristomal recurrence is a particularly ominous finding and is thought to be related to paratracheal lymph node (PTLN) metastasis or submucosal extension rather than cancer cell implantation.[67,159] The incidence of peristomal recurrence is diminished by routine pretracheal, paratracheal, and mediastinal lymph node dissection and inclusion of these lymph node areas in radiation therapy portals. Pharyngeal recurrence has the highest salvage rate, followed by nodal, pulmonary, and peristomal recurrence.[160] Investigations into the quality of life for patients with laryngeal cancer are in development. Severe psychosocial distress as a result of problems with effective communication, dysphagia, disfigurement, decreased social acceptance and thus decreased social and sexual activity, and severe financial repercussions from loss of wages and expensive treatment are all important issues.[35] Even patients with early larynx cancer experience persistent physical complaints several years following therapy.[33] In spite of these problems the majority of patients are willing to accept a total laryngectomy as treatment of their cancer. Laryngectomy patients in particular need psychosocial guidance for an extended period following cancer treatment and will benefit from improved cooperation between physicians and therapists.[37]

REFERENCES

1. al-Orieschan AT, Mahasin ZZ, Gangopadhyay K, et al: Schwannoma of the larynx: two case reports and review of the literature, *J Otolaryngol* 25(6):412-415, 1996.

2. Andryk J, Freije JE, Schultz CJ, et al: Lymphoepithelioma of the larynx, *Am J Otolaryngol* 17(1):61-63, 1996.

3. Anthony JP, Singer MI, Deschler DG, et al: Long-term functional results after pharyngoesophageal reconstruction with the radial forearm free flap, *Am J Surg* 168(5):441-445, 1994.

4. Bagwell CE: CO$_2$ laser excision of pediatric airway lesions, *J Pediatr Surg* 25(11):1152-1156, 1990.

5. Balazic J, Masera A, Poljak M: Sudden death caused by laryngeal papillomatosis, *Acta Otolaryngol Suppl (Stockh)* 527:111-113, 1997.

6. Bauman NM, Smith RJ: Recurrent respiratory papillomatosis, *Pediatr Clin North Am* 43(6):1385-1401, 1996.

7. Baxter MR: Congenital laryngomalacia, *Can J Anaesth* 41(4):332-339, 1994.

8. Benjamin B, Robb P, Clifford A, et al: Giant Teflon granuloma of the larynx, *Head Neck* 13(5):453-456, 1991.

9. Berger G, Harwood AR, Bryce DP, et al: Primary subglottic carcinoma masquerading clinically as T1 glottic carcinoma—a report of nine cases, *J Otolaryngol* 14(1):1-6, 1985.

10. Berkowitz RG: Laryngeal electromyography findings in idiopathic congenital bilateral vocal cord paralysis, *Ann Otol Rhinol Laryngol* 105(3):207-212, 1996.

11. Biavati MJ, Wood WE, Kearns DB, et al: One-stage repair of congenital laryngeal webs, *Otolaryngol Head Neck Surg* 112(3):447-452, 1995.

12. Blackwell KE, Calcaterra TC, Fu YS: Laryngeal dysplasia: epidemiology and treatment outcome, *Ann Otol Rhinol Laryngol* 104(8):596-602, 1995.

13. Blitzer A, Komisar A, Baredes S, et al: Voice failure after tracheoesophageal puncture: management with botulinum toxin, *Otolaryngol Head Neck Surg* 113(6):668-670, 1995.

14. Bough ID Jr, Chiles PJ, Fratalli MA, et al: Laryngeal chondrosarcoma: two unusual cases, *Am J Otolaryngol* 16(2):126-131, 1995.

15. Boyce SE, Meyers AD: Oral feeding after total laryngectomy, *Head Neck* 11(3):269-273, 1989.

16. Capper JW, Bailey CM, Michaels L: Squamous papillomas of the larynx in adults: a review of 63 cases, *Clin Otolaryngol* 8(2):109-119, 1983.

17. Castelijns JA, Becker M, Hermans R: Impact of cartilage invasion on treatment and prognosis of laryngeal cancer, *Eur Radiol* 6(2):156-169, 1996.

18. Castelijns JA, van den Brekel MW, Niekoop VA, et al: Imaging of the larynx, *Neuroimaging Clin N Am* 6(2):401-415, 1996.

19. Chaloryoo S: Laryngotracheoesophageal cleft, *J Med Assoc Thai* 77(4):220-224, 1994.

20. Chen JC, Holinger LD: Congenital laryngeal lesions: pathology study using serial macrosections and review of the literature, *Pediatr Pathol* 14(2):301-325, 1994.

21. Chevalier D, Piquet JJ: Subtotal laryngectomy with cricohyoidopexy for supraglottic carcinoma: review of 61 cases, *Am J Surg* 168(5):472-473, 1994.

22. Chu L, Gussack GS, Orr JB, et al: Neonatal laryngoceles: a cause for airway obstruction, *Arch Otolaryngol Head Neck Surg* 120(4):454-458, 1994.

23. Clevens RA, Esclamado RM, Hartshorn DO, et al: Voice rehabilitation after total laryngectomy and tracheoesophageal puncture using nonmuscle closure, *Ann Otol Rhinol Laryngol* 102(10):792-796, 1993.

24. Corbally MT, Fitzgerald RJ, Guiney EJ, et al: Laryngotracheo-oesophageal cleft: a plea for early diagnosis, *Eur J Pediatr Surg* 3(4):241-243, 1993.

25. Cotton RT: Prevention and management of laryngeal stenosis in infants and children, *J Pediatr Surg* 20(6):845-851, 1985.

26. Cotton RT, Myer CM III: Contemporary surgical management of laryngeal stenosis in children, *Am J Otolaryngol* 5(5):360-368, 1984.

27. Cotton RT, Seid AB: Management of the extubation problem in the premature child: anterior cricoid split as an alternative to tracheotomy, *Ann Otol Rhinol Laryngol* 89(6 Pt 1):508-511, 1980.

28. Crary MA, Glowasky AL: Using botulinum toxin A to improve speech and swallowing function following total laryngectomy, *Arch Otolaryngol Head Neck Surg* 122(7):760-763, 1996.

29. Crysdale WS: Extended laryngofissure in the management of subglottic stenosis in the young child: a preliminary report, *J Otolaryngol* 5(6):479-486, 1976.

30. Cusumano RJ, Silver CE, Brauer RJ, et al: Pectoralis myocutaneous flap for replacement of cervical esophagus, *Head Neck* 11(5):450-456, 1989.

31. Daly JF, Kwok FN: Laryngofissure and cordectomy, *Laryngoscope* 85(8):1290-1297, 1975.

32. Davidoff AM, Filston HC: Treatment of infantile subglottic hemangioma with electrocautery, *J Pediatr Surg* 27(4):436-439, 1992.

33. de Boer MF, Pruyn JF, van den Borne B, et al: Rehabilitation outcomes of long-term survivors treated for head and neck cancer, *Head Neck* 17(6):503-515, 1995.

34. Delaere P, Feenstra L: Management of acute laryngeal trauma, *Acta Otorhinolaryngol Belg* 49(4):347-349, 1995.

35. Deshmane VH, Parikh HK, Pinni S, et al: Laryngectomy: a quality of life assessment, *Indian J Cancer* 32(3):121-130, 1995.

36. Deveney CW, Benner K, Cohen J: Gastroesophageal reflux and laryngeal disease, *Arch Surg* 128(9):1021-1025; discussion 1026-1027, 1993.

37. Devins GM, Stam HJ, Koopmans JP: Psychosocial impact of laryngectomy mediated by perceived stigma and illness intrusiveness, *Can J Psychiatry* 39(10):608-616, 1994.

38. Diebold J, Audouin J, Viry B, et al: Primary lymphoplasmacytic lymphoma of the larynx: a rare localization of MALT-type lymphoma, *Ann Otol Rhinol Laryngol* 99(7 Pt 1):577-580, 1990.

39. Donnelly MJ, Timon CI, McShane DP: The role of total laryngectomy in the management of intraluminal upper airway invasion by well-differentiated thyroid carcinoma, *Ear Nose Throat J* 73(9):659-662, 1994.

40. Donovan DT, Conley J: Adenoid cystic carcinoma of the subglottic region, *Ann Otol Rhinol Laryngol* 92(5 Pt 1):491-495, 1983.

41. Eisbruch A, Thornton AF, Urba S, et al: Chemotherapy followed by accelerated fractionated radiation for larynx preservation in patients with advanced laryngeal cancer, *J Clin Oncol* 14(8):2322-2330, 1996.

42. Evans KL, Courteney-Harris R, Bailey CM, et al: Management of posterior laryngeal and laryngotracheo-esophageal clefts, *Arch Otolaryngol Head Neck Surg* 121(12):1380-1385, 1995.

43. Ferlito A, Nicolai P, Recher G, et al: Primary laryngeal malignant fibrous histiocytoma: review of the literature and report of seven cases, *Laryngoscope* 93(10):1351-1358, 1983.

44. Fine ED, Dahmas B, Arnold JE: Laryngeal hamartoma: a rare congenital abnormality, *Ann Otol Rhinol Laryngol* 104(2):87-89, 1995.

45. Fini-Storchi I, Frosini P: Laryngeal neurinoma: a case report and review, *ORL J Otorhinolaryngol Relat Spec* 59(3):182-185, 1997.

46. Foote RL, Buskirk SJ, Stanley RJ, et al: Patterns of failure after total laryngectomy for glottic carcinoma, *Cancer* 64(1):143-149, 1989.

47. Foote RL, Olsen KD, Buskirk SJ, et al: Laryngectomy alone for T3 glottic cancer, *Head Neck* 16(5):406-412, 1994.

48. Ford HR, Gardner MJ, Lynch JM: Laryngotracheal disruption from blunt pediatric neck injuries: impact of early recognition and intervention on outcome, *J Pediatr Surg* 30(2):331-334; discussion 334-335, 1995.

49. Frankel LR, Anas NG, Perkin RM, et al: Use of the anterior cricoid split operation in infants with acquired subglottic stenosis, *Crit Care Med* 12(4):395-398, 1984.

50. Froehlich P, Truy E, Stamm D, et al: Role of long-term stenting in treatment of pediatric subglottic stenosis, *Int J Pediatr Otorhinolaryngol* 27(3):273-280, 1993.

51. Gacek M, Gacek RR: Cricoarytenoid joint mobility after chronic vocal cord paralysis, *Laryngoscope* 106(12 Pt 1):1528-1530, 1996.

52. Gairola A, Bahadur S, Tandon DA: Primary subglottic carcinoma, *Indian J Cancer* 29(3):143-147, 1992.

53. Gaissert HA, Lofgren RH, Grillo HC: Upper airway compromise after inhalation injury: complex strictures of the larynx and trachea and their management, *Ann Surg* 218(5):672-678, 1993.

54. Gehanno P, Barry B, Guedon C, et al: Lateral supraglottic pharyngo-laryngectomy with arytenoidectomy, *Head Neck* 18(6):494-500, 1996.

55. Geraghty JA, Wenig BL, Smith BE, et al: Long-term follow-up of tracheoesophageal puncture results, *Ann Otol Rhinol Laryngol* 105(7):501-503, 1996.

56. Gregor RT, Oei SS, Baris G, et al: Supraglottic laryngectomy with postoperative radiation versus primary radiation in the management of supraglottic laryngeal cancer, *Am J Otolaryngol* 17(5):316-321, 1996.

57. Grewal H, Rao PM, Mukerji S, et al: Management of penetrating laryngotracheal injuries, *Head Neck* 17(6):494-502, 1995.

58. Guttenplan MD, Hendrix RA, Townsend MJ, et al: Laryngeal manifestations of gout, *Ann Otol Rhinol Laryngol* 100(11):899-902, 1991.

59. Hayes CW, Conway WF, Walsh JW, et al: Seat belt injuries: radiologic findings and clinical correlation, *Radiographics* 11(1):23-36, 1991.

60. Haylock BJ, Deutsch GP: Primary radiotherapy for subglottic carcinoma, *Clin Oncol (R Coll Radiol)* 5(3):143-146, 1993.

61. Hedrick MH, Ferro MM, Filly RA, et al: Congenital high airway obstruction syndrome (CHAOS): a potential for perinatal intervention, *J Pediatr Surg* 29(2):271-274, 1994.

62. Hengerer AS, Strome M, Jaffe BF: Injuries to the neonatal larynx from long-term endotracheal tube intubation and suggested tube modification for prevention, *Ann Otol Rhinol Laryngol* 84(6):764-770, 1975.

63. Herranz-Gonzalez J, Gavilan J, Matinez-Vidal J, et al: Complications following thyroid surgery, *Arch Otolaryngol Head Neck Surg* 117(5):516-518, 1991.

64. Hoeve LJ, Eskici O, Verwoerd CD: Therapeutic reintubation for post-intubation laryngotracheal injury in preterm infants, *Int J Pediatr Otorhinolaryngol* 31(1):7-13, 1995.

65. Hoffman HT, Brunberg JA, Winter P, et al: Arytenoid subluxation: diagnosis and treatment, *Ann Otol Rhinol Laryngol* 100(1):1-9, 1991.

66. Horowitz JB, Sasaki CT: Effect of cricopharyngeus myotomy on postlaryngectomy pharyngeal contraction pressures, *Laryngoscope* 103(2):138-140, 1993.

67. Hosal IN, Onerci M, Turan E: Peristomal recurrence, *Am J Otolaryngol* 14(3):206-208, 1993.

68. Hui Y, Wei WI, Yuen PW, et al: Primary closure of pharyngeal remnant after total laryngectomy and partial pharyngectomy: how much residual mucosa is sufficient? *Laryngoscope* 106(4):490-494, 1996.

69. Huo J, Klastsky I, Labruna A, et al: Secondary pharyngeal myotomy for tracheoesophageal speech, *Ear Nose Throat J* 74(6):405-408, 1995.

70. Isshiki N, Morita H, Okamura H, et al: Thyroplasty as a new phonosurgical technique, *Acta Otolaryngol (Stockh)* 78(5-6):451-457, 1974.

71. Iwatake H, Iida J, Minami S, et al: Transcutaneous intracordal silicon injection for unilateral vocal cord paralysis, *Acta Otolaryngol Suppl (Stockh)* 522:133-137, 1996.

72. Jani P, Koltai P, Ochi JW, et al: Surgical treatment of laryngomalacia, *J Laryngol Otol* 105(12):1040-1045, 1991.

73. Johnson JT, Myers EN, Hao SP, et al: Outcome of open surgical therapy for glottic carcinoma, *Ann Otol Rhinol Laryngol* 102(10):752-755, 1993.

74. Katsounakis J, Remy H, Vuong T, et al: Impact of magnetic resonance imaging and computed tomography on the staging of laryngeal cancer, *Eur Arch Otorhinolaryngol* 252(4):206-208, 1995.

75. Kelly SM, Gray SD: Unilateral endoscopic supraglottoplasty for severe laryngomalacia, *Arch Otolaryngol Head Neck Surg* 121(12):1351-1354, 1995.

76. Kingdom TT, Lee KC: Invasive aspergillosis of the larynx in AIDS, *Otolaryngol Head Neck Surg* 115(1):135-137, 1996.

77. Kirchner JA: Fifteenth Daniel C. Baker, Jr, memorial lecture: what have whole organ sections contributed to the treatment of laryngeal cancer? *Ann Otol Rhinol Laryngol* 98(9):661-667, 1989.

78. Kligerman J, Olivatto LO, Lima RA, et al: Elective neck dissection in the treatment of T3/T4 N0 squamous cell carcinoma of the larynx, *Am J Surg* 170(5):436-439, 1995.

79. Kooper DP, van den Broek P, Manni JJ, et al: Partial vertical laryngectomy for recurrent glottic carcinoma, *Clin Otolaryngol* 20(2):167-170, 1995.

80. Krajina Z, Lenarcic-Cepelja I, Vranesic D, et al: Investigations in exaggerated juvenile laryngeal papillomas, *Acta Otolaryngol (Stockh)* 105(5-6):483-487, 1988.

81. Laccourreye O, Brasnu D, Merite-Drancy A, et al: Cricohyoidopexy in selected infrahyoid epiglottic carcinomas presenting with pathological preepiglottic space invasion, *Arch Otolaryngol Head Neck Surg* 119(8):881-886, 1993.

82. Laccourreye O, Weinstein G, Naudo P, et al: Supracricoid partial laryngectomy after failed laryngeal radiation therapy, *Laryngoscope* 106(4):495-498, 1996.

83. Lacoste L, Karayan J, Lehuede MS, et al: A comparison of direct, indirect, and fiberoptic laryngoscopy to evaluate vocal cord paralysis after thyroid surgery, *Thyroid* 6(1):17-21, 1996.

84. Lancer JM, Syder D, Jones AS, et al: Vocal cord nodules: a review, *Clin Otolaryngol* 13(1):43-51, 1988.

85. Lancer JM, Syder D, Jones AS, et al: The outcome of different management patterns for vocal cord nodules, *J Laryngol Otol* 102(5):423-427, 1988.

86. Larson DL, Cohn AM: Management of acute laryngeal injury: a critical review, *J Trauma* 16(11):858-862, 1976.

87. Lavertu P, Guay ME, Meeker SS, et al: Secondary tracheoesophageal puncture: factors predictive of voice quality and prosthesis use, *Head Neck* 18(5):393-398, 1996.

88. Lentin R, Williams G, Sellars SL: Postlaryngectomy voice restoration—a 2-year review, *S Afr J Surg* 33(4):183-185, 1995.

89. Lerner DM, Deeb Z: Acute upper airway obstruction resulting from systemic diseases, *South Med J* 86(6):623-627, 1993.

90. Lin KY, Westra WH, Kashima HK, et al: Coinfection of HPV-11 and HPV-16 in a case of laryngeal squamous papillomas with severe dysplasia, *Laryngoscope* 107(7):942-947, 1997.

91. Lindell MM Jr, Jing BS, Fischer EP, et al: Laryngocele, *AJR Am J Roentgenol* 131(2):259-262, 1978.

92. Lindell MM Jr, Jing BS, Wallace S: Laryngeal tuberculosis, *AJR Am J Roentgenol* 129(4):677-680, 1977.

93. Lis G, Szczerbinski T, Cichocka-Jarosz E: Congenital stridor, *Pediatr Pulmonol* 20(4):220-224, 1995.

94. Lopez-Amado M, Yebra-Pimentel MT, Garcia-Sarandeses A: Cytomegalovirus causing necrotizing laryngitis in a renal and cardiac transplant recipient, *Head Neck* 18(5):455-457; discussion 457-458, 1996.

95. Luzar B, Gale N, Kambic V, et al: Human papillomavirus infection and expression of p53 and c-erbB-2 protein in laryngeal papillomas, *Acta Otolaryngol Suppl (Stockh)* 527:120-124, 1997.

96. Lydiatt WM, Shah JP, Lydiatt KM: Conservation surgery for recurrent carcinoma of the glottic larynx, *Am J Surg* 172(6):662-664, 1996.

97. MacArthur CJ, Kearns GH, Healy GB: Voice quality after laryngotracheal reconstruction, *Arch Otolaryngol Head Neck Surg* 120(6):641-647, 1994.

98. Maniglia AJ, Leder SB, Goodwin WJ Jr, et al: Tracheogastric puncture for vocal rehabilitation following total pharyngolaryngoesophagectomy, *Head Neck* 11(6):524-527, 1989.

99. Manni JJ, Mulder JJ, Schaafsma HE, et al: Inflammatory pseudotumor of the subglottis, *Eur Arch Otorhinolaryngol* 249(1):16-19, 1992.

100. Martin DS, Stith J, Awwad EE, et al: MR in neurofibromatosis of the larynx, *AJNR Am J Neuroradiol* 16(3):503-506, 1995.

101. Martin-Hirsch DP, Lannigan FJ, Irani B, et al: Oncocytic papillary cystadenomatosis of the larynx, *J Laryngol Otol* 106(7):656-658, 1992.

102. McCombe AW, Jones AS: Radiotherapy and complications of laryngectomy, *J Laryngol Otol* 107(2):130-132, 1993.

103. McLean M: Primary management of limited laryngeal cancer by radiotherapy and surgical salvage: results of 164 cases treated in a district hospital, *Clin Oncol (R Coll Radiol)* 1(2):97-100, 1989.

104. Mendelsohn M, Morris M, Gallagher R: A comparative study of speech after total laryngectomy and total laryngopharyngectomy, *Arch Otolaryngol Head Neck Surg* 119(5):508-510, 1993.

105. Meyer PR, Shum TK, Becker TS, et al: Scleroma (rhinoscleroma): a histologic immunohistochemical study with bacteriologic correlates, *Arch Pathol Lab Med* 107(7):377-383, 1983.

106. Milford CA, Mugliston TA, O'Flynn P, et al: Carcinoma arising in a pleomorphic adenoma of the epiglottis, *J Laryngol Otol* 103(3):324-327, 1989.

107. Milton CM: Sarcoidosis in ENT practice, *Clin Otolaryngol* 10(6):351-355, 1985.

108. Moe K, Wolf GT, Fisher SG, et al: Regional metastases in patients with advanced laryngeal cancer. Department of Veterans Affairs Laryngeal Cancer Study Group, *Arch Otolaryngol Head Neck Surg* 122(6):644-648, 1996.

109. Monnier P, Savary M, Chapuis G: Partial cricoid resection with primary tracheal anastomosis for subglottic stenosis in infants and children, *Laryngoscope* 103(11 Pt 1):1273-1283, 1993.

110. Nakayama M, Brandenburg JH: Clinical underestimation of laryngeal cancer: predictive indicators, *Arch Otolaryngol Head Neck Surg* 119(9):950-957, 1993.

111. Narula AA, Sheppard IJ, West K, et al: Is emergency laryngectomy a waste of time? *Am J Otolaryngol* 14(1):21-23, 1993.

112. O'Keeffe LJ, Maw AR: The dangers of minor blunt laryngeal trauma, *J Laryngol Otol* 106(4):372-373, 1992.

113. Olson NR: Skin grafting of the larynx, *Otolaryngol Head Neck Surg* 104(4):503-508, 1991.

114. Orphanidou D, Dimakou K, Latsi P, et al: Recurrent respiratory papillomatosis with malignant transformation in a young adult, *Respir Med* 90(1):53-55, 1996.

115. Osguthorpe JD: Head and neck burns: evaluation and current management, *Arch Otolaryngol Head Neck Surg* 117(9):969-974, 1991.

116. Pak MW, Woo JK, van Hasselt CA: Congenital laryngeal cysts: current approach to management, *J Laryngol Otol* 110(9):854-856, 1996.

117. Peretti G, Cappiello J, Nicolai P, et al: Endoscopic laser excisional biopsy for selected glottic carcinomas, *Laryngoscope* 104(10):1276-1279, 1994.

118. Potter CR, Sessions DG, Ogura JH: Blunt laryngotracheal trauma, *Otolaryngology* 86(6 Pt 1):ORL-909-923, 1978.

119. Prescott CA: Bifid epiglottis: a case report, *Int J Pediatr Otorhinolaryngol* 30(2):167-170, 1994.

120. Rademaker AW, Logemann JA, Pauloski BR, et al: Recovery of postoperative swallowing in patients undergoing partial laryngectomy, *Head Neck* 15(4):325-334, 1993.

121. Reidenbach MM: Normal topography of the conus elasticus: anatomical bases for the spread of laryngeal cancer, *Surg Radiol Anat* 17(2):107-111, 4-5, 1995.

122. Reuter VE, Woodruff JM: Melanoma of the larynx, *Laryngoscope* 96(4):389-393, 1986.

123. Rice DH: Vertical partial laryngectomy without tracheotomy: the use of the Cook airway exchange catheter to avoid tracheotomy, *Ann Otol Rhinol Laryngol* 105(12):933-935, 1996.

124. Roberts DN, Corbett MJ, Breen D, et al: Rhabdomyoma of the larynx: a rare cause of stridor, *J Laryngol Otol* 108(8):713-715, 1994.

125. Santos PM, Afrassiabi A, Weymuller EA Jr: Risk factors associated with prolonged intubation and laryngeal injury, *Otolaryngol Head Neck Surg* 111(4):453-459, 1994.

126. Scott JC, Jones B, Eisele DW, et al: Caustic ingestion injuries of the upper aerodigestive tract, *Laryngoscope* 102(1):1-8, 1992.

127. Seals JL, Shenefelt RE, Babin RW: Intralaryngeal nevus in a child: a case report, *Int J Pediatr Otorhinolaryngol* 12(1):55-58, 1986.

128. Seikaly H, Cuyler JP: Infantile subglottic hemangioma, *J Otolaryngol* 23(2):135-137, 1994.

129. Seikaly H, Park P: Gastroesophageal reflux prophylaxis decreases the incidence of pharyngocutaneous fistula after total laryngectomy, *Laryngoscope* 105(11):1220-1222, 1995.

130. Shaha AR, Shah JP: Carcinoma of the subglottic larynx, *Am J Surg* 144(4):456-458, 1982.

131. Shapshay SM, Rebeiz EE, Bohigian RK, et al: Benign lesions of the larynx: should the laser be used? *Laryngoscope* 100(9): 953-957, 1990.

132. Shirinian MH, Weber RS, Lippman SM, et al: Laryngeal preservation by induction chemotherapy plus radiotherapy in locally advanced head and neck cancer: the M.D. Anderson Cancer Center experience, *Head Neck* 16(1):39-44, 1994.

133. Singer MI, Hamaker RC, Blom ED, et al: Applications of the voice prosthesis during laryngectomy, *Ann Otol Rhinol Laryngol* 98:921-925, 1989.

134. Stack BC Jr, Ridley MB: Arytenoid subluxation from blunt laryngeal trauma, *Am J Otolaryngol* 15(1):68-73, 1994.

135. Suarez C, Rodrigo JP, Herranz J, et al: Complications of supraglottic laryngectomy for carcinomas of the supraglottis and the base of the tongue, *Clin Otolaryngol* 21(1):87-90, 1996.

136. Suits GW, Cohen JI, Everts EC: Near-total laryngectomy: patient selection and technical considerations, *Arch Otolaryngol Head Neck Surg* 122(5):473-475, 1996.

137. Teitel AD, MacKenzie CR, Stern R, et al: Laryngeal involvement in systemic lupus erythematosus, *Semin Arthritis Rheum* 22(3):203-214, 1992.

138. Thomas R, Kumar EV, Kameswaran M, et al: Post intubation laryngeal sequelae in an intensive care unit, *J Laryngol Otol* 109(4):313-316, 1995.

139. Thompson DM, Kasperbauer JL: Congenital cystic hygroma involving the larynx presenting as an airway emergency, *J Natl Med Assoc* 86(8):629-632, 1994.

140. Tomkinson A, Shone GR, Dingle A, et al: Pharyngocutaneous fistula following total laryngectomy and post-operative vomiting, *Clin Otolaryngol* 21(4):369-370, 1996.

141. Trudeau MD, Schuller DE, Hall DA: The effects of radiation on tracheoesophageal puncture: a retrospective study, *Arch Otolaryngol Head Neck Surg* 115(9):1116-1117, 1989.

142. Tu G, Qi Y, Tang P: Laryngeal reconstruction and survival after function-sparing laryngectomy for selected T3 and T4 lesions, *Chin Med J (Engl)* 108(6):423-427, 1995.

143. Tucker HM, Benninger MS, Roberts JK, et al: Near-total laryngectomy with epiglottic reconstruction: long-term results, *Arch Otolaryngol Head Neck Surg* 115(11):1341-1344, 1989.

144. Udaipurwala IH, Iqbal K, Jalisi M: Pharyngocutaneous fistula following laryngectomy, *JPMA J Pak Med Assoc* 45(5):130-132, 1995.

145. Verma A, Panda NK, Mehta S, et al: Post laryngectomy complications and their mode of management—an analysis of 203 cases, *Indian J Cancer* 26(4):247-254, 1989.

146. Ward RF, Jones J, Arnold JA: Surgical management of congenital saccular cysts of the larynx, *Ann Otol Rhinol Laryngol* 104(9 Pt 1):707-710, 1995.

147. Waters KA, Woo P, Mortelliti AJ, et al: Assessment of the infant airway with videorecorded flexible laryngoscopy and the objective analysis of vocal fold abduction, *Otolaryngol Head Neck Surg* 114(4):554-561, 1996.

148. Wax MK, Touma BJ, Ramadan HH: Tracheostomal stenosis after laryngectomy: incidence and predisposing factors, *Otolaryngol Head Neck Surg* 113(3):242-247, 1995.

149. Weber PC, Johnson JT, Myers EN: Impact of bilateral neck dissection on recovery following supraglottic laryngectomy, *Arch Otolaryngol Head Neck Surg* 119(1):61-64, 1993.

150. Weinstein GS, Laccourreye O, Brasnu D, et al: Reconsidering a paradigm: the spread of supraglottic carcinoma to the glottis, *Laryngoscope* 105(10):1129-1133, 1995.

151. Wenig BL, Keller AJ, Levy J, et al: Voice restoration after laryngopharyngoesophagectomy, *Otolaryngol Head Neck Surg* 101(1):11-13, 1989.

152. Wenig BM, Devaney K, Bisceglia M: Inflammatory myofibroblastic tumor of the larynx: a clinicopathologic study of eight cases simulating a malignant spindle cell neoplasm, *Cancer* 76(11):2217-2229, 1995.

153. Werkhaven J, Ossoff RH: Surgery for benign lesions of the glottis, *Otolaryngol Clin North Am* 24(5):1179-1199, 1991.

154. Werkhaven JA, Weed DT, Ossoff RH: Carbon dioxide laser serial microtrapdoor flap excision of subglottic stenosis, *Arch Otolaryngol Head Neck Surg* 119(6):676-679, 1993.

155. Wetmore RF: Fibrous histiocytoma of the larynx in a child: case report and review, *Clin Pediatr (Phila)* 26(4):200-202, 1987.

156. Weymuller EA Jr, Bishop MJ, Santos PM: Problems associated with prolonged intubation in the geriatric patient, *Otolaryngol Clin North Am* 23(6):1057-1074, 1990.

157. Wilder WM, Slagle GW, Hand AM, et al: Crohn's disease of the epiglottis, aryepiglottic folds, anus, and rectum, *J Clin Gastroenterol* 2(1):87-91, 1980.

158. Yellin SA, LaBruna A, Anand VK: Nd:YAG laser treatment for laryngeal and hypopharyngeal hemangiomas: a new technique, *Ann Otol Rhinol Laryngol* 105(7):510-515, 1996.

159. Yotakis J, Davris S, Kontozoglou T, et al: Evaluation of risk factors for stomal recurrence after total laryngectomy, *Clin Otolaryngol* 21(2):135-138, 1996.

160. Yuen AP, Ho CM, Wei WI, et al: Prognosis of recurrent laryngeal carcinoma after laryngectomy, *Head Neck* 17(6):526-530, 1995.

161. Yuen AP, Wei WI, Lam KH, et al: Thyroidectomy during laryngectomy for advanced laryngeal carcinoma—whole organ section study with long-term functional evaluation, *Clin Otolaryngol* 20(2):145-149, 1995.

162. Zalzal GH: Treatment of laryngotracheal stenosis with anterior and posterior cartilage grafts: a report of 41 children, *Arch Otolaryngol Head Neck Surg* 119(1):82-86, 1993.

163. Zalzal GH, Anon JB, Cotton RT: Epiglottoplasty for the treatment of laryngomalacia, *Ann Otol Rhinol Laryngol* 96(1 Pt 1):72-76, 1987.

164. Zbar RI, Smith RJ: Vocal fold paralysis in infants twelve months of age and younger, *Otolaryngol Head Neck Surg* 114(1):18-21, 1996.

165. Zbaren P, Greiner R, Kengelbacher M: Stoma recurrence after laryngectomy: an analysis of risk factors, *Otolaryngol Head Neck Surg* 114(4):569-575, 1996.

166. Zbaren P, Zimmermann A: Solitary plasmocytoma of the larynx, *ORL J Otorhinolaryngol Relat Spec* 57(1):50-53, 1995.

167. Zeitels SM, Kirchner JA: Hyoepiglottic ligament in supraglottic cancer, *Ann Otol Rhinol Laryngol* 104(10 Pt 1):770-775, 1995.

168. Zeitouni A, Manoukian J: Epiglottoplasty in the treatment of laryngomalacia, *J Otolaryngol* 22(1):29-33, 1993.

169. Zheng H, Li Z, Zhou S, et al: Update: laryngeal reinnervation for unilateral vocal cord paralysis with the ansa cervicalis, *Laryngoscope* 106(12 Pt 1):1522-1527, 1996.

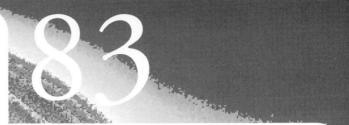

CHAPTER 83

Surgical and Nonsurgical Voice Restoration

James P. Anthony
Robert D. Foster

INTRODUCTION

Each year, over 6000 people in the United States suffer complete loss of their larynx, most often as a result of surgery for laryngeal carcinoma. For these people, successful and complete rehabilitation requires the restoration of the ability to both swallow and speak. For many laryngectomized patients, the ability to communicate verbally is more important than the ability to take food orally. In a survey on the quality of life, 20% of healthy volunteers responded that they would opt for a form of treatment (radiation therapy) that would sacrifice 20% to 30% of their full life expectancy rather than conventional therapy (laryngectomy) just to preserve normal speech.[28]

The eventual sound quality of the speech produced following laryngectomy depends primarily on (1) the type of prosthesis used and/or the degree of voice training the patient achieves, and (2) the technique used to reconstruct the pharyngoesophagus when necessary. Efforts to restore intelligible speech production have paralleled the 100-year evolution of the laryngectomy operation itself. In 1873, Billroth performed the first reported total laryngectomy.[4] That first patient was fitted with a special cannula that introduced expired air into the pharynx and produced sound from a vibrating metal membrane situated in the airstream. Three weeks after surgery the patient was able to speak with an intelligible but monotonous voice that he maintained until succumbing a few months later from recurrent carcinoma. Since that time, three principal alternatives for voice restoration have emerged: esophageal speech training, the artificial larynx, and tracheoesophageal puncture (TEP) with placement of a voice prosthesis.

When extension of a laryngeal carcinoma to the esophagus necessitates en bloc resection, the method of the pharyngoesophageal reconstruction has a significant influence on the subsequent speech results. The ideal pharyngoesophageal reconstruction would restore normal anatomy, permitting patients to produce normal phonation without aspiration and without requiring a permanent tracheostomy. Although all current reconstructive techniques fall far short of this ideal, several viable alternatives for reestablishing continuity of the upper gastrointestinal tract exist (e.g., radial forearm flap, free jejunal flap, gastric or colonic pullup), with varying degrees of effectiveness.

INDICATIONS

TECHNIQUES OF VOICE RESTORATION

Esophageal Speech

Alaryngeal voice may be produced by airflow-induced vibrations of the pharyngoesophageal mucosa either by ingested air (esophageal speech) or by shunted air (fistula or tracheoesophageal speech). First described in 1841 by Reynaud,[35] esophageal speech training became a well-established mode of rehabilitation in the era before surgical reconstruction. However, despite reports of success rates up to 68% in the literature,[45] most studies indicate that only roughly 25% of patients are able to communicate effectively.[37] The speaker swallows air into the esophagus and brings it out in small volumes for speech production (Figures 83-1 and 83-2). Because there is no longer any transnasal or transoral negative air pressure from the lungs only small amounts of air can be swallowed at any one time. A fresh intake of air is required after every four to five words,[46] and free passage of the air through the neopharynx (i.e., no stricture is essential). The voice produced is low-pitched, usually between 60 and 80 Hz, with reduced intensity and rate of speech compared with normal speech.[46] Comparatively large amounts of "jitter" (cycle-to-cycle pitch perturbation) and "shimmer" (cycle-to-cycle amplitude perturbation) are present.

With progressive improvement in the functional results using surgical reconstruction (tracheoesophageal fistula [TEF] formation), current indications for esophageal speech training are limited to patients medically unfit to tolerate operative reconstruction but who are also sufficiently motivated for the intensive voice training required. On average, 60 hours of therapeutic training are needed to develop esophageal speech.[16] Considering the age of most of these patients, the severity of their disease state, and the effort involved in the

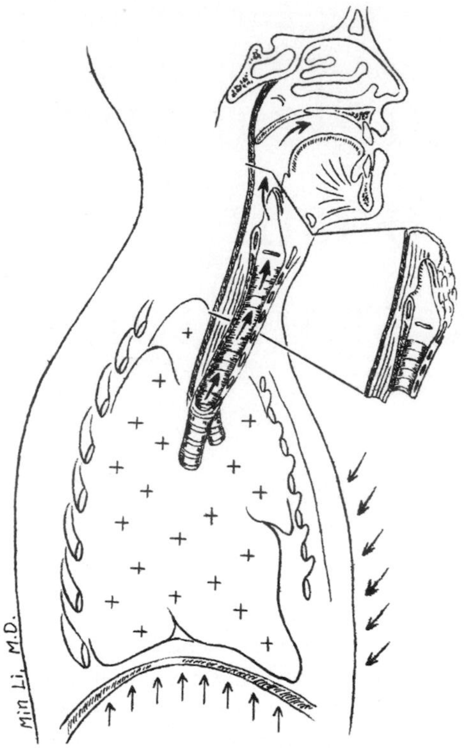

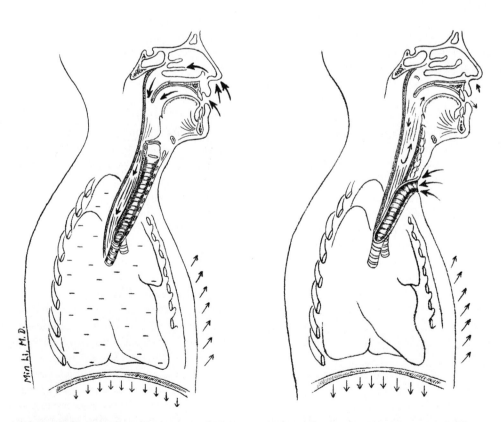

Figure 83-1. With the normal anatomy, air expired from the lungs passes through the larynx into the pharynx and oral cavity to be molded by the structures there into intelligible speech. Insert shows anatomic area affected by laryngectomy.

Figure 83-2. The negative pressure generated by the thorax during aspiration is transferred to the nose and oral cavity, pulling in air that can be used for speech. After laryngectomy, that negative pressure is no longer transferred to the oral cavity and air flow is rerouted through the tracheostomy in the neck. Esophageal speech depends on air swallowed through the mouth and nose and then expelled back out through the oral cavity since there is no connection between the airway and the oral cavity and pharynx.

rehabilitation process, it is the patient's motivation, or lack of motivation, to achieve intelligible esophageal speech that most significantly accounts for the wide variability in the long-term functional results.[20]

Artificial Larynx

The electrolarynx was introduced in the early 1940s and later transistorized to make for a lightweight, easily portable device. The instrument, however, is at best a crude vibrator. The user must learn to articulate vowels clearly with considerable exaggeration of mouth and tongue position. Without support from pulmonary air, the consonant sounds must be made in large part with the limited amount of buccal air, which requires much practice. The device must be ideally placed for optimum loudness, and phrasing must be learned, requiring the electrolarynx to be switched off at the end of each phrase to best mimic results of natural speech (Figure 83-3).

As a result of the development in laryngeal reconstructive techniques and refinements in esophageal speech training, the electrolarynx has been relegated to a minor role in the overall algorithm for voice restoration and is currently indicated when surgical reconstructive results are poor or when patients are medically unstable and/or are not sufficiently motivated for more complex approaches. The electrolarynx is, however, useful as an adjunct to delayed TEF reconstruction. During the time between laryngectomy and fistula formation, patients can benefit from use of an electrolarynx to facilitate communication.

A patient's unwillingness to proceed with voice rehabilitation following laryngectomy remains a major obstacle for all of the reconstructive methods mentioned. St. Guily et al,[50] in a prospective study of 81 patients involving all forms of postlaryngectomy voice restoration, showed a 16% total

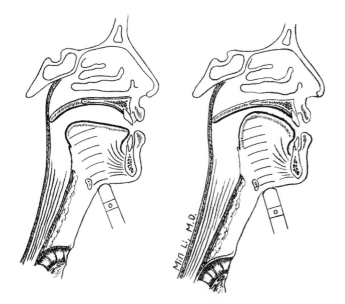

Figure 83-3. Application of the electrolarynx postlaryngectomy. Note the relative simplicity of the technique compared with esophageal speech production. Air in the oral cavity is moved by the vibratory waves.

refusal. In a prospective study of esophageal speech training, Gates et al[13] showed 25% patient refusal for reeducation, and in a long-term follow-up of 73 postlaryngectomy patients, only 50% employed methods of communication more complex than the electrolarynx.[30] Factors contributing to these failure rates (identified through patient interviews) include poor patient self image and the length and arduousness of the rehabilitation.[30] For the majority of these patients, the electrolarynx represents the least invasive and, of the three rehabilitative options considered, the easiest to learn.

Tracheoesophageal Puncture and Voice Prosthesis Placement

The addition of a pulmonary air supply in tracheoesophageal speech brings the acoustic quality of speech closer to normal compared with esophageal speech alone. This delivery of pulmonary air back into the oral cavity for speech production was achieved with the introduction of a TEF.[11] The subsequent fitting of a voice prosthesis achieves fluent, intelligible speech without the aspiration of saliva or food.

As early as the nineteenth century it was well known that if a vibrating column of exhaled air is introduced into the esophagus or pharynx, intelligible speech can be produced. All such attempts, however, ultimately failed as a result of two major complications: aspiration of saliva and food or stenosis of the shunt between the trachea and the pharynx or esophagus. For the next 100 years, many innovative techniques were developed without demonstrating a sufficient decrease in the complication rate.

In 1980, Singer and Blom[41] developed an endoscopic procedure for restoring voice production after total laryngectomy that remains the method of choice for TEF today. A one-way valve allows air to enter the esophagus when the patient exhales with the tracheostoma occluded but stops liquid and food from entering the trachea when the patient swallows. In addition, the diameter of the shunt is reliably maintained long-term. The procedure is simple to learn and is reliably accomplished in irradiated tissues. A range of other valves exists (Groningen, Provox, Panje), all of which function in a similar manner but differ in lumen size, durability, and method of insertion.

The fistula can be created either at the time of the laryngectomy (primary TEP) or at a later date (secondary TEP). Primary puncture allows for early rehabilitation. Secondary puncture is most commonly indicated when postoperative radiation therapy is anticipated or in those patients who do not achieve adequate voice production without a fistula.

Acoustic measures indicate that fistula speech more closely resembles normal speech than either esophageal or electronic speech.[16,36] In the postoperative period, an average of only 7 hours of voice therapy is required to achieve functional communication,[16] which improves the cost-effectiveness of the method compared with esophageal speech. Therefore TEP with prosthetic valve insertion is currently the method of choice for voice restoration following laryngectomy. The only contraindication to use of this procedure is the inability of the patient to tolerate the brief surgery required for secondary TEP. As with other forms of voice rehabilitation, patients have to be well-motivated and educated to gain maximum benefit from their voice prosthesis.

The simplicity and effectiveness of TEP with prosthetic valve placement has allowed this method to replace the numerous other surgical maneuvers that attempted to provide the same physiologic arrangement. Amatsu and others described a shunt between the trachea and the neopharynx to provide airflow from the tracheostomy into the oral cavity. He formed a myomucosal tube of pharynx that entered the

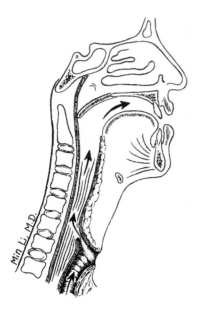

Figure 83-4. Amatsu type tracheopharyngeal fistula created with a myomucosal tube of pharyngeal wall. Expired air can pass through fistula into oral cavity to create speech.

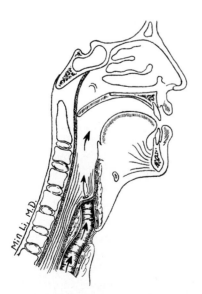

Figure 83-5. Neoglottis formation. The anterior wall of the neopharynx is sutured over the horizontally cut end of the proximal trachea. The tracheostomy attached to the neck is more distal. Expired air can pass into the oral cavity through a slit in the pharynx.

posterior wall of the trachea just above the stoma (Figure 83-4). In the neoglottis concept that arose from this, pharyngeal mucosa (or the mucosa of a jejunal free autograft or skin of a radial forearm free flap) is draped over the cut end of the trachea above the tracheostoma (Figure 83-5). A slit in the pharynx or pharynx substitute allows expired air to go through this opening in a similar fashion to air passing through the vocal cords into the mouth. Unfortunately, poor wound healing at the time of primary or secondary neoglottis reconstruction resulted in a high rate of fistula formation. Postoperative stenosis of the opening and aspiration of oral contents were also problematic in the use of this technique.

OPERATIONS

TECHNIQUES OF PHARYNGOESOPHAGEAL RECONSTRUCTION

Voice restoration has been accomplished following pharyngeal reconstruction using a variety of flaps including gastric or colonic "pullup" procedures,[49] free jejunum or colon flaps,[10] and skin/myocutaneous flaps.[52] Pedicled enteric flaps successfully reconstruct the pharyngoesophagus, but a number of disadvantages limit their use. The extensive intraabdominal dissection (with its attendant fluid shifts) and the cardiopulmonary compromise that can accompany the intrathoracic tunneling necessary represent a formidable undertaking in the typically elderly patient with head and neck cancer. As with any bowel surgery, complications (i.e., adhesions, small bowel obstruction, anastomotic disruptions) can occur and the portion of the enteric flap that must reach most superiorly to the neck anastomosis is the least well-vascularized portion of the flap, making it more susceptible to leakage, fistula formation, and late development of stricture formation. When fistulas do develop, they tend to be more difficult to treat than those in free flap reconstructions.[10,38] Gastrointestinal flaps also tolerate radiation poorly. The gastric pullup (the most common pullup procedure) disrupts the normal gastroesophageal sphincter, causing reflux gastritis in 15% of patients.[38] Finally, voice rehabilitation in these patients is problematic. When patients undergo other types of pharyngoesophageal reconstruction, the distal esophageal remnant is left in situ. This remnant is a smaller-diameter tube than the stomach and requires much less air to fill. When the gastric pullup is performed, the lack of any esophagus and the flaccidity and large air reservoir of the stomach combine to hinder the production of intelligible speech in many patients.[5,17] When such patients do acquire speech it is often low-pitched and may sound "gurgly" due to the excessive mucus production by the displaced stomach.[22]

Free jejunal reconstruction of the pharyngoesophagus for cancer of the cervical esophagus was first reported in 1959 by Seidenberg et al.[39] Since then, free jejunal reconstruction has become one of the most popular techniques for pharyngeal reconstruction. An appropriate jejunal segment of virtually any length can be harvested and reliably revascularized. If necessary, multiple jejunal loops can be used to reconstruct the entire esophagus.[8] Pharyngoesophageal reconstruction using free jejunal flaps allows the reconstructive surgeon to replace a hollow muscular tube (the pharynx) with a hollow muscular tube (the jejunum). If postoperative leaks occur, the abundant vascularity brought into the neck by this flap almost uniformly results in spontaneous closure.[38] Nevertheless, a number of disadvantages limit its use, including the need for intraabdominal surgery, the low quality of the mesenteric vessels (they tend to be fragile and short in length, <6 cm), and the relatively poor postoperative swallowing and speech function.

The donor morbidity after jejunal free flap is similar to that already outlined for pedicled enteric flaps,[10,38] and the mortality rate following free jejunal transfer is approximately 5%.[17] Although the jejunum is placed isoperistaltically, the incidence of dysphagia in our own series is at least 65%, even when excluding those patients with base of tongue resections. Unfortunately, the transferred jejunal segment continues to contract independently,[29] so that its movement is not synchronous with the contractions of the upper or lower residual native pharynx or esophagus.[27]

Prosthetic voice restoration results with free jejunum have also been disappointing. Although the jejunum contains a smaller air column and is less flaccid than the stomach or colon, it does not allow the effective mucosal apposition necessary for consistent prosthetic voice production, and the excessive mucus production can obstruct the prosthesis. Speech with the free jejunum is typically very moist and lacks volume.[25] In fact, the quality of speech after free jejunal transfer is probably inferior even to that of the gastric pullup procedure.[3,26]

Over the past 10 years, we have observed that the choice of flap reconstruction significantly influences the final speech results. Specifically, those patients who have undergone TEP with pharyngeal reconstructions that lined the pharynx with skin (i.e., the deltopectoral and pectoralis major flaps) have superior speech results compared with patients reconstructed with enteric flaps (the gastric pullup flap or free jejunum flap). Unfortunately, these pedicled skin and myocutaneous flaps have other problems relating to their reliability and excess bulk. To address this problem we began using the radial forearm free flap in 1991 as our flap of choice for patients requiring partial and full circumferential reconstructions of the pharyngoesophagus.[12]

The radial forearm flap offers the combined advantages of rapid harvest (generally about 1 hour); a long, large caliber vascular pedicle; and high flap reliability. It can also conform to virtually any size partial or full-circumference pharyngeal defect. This flap is long enough to reconstruct every defect in the cervical esophagus and will reach well into the chest. We have replaced segments of the esophagus as short as 3 cm and as long as 18 cm in length (i.e., from the base of the tongue to well below the jugular notch of the sternum). From the time of its initial description,[47] the radial free flap has had one of the highest success rates of any microvascular free flap, generally more than 95% in most series. This exceptional flap reliability is due to a combination of a large (2 to 2.5 mm) artery and several available veins in the flap for routine performance of

multiple venous anastomoses. Since most of these patients have undergone previous neck surgery and virtually all of them are irradiated, flap reliability assumes an even greater role to the ultimate success of the reconstruction than in other regions of the body.

AUTHORS' PREFERRED TECHNIQUE

Radial Forearm Free Flap with TEP and Blom-Singer Valve Insertion

The techniques used to harvest the radial forearm free flap have been well described,[47,48] and only those aspects of surgical technique related to the use of the tubed flap for pharyngoesophageal reconstruction will be addressed here.

Following a preoperative Allen's test and confirmation of patency of the palmar arch, cutaneous veins, particularly the cephalic vein, are marked on the donor site arm. The nondominant arm is used whenever possible. Exsanguination and tourniquet inflation (to 250 mm Hg) of the arm are followed by outlining of the skin island, which typically extends distally to the proximal wrist crease (Figures 83-6 and

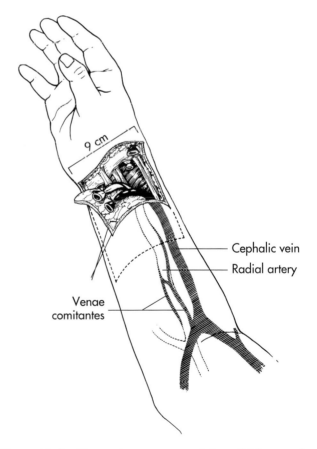

Figure 83-6. The pertinent anatomy of the radial forearm free flap for pharyngoesophageal reconstruction. Note that the distal aspect of the flap (in the area of the wrist crease) is a minimum of 9 cm in width to ensure that the flap diameter will be at least 3 cm. To achieve this 9-cm distal flap width, the flap must extend farther around the radial aspect of the wrist than conventional radial free flaps, which also allows for routine incorporation of the large cephalic vein within the flap.

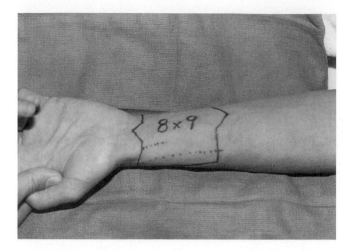

Figure 83-7. Design of a radial free flap, 8 cm long and 9 cm wide. Note the additional triangle of skin proximally and distally to be interposed during the pharyngoesophageal reconstruction to prevent stricture formation.

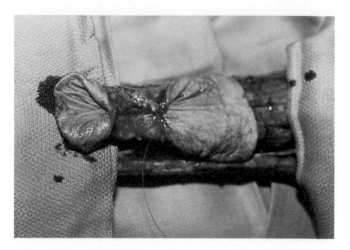

Figure 83-8. Following flap elevation and dissection of a suitably long proximal vascular pedicle, the radial free flap is tubed on itself using a running Connell stitch.

83-7). For circumferential reconstructions, the width of the skin island is kept at 9 cm throughout the length of the flap to ensure a final lumen diameter of 3 cm. This permits either end of the tubed flap to be used proximally or distally and thereby maximizes the number of neck receptor vessels that can be used. If desired, the proximal end of the radial free flap can be made even wider to improve the size match with the proximal pharyngeal lumen. For most patients, particularly women, the 9 cm wide skin island at the wrist necessitates designing the flap to extend around to the radial aspect of the wrist. Although this compromises the aesthetic appearance of the donor site to a degree, this flap design further enhances the flap's reliability by routinely including the large cephalic vein (see Figure 83-6). The sensory branches of the radial nerve should be carefully preserved during the dissection of the cephalic vein. Using this design, radial free flaps as large as 9 cm wide by 18 cm long can be safely raised without any skin loss. Obviously, when only a patch reconstruction is required, a smaller flap may be taken.

When a full-circumference pharyngoesophageal defect is being reconstructed, the ulnar and radial edges are sewn to one another with several absorbable interrupted sutures followed by a running absorbable Connell stitch (Figure 83-8). This both tubes the skin edges on themselves and inverts them inward, minimizing the possibility of leaks along the longitudinal suture line (Figure 83-9).

While the neck dissection is being completed, the ulnar and radial margins of the forearm skin are advanced to minimize the area of skin graft needed. On the radial aspect of the wound, this skin advancement has the additional benefit of re-covering the exposed sensory branches of the radial nerve, minimizing the potential for nerve irritation by the minor trauma of daily living. An unmeshed skin graft is then used to cover the wound while the tubed radial free flap continues to perfuse. When the tumor resection is completed, suitable receptor vessels for the microvascular anastomosis are identified (Figure 83-10). The recipient arteries are most commonly

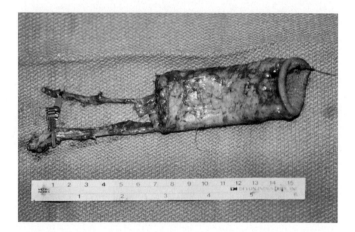

Figure 83-9. The tubed radial free flap is shown just prior to inset into the neck. Note the long vascular pedicles of the radial vessels *(below)* and the cephalic vein *(above)*. If necessary, these vessels can be separated several centimeters from each other to reach their receptor vessels in the neck.

the facial or superior thyroid arteries (high in the neck) and the transverse cervical artery (lower in the neck). The recipient veins are usually more difficult to find because they have often been removed during the neck dissection. Either the internal or external jugular vein is preferable if present. When these veins have been resected, the transverse cervical vein or the contralateral neck veins can be used. It is the ability of the radial pedicle to reach anywhere on either side of the neck (Figure 83-11), and the wide independent arcs of rotation that can be created between the cephalic vein and the radial artery, that makes the radial forearm flap the most versatile and useful flap for head and neck reconstruction.

Prior to the microvascular anastomosis, the tubed flap is inset into the defect and both upper and lower pharyngoesophageal anastomoses are constructed using a two-layer closure of 4-0 absorbable sutures. Whenever possible, a longer segment of residual pharyngeal or esophageal wall is left on one side of the resection or the other. A small segment of the radial free flap is

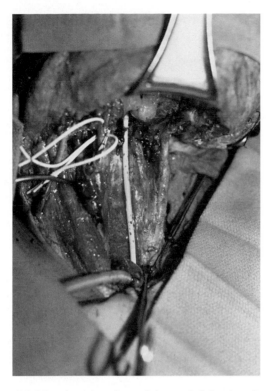

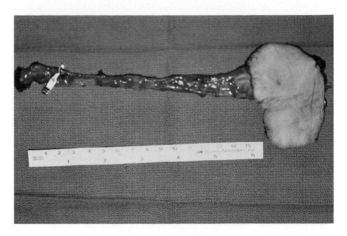

Figure 83-11. A harvested radial forearm free flap demonstrating the length of the vascular pedicle possible. If ipsilateral receptor vessels are sacrificed during the neck dissection, the radial pedicle can reliably reach vessels in the contralateral neck.

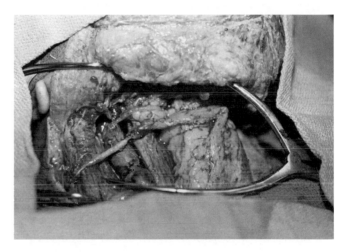

Figure 83-10. Anterior view of the neck following pharyngoesophageal resection. The defect extends from the base of the tongue to the cervical esophagus, spanned by a white feeding tube. Superiorly, the facial vessels have been isolated (encircled with vessel loops) for the planned microanastomoses.

Figure 83-12. The tubed radial free flap following insetting and microsurgical revascularization. Note the wide separation of the cephalic vein *(inferiorly)* from the radial vessels *(superiorly)*. The cephalic vein has been anastomosed to the external jugular vein, the radial vena comitans to the jugular vein, and the radial artery to the facial artery.

removed from that side, leaving the radial free flap similarly long on the opposite side. This undulating type of upper and lower anastomosis acts as a sort of Z-plasty and seems to preclude circumferential stricturing. In 1985, Harii et al[15] advocated a similar type of anastomosis and found that this dramatically decreased the rate of stricture development. Once both pharyngoesophageal anastomoses have been constructed, the flap is securely fixed within the neck and the microsurgical revascularization is performed. Two venous anastomoses (always including the cephalic vein and usually one radial vena comitans) are routinely performed. In cases in which the radial venae comitantes are very small, the cephalic vein alone can provide adequate venous drainage for the entire flap (Figure 83-12).

Postoperative monitoring is done via transcutaneous auscultation of the radial vessels through the neck skin using standard Doppler technique. The position of these vessels in the midline is verified prior to skin closure. By positioning the radial vessels in the midline, confusion with other vessels in the neck, unrelated to the flap, is avoided. Following surgery, all patients are out of bed on the first postoperative day and begin to take an oral diet at 7 to 10 days if they have not been irradiated locally, or after 2 weeks if they have been irradiated. Patients initially receive liquids and progress to a solid diet, generally within 3 to 4 weeks after surgery (Figure 83-13).

The Blom-Singer prosthesis is inserted either at the time of the laryngectomy or as a secondary procedure. Under general anesthesia, with the patient lying supine and his or her neck fully extended (Figure 83-14, *A*), a TEP is created by inserting a 14-gauge needle through the posterosuperior membranous wall of the tracheostoma, 5 mm inferior to the mucocutaneous junction, into the lumen of a rigid esophagoscope (Figure 83-14, *B*). A disposable intravenous catheter is inserted over the needle and the needle is withdrawn. The TEP tract is then dilated until a 14-Fr urethral catheter can be inserted in the tract as a stent (Figure 83-14, *C*). Three to seven days later, the urethral catheter is replaced with a Blom-Singer voice prosthesis. This acts as a one-way valve directing the exhaled air into the esophagus when the tracheostoma is occluded with a finger and preventing aspiration (Figure 83-14, *D*). The voice prosthesis must be removed periodically for cleaning and replaced. Initially, almost all patients are frightened to do so

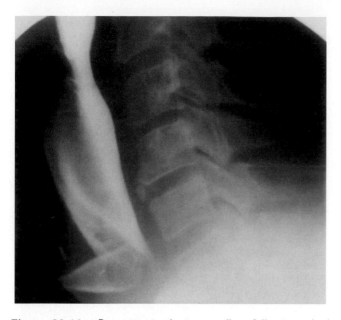

Figure 83-13. Postoperative barium swallow following tubed radial free flap reconstruction. Note that the lumen of the flap is wider than the native esophagus.

themselves, and therefore independent management is delayed until the patient consistently demonstrates the capacity to care for the prosthesis under direct supervision.

OUTCOMES

RESULTS

Long-term results after pharyngoesophageal reconstruction with the radial forearm free flap demonstrate excellent flap success rates, complication rates comparable to other popular forms of reconstruction, and superior speech results. In the largest series thus far reported (22 patients),[2] flap survival was 100%. Although 32% of the reconstructions initially leaked, all but one closed spontaneously within a few weeks. Eighty-eight percent of the patients with an intact tongue base had no dysphagia and ate a regular diet. Compared with voice-restored patients who had undergone laryngectomy with primary closure of the pharyngoesophagus, patients with a radial free flap reconstruction had similar loudness with soft

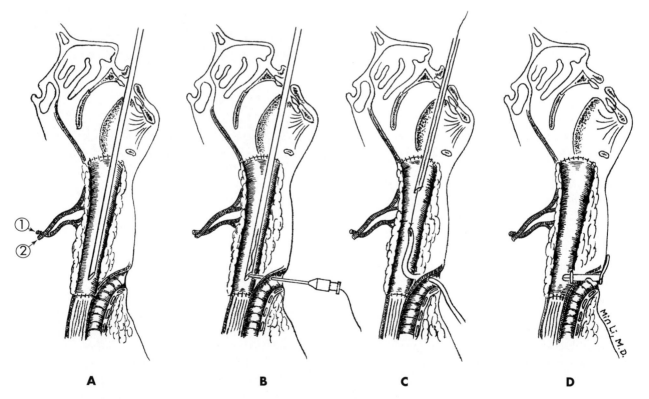

A   **B**   **C**   **D**

Figure 83-14. A, Rigid esophagoscopy for secondary tracheoesophageal puncture following pharyngoesophageal reconstruction with a tubed radial free flap. Note the orientation of the blood supply of the radial free flap; the radial vessels *(1)* and the cephalic vein *(2)*. **B,** The tracheoesophageal puncture is performed with a trocar placed through the rear wall of the trachea and maintained temporarily with a nylon thread. **C,** A no. 14 urethral catheter replaces the nylon thread, is brought out through the nose, and is secured in place. **D,** The catheter is removed and replaced by a suitably sized prosthesis (in this case, the Blom-Singer duckbill-type prosthesis). When properly fitted, the mucosal surface of the anterior esophageal wall is engaged by the flange on the prosthesis, preventing extrusion. The patient phonates by occluding the stoma with a finger, causing exhaled air to pass through the prosthesis valve into the reconstructed pharyngoesophagus.

speech (52 dB for radial patients versus 43 dB for controls) and loud speech (63 dB versus 61 dB), comparable fundamental frequencies (125 Hz versus 136 Hz), and only slightly increased jitter (5% versus 2%). In all cases a Blom-Singer prosthesis was used. All patients tested following radial free flap reconstruction achieved intelligible speech.

The results obtained with TEP (primary or secondary) in general vary considerably but are nonetheless favorable in comparison with other surgical and nonsurgical methods of voice restoration. The variability of the results may be influenced by the patient selection criteria, the type of prosthesis used, and the length of follow-up. In the immediate postoperative period, success of voice restoration has been documented ranging from 57% to 94%.[14,23] In the long-term (months or greater), success rates have been reported ranging from 37% to 93%,[18,19] with most series 80% or greater. In the largest single experience (300 patients) published thus far, the reported long-term success rate was 85%.[43]

COMPLICATIONS

As with any type of flap reconstruction, there is a small but definable risk of flap failure due to ischemia. Once flap viability is ensured, the two greatest concerns in the postoperative period are leakage at the suture line and stricture formation. Despite the additional suture line required to tube the radial forearm free flap, in 20 consecutive reconstructions with this flap, we have never observed leakage at the vertical suture line. When leaks have occurred, they usually develop at the distal esophageal suture line, just as they do in jejunal flaps.[38] The leakage rate with jejunal free flaps ranges from 15% to 40%, depending on whether or not the patient has received prior irradiation.[38,51] In our experience and that of others,[9,15] the leakage rate with tubed radial forearm flaps is somewhat higher (50% in our series of 20 patients). Fortunately, when leaks occur with either the jejunal or radial free flaps, they almost always resolve spontaneously with conservative treatment. In fact, only one of our patients has required surgical treatment of a fistula; the rest of the fistulas have closed within several weeks. Late stricture has developed in one of our circumferential radial free flap reconstructions. This compares favorably with the 15% to 22% rate of late strictures reported using free jejunal flaps,[34,38] and may partially explain the superior speech and swallowing results seen with the radial free flap.

The radial free flap does require the harvest of a skin graft from the thigh to replace the forearm flap skin (Figure 83-15). Fortunately, donor site complications on the thigh and arm are infrequent. In our own experience approximately 10% of patients have lost small areas (<15%) of their skin grafts, but all healed well without the need for further surgery. Once healing is complete, the skin coverage has proven very durable, even in manual workers. Patient acceptance of this undeniably exposed forearm donor site has been high, probably because of the patient satisfaction with the long-term results of speech and swallowing.

The reported complication rate in the literature of TEP with prosthetic insertion varies from 15% to 55%[1,7,23,40] of cases. This wide range is the result of some authors reporting only severe problems while others take into account even basic handling difficulties. Most complications, however, are mild and sufficiently motivated patients (the key element for success) are able to overcome them.

At or around the stoma site, complications include the formation of granulation tissue in the tracheoesophageal shunt[33,40] and the biodegradation of the prosthesis by microflora, particularly *Candida albicans*.[21,32] Granulation tissue at the tracheal orifice can be removed under local anesthesia using electrocautery, and the prosthesis reapplied immediately. Several antifungal regimens have been suggested as prophylactic treatment to prevent overgrowth within the prosthesis.

Most prostheses made from Silastic or polyurethane remain useful for approximately 6 months, but this interval varies from one individual to another. Over time, the prosthesis loses its resiliency and the valve function deteriorates, producing aspiration of saliva and food. As the rigidity of the material increases, greater opening pressures for phonation are required, making speech production more difficult. When these problems become sufficiently severe, the prosthesis must be replaced.

Other, relatively rare complications include fistula closure, false tract formation,[40] fistula migration,[1,33] fistula incontinence, acute inflammation in the tracheoesophageal shunt, and fistula wall necrosis.[24,33] Patients can undergo repuncture for fistula closure, false tract formation, and fistula migration. Fistula incontinence with salivary leakage around the prosthesis can be treated with silver nitrate cauterization, replacement of the prosthesis, or injection of sclerosing agents in the fistula wall (which can be repeated several times). Necrosis of the fistula wall is generally related to prior local radiotherapy. Conservative measures to achieve contraction of the fistula site are usually successful, although more severe cases may require muscle flap (pectoralis major) transposition for coverage.

Failure to achieve satisfactory speech after TEP is most commonly the result of esophageal distention with secondary spasm of the pharyngeal constrictor muscles. As a result, several procedures have been developed to address this problem, most

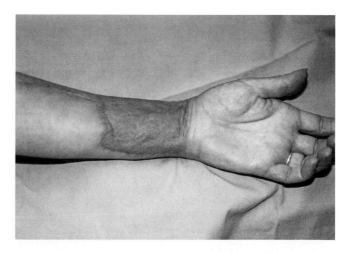

Figure 83-15. Well-healed donor site at 6 months postoperatively.

commonly pharyngeal constrictor myotomy or pharyngeal plexus denervation. Both procedures are relatively easy to perform but pharyngeal plexus neurectomy has several advantages over pharyngeal constrictor myotomy. The neurectomy does not involve an incision of the pharyngeal constrictors. The myotomy incision has been implicated in reducing the vascularity of the pharyngeal wall and therefore enhancing mucosal dehiscence and fistula formation.[44] In addition, neurectomized patients achieve a high rate of fluent TEP phonation after initial TEP failure (88% in a series of 25 patients[6]) and acquire better speech than patients treated with myotomy.[6]

Although less common, more severe complications including the progression of chronic obstructive lung disease, pneumothorax,[31] aspiration pneumonia,[1] cervical cellulitis,[1,40] and subcutaneous emphysema[42] have been described. To prevent the progression of chronic obstructive lung disease, a low-pressure type of prosthesis is preferable (Figure 83-16). Inflammatory complications caused by bacteria or fungi require temporary removal of the prosthesis and antibiotic treatment. If the problem is further complicated by mediastinitis, surgical drainage may be indicated. Subcutaneous emphysema can usually be ameliorated by discontinuing the use of the prosthesis for a few days.

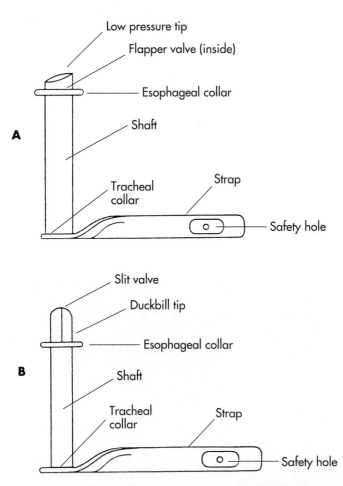

Figure 83-16. Schematic drawing of the modified low pressure prosthesis **(A)** and the duckbill-type Blom-Singer prosthesis **(B)**.

REFERENCES

1. Andrews JC, Mickel RA, Hanson DG, et al: Major complications following tracheoesophageal puncture for voice rehabilitation, *Laryngoscope* 97:562-567, 1987.

2. Anthony JP, Singer MI, Deschler DG, et al: Long-term functional results after pharyngoesophageal reconstruction with the radial forearm free flap, *Am J Surg* 168:441-445, 1994.

3. Bates GJ, McFeeter L, Coman W: Pharyngolaryngectomy and voice restoration, *Laryngoscope* 100:1025-1026, 1990.

4. Billroth CT: Ueber die erste druch Th. Billroth am menschen. Ausgefuhrte kehlkepf-extirpation und die anwendung eines kuntstlichen kahl-kopfes, *Arch Klin Chir* 17:343-356, 1874.

5. Bleach N, Perry A, Cheesman A: Surgical voice restoration with the Blom-Singer prosthesis following laryngopharyngoesophagectomy and pharyngogastric anastomosis, *Ann Orol Rhinol Laryngol* 100:142-147, 1991.

6. Blom ED, Pauloski BR, Hamaker RC: Functional outcome after surgery for prevention of pharyngospasms in tracheoesophageal speakers: Part I: speech characteristics, *Laryngoscope* 105:1093-1103, 1995.

7. Cantrell RW: The case against immediate neoglottic reconstruction, *Head Neck Surg* 10:135-138, 1988.

8. Chen HC, Tang Y, Noordhoff MS: Reconstruction of the entire esophagus with "chain flaps" in a patient with severe corrosive injury, *Plast Reconstr Surg* 84:980-984, 1990.

9. Chen HC, Tang Y, Noordhoff MS: Patch esophagoplasty with free forearm flap for oral stricture of the pharyngoesophageal junction and the cervical esophagus, *Plast Reconstr Surg* 90:45-52, 1992.

10. Coleman JJ, Searles JM, Hester TR, et al: Ten years experience with the free jejunal autograft, *Am J Surg* 154:394-398, 1987.

11. Conley JJ, DeAmesti R, Pierce MK: A new surgical technique for the vocal rehabilitation of the laryngectomized patient, *Ann Otol Rhinol Laryngol* 67:655-664, 1958.

12. Deschler DG, Doherty ET, Reed CG, et al: Tracheoesophageal voice following tubed free radial forearm flap reconstruction of the neopharynx, *Ann Otol Rhinol Laryngol* 103:929-936, 1994.

13. Gates GA, Ryan W, Cooper JC, et al: Current status of laryngectomee rehabilitation. I: results of therapy, *Am J Otolaryngol* 3:1-7, 1982.

14. Hall JG, Dahl T, Arnesen AR: Speech prostheses: failures, problems and successes. In Myers EN, editor: *New dimensions in otorhinolaryngology—head and neck surgery. Proceedings of the 13th World Congress, Miami Beach, Fla, 26-31 May 1985*, Amsterdam, 1985, Exerpta Medica, pp 418-421.

15. Harii K, Ebihara S, Ono I, et al: Pharyngoesophageal reconstruction using a fabricated forearm free flap, *Plast Reconstr Surg* 75:463-474, 1985.

16. Izdebski K, Reed CG, Ross JC, et al: Problems with tracheoesophageal fistula voice restoration in totally laryngectomized patients: a review of 95 cases, *Arch Otolaryngol Head Neck Surg* 120:840-845, 1994.

17. Jones TR, Jones NF: Advances in reconstruction of the upper aerodigestive tract and cranial base with free tissue transfer, *Clin Plast Surg* 19:819-831, 1992.

18. Kao WW, Mohr RM, Kimmel CA, et al: The outcome and techniques of primary and secondary tracheoesophageal puncture, *Arch Otolaryngol Head Neck Surg* 120:301-307, 1994.

19. Kerr AIG, Denholm S, Sanderson RJ, et al: Blom-Singer prosthesis: an 11 year experience of primary and secondary procedures, *Clin Orolaryngol* 18:184-187, 1993.

20. Lavertu P, Scott SE, Finnegan EM, et al: Secondary tracheoesophageal puncture for voice rehabilitation after laryngectomy, *Arch Otolaryngol Head Neck Surg* 115:350-355, 1989.

21. Mahieu KF, van Saene HKF, Jeroen Rosingh H, et al: *Candida* vegetations on silicone voice prostheses, *Arch Otolaryngol Head Neck Surg* 112:321-325, 1986.

22. Maniglia AJ, Leder SB, Goodwin WJ, et al: Tracheogastric puncture for vocal rehabilitation following total pharyngolaryngoesophagectomy, *Head Neck* 11:524-527, 1989.

23. Maniglia AJ, Lundy DS, Casiano RC, et al: Speech restoration and complications of primary versus secondary tracheoesophageal puncture following total laryngectomy, *Laryngoscope* 99:489-491, 1989.

24. McConnel FMS, Duck SW: Indications for tracheoesophageal puncture speech rehabilitation, *Laryngoscope* 96:1065-1068, 1986.

25. McFeeter L: Vocal rehabilitation following laryngectomy, *Aust N Z J Surg* 56:859-862, 1986.

26. McGregor IA: Fasciocutaneous flaps in intraoral reconstruction, *Clin Plast Surg* 12:453-461, 1985.

27. McKee DM, Peters CR: Reconstruction of the hypopharynx and cervical esophagus with microvascular jejunal transplants, *Clin Plast Surg* 5:305-312, 1978.

28. McNeil BJ, Weichselbaum R, Parker SG: Speech and survival tradeoffs between quality and quantity of life in laryngeal cancer, *N Engl J Med* 305:982-987, 1981.

29. Moreno-Osset E, Thomas-Ridocci M, Paris F, et al: Motor activity of esophageal substitute (stomach, jejunal, and colon segments), *Ann Thorac Surg* 41:515-519, 1986.

30. Morris HL, Smith AE, Van Demark DR, et al: Communication status following laryngectomy: the Iowa experience 1984-1987, *Ann Otol Rhinol Laryngol* 101:503-510, 1992.

31. Odland R, Adams G: Pneumothorax as a complication of tracheoesophageal voice prosthesis use, *Ann Otol Rhinol Laryngol* 97:537-541, 1988.

32. Palmer MD, Johnson AP, Elliott TSJ: Microbial colonization of Blom-Singer prostheses in postlaryngectomy patients, *Laryngoscope* 103:910-914, 1993.

33. Recher G, Pesavento G, Cristoferi V, et al: Italian experience of voice restoration after laryngectomy with tracheoesophageal puncture, *Ann Otol Rhinol Laryngol* 100:206-210, 1991.

34. Reece GP, Schusterman MA, Miller MJ, et al: Morbidity and functional outcome of free jejunal transfer reconstruction for circumferential defects of the pharynx and cervical esophagus, *Plast Reconstr Surg* 96:1307-1316, 1995.

35. Reynaud M: Observation sur une fistule aerienne, avec occlusion complete de la partie inferieure du larynx, pour servir a l'histoire de la phonation, *Gaz Med Paris* 9:583, 1841.

36. Robbins J, Fisher HE, Blom ED, et al: A comparative acoustic study of normal, esophageal, and tracheoesophageal speech production, *Speech Hear Dis* 49:202-210, 1984.

37. Ryan WJ: *How people communicate after laryngectomy.* Paper presented at ASHA Meeting, Atlanta, Ga, 1979.

38. Schusterman MA, Shestak K, Swartz WM, et al: Reconstruction of the cervical esophagus: free jejunal transfer versus gastric pull-up, *Plast Reconstr Surg* 85:16-21, 1990.

39. Seidenberg B, Rosenah SS, Hurwitt ES, et al: Immediate reconstruction of the cervical esophagus by a revascularized isolated jejunal segment, *Ann Surg* 149:162-171, 1959.

40. Silver FM, Gluckman JL, Donegan JO: Operative complications of tracheoesophageal puncture, *Laryngoscope* 95:1360-1362, 1985.

41. Singer M, Blom E: An endoscopic technique for restoration of voice after total laryngectomy, *Ann Otol Rhinol Laryngol* 89:529-533, 1980.

42. Singer MI, Blom ED, Hamaker RC: Further experience with voice restoration after total laryngectomy, *Ann Otol Rhinol Laryngol* 90:498-502, 1981.

43. Singer MI, Blom ED, Hamaker RC: Vocal rehabilitation after laryngectomy, *Otolaryngol Clin North Am* 18:605-611, 1985.

44. Singer MI, Blom ED, Hamaker RC: Pharyngeal plexus neurectomy for alaryngeal speech rehabilitation, *Laryngoscope* 96:50-54, 1986.

45. Snidecor JC: *Speech rehabilitation of the laryngectomized,* ed 2, Springfield, Ill, 1968, Charles C Thomas, pp 201-208.

46. Snidecor JC, Curry ET: Temporal and pitch aspects of superior oesophageal speech, *Ann Otol Rhinol Laryngol* 68:623-636, 1959.

47. Song R, Gao Y, Song Y, et al: The forearm flap, *Clin Plast Surg* 9:21-26, 1982.

48. Soutar DS, McGregor IA: The radial forearm free flap in intra-oral reconstruction: the experience of 60 cases, *Plast Reconstr Surg* 78:1-8, 1986.

49. Spiro RH, Bains MS, Shah JP, et al: Gastric transposition for head and neck cancer: a critical update, *Am J Surg* 162:348-352, 1991.

50. St Guily JL, Angelard B, El-Bez M, et al: Postlaryngectomy voice restoration: a prospective study in 83 patients, *Arch Otolaryngol* 118:252-255, 1992.

51. Swartz WM, Banis JC: *Head and neck microsurgery,* Baltimore, 1990, Williams and Wilkins, pp 175-186.

52. Theogaraj SD, Merritt WH, Acharya G, et al: The pectoralis major musculocutaneous island flap in single-stage reconstruction of the pharyngoesophageal region, *Plast Reconstr Surg* 65:267-276, 1980.

CHAPTER

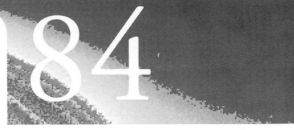

84

Salivary Gland Disorders

Jeffrey D. Wagner
John J. Coleman III

INTRODUCTION

Physicians from a variety of disciplines treat disorders involving the salivary glands. These disorders are of particular relevance to the plastic surgeon. Abnormalities of salivary gland development and anatomy may be encountered during the surgical management of congenital malformations such as hemifacial microsomia. Optimal management of traumatic facial injuries requires detailed anatomic knowledge to identify and repair potentially morbid injuries to the salivary structures. Salivary gland dysfunction due to surgery or radiation is encountered by extirpative and reconstructive head and neck surgeons. The anatomic relationship between the parotid gland and facial nerve necessitates meticulous surgical dissection during tumor extirpation or reconstructive surgery for facial reanimation. Facial cosmetic surgeons must be familiar with the anatomy of the parotid gland to prevent injury to the facial nerve during facial rejuvenation procedures.

INDICATIONS

EMBRYOLOGY

The major and minor salivary glands arise in similar embryologic fashion. The salivary glands originate at about the eighth week in the embryo as invaginations of a solid anlage of stomodeal ectoderm or pharyngeal endoderm into the underlying mesenchymal tissues. These ingrowths tubularize and arborize to form the main and terminal ductal systems and secretory acini. The oral mesenchyme regulates proliferation of cells at various sites in the developing gland, ordering them to function as secretory acinar cells producing specific enzymes or directing development of the ductal system.[40] The surrounding mesenchyme also divides the gland into lobules and envelops it to form a distinct capsule. Lymph nodes may become entrapped within parotid or submandibular glandular tissue during development.

HISTOLOGY

The basic salivary unit is similar for all salivary glands (Figure 84-1). The salivary secretory unit is composed of, from distal to proximal, acini, intercalated ducts, striated ducts, and excretory ducts. Other cells such as myoepithelial cells, oncocytes, and sebaceous cells are also found. Acinar cells are secretory and contain prominent endoplasmic reticulum, Golgi apparatus, and secretory granules. Acinar cells may secrete serous or mucinous fluids. Serous acinar cells predominate in the parotid gland, a mixture of serous and mucinous cells in the submandibular gland, and mucus-secreting cells in the sublingual and minor salivary glands. Myoepithelial cells are contractile supporting cells that lie immediately adjacent to the acini. They help moderate secretion and may help form the basement membrane.

Draining the acinus into the oral cavity is a specialized duct system. Initial drainage of the acinus is into the intercalated duct. Intercalated duct cells are lined with simple cuboidal epithelium, which has a transitional secretory and transport role. Intercalated ducts lead to striated ducts that are formed from a single layer of columnar cells. Striated duct epithelial cells are rich in mitochondria and regulate water and electrolyte content of the saliva. The intercalated ducts and striated ducts are intralobular ducts. Excretory ducts are interlobular and travel in thicker connective tissue. The excretory ducts collect and transport saliva from striated ducts into the oral cavity. Excretory ducts contain both simple columnar epithelium and stratified squamous epithelium and may help regulate the salivary osmolality.

PHYSIOLOGY

The normal salivary volume is 1,000 to 2,000 ml per day. A low basal diurnal secretory rate occurs but the vast majority of salivary volume results from stimulated secretion. Some 95% of saliva produced daily is from the parotid and submandibular glands and is predominantly serous. Sublingual and minor

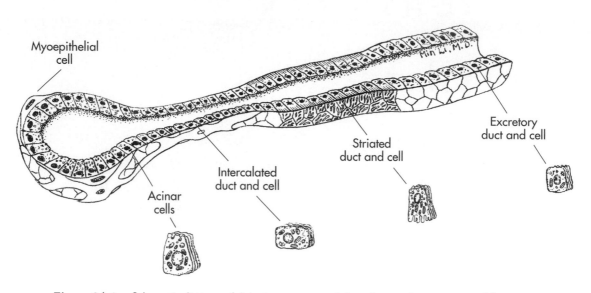

Figure 84-1. Schematic diagram of the microanatomy of the salivary unit: structure and function.

salivary glands contribute the remaining 5% of total daily secretion as mucus.

Saliva is a complex mixture of water, electrolytes, enzymes and other proteins, and several vitamins and hormones. Initial acinar production of saliva is isotonic with a high sodium/low potassium composition similar to plasma. As the saliva passes through the intercalated and striated ducts, water, sodium, and chloride are reabsorbed and potassium and bicarbonate are secreted into the saliva. Submandibular gland saliva has a relatively high calcium concentration compared with parotid gland saliva.

Saliva performs many functions within the oral cavity. Glycoprotein mucus secretions by the sublingual and minor salivary glands lubricate the oral cavity. Serous saliva clears food, cellular debris, and bacteria from the oral cavity. Salivary immunoglobulins, particularly IgA, lysozyme, and lactoperoxidase defend against a number of bacteria and viruses. Bicarbonate secretion maintains an alkaline environment, preventing growth of acidophilic bacteria. Salivary minerals such as calcium, phosphate, and magnesium help maintain the teeth against the wear of mastication and prevent caries. Amylase is secreted by the parotid and submandibular glands in zymogenic form, which is activated in the oral cavity to begin the initial stages of carbohydrate digestion.

Neural control of salivary function involves complex parasympathetic and sympathetic reflex arcs. The efferent pathway is via the parasympathetic and sympathetic autonomic nervous system. Touch, taste, and olfactory receptors send afferent signals by cranial nerves I, IV, VII, and IX to the salivatory nuclei in the brain stem, cortex, and hypothalamus. Efferent signals for both parasympathetic and sympathetic fibers arise in the hypothalamus. Preganglionic parasympathetic fibers to the parotid gland originate from the inferior salivatory nucleus and join the glossopharyngeal nerve. The tympanic branch of the glossopharyngeal nerve, known as Jacobson's nerve, enters the middle ear and anastomoses with the caroticotympanic branch carrying sympathetic fibers from the superior cervical ganglion, which tracks along the external carotid artery. This anastomosis is known as the tympanic plexus. The lesser superficial petrosal nerve arises from the tympanic plexus and travels through the temporal bone into the middle cranial fossa, exiting through the foramen ovale and joining the otic ganglion near the skull base. The parotid gland's parasympathetic preganglionic fibers synapse in the otic ganglion. The postganglionic fibers and sympathetic fibers innervate the parotid gland via the auriculotemporal nerve (Figure 84-2).

The preganglionic parasympathetic nerves to the submandibular and minor salivary glands originate in the superior salivatory nucleus of the pons. These fibers leave the brain stem as the nervus intermedius portion of the facial nerve. Fibers to the submandibular and sublingual glands travel with the chorda tympani and the lingual nerve to synapse in the submandibular ganglion (Figure 84-3). Postganglionic fibers arise in the submandibular ganglion and travel directly to the glands. The minor salivary glands receive parasympathetic fibers via the greater superficial petrosal nerve, vidian nerve, and sphenopalatine ganglion.

Parasympathetic stimuli cause secretion of mucinous saliva, whereas sympathetic stimuli increase production of serous secretions and cause myoepithelial cell contraction, which results in increased salivary flow. Factors affecting the composition and flow of saliva include the stimulated versus resting state, whole saliva versus saliva specific to one gland, patient age, drugs with cholinergic or anticholinergic side effects, diet, hormonal imbalances, irradiation, metabolic conditions such as alcoholism, cystic fibrosis, diabetes, and chronic inflammatory conditions such as Sjögren's syndrome.

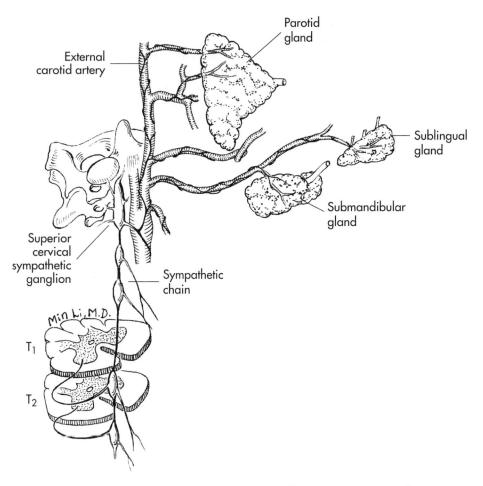

Figure 84-2. Parasympathetic innervation of the major salivary glands.

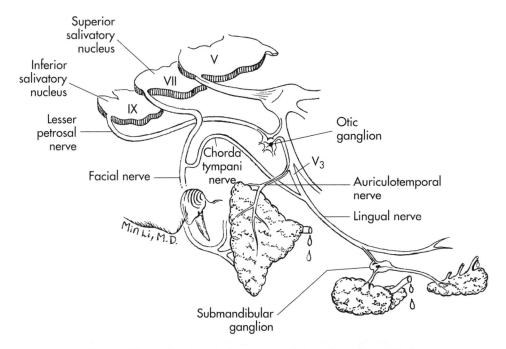

Figure 84-3. Sympathetic innervation of the major salivary glands.

ANATOMY

PAROTID GLANDS

The parotid glands are the the largest of the salivary glands. They are paired unilobular glands divided nonanatomically by the facial nerve into two surgical zones. The parotid tissue located lateral to nerve VII is designated the lateral or superficial lobe, and tissue medial to the nerve is designated the medial or deep lobe. Accessory parotid tissue may extend along the parotid duct into the buccal space.

The parotid gland is roughly pyramidal in shape and lies in the preauricular area just inferior and medial to the external auditory canal (Figure 84-4). The posterior boundaries of the parotid gland are the mastoid and tympanic processes of the temporal bone, external auditory canal, and the styloid process. The apex or tail of the gland may extend as low in the neck as the midregion of the sternocleidomastoid. Laterally the gland is covered by skin, subcutaneous fat, platysma and/or superficial musculoaponeurotic system (SMAS), and the investing parotid fascia. Medially the anterior portion of the gland lies on masseter muscle. The posterior-medial gland extends into the retromandibular area through the stylomastoid tunnel into the parapharyngeal space. The superior border is the zygomatic arch, and the inferior border is the sternocleidomastoid muscle and the posterior belly of the digastric.[41] Because the gland is encapsulated and fixed within a relatively rigid space, edema or tumors may compress the carotid sheath and interfere with function of cranial nerves VII, IX, X, and XI. Deep lobe parotid tumors may present as a parapharyngeal mass (see Figure 84-4).

The facial nerve is intimately associated with the parotid gland and is the major anatomic consideration in parotid surgery (Figure 84-5). The extratemporal portion of cranial nerve VII exits the skull through the stylomastoid foramen and passes in a superior-to-inferior, deep-to-superficial course through the gland to the lateral surface of the masseter muscle and across the zygomatic arch. Before entering the gland the facial nerve gives off three motor branches to the posterior auricular muscle, posterior belly of the digastric muscle and stylohyoid muscle.[6,60] It enters the gland lateral to the external carotid artery and posterior facial vein. The nerve then branches at an obtuse angle into an upper temporofacial division and a lower cervicofacial division. This major branch point is called the pes anserinus and is usually within 1 cm of the nerve's entrance into the gland. From this point, the nerve divides into at least five branches that innervate the muscles of facial expression. A number of common branching patterns have been described.[6,13] The zygomatic and buccal branches demonstrate multiple interconnecting patterns. The temporal and marginal mandibular branches have relatively few interconnections. Injury or

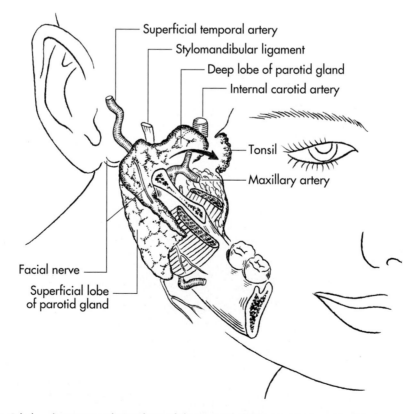

Figure 84-4. Anatomic relationships of the parotid glands to structures in the retromandibular and parapharyngeal areas. Deep lobe parotid masses may protrude into the parapharyngeal space and present as an intraoral swelling (*arrow*).

resection of these branches is more likely to result in a permanent motor deficit. The terminal branches of the facial nerve lie just deep to the investing parotid fascia over the masseter muscle and just beneath the platysma muscle in the neck.

Although the course of the facial nerve is variable, some spatial relations are important. In the adult the main trunk exits the stylomastoid foramen 1 cm superior to the tip of the mastoid process and 1 to 1.5 cm deep to its lateral surface. The nerve usually bifurcates within 2 cm of exit from the stylomastoid foramen and within 1 cm after entry into the parotid gland. The buccal branch lies along a line that connects the tragus with the midline of the upper lip. The temporal branch lies along a line from the tragus to 1.5 cm lateral to the lateral brow. The temporal branch always lies anterior to the superficial temporal vessels and just deep to the SMAS layer. It is very superficial as it crosses the zygomatic arch. Frequent anastomoses occur between the zygomatic and buccal branches within the buccal fat pad.[6] The terminal nerve branches lie just deep to the muscles of facial expression and innervate them from their deep surface. Branches of the cervicofacial division lie deep to the platysma muscle. The marginal mandibular branch of the facial nerve is found immediately lateral to the facial artery and vein near the inferior border of the body of the mandible. Posterior to the facial vessels, the ramus mandibularis usually lies cephalad to the inferior border of the mandi-

ble, but in up to 20% of cases may be located as much as 1 cm below the border.[16] Anterior to the facial vessels, the ramus mandibularis is located cephalad to the inferior mandibular border.

Drainage of parotid gland is into the parotid or Stensen's duct. The duct arises at the anterior border of the gland as a confluence of several large interlobular ducts. It runs across the lateral surface of the masseter muscle, closely accompanied by the buccal branch of the facial nerve. At the anterior surface of the masseter, the duct pierces the buccinator muscle and enters the oral cavity at the level of the second maxillary molar.

The blood supply to the parotid gland is via the terminal branches of the external carotid artery, particularly the superficial temporal and internal maxillary artery. The venous return is into the posterior facial (retromandibular) vein. A number of intraparotid and extraparotid lymph nodes receive afferent lymphatic drainage from the ear, eyelids, cheek, lacrimal glands, conjunctiva, frontal and temporal scalp, and lateral nose (Figure 84-6). Lymphatic drainage from these areas and the parotid gland itself is through the intraglandular and extraglandular parotid lymph nodes and subsequently into level II jugulodigastric nodes of the deep cervical chain. Parotid gland sensation is provided by the auriculotemporal branch of cranial nerve V and the greater auricular nerve.[41]

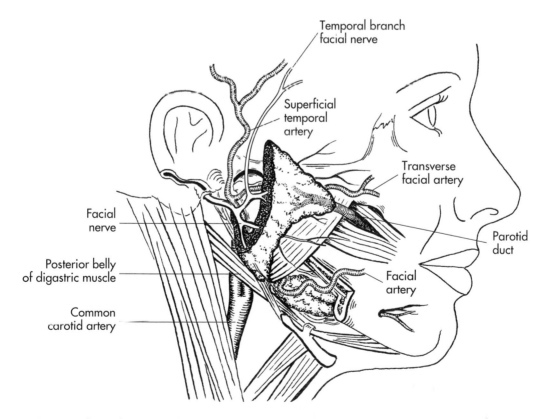

Figure 84-5. Anatomic relationships of the parotid gland to the surrounding structures. The facial nerve courses through the parotid gland parenchyma, separating the superficial and deep lobes. Note that the facial nerve is lateral to the retromandibular vein and to the terminal branches of the external carotid artery.

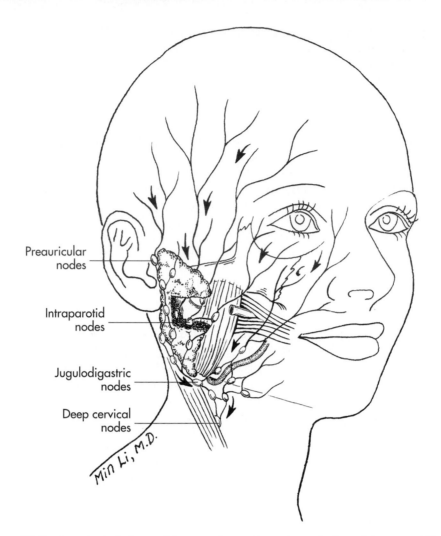

Figure 84-6. Lymphatic drainage of the upper face and anterior scalp through intraparotid lymph nodes into the jugular digastric nodes of the deep cervical lymphatics.

SUBMANDIBULAR GLAND

The submandibular glands are paired salivary glands weighing 10 to 15 grams each. The submandibular gland is a mixed seromucous gland. The glands lie below and anterior to the angle of the mandible in a triangle formed by the lower border of the mandible and the anterior and posterior bellies of the digastric muscle (Figure 84-7). The subcutaneous fat and platysma are superficial to the investing fascia of the gland. Just deep to the investing fascia lies the marginal mandibular nerve, which is immediately superficial to the facial artery and vein as these vascular structures ascend across the lateral surface of the gland. The deep surface of the gland rests on the mylohyoid and hyoglossus muscles and is closely situated to the hypoglossal and lingual nerves. At its most superior point, the gland is bordered by the lingual cortex of the body of the mandible. The submandibular, or Wharton's, duct is about 5 cm long. Wharton's duct lies on the mylohyoid and hyoglossus muscles. It runs parallel and just inferior to the lingual nerve and parallel and just superior to the hypoglossal nerve, opening into the oral cavity near the lingual frenulum.

The arterial supply to the submandibular gland is from the lingual and facial arteries. Venous drainage is through the anterior facial vein. Both the submandibular and sublingual glands receive secretomotor parasympathetic fibers from the chorda tympani and submandibular ganglion. This ganglion lies just superior and deep to the gland itself. On the surface of the submandibular gland lie several lymph nodes that drain the skin of the lower cheek, lip, floor of mouth, and oral tongue. Lymphatic drainage of the submandibular gland is into these nodes and subsequently into the level II jugulodigastric nodes.

SUBLINGUAL GLANDS

The sublingual glands are the smallest of the paired salivary glands, weighing only about 2 grams. The glands secrete a mucous saliva. They lie in the sublingual groove on the inner surface of the anterior mandible deep to the mucosa of the anterior floor of the mouth, resting directly on the mylohyoid muscle. The sublingual glands drain into the oral cavity directly via 8 to 20 short ducts that originate from the superior surface of each gland. Blood supply is from the sublingual branch of the lingual artery and the submental branch of the

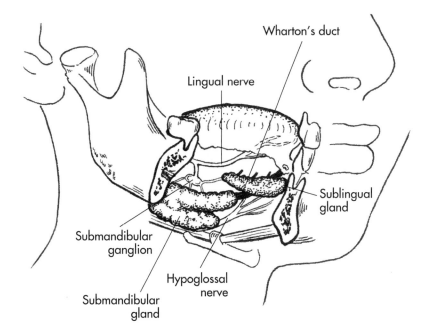

Figure 84-7. Anatomic relationships of the submandibular and sublingual glands to major structures of the submandibular triangle (note the close relationship of the hypoglossal and lingual nerves to Wharton's duct).

facial artery. Lymphatic drainage is into level I submental and submandibular cervical lymph nodes.

MINOR SALIVARY GLANDS

The minor salivary glands are estimated to number between 600 and 1,000. They are small, independent, mucus-secreting glands found throughout the oral cavity and much of the oropharynx. They are particularly abundant in the buccal, labial, palatal, and lingual areas. Each gland drains into the oral cavity through its own separate duct.

PATHOPHYSIOLOGY

NONNEOPLASTIC CONDITIONS

Sialoadenosis

Sialoadenoses are a heterogenous group of noninflammatory enlargements of the salivary glands. A variety of systemic conditions may result in salivary gland enlargement, most often of the parotid gland. Enlargement of the parotid glands may occur in patients suffering from protein and total calorie malnutrition, cirrhosis, diabetes mellitus, hypothyroidism, obesity, and drugs such as bismuth, mercury, and iodine. Histologically, acinar hypertrophy is seen with increased numbers of secretory granules. Despite this observation, sialoadenoses are usually accompanied by a decrease in salivary flow. Ultimately fatty infiltration follows and may lead to irreversible loss of function.[3] These salivary gland changes must be recognized as part of the constellation of signs and symptoms of a systemic disease rather than a problem specific to the salivary gland itself.

Infectious Disorders

Infectious disorders of the parotid gland may be viral, bacterial, mycobacterial, or fungal. Coxsackievirus, parainfluenza, cytomegalovirus, and echoviruses may cause parotitis. Mumps is a systemic viral disease with local salivary gland manifestations. The disease usually occurs in children but may be seen in adults. Clinically mumps is an acute unilateral or bilateral nonsuppurative inflammation of the parotid glands, although involvement of the submandibular, sublingual, and lacrimal glands may also occur. The tender salivary gland enlargement disappears in 7 to 10 days, leaving no salivary gland sequelae.

Bacterial salivary infections are usually the result of ductal obstruction or stasis with ascending bacterial infection by oral flora. Acute suppurative parotitis occurs with dehydration related to systemic disease, which results in decreased salivary flow and ductal stasis. About one third of cases of acute bacterial parotitis occur in the postoperative setting after major surgery, usually in elderly patients.[48] The infection is usually unilateral. Signs and symptoms include fever, cheek tenderness, trismus, and purulent discharge expressible from the parotid duct orifice. The most common pathogen is *Staphylococcus aureus,* but *Streptococcus viridans,* β-hemolytic streptococcus, and pneumococcus infections also occur. The process is initially diffuse but may progress to localized abscesses and ductal strictures, which can result in repeat episodes of acute infection known as recurrent acute parotitis. Chronic recurrent infection may ensue, characterized by recurrent attacks of low-grade inflammation with mucopurulent parotid duct discharge. A similar picture may be seen with cystic fibrosis. This condition usually manifests in the submandibular gland, which produces abnormally thick mucinous saliva. Inspissation of the abnormal saliva leads to ductal obstruction, dilatation, infection, and secondary atrophy and fibrosis.

Sialolithiasis

Calculi are one of the most common benign conditions to affect salivary glands. They occur predominantly in the submandibular gland (80%) and the parotid gland (20%), and rarely in minor salivary glands.[7] Salivary gland stones have no associated metabolic disorder. Calculi may be single or multiple. They occur in the setting of stasis of secretion, alteration in the character of secretions, and ductal strictures. The nucleus of the stone may be formed by a nidus of desquamated epithelial cells, mucus, bacteria, or the deposition of calcium salts, leading to the formation of calculi. Calculi classically present as a painful unilateral swelling of the gland with a palpable duct stone or purulent exudate through the duct. Salivary stimulation during meals increases the symptoms. Submandibular stones are usually radiopaque and solitary. Parotid stones are usually radiolucent and may be multiple and intraparenchymal. Obstruction may result in retrograde infection and present as acute or chronic bacterial sialadenitis. Salivary gland calculi are frequently recurrent because of repetitive infection, nidus formation, and disorders of salivary flow.

Congenital Disorders

Absence of the parotid gland and facial nerve may be seen in first and second branchial arch syndromes. Heterotopic salivary gland tissue and sinuses through the parotid gland may occur in first branchial cleft anomalies. These congenital disorders may present as parotid gland masses in childhood or adult life. The lesions arise when remnants of the first branchial arch become enveloped by the parotid gland during embryonic development (Figure 84-8). Mostly cystic, the lesions demonstrate squamous or pseudostratified columnar epithelium. Superimposed acute inflammation may occur.

Trauma

Salivary gland injuries are serious and frequently associated with long-term morbidity. They are often overlooked or underestimated in patients who have suffered multiple trauma. Salivary gland trauma is often associated with injuries involving the overlying skin, teeth, oral cavity, and facial skeletal structures. Mechanisms of parotid gland injury include lacerations, avulsions (especially bite wounds), and blunt injuries. Complications of unrecognized injury include pseudocyst and salivary fistula. Both are caused by unrepaired transection of the main duct of the gland.

Mucoceles

Mucoceles are mucus-retention cysts or pseudocysts resulting from ductal rupture and localized extravasation. They are usually seen on the lower lip but may occur anywhere in the mouth. A mucus-retention cyst resulting from blockage of the sublingual duct with true cyst formation is called a ranula.

Granulomatous Inflammation

Sarcoidosis affects the parotid gland in approximately 5% of cases. Usually multiple salivary and lacrimal glands are involved by the granulomatous process (Heerfordt's disease).[39] Histologically, noncaseating granulomas are found within the glands. Stains and cultures for infectious agents are negative. Facial nerve palsy may be seen with this syndrome. Granulomatous involvement of the salivary glands may also be seen with mycobacterial infections. Both typical and atypical mycobacterial infections occur, most commonly in children or immunosuppressed hosts.

Autoimmune Disorders

A variety of autoimmune disorders may affect the salivary glands. Mikulicz described bilateral enlargement of the salivary and lacrimal glands in a nonspecific syndrome associated with several diseases including leukemia, lymphoma, and tuberculosis. A more distinct description of salivary gland changes seen in these disorders and autoimmune diseases is the benign lymphoepithelial lesion (BLEL).[28] This may be viewed as the end stage of a chronic inflammatory process initiated by early injury to the gland caused by ductal obstruction or other etiology.[3] Histologically the lesion shows almost total replacement of acinar and duct epithelium with a chronic inflammatory infiltrate.

BLEL may present as an isolated unilateral or bilateral phenomenon. There is an equal sex distribution unless it occurs as part of a systemic autoimmune disease with a female predominance such as Sjögren's syndrome. Sjögren's syndrome includes keratoconjunctivitis sicca, resulting from acinar atrophy and chronic inflammation of the lacrimal gland, and xerostomia from a similar process in the salivary glands associated with frequent salivary gland enlargement. BLEL may also occur with other collagen vascular diseases such as rheumatoid arthritis or scleroderma. Serologic studies reveal elevated antinuclear antibody titers, rheumatoid factor, and polyclonal gammopathy in many patients. In Sjögren's syndrome the lesion affects all salivary glands and the diagnosis can be made from lower lip biopsy with examination of a minor salivary gland. BLEL is seen frequently in patients suffering from human immunodeficiency virus (HIV) infection.[50]

Malignant degeneration of the epithelial and lymphatic components of the salivary gland lesion in BLEL has been described. An increased incidence of lymphoma is associated

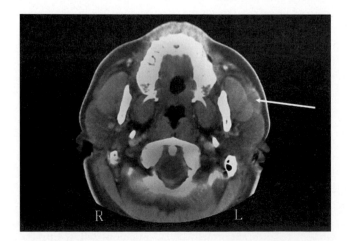

Figure 84-8. First branchial cleft cyst remnant presenting as a left parotid mass, as demonstrated on CT scan (arrow).

with Sjögren's syndrome. Rarely, anaplastic carcinomatous transformation may occur with BLEL. This rare disorder has a racial predisposition for Eskimos and American Indians.[29]

Necrotizing Sialometaplasia

Sialometaplasia is an unusual benign disorder caused by salivary tissue injury, which induces a metaplastic tissue repair process. The cause is uncertain but some cases have been associated with ill-fitting dentures and other trauma. Similar lesions in major salivary glands may be seen following trauma or surgery. The lesion usually presents as an ulcerated nodule of the palate that mimics carcinoma clinically and pathologically. Histologically, necrotizing sialometaplasia shows an intralobular infarct-like necrosis and extensive squamous metaplasia.[1] Residual ductal epithelium and inflammatory-induced atypia can lead to the erroneous diagnosis of mucoepidermoid or squamous cell carcinoma.

NEOPLASTIC DISORDERS

Theories of Oncogenesis

Salivary gland tumors are an extremely heterogenous collection of tumors with respect to histologic and morphologic findings. The relatively rare nature of these tumors, coupled with the complexity of proper classification, has made salivary gland diagnoses difficult for both surgeon and pathologist. Controversy surrounds the putative cells of origin, tumor grouping, and clinical staging. There has been a historical

lack of a single clearly defined, widely accepted classification system for salivary gland tumors. The World Health Organization classification of salivary tumors is found in Box 84-1.[49]

Benign and malignant tumors of major and minor salivary glands originate primarily from the epithelial cells and are therefore carcinomas. Sarcomas rarely may arise from mesenchymal tissues. Two basic theories have been proposed to account for the development of salivary gland neoplasia. In the first theory, dedifferentiation, mature cellular elements of the salivary unit respond to an oncogenic stimulus, resulting in benign or malignant tumors whose structure and behavior are similar to the highly specialized precursor cell. Acinous cell carcinoma would therefore arise from acinar cells, squamous cell carcinoma from the squamous cells of the excretory duct, and adenocarcinoma from the fully differentiated intercalated duct cells.

The bicellular theory of origin proposed by Eversole suggests that neoplasms arise from the two types of stem or reserve cells.[20] When a reserve cell that still has capacity to synthesize DNA is affected by an oncogenic stimulus, the resulting neoplasm is malignant. When the oncogenic event occurs further down the sequence of cellular differentiation, the tumor is benign. The basal cells of the excretory duct may be transformed into low-or high grade mucoepidermoid cancers or squamous cell cancers depending on the point at which the oncogenic stimulus occurs. When the reserve cells of the intercalated ducts are transformed after they have begun

---

Box 84-1.
The World Health Organization Classification of Salivary Tumors[49]

Adenomas
Myoepithelioma (myoepithelial adenoma)
Warthin's tumor (adenolymphoma)
Oncocytoma (oncocytic adenoma)
Sebaceous adenoma
Inverted ductal papilloma
Sialadenoma papilliferum
Papillary cystadenoma
Carcinomas
Mucoepidermoid carcinoma
Epithelial-myoepithelial carcinoma
Papillary cystadenocarcinoma
Oncocytic carcinoma
Adenocarcinoma
Squamous cell carcinoma
Undifferentiated carcinoma
Nonepithelial tumors
Secondary tumors
Tumor-like lesions
Oncocytosis
Cystic lymphoid hyperplasia in AIDS
Pleomorphic adenoma
Basal cell carcinoma
Canalicular adenoma

Sebaceous adenoma
Ductal papilloma
Intraductal papilloma
Cystadenoma
Mucinous cystadenoma
Acinic cell carcinoma
Adenoid cystic carcinoma
Sebaceous carcinoma
Mucinous adenocarcinoma
Salivary duct carcinoma
Salivary gland cysts
Small cell carcinoma
Other carcinomas
Malignant lymphomas
Unclassified tumors
Sialadenosis
Benign lymphoepithelial lesion
Necrotizing sialometaplasia (salivary gland infarction)
Chronic sclerosing sialadenitis of submandibular gland
Polymorphous low-grade adenocarcinoma (terminal duct adenocarcinoma)
Malignant myoepithelioma (myoepithelial carcinoma)
Carcinoma in pleomorphic adenoma (malignant mixed tumor)

differentiation toward striated duct cells they become onco-cytic tumors. Acinous cell carcinomas arise from the cells that would normally differentiate into acinar cells. Pleomorphic adenomas and adenocarcinomas arise from aberrant differenti-ation of the intercalated duct cells.

The majority of salivary gland neoplasms, both malignant and benign, occur in the parotid gland. Tumors of the minor salivary glands, in contrast with those of the major salivary glands, are more likely to be malignant. Approximately 20% of parotid gland tumors, 50% of submandibular gland tumors, and 70% of minor salivary gland tumors are malignant. Histological features and stage rather than site of origin are the main determinants of clinical outcome. The relative frequency of salivary gland tumors by site is shown in Table 84-1. The relative frequency of salivary gland malignancies by site is shown in Table 84-2.

Table 84-1.
Relative Frequency of Salivary Gland Tumors by Site

HISTOLOGIC TYPE	ALL SALIVARY GLANDS (%)	PAROTID GLAND (%)	SUBMANDIBULAR GLAND (%)	MINOR GLANDS (%)
Pleomorphic adenoma	43	40-70	43-60	40-53
Monomorphic adenoma	12	3-20	—	3
Mucoepidermoid carcinoma	12	12-21	4-11	16-45
Adenoid cystic carcinoma	6	2-8	15-19	20-24
Adenocarcinoma	3	4-11	7	18
Squamous cell carcinoma	2	3-5	7	—
Acinous cell carcinoma	2	2-3	1	6
Undifferentiated carcinoma	1	1	—	1
Carcinoma ex pleomorphic adenoma	3	3	3-11	3

Adapted from Jurkiewicz MJ, Krizek TJ, Mathes SJ, et al: Salivary gland disorders, *Plast Surg* 1:379-417, 1990.

Table 84-2.
Relative Frequency of Salivary Gland Malignancies by Site

HISTOLOGIC TYPE	ALL SALIVARY GLANDS (%)	PAROTID GLAND (%)	SUBMANDIBULAR GLAND (%)	MINOR GLANDS (%)
Mucoepidermoid carcinoma				
High-grade	10	21-50	25	11
Low-grade	18	—	—	—
Adenoid cystic carcinoma	15	17-29	31-41	14-25
Adenocarcinoma	13	22	7-16	33
Squamous cell carcinoma	6	3	5	—
Acinous cell carcinoma	6-8	12-15	—	—
Undifferentiated carcinoma	12	5	7	1
Carcinoma ex pleomorphic adenoma	12	5	11	4

Adapted from Jurkiewicz MJ, Krizek TJ, Mathes SJ, et al: Salivary gland disorders, *Plast Surg* 1:379-417, 1990.

BENIGN TUMORS

Monomorphic Adenoma

Monomorphic adenomas are benign neoplastic growths composed entirely of a single epithelial cell type.[26] They are benign growths in which the epithelium forms a regular (usually glandular) pattern without mesenchymal tissue characteristics of the pleomorphic adenoma. Monomorphic adenomas include the papillary cystadenoma lymphomatosum (Warthin's tumor), the oxyphilic adenoma (oncocytoma), and a group of rarer lesions that resemble benign dermal appendage tumors (basal cell adenoma, sebaceous adenoma, myoepithelioma, intraductal papilloma, and sialadenoma papilliferum). Monomorphic adenomas originate from the intercalated duct cell, and account for 4% to 8% of salivary gland neoplasms. Monomorphic adenomas have a propensity toward multicentricity. They have the capacity to transform into pleomorphic adenomas.

Papillary Cystadenoma Lymphomatosum

Warthin's tumor is the most common of the monomorphic adenomas. It is a benign tumor with neoplastic duct epithelium and a prominent lymphoid element. It occurs in the parotid gland and accounts for 6% to 10% of all parotid tumors. It may also occur in heterotopic salivary tissue.[11] The parotid gland develops by epithelial budding, which surrounds the facial nerve and rudimentary lymph nodes. Lymph node aggregates may envelop developing salivary tissue within the capsule of the gland. When the lymphoid-encapsulated epithelial tissue is subjected to oncogenic stimulus, Warthin's tumors occur. Warthin's tumors have a high incidence of multicentricity and bilaterality (approximately 10%), which explains the tendency for local recurrence. There is a 5:1 male gender ratio predominance. Most patients (>90%) are smokers. The usual presentation is an asymptomatic mass in the tail of the parotid gland at the angle of the mandible.

Oncocytomas

Oncocytomas are unusual lesions accounting for about 1% of salivary gland tumors. Oncocytosis is a normal degenerative change in the salivary glands that occurs with age. Oncocytes contain defective mitochondria that undergo hyperplasia to give the cell its characteristic eosinophilic histologic appearance. The origin of the neoplastic cell is probably the striated duct. Oncocytoma is differentiated from Warthin's tumor by the lack of a lymphoid element. The tumor is benign and occurs most frequently in the parotid gland. Histologic differentiation of benign from malignant oncocytoma is difficult, and clinical behavior usually determines the diagnosis.

Pleomorphic Adenoma

The pleomorphic adenoma (benign mixed tumor) is the most common salivary gland tumor.[53] The tumor is composed of benign epithelial cells surrounded by myoepithelial cells interspersed with areas of myxoid or chondroid stroma

(Figure 84-9). The proportions of cellular and myxoid areas may vary considerably and do not predict malignancy. The neoplastic elements of pleomorphic adenomas are derived from the reserve cell of the intercalated ducts, which may differentiate into either myoepithelial or epithelial cells. Both cells may participate in the neoplasia of pleomorphic adenoma, the epithelial cell providing the cellular proliferation and the myoepithelial cell the mesenchymal stroma.

Pleomorphic adenomas usually present as a solitary painless mass. Most pleomorphic adenomas occur in the parotid gland, and 70% of parotid tumors are pleomorphic adenomas. Most occur in the tail of the parotid gland, but up to 10% may involve the deep lobe. There is a slight female to male predominance and the tumor usually presents in the fifth decade. The tumors clinically appear to be well encapsulated and grow slowly. However, there is frequently extension of pseudopods beyond the palpable and visible tumor mass. This morphologic characteristic increases the risk of recurrent disease after resection. Recurrent pleomorphic adenoma frequently presents in a nodular multifocal pattern resulting from the seeding of the surgical bed by rupture of tumor capsule.

Benign Lymphoepithelial Lesions

BLEL is a disease process characterized histologically by replacement of salivary gland parenchyma with lymphoid tissue containing epithelial islands. The disease may be diffuse or focal, encapsulated or nonencapsulated. Infiltration of lymphocytes and plasma cells is progressive until the parenchyma is entirely replaced and only ductal remnants remain. A cystic pattern may be seen.[50] The differential diagnosis between BLEL and primary lymphomas of the salivary glands may be difficult. In BLEL the cells are well differentiated and do not invade the salivary gland capsule and there is no involvement of adjacent lymph nodes or distant sites. (See also the section on Autoimmune Disorders.)

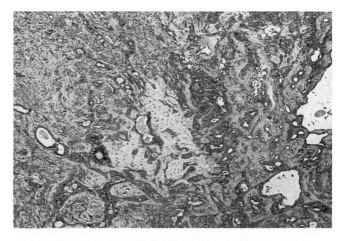

Figure 84-9. Characteristic histologic appearance of pleomorphic adenoma (benign mixed tumor). Note areas of benign cellular neoplasia interspersed with areas of myxoid stroma. (×40.)

MALIGNANT NEOPLASIA

Acinic Cell Carcinoma

Acinic cell carcinoma arises from the reserve cell of the intercalated duct. Nearly all cases arise in the parotid gland; only rarely are the submandibular or minor salivary glands involved. Acinic cell carcinomas account for 2% to 4% of all parotid gland tumors.[53] Approximately 3% are bilateral. Acinic cell carcinomas behave as low-grade malignant tumors in that they have a strong tendency to recur locally. Aggressive lesions may be locally extensive.

Adenoid Cystic Carcinoma

Adenoid cystic carcinoma is the most common malignant tumor of the submandibular, sublingual, and minor salivary glands, but accounts for only about 15% of parotid gland cancers. Cell of origin is the intercalated duct reserve cell. These tumors are also known as cylindromas because of the cribriform pattern sometimes seen histologically (Figure 84-10). Adenoid cystic carcinomas vary considerably in their histologic appearance. Perzin and associates classified adenoid cystic carcinomas according to their predominant histologic pattern: tubular, cribriform, or solid.[44] Tubular differentiation carried the most favorable prognosis, whereas those consisting predominantly of solid nests were worse. Adenoid cystic carcinomas tend to grow slowly and invade locally. They are characterized by invasion beyond the palpable and visible mass. Histologic evidence of perineural invasion is seen in most cases. More than any other salivary gland tumor, adenoid cystic carcinoma presents with pain and facial nerve paralysis.

Adenocarcinoma

Adenocarcinomas of the salivary gland also arise from the stem cell of the intercalated duct. They account for about 13% of all salivary gland malignancies, being somewhat more common in the parotid and minor salivary glands than the submandibular gland. They are aggressive tumors with a variable propensity for local recurrence, regional lymph node metastasis, and dissemination to lungs, bone, and liver. Behavior of individual tumors correlates somewhat with histologic grade. High-grade lesions have a trabecular histologic appearance. Polymorphic or papillary histology generally indicates a lower grade tumor.[19] The course may be indolent and progressive with development of late hematogenous metastases and local failure.

Malignant Mixed Tumor (Carcinoma Ex Pleomorphic Adenoma)

Carcinoma ex pleomorphic adenoma usually is associated with pleomorphic adenoma. Clinical presentation may be microscopic evidence of a malignancy involving a pleomorphic adenoma or, more commonly, primary or recurrent pleomorphic adenoma of long duration that undergoes rapid growth and is found to be malignant. The risk of malignancy in primary pleomorphic adenoma is less than 10% but recurrent pleomorphic adenomas are more likely to undergo malignant degeneration. Malignant mixed tumors account for 11% of all salivary gland malignancies and 5% to 18% of parotid gland malignancies.[56,57] The progenitor cell, similar to pleomorphic adenoma, is probably the intercalated duct cell. Generally, only the epithelial component is malignant.

Mucoepidermoid Carcinoma

Mucoepidermoid carcinoma is the most common parotid gland cancer and second to adenoid cystic carcinoma in the submandibular and minor salivary glands.[58] Mucoepidermoid carcinomas occur commonly in the fifth decade of life, although it is also the most common salivary gland tumor in children. Female gender predominance is 2.4:1. Mucoepidermoid carcinomas arise from the excretory duct system with their progenitor cells being the basal cells of the excretory ducts. Mucoepidermoid carcinoma is composed of mixed epidermoid and mucous secretory malignant cells (Figure 84-11).

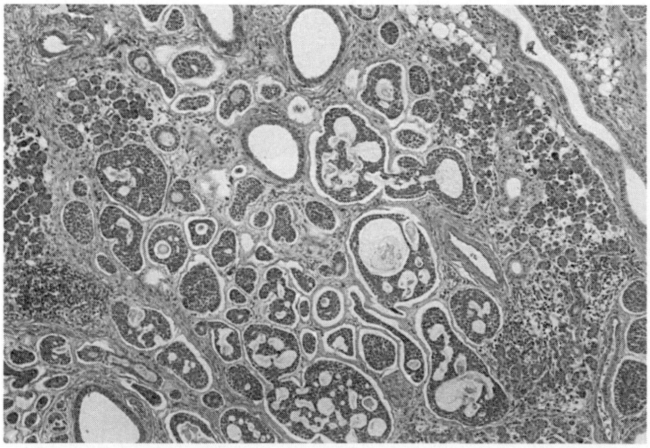

Figure 84-10. Adenoid cystic carcinoma. Characteristic histologic finding of the cribriform or cylindromatous subtype. (×40.)

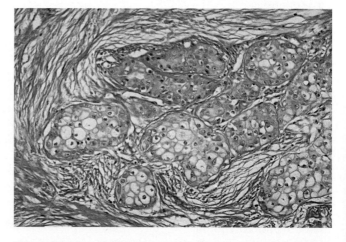

Figure 84-11. Mucoepidermoid carcinoma. Note characteristic histologic appearance with mixed epidermoid and mucus-secreting malignant cells. (×100.)

Squamous Cell Carcinoma

True squamous cell carcinoma of salivary gland origin is rare, accounting for only 1% of salivary gland malignancies. It is a diagnosis of exclusion after cutaneous squamous cell carcinomas, which could potentially metastasize to the salivary gland lymph nodes, have been ruled out.[56] When present it arises from the basal cell of the excretory duct. Strong association with tobacco use has been described. Squamous cell carcinoma of the salivary glands is a high-grade malignancy characterized by perineural invasion, regional and distant metastatic disease, and local recurrence.

Lymphoma

Primary malignant lymphomas of the salivary glands are rare, constituting only 4% to 5% of extranodal lymphomas. Parotid glands are involved in the usual instance. Patients are typically in the sixth or seventh decade of life. The majority of lymphomas of the salivary glands are of the non-Hodgkin's nodular type followed by diffuse large cell lymphomas.[23] The histologic and clinical criteria for differentiating lymphoma and benign lymphoepithelial lesions have been discussed.

Metastatic Carcinoma to the Salivary Glands

Metastases to the major salivary glands may occur by lymphatic spread, hematogenous dissemination, or contiguous extension.[5] Contiguous spread is most commonly seen with locally invasive or advanced overlying tumors of the skin (Figure 84-12). The majority of lymphatic and hematogenous

metastases occur in the parotid glands. The parotid gland contains a rich network of intercommunicating lymphatic vessels and periparotid and intraparotid lymph nodes (see Figure 84-6) that collects lymphatic drainage of the anterior scalp, cheeks, external ear, eyelids, and lateral nose. Cutaneous squamous cell carcinoma and melanoma arising in these areas are the most frequent metastatic tumors to parotid lymph nodes, each comprising about 40% of metastatic tumors. Occasionally, squamous cell carcinomas of the palate, tonsil, and nasopharynx are the sites of origin of deep lobe parotid gland metastases. Hematogenous metastatic carcinoma to the parotid gland arises most commonly from the primary tumors in the lung, breast, kidney, or gastrointestinal tract.

Salivary Gland Disorders in Children

Fewer than 5% of all tumors of the salivary glands occur in children and young adults. Determination of the true incidence of salivary gland tumors is confounded by the variation in disease patterns during the different periods of childhood and the inclusion of vascular tumors in many series. The ratio of benign to malignant lesions varies greatly with age and depends on whether hemangioma is considered part of the neoplastic process. In reality, the true rate of malignancy is unknown.

Hemangioma of the salivary gland is usually cited as the most common pediatric salivary neoplasm, accounting for up to 60% of lesions.[3] It occurs in infants and children, first presenting at an average age of 9 months. The majority

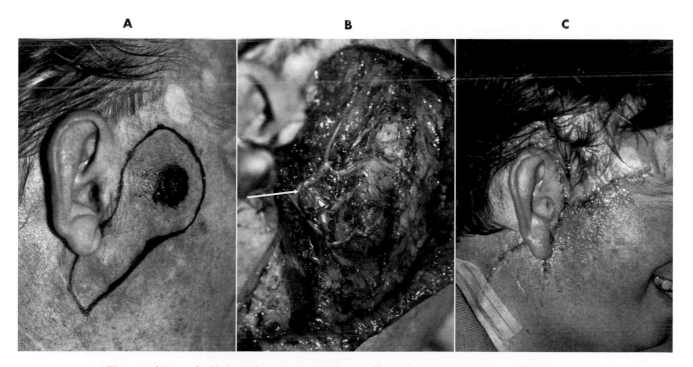

Figure 84-12. **A,** High-grade cutaneous malignant fibrous histiocytoma with contiguous deep invasion of the parotid gland and dermal metastases, marked for wide excision and parotidectomy. **B,** Superficial parotidectomy demonstrating intact facial nerve *(arrow)*. **C,** Postoperative, after closure with cervical facial rotation advancement flap.

occur in the parotid gland and are clinically evident before 2 years of age. Hemangiomas may be multiple or solitary. Typical lesions are asymptomatic, soft, compressible masses that increase in size when the child cries (Figure 84-13). Occasionally, there is an overlying telangiectasia, but usually the vascular neoplasm is confined to the gland beneath its capsule, replacing normal salivary gland parenchyma. Lymphangiomas and mixed hemangiolymphangiomas are also common pediatric salivary gland tumors. They present in similar fashion.

If vascular neoplasms are excluded and only solid tumors are considered, the frequency of malignancy in children is higher than in adults. Schuller and McCabe calculated from collected series that in any child the risk of malignancy from a solid tumor of the salivary gland is 35%.[47] Mucoepidermoid carcinoma is the most common malignancy, accounting for 40% to 50% of observed tumors. It occurs predominantly in adolescents.

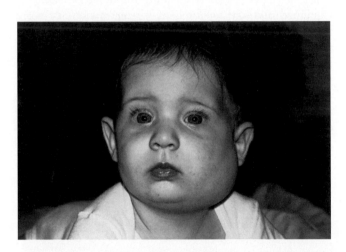

Figure 84-13. A 1-year-old girl with large parotid hemangioma. The tumor resolved spontaneously without therapy by age 3.

APPROACH TO THE PATIENT

The clinician's major goal in the evaluation of a patient with a salivary gland disorder is to determine or exclude the diagnosis of malignancy. The most important questions related to salivary gland problems are whether or not a mass is malignant, primary or metastatic, and what the extent of surgical resection should be.

HISTORY

The patient with a salivary gland mass (usually a parotid mass) is equally likely to be a man or woman, age of 30 to 50 years for benign neoplasms and 50 to 60 years for malignant tumors. The lesion is usually asymptomatic, mobile, nontender, discrete, and less than 3 cm in diameter (Figure 84-14). It is common to find a history of a mass for greater than 1 year. Masses may be subtle, such as asymmetry of the earlobe. Deep lobe parotid tumors may not present with a visible mass at all but with a sore throat or dysphagia as they enlarge through the parapharyngeal space.

Infectious, autoimmune, or neoplastic involvement of the parotid gland may present as a diffuse mass. History is useful in distinguishing inflammatory from neoplastic masses and of some benefit in differentiating between benign and malignant neoplasms. Complaints of diffuse swelling or sudden onset with pain and systemic symptoms of infection are most consistent with an inflammatory condition. A history of predisposing factors such as a postoperative state, previous mycobacterial infection, or exposure to cats may be suggestive of an inflammatory or infectious condition.

Swelling after an infectious episode or in association with food ingestion is characteristic of duct obstruction. This occurs more commonly in the submandibular gland than in the parotid gland. A number of diffuse parotid gland enlargements

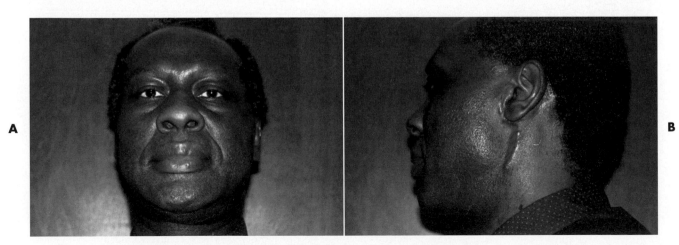

Figure 84-14. Patient with a typical parotid gland mass. **A,** Frontal view. **B,** Lateral view. Mass is subtle and barely visible on frontal view.

may be associated with connective tissue diseases. A careful history should be directed at associated features such as arthralgias, skin rashes, urethritis, ocular problems, xerostomia, and the constellation of symptoms peculiar to autoimmune diseases. A history of radiation to the head and neck is important in the consideration of neoplasia. A history of previous salivary gland tumors, particularly contralateral tumors such as Warthin's tumor or acinic cell cancer, should be sought. A history of previous cutaneous malignancies, particularly melanoma or squamous cell carcinoma in the areas drained by the lymph nodes of the parotid gland, is of obvious relevance.

Pain in association with a discrete mass is an important symptom of malignancy.[56] It occurs in approximately 12% of patients with parotid cancers and is very rare in benign lesions. Paresthesias in the distribution of the trigeminal nerve suggest perineural invasion by a high-grade malignancy.

PHYSICAL EXAMINATION

Careful examination of the salivary glands, neck, and cranial nerve function is an important key to the diagnosis of parotid gland tumors. The gland lies in the preauricular area but also extends below the lobule of the ear and sometimes into the retroauricular area. The tail of the parotid gland may extend low in the neck, particularly in elderly patients (Figure 84-15). A discrete, firm, mobile mass is the most common presentation for parotid gland tumors. Limited mobility is seen in about 15% of patients, fixation to the underlying master or pterygoid musculature in about 17%, and skin ulceration in 9%. Benign

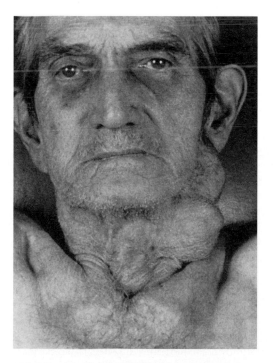

Figure 84-15. Large parotid gland mass demonstrating the lower extent of the parotid gland in the midneck. (From Jurkiewicz MJ, Krizek TJ, Mathes SJ, et al: *Plast Surg* 1:379-417, 1990.)

lesions, even those of large size, are usually mobile and are rarely locally invasive.

Several normal structures are sometimes confused with parotid masses (Figure 84-16). Normal anatomic structures sometimes simulating parotid gland masses include the hypertrophic masseter muscle, the mandibular coronoid process and condyle, prominent angle of the mandible, transverse process of the second cervical vertebra, and occasionally the mastoid process. A calcified carotid bulb or prominent hyoid bone is sometimes confused with submandibular gland masses. In these cases, computed tomography (CT) or magnetic resonance imaging (MRI) delineates the true nature and location of the mass.

Inspection of the skin of the anterolateral scalp, eyelids, conjunctiva, lacrimal glands, ears, cheek, and nose is important as a search for primary cutaneous carcinomas, which may produce parotid nodal metastases. For the submandibular gland, intraoral examination of the tongue, floor of mouth, and skin of the lower cheek and lip is pertinent.

Facial nerve weakness is indicative of malignancy.[17,56] Complete palsy of the nerve is noted in up to 10% of cancers, but careful examination of the entire distribution of the facial nerve shows some evidence of dysfunction in up to 25% of cases. Facial nerve paralysis is almost never seen with benign tumors in the absence of associated trauma or sudden hemorrhage into the mass. Facial nerve weakness at presentation is a poor prognostic sign associated with a 5-year survival of 26% and a 10-year survival of only 12%.

Examination of the lymph node–bearing areas of the neck for metastases is necessary in the assessment of salivary gland masses. Cervical node metastases are present in approximately 25% of parotid gland malignancies. Examination of axillary and inguinal lymph node basins and the abdomen for splenomegaly may indicate a systemic lymphoreticular disorder presenting with incidental salivary gland enlargement.

Intraoral inspection and bimanual palpation are necessary to assess for deep parotid tumors or those arising in the parapharyngeal space. The palate and intraoral mucosa should be examined for a submucosal mass suggestive of a tumor of minor salivary gland origin. Trismus may occur if cancer of the parotid gland extends into the infratemporal fossa to involve the pterygoid muscles. The ear canals, nasopharynx, cranial nerves, neck, and skin should be examined to detect extensive spread of any tumor. Skin involvement is relatively rare and is usually associated with advanced parotid malignancies. Cranial neuropathies also suggest advanced disease and can occur in patients with parapharyngeal space involvement from extension of a parotid or minor salivary gland cancer. Signs of cranial neuropathy include hoarseness (cranial nerve X), aspiration (IX, X), shoulder dysfunction (XI), and hemitongue atrophy (XII).

In case of trauma, thorough inspection of the injury site with anticipation of potential injuries is the cornerstone of diagnosis. The physician must assess the status of the regional skin, oral cavity, dental structures, and facial skeleton, with an initial emphasis on physical examination and reliance on radiographic studies for confirmation and detail. The muscles

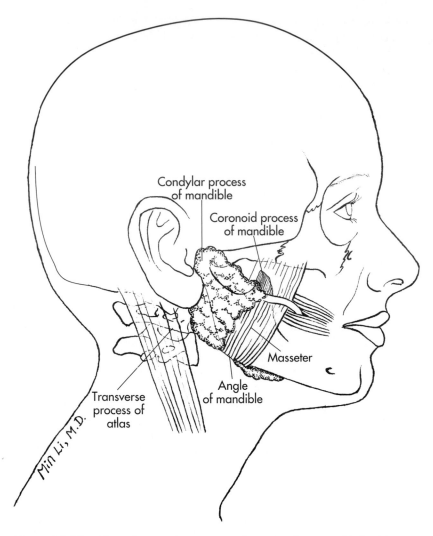

Condylar process of mandible

Coronoid process of mandible

Masseter

Angle of mandible

Transverse process of atlas

Min Li, M.D.

Figure 84-16. Normal anatomic structures that may mimic parotid gland tumors.

of facial expression and mastication are inspected for laceration or tissue loss. The salivary gland parenchyma and ducts are inspected for evidence of injury. The most critical steps involve the evaluation of the salivary gland ducts (Stensen's or Wharton's) for evidence of laceration or transection. Laceration of salivary ducts usually results in the presence of saliva in the wound. If in doubt, cannulation of the duct through the intraoral orifice with a lacrimal probe or plastic catheter will confirm the integrity of the duct. Injection of a small amount of methylene blue may also be helpful. In rare cases, contrast sialography can be utilized.

Assessment of facial nerve function includes attention to the areas of peripheral motor innervation. Branches of the facial nerve should be evaluated separately and the patient should be asked to smile, show the teeth, raise the forehead, close the eyes, pucker the lips, and blow. Sensation and motor function of the tongue should be assessed to evaluate the integrity of the hypoglossal and lingual nerves. Local anesthetic should not be injected to facilitate probing of the wounds, since this

may hamper identification of the nerve ends with the nerve stimulator. If necessary, penetrating wounds should be cleansed and evaluated in the operating room. Exploration of penetrating injuries with the possibility of motor nerve injury should be performed within the first 48 hours to take advantage of the ability to stimulate the distal portion of the nerve electrically.

PREOPERATIVE TESTS

LABORATORY STUDIES

Hematologic and serologic studies are of little value in the evaluation of salivary gland tumors. The exception is when autoimmune or inflammatory disorders are suspected. In these cases tests for rheumatoid factor, antinuclear antibody, sedimentation rate, and blood counts may be useful.

RADIOLOGIC EVALUATION

Sialography

Contrast sialography is seldom indicated in the evaluation of suspected salivary gland neoplasms, but can be useful in demonstrating ductal strictures and parenchymal destruction associated with salivary gland calculi or strictures. The potential problem with contrast sialography in the setting of suspected ductal obstruction is the possibility of inciting an inflammatory or infectious episode by injecting contaminated material under pressure into the duct system. Normally the ductal system will fill to the intercalated ducts. Radiolucent calculi will be seen as a bubble in the duct. Radiopaque calculi will be seen on plain film prior to contrast injection. Salivary gland neoplasms will distort the ductal architecture and leave areas of gland devoid of contrast material.[27]

Computed Tomography

CT scans may be helpful in evaluating the patient with a parotid gland mass. Parotid tissue is more radiolucent than adjacent muscles but more dense than fat planes in the subcutaneous tissue, infratemporal fossa, and parapharyngeal space. Use of intravenous contrast allows separation of parotid tissue from adjacent lymph nodes and vascular structures. CT scan is extremely sensitive for detection of the presence of a salivary gland mass. CT imaging can precisely localize the mass and estimate its size and local extension. Several characteristic CT appearances of salivary gland tumors are useful; round, smoothly outlined masses are likely to be benign, whereas lobulated, well-outlined masses and infiltrating masses with poorly defined margins are likely to be malignant[8] (Figure 84-17). CT cannot definitively differentiate between a benign and malignant mass, both of which may be encapsulated. Similarly CT cannot distinguish between an inflammatory and a malignant mass, both of which may be infiltrative. The facial nerve cannot be identified on CT scan, but an estimate of its location can be made by comparing the location of the retromandibular vein and the stylomastoid foramen.[46] Cervical lymph nodes with a long axis diameter greater than 1.5 cm, with ill-defined borders, or with a central lucency suggest metastases.[34]

CT is often helpful in evaluating submandibular triangle lesions. Differentiation of low-lying parotid or submandibular glands from lymph nodes is provided. The recent introduction of spiral (volumetric) CT coupled with intravenous contrast enables an entire vascular territory to be imaged within a 30-second breath hold. The short time frees the resulting images from ventilatory misregistration. Spiral CT is therefore quicker and results in smoother three-dimensional renderings from numerous views with diminished artifact.

Magnetic Resonance Imaging

MRI has several advantages over CT. It does not involve ionizing radiation, imaging in multiple orientations is possible, and it provides superior soft tissue detail.[10] Disadvantages include higher cost and sensitivity to motion artifact.

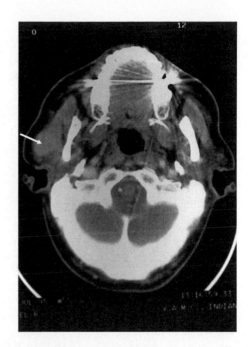

Figure 84-17. Right parotid gland mass demonstrated by CT scan *(arrow)*. Features of this squamous cell carcinoma consistent with malignancy include invasion of the masseter muscle and poorly defined margins.

MRI has several other specific advantages over CT scanning. Very sharp definition of tumor margins is often possible. T1 and T2 weighted images can be suggestive of the nature of the salivary mass.[31] High-grade malignancies tend to have low signal intensity on both T1 and T2 weighted images, whereas benign tumors have low T1 and high T2 signal intensities (Figure 84-18). Other MRI findings suggestive of malignancy include a heterogenous signal, soft tissue invasion, lymphadenopathy, and enlargement of the facial nerve. Malignancies generally enhance with gadolinium contrast as opposed to the poor enhancement seen with benign tumors.

MRI is sometimes helpful in delineating the relationship between the tumor and the facial nerve. Capability of MRI to detect different signal intensities of fat, nerve, cerebrospinal fluid, and brain allows for assessment of perineural spread of tumor.[35,37] The high intensity of surrounding fat is often replaced with tumor signals similar to those on T1 weighted images. Trigeminal nerve involvement is suggested by thickening of the nerve itself, expansion of foramen ovale, and atrophy of the muscles of mastication.

Magnetic resonance angiography (MRA) generates signal relative to stationary views, providing a unique opportunity to obtain quantitative flow data. The major advantage of MRA is that it does not require intravenous contrast or catheters. MRA is useful for large tumors when it is particularly important to know the anatomy of the nearby major vessels such as the carotid artery. Because of the indirect nature of this assessment, MRA is not as precise as conventional angiography.

In summary, both CT and MRI can precisely distinguish tumors from surrounding tissue. Both techniques are

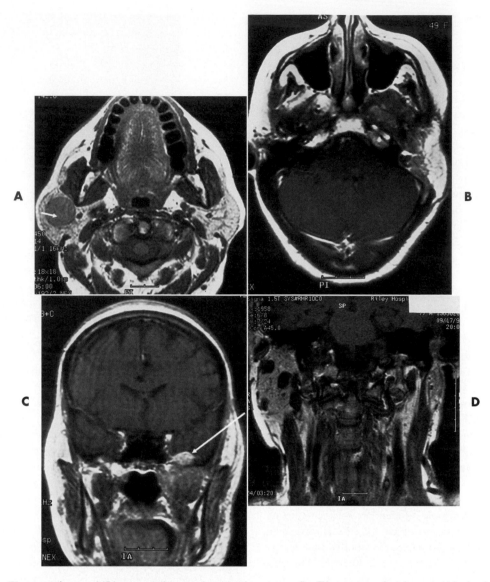

Figure 84-18. MRI scans of several parotid tumors. **A,** T1 images of right parotid gland pleomorphic adenoma *(arrow)*. **B** and **C,** Axial and coronal images, respectively, of a left parotid deep lobe carcinoma ex pleomorphic adenoma. Note skull base invasion on coronal view *(arrow)*. **D,** Multifocal tumor nodules in right parotid gland (lymphoma).

valuable in delineating the location, extent, and extraglandular extension of tumors. MRI provides superior soft tissue detail with respect to the facial nerve and deep lobe tumors. Neither technique can be relied on to differentiate malignant from benign tumors. With respect to cost-effectiveness, CT scan might be considered as an initial imaging modality choice.

Nuclear Medicine Imaging

Because of the superiority of CT and MRI, radionuclide imaging plays a minor role in management of salivary tumors. Radionuclide imaging may be used to detect certain neoplasms in patients who are poor surgical risks. Both oncocytoma and Warthin's tumors preferentially concentrate technetium 99m. An area of increased activity in the parotid gland may add credence to a presumptive diagnosis or may indicate bilateral

involvement. Other tumors may also show increased uptake, including some malignancies.[31]

Angiography

Contrast angiography is used to predict the involvement or proximity of the internal carotid artery to locally extensive tumors (Figure 84-19). The test is also used to predict the potential for neurologic morbidity following surgery of the internal carotid artery.[15] The test is only recommended for patients in whom surgery is planned on tumors intimately associated with the internal carotid artery, possibly necessitating sacrifice of the vessel. In this situation a balloon occlusion test is performed with balloon occlusion of the proximal internal carotid artery. The patient's mental status and motor function are continuously monitored to predict the adequacy of collateral cerebral

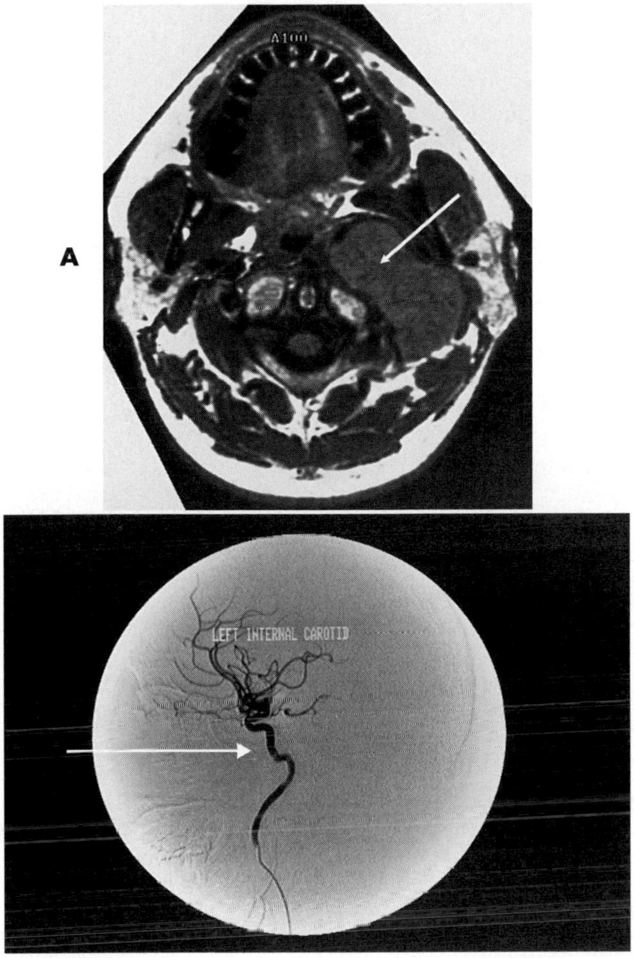

Figure 84-19. **A,** MRI scan demonstrating a large parapharyngeal space tumor *(arrow)*. **B,** Carotid angiogram demonstrating posterior displacement of left internal carotid artery by the mass. No vascular invasion is noted. The tumor was a benign ganglioneuroma.

perfusion. Mild systemic hypotension or xenon cerebral blood flow scans can be added to further classify risk of internal carotid artery ligation.

MANAGEMENT OF SALIVARY GLAND DISORDERS

Accurate diagnosis is essential to plan appropriate therapy. After the diagnosis is made, treatment planning can be focused to eradicate or palliate the disorder. Surgery is essential to the

diagnosis and management of most benign and malignant neoplasms and many congenital and inflammatory disorders of the salivary glands. This is because of the need for tissue to establish histologic diagnosis, the lack of effective nonsurgical therapies (even for benign neoplasia), and the chronic recurrent nature of many inflammatory conditions.

The initial goal of surgical treatment of the salivary gland mass is usually to establish or confirm the diagnosis. In many instances, this will be followed by a series of intraoperative decisions regarding treatment of benign and malignant neoplasia. The second goal is surgical eradication of the salivary pathology. The third goal is preservation (or restoration) of function. Cases requiring facial nerve sacrifice may involve adjunctive reconstructive procedures.

Preoperative discussion with the patient about to undergo surgery of the salivary glands must include discussion of a natural history of the disease process being treated. Typically, the patient undergoing parotid or submandibular gland resection will need to be counseled on the need for surgery and intraoperative decision making based on extent of the tumor, frozen sections, and other findings such as involvement of the facial nerve or other surrounding structures that may need to be resected. The possible need for facial nerve sacrifice must be explained. The possible need for facial nerve rehabilitative procedures such as nerve repair, grafting, tarsorrhaphy, and other reconstructive procedures should be discussed with the patient in advance. The course of functional recovery should also be discussed. If malignancy is a possibility, the patient should be counseled regarding the possibility of neck dissection, including sacrifice of the sternocleidomastoid muscle and the spinal accessory nerve. With parotidectomy, a contour deformity is expected. Paresthesias or numbness of the anterior portion of the ear and preauricular cheek skin is common after parotidectomy. Auriculotemporal or Frey's syndrome may occur in 15% to 20% of patients undergoing parotidectomy. Placement of incisions and expected scars should be discussed with the patient. The possibility of tumor recurrence will depend on histology, grade, and stage of the tumor, which are often not known until final pathologic evaluation of the surgical specimen. Nonetheless, possible recurrence of malignancy, as well as the possible need for adjuvant therapy, should be discussed in these cases. It is not possible to foresee all surgical maneuvers that must be made, particularly in cases involving surgery for malignancy. Informed consent should reflect clear understanding of these issues by the patient.

BIOPSY TECHNIQUES

Histologic diagnosis determines management of salivary gland tumors. Because most tumors arise in the superficial lobe of the parotid gland and are in relatively close proximity to the facial nerve or its terminal branches, the safest and most definitive method of obtaining adequate tissue for diagnosis is superficial parotidectomy. The preferred method of biopsy for tumors of the sublingual, submandibular, or minor salivary glands is complete gland excision. Excisional biopsy and enucleation are dangerous because they increase the risk of recurrence of benign tumors, jeopardize the facial nerve, and may contaminate the surgical field with malignant cells.

Certain situations may warrant an open biopsy without formal dissection. Examples of these unusual cases are patients who are poor surgical risks, when a diagnosis is important to avoid surgery, and suspected cases of inoperable malignancy, such as lymphoma or metastatic disease. Intraoral biopsy of a parapharyngeal space mass is not recommended due to the possibility of tumor implantation, bleeding, or infection. When open biopsy is used, the incision must be well planned so that an adequate margin of skin and soft tissue may be excised at the time of definitive resection without unnecessary sacrifice of surrounding structures.

FINE-NEEDLE ASPIRATION BIOPSY

Fine-needle aspiration has a sensitivity of up to 95% in salivary gland malignancies.[63] Specificity is lower due to the difficulty in differentiating among the many types of malignant tumors. The reasons for diagnostic failure include inadequate specimen, sampling error, and inexperience of the cytopathologist.[62]

The decision to operate on a patient with a salivary gland neoplasm is not usually affected by fine-needle aspiration biopsy because the presence of tumor is an indication for surgical removal. Furthermore, fine-needle aspiration biopsy does not provide the surgeon with information on the location or extent of the tumor. Fine-needle aspiration biopsy should not be done when the treatment course will not be affected by the results.

There are several situations in which fine-needle aspiration biopsy may be of value. Preoperative planning and counseling of the patient is enhanced, particularly with respect to the possibility of facial nerve sacrifice and neck dissection when a diagnosis of high-grade cancer is obtained. The diagnosis of a benign process such as Warthin's tumor in a high-risk patient may aid in deciding not to pursue surgical treatment. Patients with metastatic tumors such as melanoma or distant metastasis from lung or renal cell cancer may benefit from information provided by fine-needle aspiration biopsy. However, surgery should not be excluded on the basis of negative fine-needle aspiration biopsy if the patient has a clinically suspicious mass. Further investigation is necessary when the clinician is highly suspicious of neoplasm but fine-needle aspirate is nondiagnostic or negative.

FROZEN SECTION BIOPSY

Many surgeons rely on intraoperative frozen section biopsy to guide intraoperative decision making. The purpose of frozen section is to provide information that allows the surgeon to make an immediate decision about operative management. Frozen section analysis is most useful for determining lymph node metastasis, surgical margins, and perineural invasion.

The accuracy of frozen section analysis for diagnoses of salivary gland masses has been questioned. Hillel and Fee reported an average accuracy rate of 93% and a false-negative rate of 5%.[32] Other authors have reported accuracy rates varying from 65% to 86%.[30] Caution must be taken not to perform inappropriate procedures based on fine-needle aspiration or frozen section diagnosis. Weaknesses of fine-needle aspiration biopsy and frozen section are similar, and one technique should not be relied on to verify the other in equivocal cases.

If there is question about the tissue diagnosis of malignancy at the time of superficial parotidectomy, two approaches can be taken. The procedure can be terminated and a subsequent total parotidectomy can be performed several days later. Alternatively, if there is no clinical involvement of the facial nerve, a conservative facial nerve–sparing total parotidectomy may be performed if the suspicion of malignancy is high.

MANAGEMENT OF NONNEOPLASTIC SALIVARY GLAND DISORDERS

Treatment of the sialoadenoses, autoimmune and self-limited viral enlargements of the salivary glands is generally nonsurgical. When possible, treatment is directed at correction of the underlying problems (i.e., malnutrition, alcoholism, iodine intoxication, or hypothyroidism). These diagnoses are usually strongly suggested by history and physical examination. Rarely, patients with Sjögren's syndrome, sarcoidosis, or other autoimmune disorders have chronic parotid or submandibular gland enlargement that becomes symptomatic. In these cases surgical excision may be indicated.

Mucoceles of the minor salivary glands or sublingual glands usually recur after spontaneous rupture or simple surgical drainage. The treatment of choice is surgical excision.

Necrotizing sialometaplasia of the minor salivary glands usually presents as a worrisome lesion suspicious for malignancy. The diagnostic dilemma usually requires generous biopsy or excision to rule out malignancy. This maneuver provides tissue for diagnosis and is also curative.

Type I branchial cleft anomalies also typically present the dilemma of benign versus malignant mass. Imaging and fine-needle aspiration biopsy usually suggest a benign process. Superficial parotidectomy serves as the definitive diagnostic procedure and therapy.

BLEL is a nonspecific description of salivary gland histologic changes seen in a number of disorders. In most cases the salivary manifestations are limited to the parotid gland and are relatively asymptomatic. End stage degeneration may occasionally result in xerostomia. BLEL associated with HIV infection is occasionally symptomatic and generally not affected by medical management. Surgical therapy is sometimes indicated. Aspiration, limited parotidectomy, and simple enucleation of the cysts are effective palliative measures.[50] Sialogogues may be effective palliative measures for treating xerostomia.

MANAGEMENT OF ACUTE AND CHRONIC SALIVARY GLAND INFECTION

Salivary gland infections are usually related to ductal obstruction: either discrete obstruction by stones or related to stasis and inspissation of secretions. Surgery on the obstructed duct itself is rarely successful as definitive treatment. A few patients who present with obvious ductal calculi near the duct orifice that are palpable intraorally may be managed by marsupialization of the duct and resection of the stone. Most cases of ductal obstruction will require surgery on the gland parenchyma rather than the duct.

Acute parotitis or submandibular gland infection may be successfully treated by hydration and antibiotics against the most common causative organisms. In the usual case, the remedy is a penicillinase-resistant penicillin or cephalosporin. Atypical infections, such as mycobacterial infections, may require prolonged courses of multiple drugs. Gland massage, warm packs, and elevation of the head are adjuvant maneuvers. Patients who do not respond to medical maneuvers should be suspected of having a salivary gland abscess. CT or MRI will confirm the presence and extent of an abscess. Drainage of a parotid gland abscess requires raising a flap in front of the ear similar to parotidectomy. The parotid gland parenchyma is opened by blunt dissection along the plane of the facial nerve, with effort made to break up the numerous vertical fascial septa throughout the parotid gland. A drain is left in the wound and antibiotic therapy is continued. The submandibular gland may be approached for drainage directly through a cervical incision made below the ramus mandibularis of the facial nerve. Attempts to resect an infected salivary gland should be delayed until after resolution of the acute infection.

Chronic parotitis is defined as two or more episodes of acute parotitis with or without obvious ductal obstruction. Purulent secretions are usually expressible from the salivary duct. Acute or subacute episodes are again treated with hydration, gentle milking of the duct, and antibiotics. Sialography may be performed in the subacute setting and may show multiple areas of ductal obstruction. Treatment is with facial nerve–sparing total parotidectomy after resolution of the acute episode. Submandibular gland excision is indicated for recurrent infectious sialadenitis of the submandibular gland.

MANAGEMENT OF PAROTID GLAND NEOPLASIA

The definitive therapy for salivary gland neoplasia is surgical resection. This holds for parotid, submandibular, and minor salivary gland tumors. There is no effective medical treatment, even for benign neoplasia. Radiotherapy and chemotherapy may be effective as adjuvant or palliative measures, but should not be considered as definitive treatment for resectable salivary gland neoplasia. Thus, for both diagnosis and therapy, surgery is usually necessary.

In selected cases observation of a tumor may be appropriate. Observation of a salivary gland mass is usually limited to patients at high risk for surgery who are believed to have a high likelihood by imaging or fine-needle aspiration biopsy of harboring a benign tumor such as Warthin's tumor or pleomorphic adenoma. The finite risk of malignant degeneration must be discussed with the patient.

The hallmark of surgical management of salivary gland tumors is complete removal of the neoplastic lesion with a margin of normal tissue. Because the facial nerve traverses the parotid gland, the usual oncologic rule of en bloc resection of the entire affected area is not possible without nerve sacrifice. The predominance of benign tumors and the predilection of both benign and malignant tumors for the lateral parotid tissue allow preservation of the nerve in most cases. This is not always possible in larger or recurrent benign tumors or many malignancies. The surgeon must decide whether or not to preserve this functionally important nerve and how to rehabilitate the face if nerve sacrifice is required. Factors important in this decision are the preoperative functional status of the nerve, extent of the tumor and its location with respect to the nerve, histologic type, perineural spread or encasement, and radiosensitivity of the tumor. Facial nerve weakness or paralysis is occasionally due to benign parotid lesions, so histologic confirmation of malignancy must be made prior to nerve sacrifice.

The preferred treatment of parotid tumors, both benign and malignant, is complete excision with preservation of a normal functioning facial nerve. Even if tumor is adjacent to the nerve, as long as tumor does not directly infiltrate or encase it, every attempt is made to preserve the nerve. If the nerve function is normal preoperatively, normal function can usually be expected to return postoperatively, even after radiotherapy. For many malignancies, long-term tumor cure rates appear equivalent whether the facial nerve is resected or not as long as postoperative radiotherapy is administered.[9,52,59] However, the efficacy of postoperative radiation therapy should not breed complacency about complete removal of all gross tumor.

About 10% to 20% of malignant tumors present with facial nerve weakness or paralysis. Most surgeons agree the nerve should be sacrificed in this situation. Other relative indications for facial nerve sacrifice include histologically demonstrated perineural invasion or a malignant tumor that cannot be separated from the nerve. Both adenoid cystic carcinomas and, to a lesser extent, squamous cell carcinomas have a propensity for perineural invasion. For this reason the facial nerve is more often sacrificed with these tumor types than others. If the tumor is small and situated such that complete resection of the tumor with normal cuff of tissue can be accomplished while leaving the nerve intact, it is reasonable to preserve the nerve. For larger tumors, radical parotidectomy with planned facial nerve sacrifice is preferable. Frozen section confirmation of negative nerve margins should be obtained.

MANAGEMENT OF BENIGN NEOPLASMS

Common benign tumors include pleomorphic adenoma, monomorphic adenoma, Warthin's tumor, and oncocytomas. Enucleation of these tumors is not considered adequate therapy because of the high incidence of recurrence due to pseudopod extension beyond the clinically obvious capsule of the tumor. For benign tumors located in the superficial lobe of the parotid gland, superficial parotidectomy or lateral lobectomy with preservation of the facial nerve is adequate therapy. Since 75% of benign tumors, particularly Warthin's tumor and pleomorphic adenomas, are in the superficial lobe, this operation is adequate. Only about 25% of tumors will originate in or extend into the deep lobe. In these cases, conservative total parotidectomy with facial nerve preservation is indicated. In patients in whom there is clinical suspicion of malignancy or doubt concerning frozen section diagnosis, conservative total parotidectomy should be considered.

Recurrence of benign tumors is also ideally treated with surgical reexcision. Multicentric cutaneous and subcutaneous nodules are typical for recurrences of benign mixed tumors.

Wide excision with preservation of the facial nerve should be attempted. Occasionally, overlying skin or the nerve must be resected and reconstruction may be necessary. Adjuvant radiation therapy may be useful for preventing recurrences.[14]

MALIGNANT TUMOR STAGING

Staging of salivary gland malignancy is important to provide an accurate description of the disease, a method of communication, and prognostication for treatment planning. In the *Manual for Staging of Cancer* the TNM system is outlined (Box 84-2). Information with respect to the grade of the tumor coupled with accurate staging is of primary importance to the surgeon in deciding the extent of the operation, adjuvant treatment, and prognosis for the patient. General guidelines for treatment of malignant neoplasms of the parotid and submandibular glands are outlined in Table 84-3.

T delineates the tumor stage, with size the distinguishing characteristic among lesions; *N* denotes the status of regional cervical lymph nodes; and *M* denotes the presence or absence

---

Box 84-2.
Clinical Staging of Salivary Gland Tumors

PRIMARY TUMOR (T)

TX — Primary tumor cannot be assessed

T0 — No evidence of primary tumor

T1 — Tumor 2 cm or less in greatest dimension

T2 — Tumor more than 2 cm but not more than 4 cm in greatest dimension

T3 — Tumor more than 4 cm but not more than 6 cm in greatest dimension

T4 — Tumor more than 6 cm in greatest dimension

Note: All categories are subdivided: (a) no local extension; (b) local extension. Local extension is clinical or macroscopic evidence or invasion of skin, soft tissues, bone, or nerve. Microscopic evidence alone is not local extension for classification purposes.

REGIONAL LYMPH NODES (N)

NX — Regional lymph nodes cannot be assessed

N0 — No regional lymph node metastasis

N1 — Metastasis in a single ipsilateral lymph node, 3 cm or less in greatest dimension

N2 — Metastasis in a single ipsilateral lymph node, more than 3 cm but not more than 6 cm in greatest dimension, or in multiple ipsilateral lymph nodes, none more than 6 cm in greatest dimension; or in bilateral or contralateral lymph nodes, none more than 6 cm in greatest dimension

N2a — Metastasis in single ipsilateral lymph node more than 3 cm but not more than 6 cm in greatest dimension

N2b — Metastasis in multiple ipsilateral lymph nodes, none more than 6 cm in greatest dimension

N2c — Metastasis in bilateral or contralateral lymph nodes, none more than 6 cm in greatest dimension

N3 — Metastasis in a lymph node more than 6 cm in greatest dimension

DISTANT METASTASIS (M)

MX — Presence of distant metastasis cannot be assessed

M0 — No distant metastasis

M1 — Distant metastasis

STAGE GROUPING

Stage	T	N	M
Stage I	T1a	N0	M0
	T2a	N0	M0
Stage II	T1b	N0	M0
	T2b	N0	M0
	T3a	N0	M0
Stage III	T3b	N0	M0
	T4a	N0	M0
	Any T (except Tb4)	N1	M0
Stage IV	T4b	Any N	M0
	Any T	N2, N3	M0
	Any T	Any N	M1

Adapted from the American Joint Committee on Cancer: Beahrs OH, Henson DE, Hutter RVP, et al, editors: *Manual for staging of cancer*, ed 4, Philadelphia, 1993, JB Lippincott.

Table 84-3.
Guidelines for Treatment of Salivary Gland Malignancy

| | TREATMENT GROUP | | | |
	I	II	III	IV
TUMOR **Stage/Grade**	T1 and T2 low-grade, N0 Low-grade Mucoepidermoid Acinous cell	T1 and T2 high-grade, N0 Adenocarcinoma Malignant mixed Undifferentiated Squamous cell	T3, N0 or N+ Recurrences, any tumors not in Group IV	T4, N0 or N+
TREATMENT **Parotid Gland**	Superficial or total parotidectomy Preservation of CN-VII	Total parotidectomy with preservation of CN-VII, unless involved Supraomohyoid neck dissection	Radical parotidectomy (sacrifice of CN-VII with immediate reconstruction) Complete neck dissection for N+ neck Supraomohyoid neck dissection for N0 neck	Radical parotidectomy with resection of skin, mandible, muscles, mastoid tip, as indicated. Sacrifice of CN-VII with immediate reconstruction, possible flap reconstruction Complete neck dissection
		Consider postoperative radiation therapy for close margins, perineural invasion, or occult N+	Postoperative irradiation for high-grade, close margins, occult N+, or perineural invasion	Postoperative irradiation
Submandibular **Gland**	Submandibular triangle resection	Supraomohyoid neck dissection Preserve nerves unless involved Postoperative radiation therapy	Complete neck dissection to include 12th nerve and lingual nerve Postoperative radiation therapy	Complete neck dissection, with resection of skin, nerves, mandible, tongue, as indicated Possible flap reconstruction Postoperative irradiation

of distant metastatic disease. Also incorporated into the staging system is involvement of surrounding musculoskeletal structures, skin, or the facial nerve, denoted as the *b* substage. Local recurrence, cervical metastases, and distant metastatic disease all increase with higher stage disease.

Tumor grade is also important in therapeutic decision making. Tumors of low-grade malignancy include acinic cell carcinoma, low-grade adenocarcinoma, and low-or intermediate-grade mucoepidermoid carcinoma. These tumors have a low risk for local recurrence and regional and distant metastasis. High-grade malignancies include high-grade mucoepidermoid carcinoma, squamous cell carcinoma, undifferentiated tumors, carcinoma ex pleomorphic adenoma, high-grade adenocarcinomas, and adenoid cystic carcinoma. High-grade malignancies have a higher risk of local recurrences and regional nodal and distant organ metastases.

Treatment of the primary tumor is guided by tumor histology, size, and extent.[33] In general, treatment of low-grade neoplasms is by facial nerve–sparing total parotidectomy. Small tumors in this category may be managed by superficial parotidectomy if localized to the superficial lobe and histologically clear margins can be obtained.

High-grade malignancies include high-grade mucoepidermoid carcinoma, squamous cell carcinoma, high-grade adenocarcinoma, malignant mixed tumors, adenoid cystic carcinoma, and undifferentiated carcinoma. Surgery of small tumors is ideally by facial nerve–sparing total parotidectomy. For T1 and T2 lesions this is usually possible. Consideration should be given to elective treatment of the cervical lymph nodes in high-grade mucoepidermoid carcinoma, undifferentiated carcinoma, squamous cell carcinoma, and malignant mixed tumors. High-grade tumors should also receive adjuvant radiation therapy.

Most T3 and T4 salivary gland malignancies are of high-grade histology. With these larger cancers, preservation of the facial nerve usually will not be possible. The same is true of most cases of recurrent salivary gland carcinoma. Radical or extended parotidectomy should be performed when it is the only method of removal of all tumor with a clear margin and minimal violation of the neoplasm. This is usually necessary in large deep lobe malignancies, cancers with extraparotid extension, recurrent malignancy, and diffuse malignancies. When the neoplasm is discrete and involves only a branch of the facial nerve, the entire nerve may not need to be sacrificed if a clear margin can be obtained with a subtotal resection of the nerve. If malignancy invades beyond the capsule of the gland, consideration must be given to the resectability of the lesion. Preoperative imaging is recommended in these cases. Local extension into the skin, masseter, pterygoid muscles, or mandible dictates wide resection to include these structures. Selected extensive tumors may be amenable to intracranial/extracranial approach. In advanced stage salivary gland malignancy, treatment considerations should include the regional lymph nodes and adjuvant radiation therapy.

MANAGEMENT OF REGIONAL LYMPH NODES IN SALIVARY GLAND MALIGNANCIES

Therapeutic neck dissection for clinically involved lymph nodes should be performed at the time of surgical treatment of the primary tumor. With clinically involved lymph nodes, neck dissection should be comprehensive, either the modified or radical type depending on the surgeon's ability to extirpate all gross disease while preserving functional structure such as the spinal accessory nerve and/or sternocleidomastoid muscle.

The management of the clinically negative neck is more controversial. The options for management of the N0 neck in patients with cancers of the salivary gland include observation with treatment when occult disease becomes clinically obvious, elective neck dissection, and radiation therapy. Due to the relative scarcity of data and multitude of histologic types, it is difficult to make sound conclusions on efficacy of elective neck treatment in patients with cancers of the salivary gland. Decisions regarding elective management of N0 neck are usually based on the stage and grade of tumor, presence of perineural invasion, and the perceived need for adjuvant radiation therapy of the primary site.[21]

Elective treatment of the clinically negative neck should be reserved for malignancies with a high risk of subclinical lymph node metastases. It is generally accepted that patients with low-grade malignant lesions of the major salivary glands do not require nodal dissections at the time of initial operation. Acinic cell and low-and intermediate-grade mucoepidermoid carcinomas have a low risk of occult lymph node metastases. Similarly, T1 and T2 lesions rarely require elective management of the neck. T3 and T4 lesions are at higher risk. Usual indications for elective cervical lymphadenectomy in N0 salivary gland cancer include squamous cell carcinoma, high-grade mucoepidermoid carcinoma, undifferentiated carcinoma, carcinoma ex pleomorphic adenoma, and high-grade adenocarcinoma. Comprehensive modified neck dissection is reasonable, but most surgeons limit the extent of resection to an upper jugular chain sampling of level I, II, and III lymph nodes for parotid gland carcinoma and a supraomohyoid neck dissection for submandibular gland carcinoma.

Radiation therapy is effective as adjuvant treatment in salivary gland cancer for improving local control. It can be a viable option for treatment of the clinically negative neck in patients at high risk for occult neck metastasis.

A special situation is the question of parotidectomy for lymph node metastases for cancer of the skin, scalp, conjunctiva, or cheek. Anatomic studies show the majority of lymph node tissue in the parotid gland lies superficial to the facial nerve and can be removed by lateral parotidectomy. However, some lymph node tissue does exist in the deep lobe of the parotid gland. If clinically evident lymph node metastases are present in the parotid gland or neck from a cutaneous malignancy, total parotidectomy should probably be performed. Elective parotidectomy is generally not indicated for most cutaneous squamous cell or basal cell carcinomas unless contiguously invasive into the parotid gland. The role of elective parotidectomy in malignant melanoma is more controversial. Lateral parotidectomy may be considered when drainage is demonstrated to the parotid nodes from an intermediate depth cutaneous melanoma of the head and neck, either as an elective procedure or as an aid in removing the intraparotid sentinel lymph node for analysis. In this situation, lymphoscintigraphy is recommended to accurately predict lymphatic drainage patterns.

Adjuvant Therapy for Salivary Gland Malignancies

Adjuvant radiation therapy after resection of high-grade, locally extensive, or recurrent salivary gland carcinomas should be considered.[9,52,59] Radiation therapy should not be expected to compensate for inadequate surgery. The first operation and first course of radiotherapy provide the best and often the only chance to control salivary malignancy. Planned postoperative radiation therapy probably gives the best chance for local control but does not seem to alter survival. This is primarily due to failure in preventing distant metastatic disease. Indications for postoperative radiation therapy in cancer of the major and minor salivary glands include positive surgical margins, cancer close to the facial nerve, high-grade malignancy (e.g., high-grade adenocarcinoma or mucoepidermoid carcinoma, malignant mixed tumor, undifferentiated carcinoma, squamous cell carcinoma, and adenoid cystic carcinoma), perineural spread of tumor, presence of cervical metastatic disease, recurrent cancer, and locally extensive cancers. Radiation therapy should not be considered as a primary therapeutic alternative for surgically resectable salivary gland carcinoma. Radiotherapy, in particular, neutron beam irradiation, should be considered for inoperable salivary tumors for palliative considerations.[36]

The role of chemotherapy in cancer of the salivary glands is unclear. Adenoid cystic carcinoma has been the cancer most commonly treated with systemic agents. Response rates of 40% to 50% have been noted. Cisplatin, doxorubicin, and fluorouracil are active agents against adenoid cystic carcinoma, malignant mixed tumor, adenocarcinoma, and acinic cell carcinoma. Mucoepidermoid carcinoma and squamous cell carcinoma seem to respond best to cisplatin, methotrexate, and fluorouracil. Despite these findings it remains unproven that response rates to chemotherapy translate into improved survival or quality of life. Chemotherapy is considered palliative and generally investigational in the management of salivary gland malignancies at this time.

MANAGEMENT OF PEDIATRIC SALIVARY GLAND DISORDERS

Evaluation of the pediatric patient with a salivary gland mass depends on history and physical examination. Vascular lesions consistent with hemangioma or lymphangioma can usually be observed. Indications for surgical treatment of these lesions include severe deformity, rapid growth that endangers the airway or upper aerodigestive tract, hemorrhage, or infection. Mumps, cystic fibrosis, sialadenitis, cat-scratch disease, and mycobacterial infection may cause unilateral or bilateral salivary gland enlargement with or without systemic symptoms. Congenital masses may include first branchial cleft cyst. These anomalies are rare but may simulate a parotid mass. Management of solid salivary gland tumors in children is similar to adults, usually requiring surgery for both diagnosis and therapy.

MANAGEMENT OF SALIVARY GLAND TRAUMA

Management of salivary gland trauma follows the principles of tissue debridement and repair for any traumatic tissue injury. Special considerations in management of salivary glands are the potential for salivary fistula related to major duct disruption and facial nerve injury. Most injuries are penetrating in nature but blunt injuries can occur. Diagnostic maneuvers have been previously outlined. Identification of facial nerve injuries is ideally by physical examination. Unresponsive or uncooperative patients and those identified as having facial nerve deficits will require exploration of the wound in the operating room under general anesthesia. Local anesthetics should be avoided because of their adverse affect on the ability to locate the transected nerve ends. The distal nerve end is usually electrically responsive for 48 to 72 hours and then becomes unresponsive.

In general any major nerve branch laceration should be repaired primarily. Nerve grafts may be necessary in avulsion injuries. Exception to the general rule of exploration and repair may sometimes be considered with lacerations of the nerve distal to the lateral canthus of the eye. Numerous branches occur in this region between the buccal and zygomatic branches, and prognosis for return of function for laceration of distal nerve in the cheek branches in this area is generally good. Lacerations of the temporal and marginal mandibular branch should generally be repaired regardless of their location. Use of the operating microscope facilitates surgical repair of the facial nerve. The principles of atraumatic handling, tension-free anastomosis, and minimal number of approximating sutures should be adhered to.

Ductal lacerations should be suspected if weakness of the buccal branch of the facial nerve is noted or if a cheek hematoma is seen. Laceration of Stensen's duct should be repaired by direct end-to-end anastomosis of the lacerated duct over a Silastic stent (Figure 84-20). The stent is removed in 10 to 14 days.

Debridement of salivary injuries is important. Wounds needing debridement include human and animal bites, blast injuries such as gunshot wounds, and high-pressure injection injuries. Heavily contaminated wounds may require delayed closure. In the case of a destroyed submandibular or parotid gland, total glandular resection may be necessary.

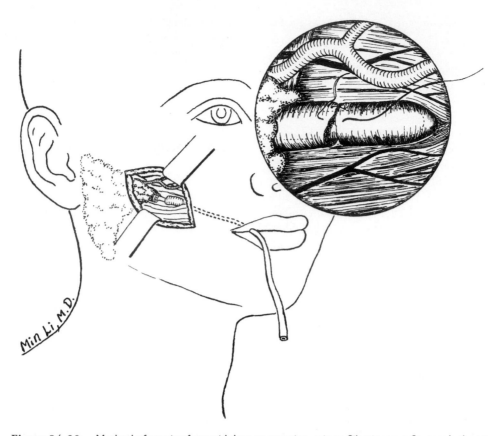

Figure 84-20. Method of repair of parotid duct transection using a Silastic stent. Stensen's duct is cannulated transorally. The stent is brought into the cheek wound and threaded into the proximal duct, which is identified by the presence of saliva. Anastomosis is performed with 8.0 monofilament suture. Stent is pulled after 14 days.

OPERATIONS

Surgery of the parotid gland and other salivary glands has evolved over the last 150 years and parallels the advent of general anesthesia.[38] The earliest surgical procedures directed at the salivary glands involved the excision of ranula and removal of calculi transorally. In 1802 Bertrand outlined the first surgical approach to parotidectomy for tumor treatment. Today's modern techniques of surgery are the result of accumulated wisdom of many surgeons over the years. Accompanying the refinements in surgery has been a more thorough understanding of the clinical behavior of salivary gland neoplasms.

Surgery of the salivary glands requires advanced familiarity with the anatomy of the retromandibular, viscerovertebral, and cervical regions. The operations of superficial, total, and extended parotidectomy as well as submandibular dissection will be discussed.

SUPERFICIAL PAROTIDECTOMY

The aspect of salivary gland surgery of greatest challenge to the surgeon is performance of a parotidectomy without facial nerve injury. Techniques have been described to allow rapid and safe parotidectomy.[61] Careful positioning of the patient, thorough exposure of the anatomy, and meticulous dissection around the facial nerve and its branches will provide dividends, regardless of the technique chosen by the surgeon.

Parotidectomy is performed under general anesthesia. The endotracheal tube and other monitoring devices are positioned to allow an unobstructed view of the ipsilateral face. The head of the bed is elevated 10 to 15 degrees to minimize venous bleeding in the operative field. Face, ear, lateral scalp, and the entire neck are exposed with a head drape. The authors prefer to inject a small volume of dilute epinephrine in the subcutaneous plane to minimize bleeding from the skin flap edges. A preauricular incision is carried from above the zygomatic arch extending around the ear lobe as a postauricular lazy S or Y extension. These extensions allow easy access to the mastoid and cartilaginous portions of the external auditory canal. The incision is marked with the head in anatomic position to allow placement in the natural skin creases. The lower limb is extended into the neck along the anterior border of the sternocleidomastoid muscle. If resection of skin overlying the gland is necessary, the incision should be positioned to permit this.

The skin flap is raised in the preauricular region from posterior to anterior just above the preparotid fascia. Traction with skin hooks identifies this distinct plane readily (Figure 84-21, *A*). Use of a face lift scissors facilitates the dissection.

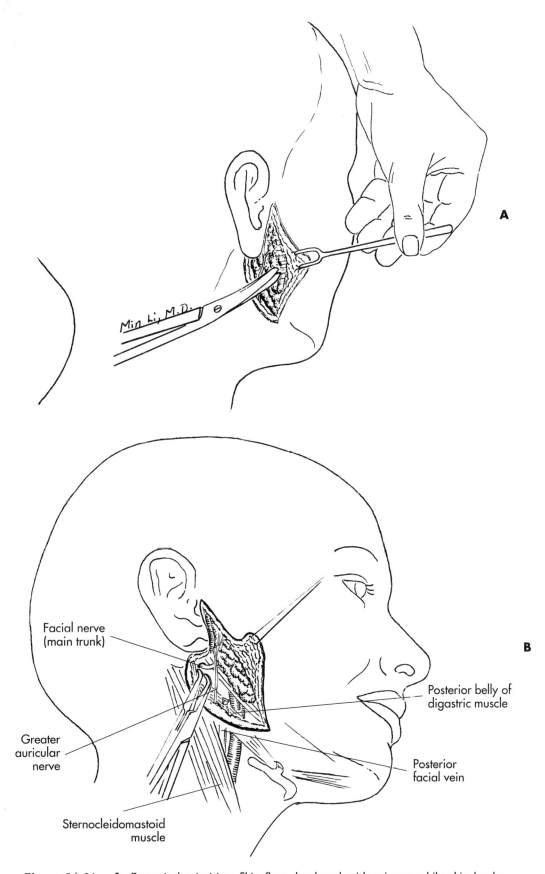

Figure 84-21. A, Preauricular incision. Skin flaps developed with scissors while skin hooks retract. **B,** Development of the plane between the posterior belly of the digastric muscle, parotid gland and between the perichondrium of the external auditory canal identifies the trunk of the facial nerve exiting the stylomastoid foramen.

Continued

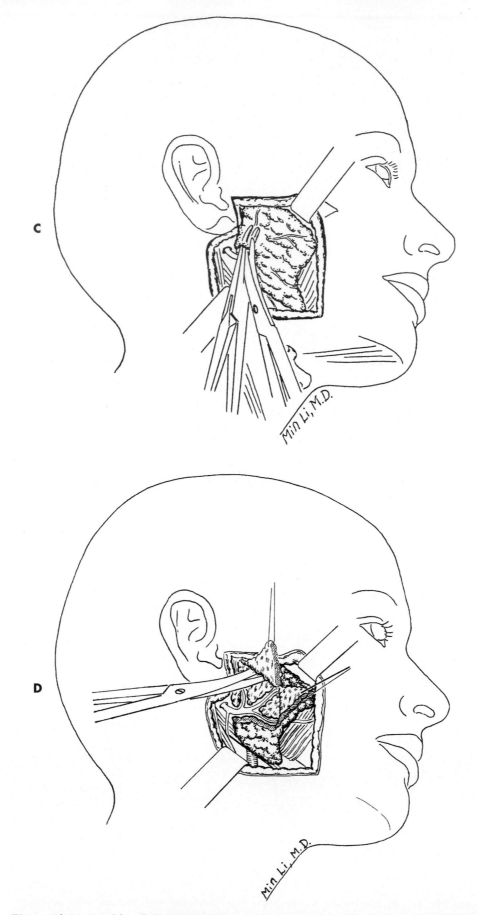

Figure 84-21, cont'd. C, Dissection lateral to the facial nerve with a fine-tipped hemostat and division of the overlying glandular parenchyma with scissors to identify the pes anserinus. **D,** Dissection of the remaining branches of the temporal facial division of the nerve. The lower division has already been dissected free. Stensen's duct is ligated as it pierces the buccal fat pad.

Continued

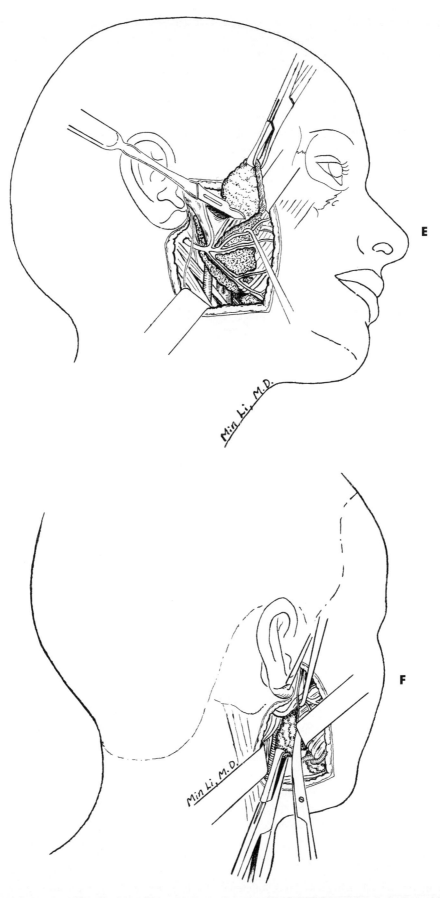

Figure 84-21, cont'd. **E,** Completion of dissection over the terminal branches is facilitated by medial retraction on the specimen. **F,** Total parotidectomy is performed by gentle retraction on the facial nerve branches and dissection of the deep lobe from the retromandibular space.

Care must be taken as the gland thins out over the masseter muscle and zygoma to prevent injury to the peripheral branches of the nerve exiting the substance of the gland in this superficial location. Hemostasis is obtained with bipolar electrocautery.

The parotid gland may extend variable distances into the neck. Therefore exposure of the sternocleidomastoid muscle is necessary. The posterolateral skin flap over the sternocleidomastoid muscle is raised sharply with a knife. In most cases the greater auricular nerve and posterior facial vein must be divided at this point. The dense fibrous attachments of the parotid gland to the anterior border of the sternocleidomastoid muscle must be divided sharply. This exposes the posterior belly of the digastric muscle. The trough between the gland and the digastric muscle is deepened along the superior and anterior edge of the posterior belly of the digastric muscle to allow exposure of the main trunk of the facial nerve (Figure 84-21, *B*).

Next, the dissection proceeds to the preauricular area. There is a distinct and relatively avascular plane between the perichondrium of the external auditory canal and the posterior fascial envelopment of the parotid gland. This interval is entered by sharp dissection and opened by blunt dissection. Annoying bleeding occurs if dissection is too far anterior or posterior from this plane. The preauricular dissection plane is developed medially. Retraction on the divided portion of the preauricular gland anteriorly and superiorly facilitates this dissection.

The major goal at this point is identification of the facial nerve trunk. Two major approaches are available to identify the nerve (i.e., identification of the main trunk posteriorly or of peripheral branches anteriorly with retrograde dissection toward the trunk). For most parotidectomies, particularly superficial lobectomy, identification of the main trunk is safe and convenient. This technique requires good exposure of the mastoid, digastric, and cartilaginous auditory canal. The main trunk of the nerve is found approximately 1.5 cm inferior to and 1 cm deep to the tip of the mastoid process. The cartilaginous portion of the external auditory canal forms a point at its bony junction with the skull, the so-called tragal pointer. The tragal pointer indicates the main trunk of the nerve is leaving the stylomastoid foramen within 5 to 6 mm. The stylomastoid foramen and the main trunk of the facial nerve can also be located by finding the tympanomastoid fissure. This is the suture line between the posterior bony hard auditory canal and the mastoid portion of the temporal bone. The nerve lies 6 to 8 mm below the inferior end of this suture line. Careful dissection in this small area with a fine hemostat in the direction of the facial nerve will separate the soft tissues until the glistening white facial nerve is identified (Figure 84-21, *B*). Although not necessary, a nerve stimulator is sometimes useful.

Occasionally the tumor may be sitting over the main trunk of the facial nerve or previous surgery may obscure the anatomy. A common approach to identifying the facial nerve in this instance is to follow the posterior facial vein superiorly as it enters the parotid gland. The surgeon can find the marginal mandibular branch of the nerve crossing just superficial to the facial vein, and follow it retrograde to the main trunk. Another technique that is useful for patients who have had previous surgery or recurrent tumor in the area of the main trunk is removal of the mastoid tip and identification of the nerve as it exits the stylomastoid foramen. The mastoid tip can be removed using an osteotomy or an otologic drill. This allows identification of the facial nerve in a nonoperated area. Another useful landmark is the buccal branch as it runs parallel to the parotid duct at the midportion of the anterior border of the masseter muscle.

Once a peripheral branch or the main trunk of the facial nerve is identified, a tunnel is created just above the nerve and the parotid tissue is incised, splitting the gland toward the pes anserinus (Figure 84-21, *C*). At this point, the facial nerve branches are identified and dissected both retrograde and anterograde. Bipolar electrocautery is helpful in preventing injury to the nerve branches. A nerve stimulator provides a relatively atraumatic method of identifying small branches. As the tunnel is created between the nerve and the gland, a knife or bipolar electrocautery divides the overlying parotid tissue. Once the first branch is completely dissected to its point of exit from the gland, the surgeon returns to find the adjacent branch (Figure 84-21, *D*). This pattern is repeated until all nerves and branches are exposed (Figure 84-21, *E*). The gland is resected from the underlying facial nerve by serial identification of each nerve branch until the entire superficial portion of the gland is freed from the most inferior branch of the facial nerve. Care should be taken to preserve the anastomoses between the buccal and cervicomandibular branches. Stensen's duct will be found closely applied to the buccal branch and should be divided and ligated.

TOTAL PAROTIDECTOMY

The majority of tumors in the parotid gland arise in the superficial portion of the gland and are satisfactorily managed by lateral parotidectomy. About 10% to 12% of tumors will lie at least partially in the deep portion of the gland medial to the facial nerve. Smaller tumors involving the deep lobe can generally be removed by the standard external approach, preserving the facial nerve branches. When total parotidectomy with preservation of the facial nerve is indicated, the superficial gland is first removed as described previously. The exposed branches of the facial nerve are then dissected from the deep lobe by gentle retraction of the main trunk of the nerve laterally with a nerve hook or vessel loops (Figure 84-21, *F*). The deep lobe tissue along with the tumor is then dissected from the mandible and stylomandibular membrane by diligent mobilization of the gland from all four sides and its deep attachments. Sometimes the tissue will be removed in a piecemeal fashion. Dissection should be patient and under direct vision to avoid bleeding from the numerous branches of the internal maxillary artery and the pterygoid venous plexus.

EXTENDED PAROTIDECTOMY

The previously described procedures suffice for benign or small malignant tumors that are confined to the described portions of the parotid gland. When the tumor invades various planes or is very large, the surgeon often must use a combination of methods to ensure that complete removal of the tumor with a margin of normal tissue is achieved. The extent of surgery is determined by the extent of the tumor, and therefore there is no standard approach in these situations. In cases of extensive malignancy, the facial nerve must be sacrificed. Sometimes this is also necessary in rare cases of multiple recurrences of a benign mixed tumor that surrounds and encases the nerve. When the facial nerve is resected, frozen sections of the proximal and distal stumps are obtained to rule out perineural spread. The nerve is resected back to clear margins. Malignant tumors invasive of the muscles of mastication or mandible will require en bloc resection of these structures. The surgeon should excise overlying skin if the tumor is adherent to the dermis. Facial nerve reconstruction is carried out at the time of primary resection. Soft tissue and/or bony reconstruction of the resected mandible or surrounding tissues may be necessary.

SUBMANDIBULAR GLAND RESECTION

Positioning and preparation of the patient are similar to the parotidectomy operation. The planned skin incision is made in a natural neck skin crease 3 to 4 cm inferior to the caudal border of the mandible, extending from the hyoid bone posteriorly toward the angle of the mandible (Figure 84-22, A). This incision is a natural extension of the inferior portion of a parotidectomy incision. Subplatysmal flaps are raised superiorly and inferiorly. The anterior facial vessels, the anterior belly of the digastric muscle, and the anterior border of the sternocleidomastoid muscle are identified. The marginal mandibular nerve runs immediately superficial to the anterior facial vessels. Positive identification of this branch is the best method to ensure its preservation. Use of a nerve stimulator is helpful in some cases. The facial vessels are ligated just below the level of the marginal mandibular branch. The ligature can be left long and used to retract the nerve superiorly away from the field (Figure 84-22, B).

Incision of the investing fascia of the submandibular triangle exposes the gland. A clamp is used to grasp the gland and retract it downward from its bed beneath the mandibular border. The posterior margin of the mylohyoid muscle is retracted anteriorly. The gland is retracted to expose the vital structures of the floor of the submandibular triangle (i.e., the lingual nerve, Wharton's duct, and the hypoglossal nerve, which lie on the hyoglossus muscle) (Figure 84-22, C). These structures lie, in order, from posterior superior to anterior inferior: lingual nerve, Wharton's duct, and hypoglossal nerve. The submandibular ganglion with its venous plexus is ligated and divided from the lingual nerve. Wharton's duct is divided and ligated. The hypoglossal nerve is identified and preserved as the inferior border of the submandibular gland is dissected free (Figure 84-22, D). The facial artery and facial vein stump must again be ligated and divided at the level of the posterior belly of the digastric muscle to remove the specimen.

In cases of suspected or proven submandibular gland malignancy, supraomohyoid lymphadenectomy (cervical nodal levels I, II, and III) is performed to provide both diagnosis and therapy. Large or recurrent malignancies sometimes invade the bony cortex of the mandible or skeletal muscle of the tongue or neck. If so, these structures are resected en bloc with the lesion.

EXCISION OF MINOR SALIVARY GLAND TUMORS

There are many minor salivary glands in the oral cavity and oral pharynx. Preferred treatment of minor salivary gland tumors is wide surgical excision. CT scanning is useful for formulating an operative plan and assessing bony invasion (Figure 84-23). Resection of minor salivary gland tumors must be planned on an individual basis, taking into account the location, histology, and size of the tumor. Certain principles should be followed. The diagnosis should be certain before a radical procedure aimed at malignancy is performed. In most cases this means an incisional or excisional biopsy of the tumor with permanent pathology. Malignant tumors should be resected with clear histologic margins. Adjacent bone, mucosa, or muscle may need to be resected to obtain adequate margins. Adequate exposure is essential. Immediate reconstruction of surgical defects is desirable. Depending on the location of the tumor, and size of the defect, prosthetic obturators or autogenous tissue reconstruction may be indicated.

Malignancy is more likely in minor salivary gland tumors than in the major salivary glands. The most common tumor types are adenoid cystic carcinoma followed by adenocarcinoma. Because these histologic types have a low risk of regional metastases and a relatively high risk of distant metastases, elective neck dissection of the N0 neck is generally not warranted. Postoperative radiation therapy is employed for indications similar to the major salivary gland tumor sites.

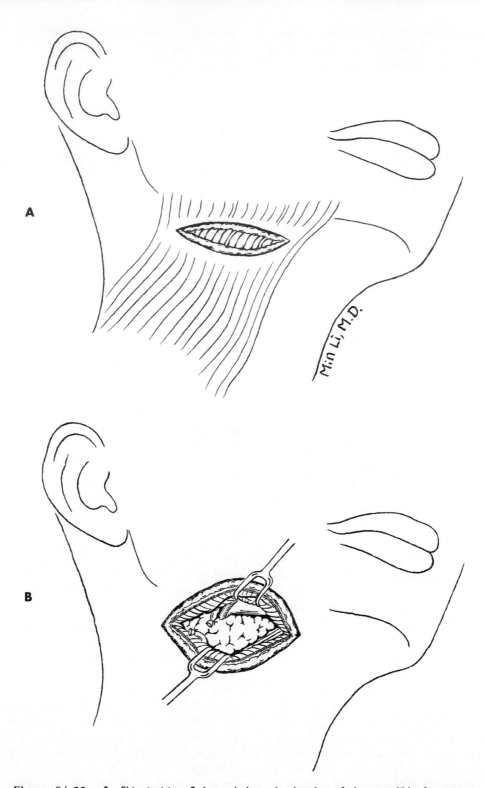

Figure 84-22. **A,** Skin incision 3-4 cm below the border of the mandible for access to the submandibular triangle. **B,** Ligation of the facial artery and vein. The ramus mandibularis lies just superficial to the facial vessels on the deep surface of the platysma.

Continued

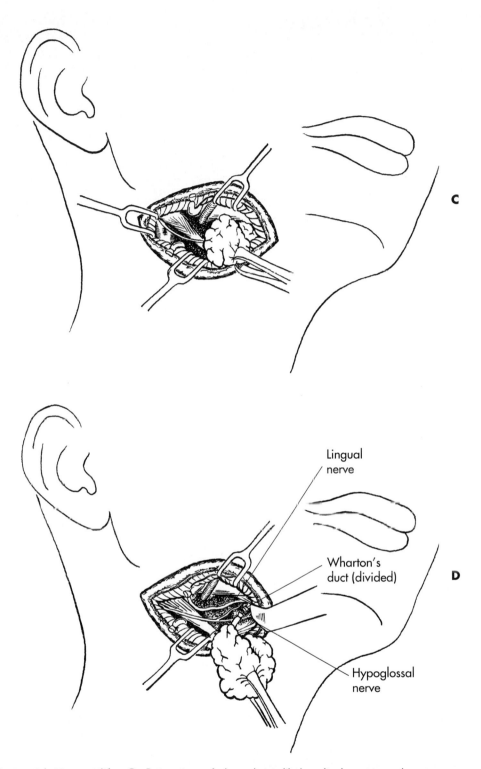

Figure 84-22, cont'd. C, Retraction of the submandibular gland exposes the structures of the submandibular triangle (from superiorly to inferiorly): lingual nerve, Wharton's duct, and hypoglossal nerve. **D,** The submandibular ganglion has been divided from the lingual nerve. Wharton's duct is divided. The lingual and hypoglossal nerves lie on the hyoglossus muscle.

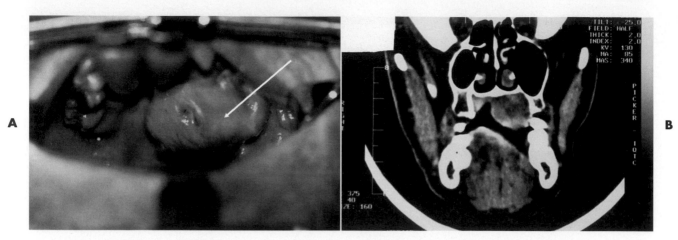

Figure 84-23.   A, Minor salivary low-grade adenocarcinoma arising from the mucosa of the hard palate *(arrow)*. **B,** CT scan demonstrates no bone invasion.

PARAPHARYNGEAL SPACE TUMORS

Tumors involving the parapharyngeal or retromandibular space can be exposed using a submandibular approach or by osteotomy of the mandibular ramus with reflection of the mandible superiorly. The submandibular approach involves resection of the Level I lymph nodes and submandibular gland from the submandibular triangle. Following submandibular gland excision, a superficial parotidectomy may be necessary to identify and preserve the facial nerve. The stylomandibular ligament is then incised and detached from the mandible. This allows for anterior dislocation of the mandible to improve access to the parapharyngeal space. This approach usually provides sufficient exposure so that most tumors can then be dissected from the parapharyngeal space.

For larger tumors or those encroaching on the carotid sheath, the authors prefer extensive exposure of the parapharyngeal space afforded by a mandibular ramus osteotomy. The facial nerve is identified and a superficial parotidectomy is performed. The marginal mandibular branch is retracted superiorly and, using a periosteal elevator, the surgeon elevates the masseter muscle from the angle of the mandible. A vertical ramus or step cut osteotomy at the angle of the mandible is then performed, with care taken to preserve the inferior alveolar nerve. The internal pterygoid muscle is detached and the posterior bony segment reflected laterally. This allows exposure to the parapharyngeal space for direct visualization of the tumor. After removal of the tumor, the mandible is reapproximated with plates and screws.

POSTOPERATIVE MANAGEMENT

At the completion of the procedure while the facial nerve is still exposed, it is helpful to stimulate it electrically to determine if there will be an early nerve deficit. It is also important to confirm that each branch is intact so the patient can be told that a complete recovery is to be anticipated even in the presence of initial nerve weakness. The wound is irrigated and a closed suction drain is placed. The wound is closed in layers and the drain is left until output diminishes, usually in 24 to 72 hours. The head of the bed is elevated to prevent postoperative edema. Compressive wraps and dressings are generally not placed to avoid pressure to the skin flaps and to allow direct visualization of the wound in case bleeding should develop.

If the facial nerve has been resected, protection of the eye must be ensured. Eye closure should be assessed immediately. If compromised, the patient is educated on eye protection maneuvers and lubrication eye drops are started. Depending on the expected time course of recovery, temporary eye taping and lubrication may suffice until return of function. Longer delays are probably better managed by placement of a gold weight to aid in eye closure.

ADJUNCTIVE PROCEDURES

FACIAL NERVE RECONSTRUCTION

Resected facial nerve stumps should be confirmed free of tumor by frozen section. It is usually possible to obtain negative margins in the extracranial segment of the nerve or at least in the mastoid segment. Rarely a tumor will require resection of the nerve into the tympanic segment to obtain clear margins.

When the facial nerve is transected, direct approximation of the nerve (epineural neurorrhaphy) at the time of surgery is the procedure of choice. When primary repair is not possible, the second choice is interpositional nerve grafting. The sural nerve or opposite greater auricular nerve is the donor tissue of choice. All divided branches should be grafted if possible.

Occasionally there may be a patient in whom a proximal nerve stump is unavailable for grafting. If reconstruction is undertaken within 2 years of nerve division, grafting of the proximal portion of another cranial nerve to the facial nerve is the third best choice. The ideal donor is cross facial nerve grafting from a buccal branch of the contralateral facial nerve. This provides the best potential for return of spontaneous movement. If unavailable, the next option is hypoglossal to facial nerve transfer or graft.

When improvement is desired in a long-standing facial paralysis, disuse muscle atrophy makes reinnervation procedures unsatisfactory. In these cases the traditional treatment has been with static fascial slings or dynamic temporalis or masseter muscle transfers. More recently, vascularized reinnervated free muscle reanimation procedures such as the gracilis or pectoralis minor transverse have produced good outcomes. These are performed as two-stage procedures with cross facial nerve grafting to a contralateral buccal facial nerve branch. Several months are allowed for nerve regeneration, followed by a vascularized muscle transfer and nerve anastomosis to provide reanimation of the opposite face.

Protection of the eye in the patient with resected or newly reconstructed facial nerve is paramount. Options include a partial lateral tarsorrhaphy, placement of upper lid gold weight, lid taping, and implantable springs. The authors' preferred method is placement of a gold weight that can be removed later if return of function occurs.

Return of animation to the forehead and lower lip after nerve reconstructive procedures is frequently unsatisfactory. Unilateral brow lift is effective for paralysis of the temporal branch of the facial nerve. Lower lip drooling can be controlled by vertical wedge resection of the adynamic lower lip with advancement of functional contralateral lower lip orbicularis muscle.

OUTCOMES

The outcome of management of salivary gland disorders is dependent on many factors, including the natural history of the disease process, the treatment modalities employed, and the general medical condition of the patient. Because salivary gland disorders comprise a broad range of inflammatory, infectious, and neoplastic disorders, the outcomes are generally most dependent on the nature and extent of the disease process.

SURGICAL OUTCOMES

Parotidectomy

Parotidectomy can be done with little morbidity and essentially no mortality. The most serious complication of parotid resection is damage to the facial nerve. Temporary paresis of a portion or all of the facial nerve may occur after ligation of the branch of the stylomastoid artery adjacent to the nerve trunk. Even when the nerve is not resected, many patients can expect temporary weakness at some or all branches. In cases of

temporary nerve damage return of function usually is complete and occurs within 6 to 12 weeks. Permanent injury to the nerve during complete facial nerve exposure with attempts at preservation ranges from 1% to 2%, but may be as high as 10%. Most commonly injured branches are the marginal mandibular and temporal branches.

Dysesthesia over the anterior portion of the ear occurs when the great auricular nerve is divided. This occurs in essentially 100% of patients, but most patients adapt to this loss of sensation.

With even a superficial parotidectomy a contour deformity is to be expected. This consists of a noticeable depression of the preauricular cheek with prominence of the angle of the mandible on the operated side. Rehabilitation of the contour deformities can be successful with the use of vascularized free tissue transfers such as the scapula flap or, in mild cases, nonvascularized dermal grafts.

Auriculotemporal or Frey's syndrome occurs in 15% to 20% of patients undergoing parotidectomy. This phenomenon results from aberrant regeneration of auriculotemporal nerve fibers into sweat glands of the skin. The problem is aggravated by thin surgical flaps over the parotid gland. Gustatory sweating is the hallmark symptom of the condition. The diagnosis is confirmed by the starch iodine test or thermography. Control of auriculotemporal syndrome may be accomplished with a 20% aluminum chloride solution applied daily to the affected area, or with anticholinergics such as glycopyrrolate. Severe cases can be corrected by interposition of a vascularized superficial temporal fascial flap or excision of the overlying skin.[2]

Uncommon sequelae of parotidectomy include seroma, hematoma, and infection. Each of these complications should occur with 1% to 2% frequency. Wound flap necrosis is rare but may occur in reoperative parotid surgery, particularly when radiation has been previously used.

Unilateral parotidectomy or submandibular gland excision usually does not cause symptomatic xerostomia when the remaining salivary glands are normal or functional. Profound xerostomia and its sequelae may follow bilateral parotid gland excision or irradiation.

OUTCOMES FOR SPECIFIC DISEASE PROCESSES

Sialoadenoses generally affect the parotid gland as a manifestation of systemic conditions. Atrophy of the gland parenchyma and fatty infiltration is sometimes followed by an irreversible loss of secretory function. The salivary gland symptoms should be recognized as part of the constellation of signs and symptoms of a systemic disease rather than a specific salivary gland disorder.

CONGENITAL DISORDERS

Congenital disorders presenting as parotid gland masses in childhood or adult life sometimes pose diagnostic dilemmas.

Surgical excision, usually accomplished by lateral parotidectomy, is both diagnostic and curative.

INFECTION

Acute sialadenitis is usually treated medically. Nonoperative measures consisting of hydration, intravenous antibiotics, and oral hygiene are successful in the majority of cases. Recognition and aggressive medical management usually resolve the initial infection. The need for surgical drainage is uncommon.

Chronic sialadenitis may follow an acute attack of suppurative sialadenitis, presenting as persistent or recurrent periods of salivary swelling. In this situation, medical treatment is usually not effective. Complete surgical removal of the involved salivary gland and its corresponding duct, sparing the facial nerve, is curative.

SIALOLITHIASIS

The presence of a salivary calculus is often associated with an underlying salivary infection. In most situations, the problem presents as recurrent chronic parotitis. Occasionally patients will present with a stone that is palpable in the salivary duct. These are the few patients who may benefit from simple sialolithotomy. The success of this procedure is often impeded by the fact that 65% of all stones are deep in the substance of the gland.[7] Most cases of sialolithiasis are best treated by total salivary gland resection with nerve preservation, which is curative.

NECROTIZING SIALOMETAPLASIA

Necrotizing sialometaplasia is a benign, self-limited disorder. The major dilemma is usually diagnostic and differentiation from malignant disorders can be difficult. Complete excision is often necessary for diagnosis. Excision and observation without treatment both appear to be curative.

TRAUMA

Most salivary gland injuries are seen in association with penetrating wounds of the cheek. Injuries may occur to the salivary duct or the facial nerve. Those involving Stensen's duct pose the most serious problems. Laceration of minor ductal structures rarely causes morbidity. There may be temporary salivary leakage, which ceases when the wound heals. Unrecognized lacerations involving Stensen's duct are associated with a salivary fistula rate over 50%. Salivary fistula and sialoceles after parotid trauma usually resolve in 1 to 4 weeks with conservative therapy consisting of aspirations, pressure dressings, and antisialogogues.[43]

Recognized lacerations repaired immediately over a stent heal well. Rarely, ductal stenosis may ensue. If anastomotic structures are near the orifice, dilatation or ductal reconstruction can be effective. Resistant cases associated with bouts of infection may require salivary gland resection.

SALIVARY GLAND IRRADIATION

Radiation injures the salivary gland secretory unit. When the parotid or submandibular salivary glands are included in radiation therapy fields, xerostomia is a sequela. After 1,000 rads the saliva becomes viscous and loses its lubricating property because of the loss of serous secretory activity caused by damage to secretory organelles. If at least one major salivary gland is spared the full dosage, hyperplasia of the residual secretory cell population occurs after several months and symptoms may be temporary. Otherwise, xerostomia due to total salivary gland irradiation is permanent. Sialogogues may be useful for increasing salivary flow in this situation.

External irradiation is carcinogenic. There is potential for malignant neoplasms or transformation of benign neoplasms to occur as a late sequela of radiation therapy. Epidemiologic studies have shown that both benign and malignant salivary gland tumors are seen more frequently with a history of radiation.[4] For this reason irradiation of benign conditions such as primary pleomorphic adenoma is generally not condoned, especially in young patients.

BENIGN NEOPLASMS/WARTHIN'S TUMOR

Surgical treatment of Warthin's tumor with superficial parotidectomy for lesions of the superficial lobe and total conservative parotidectomy sparing the facial nerve for tumors involving the deep lobe is curative. Because of the tumor's propensity toward bilaterality and multicentricity, recurrence rates are difficult to determine precisely. The tumor does not metastasize. Malignant degeneration occurs in approximately 0.3% of patients. Observation of carefully selected poor surgical risk patients confirmed to have Warthin's tumors is a reasonable option.

PLEOMORPHIC ADENOMAS

Appropriate surgical treatment of pleomorphic adenomas by superficial parotidectomy or conservative total parotidectomy with clear margins results in a recurrence rate of 1% to 5%. Recurrences are frequently multifocal and difficult to treat. Repeat surgical excision with facial nerve preservation is the treatment of choice, if possible. In some cases of recurrent tumor the facial nerve may need to be sacrificed. Surgical therapy of recurrent pleomorphic adenoma is much less satisfactory, with recurrence rates of up to 50%. Adjuvant radiation therapy may decrease the subsequent recurrence rates.[14] The incidence of malignant transformation of pleomorphic adenomas is approximately 2% to 10%. For this reason, observation of these lesions is generally not advisable.

MONOMORPHIC ADENOMAS

Biologically, monomorphic adenomas behave similarly to benign mixed tumors. Recurrences are described but are relatively rare if adequate initial excision is performed. Although a malignant form of monomorphic tumor is not well documented, a relationship to adenoid cystic carcinoma is histogenetically possible.

MALIGNANT NEOPLASMS

General Prognostic Factors for Salivary Gland Malignancy

Major determinates of survival for malignant salivary gland neoplasms are tumor histology and clinical stage.[53] Five- and 10-year survival rates among patients with parotid cancer according to histologic types are found in Table 84-4. Survival correlates most closely with the clinical stage. A poor prognosis is therefore associated with increasing tumor size, regional lymph node metastases, and distant metastases. Poor prognosis is also associated with the presence of high-grade neoplasia, perineural involvement, locally extensive disease, pain, advanced age, and facial nerve paralysis. Relationship between tumor stage and grade and survival is illustrated in Figure 84-24.

Several tumor markers are under investigation as potential prognostic markers in salivary gland malignancy. Examples include neural cell adhesion molecules (N-CAMs) and Ki-67 in adenoid cystic carcinoma and p53 gene mutations in malignant transformation of pleomorphic adenomas.[25,42,45] These and other tumor markers may become important in the management of salivary gland malignancies in the future.

Acinic Cell Carcinoma

Acinic cell carcinomas behave as low-grade malignancies. They have a strong tendency to recur locally and aggressive lesions may be locally extensive. Tumors are often slow growing and long follow-up periods are necessary to determine survival. Five-year survival does not guarantee cure. Lymph node metastases are infrequent (approximately 10% of cases at

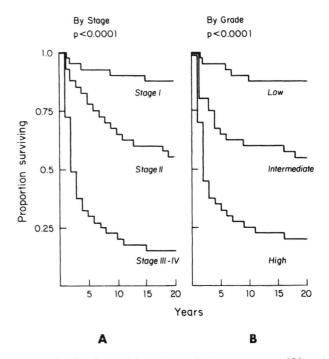

Figure 84-24. Survival by salivary gland tumor stage **(A)** and grade **(B)**. (From Spiro RH, Armstrong J, Harrison L, et al: *Arch Otolaryngol Head Neck Surg* 115:316-320, 1989.)

Table 84-4.
Five- and 10-Year Survival Rates among Patients with Parotid Carcinoma

TUMOR HISTORY	ENEROTH[18] 5-YEAR/10-YEAR (%)		SPIRO ET AL[56] 5-YEAR/10-YEAR (%)		FU ET AL[24] 5-YEAR/10-YEAR (%)		CONLEY[12] 5-YEAR/10-YEAR (%)	
Mucoepidermoid					97	95		
Low-grade	97	97	92	90	—	—	94	94
High-grade	56	54	49	42	—	—	35	28
Acinous cell	90	80	—	—	80	80	86	
Adenoid cystic	75	60	45	28	65	29	82	77
Adenocarcinoma	75	60	—	—	72	62	49	41
Malignant Mixed	50	30	63	39	—	—	77	
Squamous cell	—	—	—	—	57	57	42	—
Undifferentiated	30	25	—	—	44	22	30	—

presentation) but may occur in up to 30% of recurrent cases.[54] Hematogenous dissemination to lung and bone may occur up to 10 to 15 years after presentation.

Adenoid Cystic Carcinoma

Adenoid cystic carcinoma is considered a high-grade malignancy. It is characterized by histologic evidence of perineural invasion in most cases. Neural invasion beyond the gross confines of the lesion is often responsible for direct invasion of the central nervous system or bone. Involvement of regional lymph nodes is found in 10% to 15% of cases but is often by direct extension. Distant metastases to lung and bone may occur late in the course of the disease (approximately 40% of cases). Similar to acinic cell carcinoma, distant metastases may be relatively asymptomatic. Death is usually the result of local progression of disease into the cranial cavity by perineural extension rather than disseminated disease.

The histologic growth pattern of adenoid cystic carcinomas appears to correlate with outcome.[44,55] Solid growth patterns have a recurrence rate up to 100%, while tubular growth patterns recur in approximately 60%. In general, the prognosis for adenoid cystic carcinoma is poor. Although 5-year survival may be as high as 80%, 10-year survival rates are 30% to 50%. Adenoid cystic carcinomas arising in the submandibular gland are the most lethal.

Adenocarcinomas

Adenocarcinomas also vary in histologic pattern and grade, both of which correlate with survival.[19] High-grade lesions are characterized by a trabecular histologic appearance and have a 5-year survival rate of only approximately 20%. Well-differentiated papillary adenocarcinomas are relatively indolent, with an approximately 75% 5-year survival rate. As with other low-grade tumors, the course of patients with adenocarcinoma may be indolent and progressive with the development of late hematogenous metastases and local failure.

Malignant Mixed Tumor

Malignant mixed tumors are generally high-grade malignancies. They are characterized by high rates of regional lymph node metastases (25% to 50%) and local recurrence (50%) and distant metastatic disease (30%). Five- and 10-year survival rates with aggressive therapy are 50% to 75% and 30% to 40%, respectively.[56,57]

Mucoepidermoid Carcinoma

For mucoepidermoid carcinoma, stage and survival correlate closely with histologic grade.[22,58] Low-grade lesions have predominantly mucoid differentiation, whereas high-grade tumors are predominantly epidermoid. Low-grade lesions have a 15% to 20% recurrence compared with 60% to 70% for high-grade tumors. Regional lymph node metastases are rare in low-grade lesions but occur in up to 60% of high-grade tumors. Distant metastases are seen in approximately 30% of high-grade lesions, with skin, lung, bone, and brain being the most common sites. As with other salivary gland malignancies, the late appearance of distant metastatic lesions may occur in the absence of local or regional recurrence.

Squamous Cell Carcinoma

Squamous cell carcinomas of the salivary glands are high-grade malignancies. Salivary squamous cell carcinoma is locally aggressive, and local regional failure is a common sequela. Most tumors present in advanced stages. Perineural invasion and a high incidence (>50%) of cervical lymph node metastases occur.[56] Distant metastases are also common. Control of small tumors can be achieved if surgical margins are negative and the facial nerve not involved. Survival is approximately 75% for Stage I and 10% to 20% for Stages II and III at 10 years.

Lymphoma

Patients with salivary lymphoma generally undergo surgery only for diagnosis and occasionally for staging. Definitive treatment is by chemotherapy for disseminated lymphomas. Radiotherapy has a role for management of isolated salivary gland involvement. Five-year survival rates are approximately 30% to 40%.

Metastatic Carcinomas to the Salivary Glands

Metastatic neoplasms involving the salivary glands may represent Stage IV disease related to primary tumors in the lung, breast, kidney, or GI tract. In these situations prognosis is extremely grave, with survival rates of less than 10%. Regional lymph node metastases involving the salivary glands from cutaneous squamous cell carcinoma or melanoma also carry a poor prognosis. Despite aggressive therapy with radical lymphadenectomy and radiation therapy, 5-year survivals are only 25% to 35%.

Submandibular Gland Resection

Submandibular gland resection carries little morbidity and essentially no mortality. Potential for injury to the marginal mandibular nerve branch exists but should be avoidable in straightforward cases. A slight asymmetry to the upper neck contour may be seen after unilateral submandibular gland resection. Injury to the lingual and hypoglossal nerves may occur, resulting in loss of sensation, taste, and/or movement to the ipsilateral hemitongue. Functional deficits are expected when en bloc resection for advanced malignancy necessitates sacrifice of these structures.

Facial Nerve Reconstructive Procedures

Typical return of function after primary nerve anastomosis is a House Grade II to III.[9] Usually there will be some return of facial tone in 2 to 4 months followed by a gradual return of voluntary movement over the next year. Best results can be expected in the midface and poorer results for the lower lip and forehead. Voluntary and involuntary movement will improve for a year or more but may be accompanied by increasing synkinesis that detracts from the final functional result. This occurs because there is no consistent topographic representation of fibers in the facial nerve.

The average outcome of nerve grafting is somewhat worse than primary anastomosis, typically a House Grade III to IV.[9] The typical result is near-normal symmetry at rest with good eye closure but usually with considerable synkinesis and mass movement. Typical results of facial hypoglossal anastomosis include good tone and symmetry at rest. Some voluntary movement is usually achieved, but frequent involuntary motion degrades the final result.

The theoretic reason for the advantage of primary anastomosis over grafting is that there is only one anastomosis for the nerve fibers to grow through rather than two. About 50% to 80% of nerve fibers are lost at each anastomosis, accounting for a less complete return of function. Radiation therapy is not generally thought to significantly decrease the outcome of facial nerve reconstructive procedures.

COST

Cost of care studies for salivary gland disorders and their management have not been performed. Because salivary gland disorders frequently require surgery for diagnosis and definitive therapy and because many disease processes are malignant and involve sacrifice of functional structures with need for rehabilitation and adjunctive therapy, the cost for dealing with this group of diseases can be very high. Nonetheless, several important points in the decision-making algorithm present opportunities to optimize cost-effectiveness in the care of salivary gland disorders. Specifically, these include diagnostic imaging and biopsy procedures.

Diagnostic Imaging
Imaging studies can be invaluable in assessing deep lobe parotid tumors, large tumors, and the extent of invasion of nearby structures. However, routine use of CT or MRI is unnecessary. Imaging studies cannot provide definitive diagnosis. The extent of most salivary tumors is evident by clinical examination. Furthermore, decisions regarding the facial nerve are rarely altered by the results of a scan. Although it is recognized that the selective use of CT, MRI, and nuclear imaging studies is occasionally valuable in assessing salivary malignancies, their routine use should be condemned. Imaging studies should only be used when the information they provide is likely to be useful in planning further investigations or treatments. CT scan is recommended as an initial imaging choice in most instances, because it is cheaper than MRI.

Diagnosis
Over the past 10 years, fine-needle aspiration biopsy of salivary lesions has become a common part of the initial assessment prior to surgery. In skilled hands, only rarely are false-negatives or false-positives encountered. Fine-needle aspiration biopsy is sometimes useful in treatment planning. However, most salivary masses require surgical treatment. A fine-needle aspiration biopsy that does not fit the clinical picture or is inadequate should be repeated and if necessary followed by an appropriate surgical procedure. Delays in surgical therapy based on a fine-needle aspiration biopsy that does not correlate with the clinical picture or is inadequate can be costly in both outcome and expense.

Adjuvant Therapy
Extensive surgical procedures are usually not indicated for most patients with low-grade or early-stage salivary malignancies. In contrast, advanced and poorly differentiated malignancies require a more aggressive multidisciplinary approach. The first operation and the first course of radiotherapy provide the best and often the only chance to control salivary gland malignancy. Mature surgical judgment and experience are important in advanced cases of salivary gland disease. Early referral to centers experienced in the management of advanced malignancies is likely to be the most appropriate and cost-effective approach.

REFERENCES

1. Abrams AM, Melrose RJ, Howell FV: Necrotizing sialometaplasia: a disease simulating malignancy, *Cancer* 32:130, 1973.
2. Allison GR, Rappaport I: Prevention of Frey's syndrome with superficial musculoaponeurotic system interposition, *Am J Surg* 166:407-410, 1993.
3. Batsakis JG: *Tumors of the head and neck: clinical and pathological considerations,* Baltimore, 1979, Williams & Wilkins.
4. Belsky JL, Takechi N, Yamamoto T, et al: Salivary gland neoplasms following atomic radiation: additional cases and reanalysis of combined data in a fixed population 1957-1970, *Cancer* 35:555, 1975.
5. Bergensen PJ, Kennedy PJ, Kneale KL: Metastatic tumors of the parotid region, *Aust N Z J Surg* 57:23-26, 1987.
6. Bernstein L, Nelson RH: Surgical anatomy of the extraparotid distribution of the facial nerve, *Arch Otolaryngol Head Neck Surg* 110:117, 1984.
7. Blatt IM: Studies in sialolithiasis. III. Pathogenesis, diagnosis and treatment, *South Med J* 57:723, 1964.
8. Bryne MN, Spector JG, Garvin CF, et al: Preoperative assessment of parotid masses: a comparative evaluation of radiologic techniques to histopathologic diagnosis, *Laryngoscope* 99:284-292, 1989.
9. Calhoun KH: Management of the facial nerve in parotid malignancies, *Proceedings of the 4th International Conference on Head and Neck Cancer*, Madison, Wis, 1996, Omnipress, pp 712-718.
10. Casselman JW, Mancuso A: Major salivary gland masses: comparison of MR imaging and CT, *Radiology* 165:183-189, 1987.
11. Chaudhry AP, Gorlin RJ: Papillary cystadenoma lymphomatosum (adenolymphoma): a review of the literature, *Am J Surg* 95:923, 1958.
12. Conley J: *Salivary glands and the facial nerve,* New York, 1975, Grune & Stratton.

13. Davis RA, Anson BJ, Budinger JM, et al: Surgical anatomy of the facial nerve and parotid gland based upon a study of 350 cervicofacial halves, *Surg Gynecol Obstet* 102:385, 1956.

14. Dawson MB, Orr FR: Long-term results of local excision and radiotherapy in pleomorphic adenoma of the parotid, *Rad Oncol Biol Phys* 11:451-455, 1985.

15. deVries EJ, Sekhar LN, Janecka IP, et al: Elective resection of the internal carotid artery without reconstruction, *Laryngoscope* 98:960-966, 1988.

16. Dingman RO, Grabb WC: Surgical anatomy of the mandibular ramus of the facial nerve based on the dissection of 100 facial halves, *Plast Reconstr Surg* 29:266, 1962.

17. Eneroth CM: Facial paralysis: a criterion of malignancy in parotid tumors, *Arch Otol* 95:300-304, 1972.

18. Eneroth CM: Histological and clinical aspects of parotid tumors, *Acta Otolaryngol (Suppl)* 191:1, 1964.

19. Evans HL, Batsakis JG: Polymorphous low-grade adenocarcinoma of minor salivary glands: a study of 14 cases of a distinctive neoplasm, *Cancer* 53:935, 1984.

20. Eversole LR: Histogenic classification of salivary tumors, *Arch Pathol* 92:433, 1971.

21. Frankenthaler RA, et al: Predicting occult lymph node metastasis in parotid cancer, *Arch Otolaryngol Head Neck Surg* 119(5):517-520, 1993.

22. Frazell EL: Clinical aspects of tumors of the major salivary glands, *Cancer* 7:637, 1954.

23. Freeman C, Berg JW, Cutler SJ: Occurrence and prognosis of extra-nodal lymphomas, *Cancer* 29:252-260, 1972.

24. Fu KK, Leibel SA, Levine ML: Carcinoma of the major and minor salivary glands, *Cancer* 40:2882, 1977.

25. Gadour-Edwards R, Kapadia SB, Barnes L, et al: Neural cell adhesion molecule in adenoid cystic carcinoma invading the skull base, *Otolaryngol Head Neck Surg* 117:453-458, 1997.

26. Gardner DG, Daley TD: The use of the terms monomorphic adenoma, basal cell adenoma, and canalicular adenoma as applied to salivary gland tumors, *Oral Surg* 56:608, 1983.

27. Gates GA: Sialography and scanning of the salivary glands, *Otolaryngol Clin North Am* 10:379, 1977.

28. Godwin JT: Benign lymphoepithelial lesion of the parotid gland (adenolymphoma, chronic inflammation, lymphoepithelioma, lymphocystic tumor, Mikulicz disease): report of 11 cases, *Cancer* 5:1089, 1952.

29. Hanji D, Gohao L: Malignant lymphoepithelial lesions of the salivary glands with anaplastic carcinomatous change: report of nine cases and review of the literature, *Cancer* 52:2245, 1983.

30. Heller KS, Attie JW, Dubner S: Accuracy of frozen section in the evaluation of salivary gland neoplasms, *Am J Surg* 166:424-427, 1993.

31. Higashi T, Shindo J, Everhar TR, et al: Technetium-99m pertechnetate and gallium-67 imaging in salivary gland disease, *Clin Nucl Med* 14:504-514, 1989.

32. Hillel AD, Fee WE, Jr: Evaluation of frozen section in parotid gland surgery, *Arch Otolaryngol* 109:230-232, 1983.

33. Johns ME: Parotid cancer: a rational basis for treatment, *Head Neck Surg* 3:132-144, 1980.

34. Krol G, Strong E: Computed tomography in head and neck malignancies, *Comp Plast Surg* 13:475-491, 1986.

35. Laine FJ, Braun IF, Jensen ME, et al: Perineural tumor extension through the foramen ovale: evaluation with MR imaging, *Radiology* 174:65-71, 1990.

36. Laramore GE, Krall JM, Griffin TW, et al: Neutron versus photon irradiation for unresectable salivary gland tumors: final report of an RTOG-MRC randomized clinical trial, *Int J Radiat Oncol Biol Phys* 27:235-240, 1993.

37. Mandelblatt SM, Braun IF, Davis P, et al: Parotid masses: magnetic resonance imaging, *Radiology* 163:411-414, 1987.

38. Micheli-Pelligrini VC, Polayes IM: Historical background. In Rankow RM, Polayes IM, editors: *Diseases of the salivary glands*, Philadelphia, 1976, WB Saunders, pp 1-16.

39. Miglets AW, Viall JH, Kataria YP: Sarcoidosis of the head and neck, *Laryngoscope* 87:2038, 1977.

40. Moss-Salentijn L, Moss ML: Developmental and functional anatomy. In Rankow RM, Polayes IM, editors: *Diseases of salivary glands*, Philadelphia, 1976, WB Saunders.

41. Netter FH: Digestive system: part I, upper digestive tract. In *The CIBA collection of medical illustrations*, vol 3, New York, 1978, RR Donnelley & Sons.

42. Nordgard S, Franzen G, Boysen M, et al: Ki-67 as a prognostic marker in adenoid cystic carcinoma assessed with the monoclonal antibody M1B1 in paraffin sections, *Laryngoscope* 107:531-536, 1997.

43. Parekh D, Calezerson MB, Stewart M, et al: Posttraumatic parotid fistulae and sialoceles: a prospective study of conservative management in 51 cases, *Ann Surg* 209:105-111, 1989.

44. Perzin KH, Gullane P, Clairmont AC: Adenoid cystic carcinomas arising in salivary glands, *Cancer* 42:265, 1978.

45. Righi PD, Li YQ, Deutsch M, et al: The role of the p53 gene in the malignant transformation of pleomorphic adenomas of the parotid gland, *Anticancer Res* 14:2253-2258, 1994.

46. Russell EJ: The radiologic approach to malignant tumors of the head and neck with emphasis on computed tomography, *Clin Plast Surg* 12:343-374, 1985.

47. Schuller DE, McCabe BF: Salivary gland neoplasms in children, *Otolaryngol Clin North Am* 10:399, 1977.

48. Schwartz AW, Devine KN, Beahrs OH: Acute postoperative parotitis ("surgical mumps"), *Plast Reconstr Surg* 25:51-58, 1966.

49. Seifert G, Sobin LH: The World Health Organization's histological classification of salivary gland tumors, *Cancer* 70:379-385, 1992.

50. Shaha AR, DiMaio T, Webber C, et al: Benign lymphoepithelial lesions of the parotid, *Am J Surg* 166:403-406, 1993.

51. Som PM, Biller HF: High-grade malignancies of the parotid gland: identification with magnetic resonance imaging, *Radiology* 163:823-826, 1989.

52. Spiro IJ, Wang CC, Montgomery WW: Carcinoma of the parotid gland: analysis of treatment results and patterns of failure after combined surgery and radiation therapy, *Cancer* 71(9):2699-2705, 1993.

53. Spiro RH: Salivary neoplasms: overview of a 35-year experience with 2,807 patients, *Head Neck Surg* 8:177-184, 1986.

54. Spiro RH, Huvos AG, Strong EW: Acinic cell carcinoma of the salivary origin: a clinicopathologic study of 67 cases, *Cancer* 41:924, 1978.

55. Spiro RH, Huvos AG, Strong EW: Adenoid cystic carcinoma: factors influencing survival, *Am J Surg* 138:579, 1979.

56. Spiro RH, Huvos AG, Strong EW: Cancer of the parotid gland: a clinicopathologic study of 288 primary cases, *Am J Surg* 130:452, 1975.

57. Spiro RH, Huvos AG, Strong EW: Malignant mixed tumor of salivary origin: a clinicopathologic study of 146 cases, *Cancer* 39:388, 1977.

58. Spiro RH, et al: Mucoepidermoid carcinoma of salivary gland origin: a clinicopathologic study of 367 cases, *Am J Surg* 136:461, 1978.

59. Toonkel LM, Guha S, Dembrow V: Radiotherapy for parotid cancer, *Ann Surg Oncol* 1(6):468-472, 1994.

60. Warwick KR, Williams PL, editors: *Gray's anatomy, 35th Br,* Philadelphia, 1973, WB Saunders.

61. Woods JE: Parotidectomy: points of technique for brief and safe operation, *Am J Surg* 145:678-683, 1983.

62. Zakowski MF: Fine-needle aspiration cytology of tumors: diagnostic accuracy and potential pitfalls [Review], *Cancer Invest* 12(5):505-515, 1994.

63. Zurrida S, et al: Fine-needle aspiration of parotid masses, *Cancer* 72(8):2306-2311, 1993.

The Maxilla and Midface

David L. Larson

INTRODUCTION

The nose, nasal cavities, and sinuses are the principal anatomic structures of the middle third of the midface. That simple statement is deceiving because it masks an extremely complex group of anatomic structures that, while providing characteristic and well-recognized form to the face, also facilitates function, which is poorly understood and minimally described. Although one can breathe and smell without a nose, without restoration of the external nose (via reconstruction or a prosthesis), a patient would be severely restricted in social interaction with the surrounding world. Reconstruction of the external nose and craniofacial surgery are addressed in later chapters; however, it is important that the surgeon has an understanding of the benign and malignant diseases of the nasal cavity and sinuses and their surgical treatment.

INDICATION

THE PROBLEM

The maxillary sinus is an evagination of nasal mucosa into the maxillary bone.[2,7] The associated sinuses—the ethmoid, frontal, and sphenoid—similarly invade the skull bones that bear their names (Figure 85-1, *A* and *B*). Although none of the sinuses have any known unique physiologic function, they are air-bearing cavities that can quietly harbor significant disease. This is the reason that early disease is so rarely identified. It is only with extension into neighboring structures such as the eye, brain, skin, or teeth that the patient or physician is stirred to action (Figure 85-2). Most of the diseases that afflict the sinuses arise from the mucosa and expand slowly, producing "cold" symptoms and unilateral nasal obstruction, which only worsened despite traditional "cold" treatments.[9] These may be the only symptoms experienced until invasion of the periorbital tissue, extension into the anterior or middle cranial fossa, dental displacement from palatal involvement, cranial nerve alteration, or distortion of facial anatomy dictates a computed tomography (CT) or magnetic resonance imaging (MRI) scan. The scan may reveal an unresectable tumor; more often than not, however, the tumor is so large when discovered that definitive treatment involves both removal of the bony structure of the midface (including the orbital contents) and postoperative radiotherapy. Although some infectious processes may alter midface form, the most common (>80%) destructive process of the paranasal sinuses is squamous cell carcinoma (SCC) because of the broad epithelial expanse of the maxilla, nose, nasal vestibule, and septum, and the frequent exposure to carcinogenic agents.[1] The most common source of distant metastases to the sinuses is renal carcinoma. Risk factors for development of this disease include smoking and exposure to wood, nickel, chromium, or radium. SCC most commonly occurs "de novo," but may occasionally be associated with an inverting papilloma. This papilloma, which usually arises from the lateral wall of the nose, is in itself a benign tumor.[4,5,8] It can expand within the closed space of a sinus and cause "pressure" necrosis of bone but rarely requires reconstruction after excision. There are other, much less common nonsquamous cancers of the sinuses (e.g., adenoid, cystic, carcinoma, and adenocarcinoma), but their treatment is much the same as SCC. Radiation is frequently required after the surgical treatment of sinus cancer.[1] Juvenile nasopharyngeal angiofibroma and midline granulomatous destructive lesions, although benign, can be just as challenging to manage as a cancer because of their location and resistance to medical therapy.

Work-up of a patient with SCC of the maxillary or associated sinuses includes a history and physical examination, paying particular attention to the eye and cranial nerves. An ophthalmology consult is best obtained to determine the status of both the involved side and the normal side, since the remaining eye may be the only source of vision once definitive therapy of the sinus cancer has occurred. Plane films of the facial bones, a CT scan to determine bone destruction, and an MRI study to evaluate soft tissue and intracranial extension are all important aspects of the preoperative evaluation. Biopsy is usually performed in the operating room under general anesthesia, where bleeding can be controlled and patient comfort ensured.

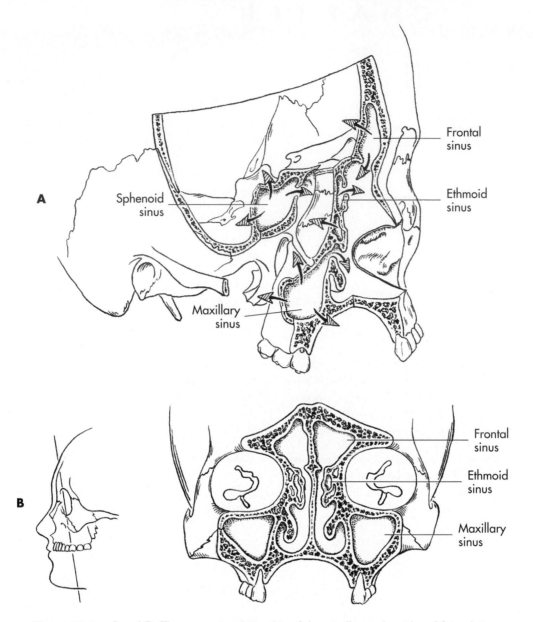

A

Sphenoid
sinus

Maxillary
sinus

Frontal
sinus

Ethmoid
sinus

B

Frontal
sinus

Ethmoid
sinus

Maxillary
sinus

Figure 85-1. **A** and **B,** The anatomic relationship of the maxillary, ethmoid, and frontal sinuses shows how disease of one can extend into another. Surgical procedures of one sinus often violate another.   *Continued*

Classically, tumors below Ohngren's line (Figure 85-3), so-called infrastructure tumors, have a better prognosis but are uncommon. Suprastructure tumors above the line involve the roof of the sinus and the lateral wall of the nose, and impinge on or invade the periorbita. The suprastructure tumors, which may also involve the infrastructure area, are seen most frequently.

Treatment of SCC of the maxilla is surgical and involves some form of maxillectomy.[12] In most cases, the surgery is combined with postoperative external beam radiation therapy. Preoperative radiation is usually not performed, since the exact extent (and therefore radiation fields) cannot be determined until the time of surgery. Also large "boost" doses of radiation can be more accurately delivered in the

postoperative setting. Radiation is not without its own problems. Complications from the radiotherapy include vision impairment, brain or bone necrosis, trismus, hearing loss, and pituitary insufficiency. The incidence and severity of these major side effects are determined by the extent of disease, dosage, and treatment technique of the radiotherapist. When radiotherapy is chosen as definitive therapy, perioperative dose planning with three-dimensional CT scanning software will improve the accuracy of the therapy and decrease the incidence of complications.

SCC of the sinus is a deadly disease, and in spite of the best treatment, many patients will die from local recurrence.[1,2,12] If the primary tumor has associated adenopathy in the neck, the mortality rate is greater than 90%.

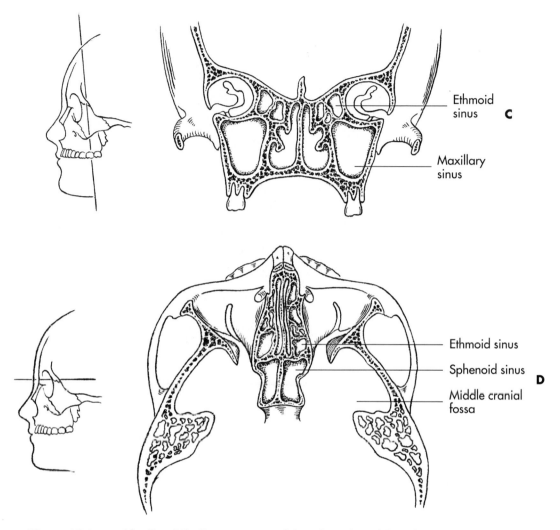

Ethmoid
sinus **C**

Maxillary
sinus

Ethmoid sinus

Sphenoid sinus **D**

Middle cranial
fossa

Figure 85-1, *cont'd.* C and **D,** Demonstration of the relationship of the ethmoid sinus to the anterior cranial fossa. Tumors of the high ethmoid cells can invade the cribriform fossa and must be removed by a combined intracranial and extracranial approach.

TUMOR MANAGEMENT

There are a number of factors that help to determine the best therapy for a given patient.

Tumor Type and Grade

Benign and low-grade tumors are usually treated successfully with surgery alone. Reconstruction with a skin graft and a dental appliance is usually adequate. SCC of the sinus, however, frequently presents with higher grade histology, is extensive, and requires a well-designed plan of ablation that may include orbital exenteration, craniotomy, and a composite reconstruction to separate intracranial structures from the nasal passages. Consideration must also be given to adjunctive

radiation therapy and neoadjuvant chemotherapy, the latter more commonly used for adenoid cystic carcinoma or adenocarcinoma.

Stage of the Tumor

Unlike most sites where size is the main criterion for staging, location within the sinuses is an important part of staging of this disease. Obviously extensive, late-stage disease carries a poor prognosis. The treatment must be appropriate for the potential for cure and for its impact on the patient's quality of life. Contraindications to maxillectomy include invasion into life-threatening structures such as the cavernous sinus and base of the skull. Local recurrence after appropriate therapy (e.g., "clean" resection plus radiation therapy) is believed by many

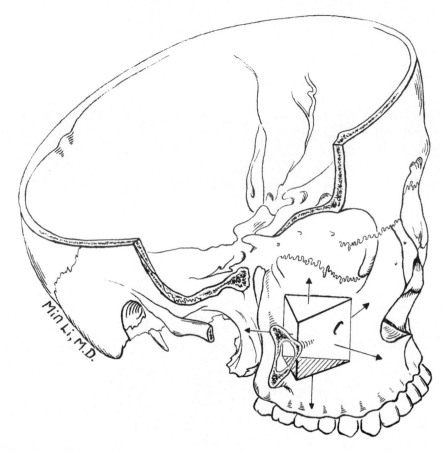

Figure 85-2. The "box" of the maxillary sinus can produce a variety of symptoms depending on the direction of extension of the disease.

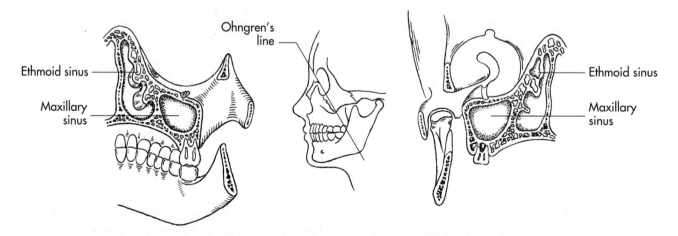

Figure 85-3. Ohngren's line is a theoretic plane that joins the medial canthus of the eye with the angle of the mandible. Tumors below the line are considered infrastructure and carry a better prognosis than those above, where suprastructure tumors are found.

to be a contraindication to surgery. Recent advances in craniofacial techniques and reconstruction have improved survival after recurrence.

Facilities Available

Ideally, definitive treatment should be carried out in a medical center capable of the full scope of sophisticated treatment noted above; surgery, radiotherapy, medical oncology, prosthetic skills, and facilities should be equally excellent. None of these treatments should be done on an itinerant basis. The first time a patient receives surgery and radiotherapy is the best opportunity he or she has to be cured; if treatment cannot be done properly, referral is mandatory.

Surgery versus Radiation

Almost all of these tumors are extensive, and the surgical goal is to obtain clean margins around the tumor. Since tissue planes are usually destroyed in the resection, and "clean" margins are only rarely obtained, postoperative radiotherapy is usually appropriate.[1] The advantage of postoperative adjuvant radiotherapy over preoperative or definitive radiation is that it will allow the radiotherapist a more detailed mapping of where tumor was located; it also "sterilizes" the microscopic seeds of tumor left from the ablation. Since there is no known effective agent or combination of agents for this disease, chemotherapy for SCC should be given only on protocol. Neoadjuvant chemotherapy and preoperative radiotherapy protocols have been promising in larynx preservation but have not yet been applied to paranasal sinus lesions.

Patient Desires

Although the surgeon may have decided what the best therapy will be, a realistic discussion with the patient concerning the possible outcomes of therapy is crucial to successful patient management. This is discussed in detail in the next section.

INFORMED CONSENT

As with all cancers, the patient must be informed of the diagnosis and the consequences if not treated. In the latter case, malignant tumors of the midface will cause pain and/or compromise of function (e.g., loss of vision, altered dentition), meningitis, and death, or at the very least will become a significant hygiene problem. If untreated, a potentially resectable tumor can become unresectable. Informed consent in cases of cancer of the sinuses must include a description of the process and its impact on the normal structures of the midface. The most important anatomic relationships are those of the sinus, eye, dura, and brain. If the tumor may possibly involve the eye, the patient must understand that this structure may be sacrificed in order to excise all of the tumor. The patient must also understand that definitive, therapeutic, and adjuvant postoperative radiotherapy may all result in loss of function of the eye by decreasing its lubrication or by cataract or corneal injury. Surgery, usually followed by radiation therapy, is the treatment of choice. If the tumor is low or lateral (infrastructure) in the maxilla, surgery may be all that is required. If the tumor obviously invades the orbit, causing distortion of facial features and visual disturbance, an orbital exenteration and radical maxillectomy followed by radiation therapy are most appropriate.

CT and MRI studies that are equivocal regarding tumor presence in the floor of the orbit/periorbita may represent inspissated mucosal drainage and edematous mucosal lining on the roof of the sinus. Obviously, in this case the orbit and its contents may be preserved. If the tumor is truly invading the floor of the orbit without invading the periorbita, the bone must be taken and the floor must be reconstructed with some vascularized tissue to support the orbit and prevent diplopia. Postoperative radiation likely to be given in this setting will, of necessity, include the reconstruction and a portion of the orbital contents in the radiation field. The morbidity of orbital preservation followed by radiation includes blindness, cataracts, diplopia, pain, keratoses, and

local recurrence from an inadequate resection.[11] If the periorbita is actually invaded, the orbital contents must be sacrificed, since clear margins with preservation of function can never be obtained in this setting. Palliative orbital exenteration should be extremely uncommon.

The real problem of informed consent arises when the floor must be sacrificed and an attempt is made to preserve the contents of the orbit. A number of long-term studies have demonstrated that the end result of an eye submitted to radiation in this setting is at least a significant compromise of function, if not total loss.[11] The patient must be made aware of this possibility and should discuss his or her desires with the surgeon if this intraoperative decision must be made. It has been my experience that, even with the presence of normal or corrected normal vision in the opposite eye, patients will opt for doing everything possible to preserve function on the affected side. The reader is directed to the references in the bibliography for more detailed information about this conundrum of maxillary cancer surgery.[3,11]

OPERATIONS

EVOLUTION OF MODERN SURGICAL TECHNIQUES

Although the maxillectomy operation has been in existence since the last century, the development of appropriate and safe surgical resections has only come about within the last few decades. As with many surgical procedures, this evolution has been related to the development of modern anesthesia and blood and fluid replacement. These improvements, combined with radiologic techniques that can identify the location and degree of destruction of the tumor, give the surgeon the ability to plan an appropriate extirpation. The advent of craniofacial and base of skull surgery, which allowed the ablative surgeon a safe approach to previously inaccessible structures, and the ability of the reconstructive surgeon to seal intracranial cavities from the airway have revolutionized surgery in this complex anatomic region.

Operations of the Maxilla and Midface

The most common disorder of the maxillary sinus is infection. The mucosal lining of the sinus leading to the nose can become inflamed from trauma, allergy, or infection obstructing the only pathways for secretions to drain. If not relieved by oral decongestants or topical sprays, the maxilla must have a new passage created by means of a nasoantral window (Figure 85-4) or endoscopic sinus surgery may be indicated if there are discrete areas of obstruction or polyps.

Surgical Approaches

Surgery remains the cornerstone for the management of all tumors of the nose and paranasal sinuses and most persistent inflammatory conditions. There are many operations and techniques described to resect any part of the midface. These involve exposing and resecting involved tissue using a combination of external incisions and osteotomies. There are three soft tissue, transfacial approaches that have evolved:

1. The *lateral rhinotomy,* which provides excellent exposure for the medial maxillectomy (Figure 85-5, *A*) and can be extended into the upper lip to gain access to the maxilla

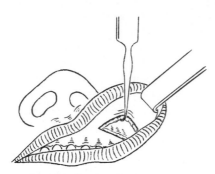

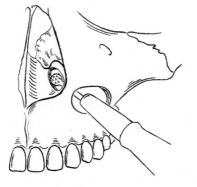

Figure 85-4. In order to provide drainage to the maxillary sinus, a window is created into the floor of the nose by way of the anterior wall of the sinus. Reconstruction of the anterior wall is not necessary.

(Figure 85-5, *B*) and into the glabellar and show area to access the maxilla and ethmoids. The incision falls in the nasolabial crease and a subciliary incision provides lateral access until the status of the orbital contents can be made intraoperatively. This is the most common incision for maxillary surgery (Figure 85-5, *A* to *C*).

2. The *total rhinotomy* is used to approach the midline, cribriform plate, and bilateral ethmoid disease and is frequently combined with a craniofacial resection and craniotomy (Figure 85-5, *E*).

3. The *midface degloving incision* provides the advantage of avoiding facial incisions by making a large gingivobuccal incision extending from one maxillary tuberosity to the opposite tuberosity. This incision is then connected to a transfixion incision in the columella and intercartilaginous incisions of the nasal cartilages. Although this does provide good visualization for the infrastructure of the maxilla, it compromises exposure of the anterior ethmoid, high in the nose, and anterior base-of-skull areas (Figure 85-6).

SURGICAL OPERATIONS OF THE SINUSES. Since the maxilla is the primary source of pathology, bony surgery in this area involves some form of maxillectomy for exposure or resection, including medial, suprastructure, infrastructure, and radical maxillectomy. These may be extended to include exenteration of the orbital contents, infratemporal fossa dissection, craniofacial resection, total palatectomy, and rhinectomy.

Medial Maxillectomy. The medial maxillectomy (Figure 85-7) is commonly used for benign tumors and low-grade malignancies that involve the lateral wall of the nose. It is easily combined with craniofacial resection and suprastructure maxillectomy whether or not the orbital is exenterated. It can also be used to access a posteriorly placed tumor such as an

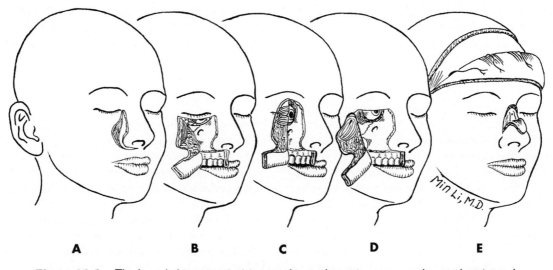

A   B   C   D   E

Figure 85-5. The lateral rhinotomy incision can be used to gain access to the nasal cavity and septum by extending to the medial canthus **(A),** can be extended to the orbital margins either inferiorly or superiorly for access to the globe or ethmoid **(B to D),** or can be combined with a craniotomy for intracranial extension **(E).**

angiofibroma that originates from the posterior aspect of the maxilla. The only real potential complication of this operation is stenosis of the nasolacrimal duct.[6,10]

Suprastructure Maxillectomy. As its name implies, the suprastructure maxillectomy (Figure 85-8) addresses tumors in the sinus that involve the orbit and may have intracranial extension. The incision is along the nasolabial sulcus and extends laterally to include the orbit and its contents and the ethmoid complex (see Figure 85-5, *C*).

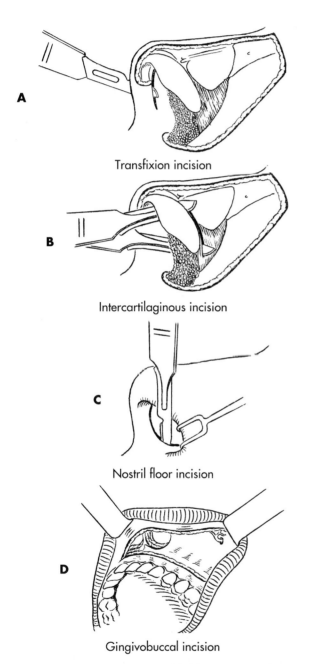

Transfixion incision

Intercartilaginous incision

Nostril floor incision

Gingivobuccal incision

Figure 85-6. In order to avoid facial incisions and gain access to nasal tumors and the sinuses, the facial degloving approach is used. A transfixion incision **(A)** is combined with an intercartilaginous incision **(B)**, a nostril floor incision **(C)**, and a gingivobuccal incision **(D)** to expose the midfacial skeleton after subperiosteal dissection over the maxillas.

Infrastructure Maxillectomy. The infrastructure maxillectomy (Figure 85-9) is probably the least common procedure since it is employed when the tumor is confined to the floor of the antrum, hard palate, or superior alveolar ridge. This can be performed through an intraoral approach and repaired with a skin graft to line the exposed buccal soft tissues and remaining maxillary sinus or the sinus mucosa can be left intact on its bony vault. A temporary prosthesis will hopefully limit the extent of wound contraction and allow the subsequent construction of a permanent denture to obturate the defect and replace the missing palate, alveolus, and teeth.

Maxillectomy with Preservation of the Orbital Contents (Figure 85-10). When the status of the floor of the orbit and periorbita are uncertain, the surgeon elevates the facial flap and explores the floor of the orbit for invasion. If the bone is violated by tumor, but the periorbita is intact, the bony floor is removed and reconstruction is performed with a split-thickness skin graft placed on the periorbita. This usually will be adequate to support the globe and orbital structures satisfactorily. If, however, the periorbita is involved with tumor, orbital exenteration is indicated even though the glove may not be violated for both oncologic and functional reasons. In such cases, adjuvant radiotherapy to the orbit will doubtless alter function of the eye, if not produce blindness, xerophthalmia, and pain. Furthermore, although reconstructive techniques may approximate normal appearance of the orbit, the intricate functions of the extraocular muscles, lacrimal drainage system, and other structures of the orbit are presently impossible to recreate.

Radical Maxillectomy. A radical maxillectomy (Figures 85-5, *C*, and 85-11) is the indicated operation for an advanced cancer of the maxillary sinus. It includes en bloc removal of the maxilla, the lower half of the ethmoid sinus, and the pterygoid plates and extends posterior to the pterygoid muscles and superiorly to the roof of the orbit, thereby including orbital exenteration.

Infratemporal Fossa Dissection. When tumor extends laterally, the zygomatic arch and the temporomandibular joint must be removed, as well as the pterygoids and sometimes temporalis muscles. On occasion, it is actually necessary to split the mandible to gain access to the area. This should be used for benign or low-grade tumors, sarcomas, and very occasionally invasive epithelial or salivary carcinomas whose epicenter is lateral.

Craniofacial Resection. A craniofacial resection (Figures 85-5, *C* and 85-12) is best used with the frontal craniotomy as the first step to evaluate anterior or middle fossa extension and thereby determine resectability of a sinus tumor. In this way, tumor invasion of the dura, cavernous sinus, and even the frontal lobe can be evaluated and, if reasonable, be resected prior to the midface/maxillary resection, obtaining safe visible cuts from both above and below for the en bloc resection.

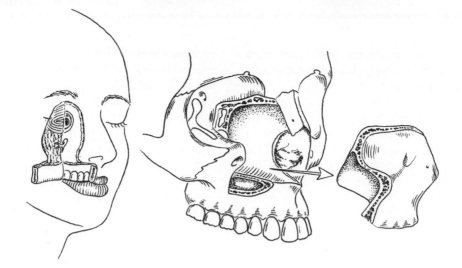

Figure 85-7. The medial maxillectomy is used to remove the anterior and middle ethmoid sinus cells en bloc. Using an extended lateral rhinotomy incision (see Figure 85-5, *A*), the periorbita is dissected laterally and the lateral wall of the nose is cut inferiorly, posteriorly, and superiorly and combined with bony cuts of the lamina papyracea and removal of the anterior wall of the maxilla sinus.

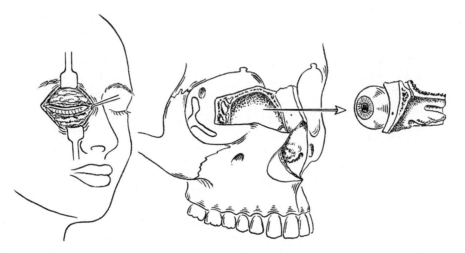

Figure 85-8. Suprastructure maxillectomy demonstrating removal of the anterosuperior portions of the maxilla and orbit.

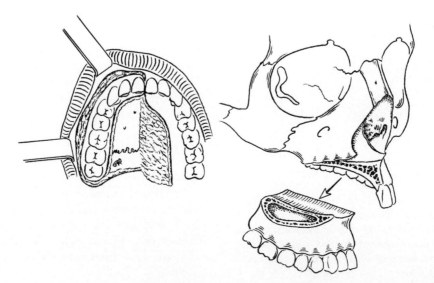

Figure 85-9. Infrastructure maxillectomy is an intraoral operation that does not require a lip incision and removes the floor of the sinus and half of the hard palate.

RECONSTRUCTION. Many of the previously mentioned operations require no reconstruction other than plating of osteotomies used to gain access and closure of the soft tissue (e.g., medial maxillectomy, lateral rhinotomy). In the event that the palate is removed but the bony floor of the orbit is preserved, a skin graft is usually sufficient to reline the buccal area. Reconstruction of the radical maxillectomy defect, previously done most frequently with a skin graft, is now often approached by three-dimensional reconstruction with a microvascular flap to restore the soft tissue defect. If the tumor dictated intracranial extension, a pericranial flap or free tissue transfer of muscle (rectus abdominis or latissimus) to seal off the dural defect from the nasal cavity is indicated. More elaborate reconstruction may occasionally be contraindicated because of the need for adjunctive x-ray therapy and/or chemotherapy and the patient's poor prognosis.

The real challenge and clinical discretion come when attempting to reconstruct the bony floor of the orbit in the face of intact periorbita and its contents. Vascularized bone with associated soft tissue for coverage of the bone is ideal in this

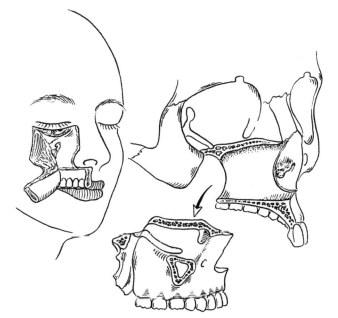

Figure 85-10. Maxillectomy with preservation of orbital contents. Bone cuts are outlined on the palate, orbit, and zygoma or malar bone, and the resultant defect is reconstructed with a skin graft on the facial flap and the periosteal envelope of the orbital floor if the bony floor was removed.

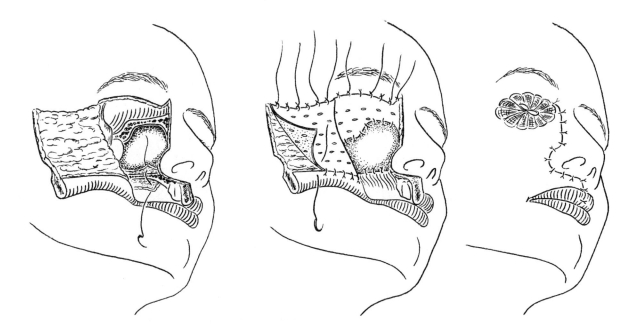

Figure 85-11. The radical maxillectomy includes the lateral rhinotomy with a lateral extension to include the upper lip (see Figure 85-5, *C* and *D*) and the bony cuts through the ethmoids, malar bone, and half of the palate to produce the defect shown. This may be reconstructed with a skin graft, temporalis flap, or free tissue transfer.

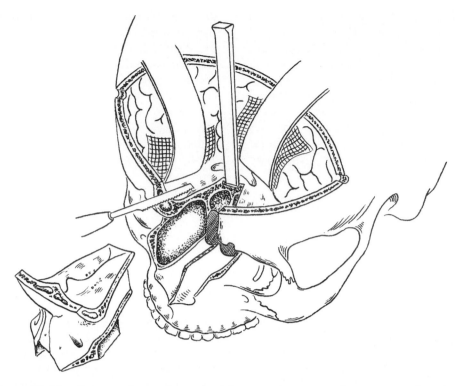

Figure 85-12. Bone cuts for craniotomy and frontonasal osteotomy for exposure of combined craniofacial resection. These skin and bone cuts allow access to the anterior cranial base for resection of tumors of the high ethmoids and olfactory tract.

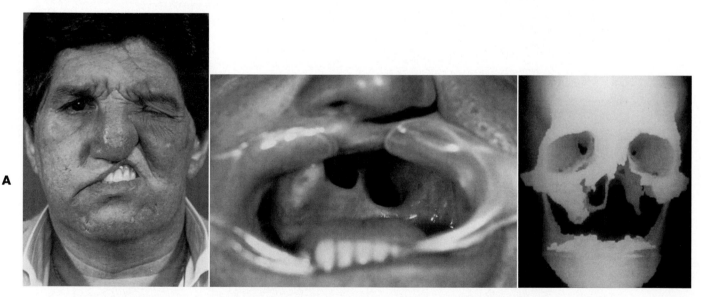

A

B,

Figure 85-13. An example of the complexity of palatal and midface reconstruction. **A** and **B,** Near total palatectomy and left maxillectomy followed by radiation therapy for squamous cell carcinoma. Orbital contents subsequently had to be removed because radiated eye was nonfunctional and painful. **C,** CT demonstrates bone defect.   *Continued*

setting, since the patient will need radiation if he or she has not already had it, and nonvascularized tissue in the setting of high-dose adjuvant radiotherapy has an unacceptably high risk of failure.

An osteocutaneous flap of the scapula or fibula is useful in this area, although the arc of rotation with the conventional skin-bone design is somewhat limited once the bone is secured. Use of the bipedicle osteocutaneous scapula flap or of two free flaps—fibula for the bone and radial forearm or lateral arm for the soft tissue coverage—may obviate this problem. Such modifications allow true customization of the defect of the patient but add time to the procedure (Figure 85-13).

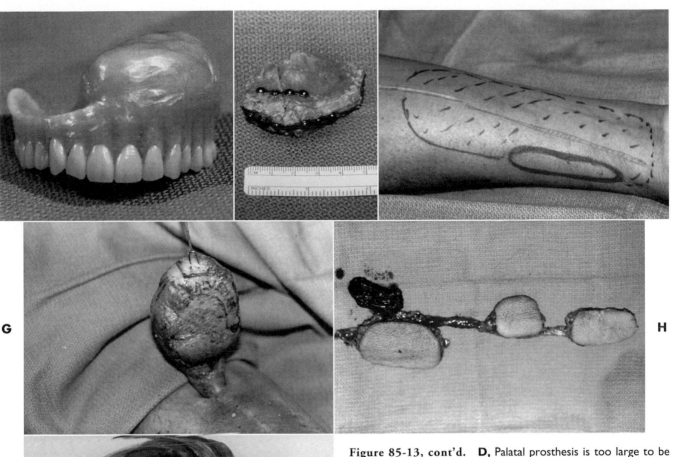

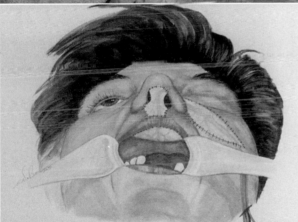

Figure 85-13, cont'd. **D,** Palatal prosthesis is too large to be supported by remaining tissue of palatal ledge on the contralateral side. **E** and **F,** Customization of the palatal reconstruction on forearm by wrapping forearm fascia around the bone graft and covering with a skin graft. **G,** Flap is transferred from forearm by microvascular anastomosis to provide new palate and fresh tissue to alveolus. **H,** Opposite forearm flap divided to reconstruct alveolar ridge, columella, and soft tissue deficit of the midface. **I,** Schematic of inset of soft tissue flaps from **(H)** used for reconstruction. (Courtesy Hani Matloub, MD, N. John Yousif, MD, and James R. Sanger, MD.)

REFERENCES

1. Jiang GI, Ang KK, Peters LJ, et al: Maxillary sinus carcinomas: natural history and results of postoperative radiotherapy, *Radiother Oncol* 21:193-200, 1991.

2. Kraus DH, Sterman BM, Levine HL, et al: Factors influencing survival in ethmoid sinus cancer, *Arch Otolaryngol Head Neck Surg* 118:367-372, 1992.

3. Larson DL, Christ JE, Jesse RH: Preservation of the orbital contents in cancer of the maxillary sinus, *Arch Otolaryngol Head Neck Surg* 118:370-372, 1982.

4. Myers EN, Fernau JL, Johnson JT, et al: Management of inverted papilloma, *Laryngoscope* 100:481-490, 1990.

5. Mickelson SA, Nichols RD: Denker rhinotomy for inverted papilloma of the nose and paranasal sinuses, *Henry Ford Med J* 38:21-24, 1990.

6. Osguthorpe D, Weisman RA: "Medical maxillectomy" for lateral nasal wall neoplasms, *Arch Otolaryngol Head Neck Surg* 117:751-756, 1991.

7. Pearson BW: The surgical anatomy of maxillectomy, *Surg Clin North Am* 4:701-721, 1977.

8. Phillips P, Gustafson RO, Facer GW: The clinical behavior of inverting papilloma of the nose and paranasal sinuses: report of 112 cases and review of the literature, *Laryngoscope* 100:463-469, 1990.

9. Robin PE, Powell DJ: Diagnostic errors in cancers of the nasal cavity and paranasal sinuses: the essential role of surgery, *Arch Otolaryngol Head Neck Surg* 107:138-142, 1981.

10. Session RB, Larson DL: En bloc ethmoidectomy and medial maxillectomy, *Arch Otolaryngol Head Neck Surg* 103:195-202, 1977.

11. Stern SJ, Goepfert H, Clayman G, et al: Orbital preservation in maxillectomy, *Otolaryngol Head Neck Surg* 109:111-115, 1993.

12. Weymueller EA, Reardon EJ, Nash D: A comparison of treatment modalities in carcinoma of the maxillary antrum, *Arch Otolaryngol Head Neck Surg* 106:625-629, 1980.

CHAPTER

Midface Reconstruction

86

John J. Coleman III

INTRODUCTION

The midface, whose structures are roughly $12 \times 6 \times 6$ cm in an adult, occupies the paired volumes and comprises the tissues between the orbit (bottom or top) and the palate. It is a complex anatomic and functional region that initiates the process of respiration, modulates its corollary functions (i.e., voice, taste, and smell), impacts on alimentation, and presents to the world a key part of the human being's appearance. There are a number of ways to perceive the appearance and function of the midface. Situated between the eyes, mediators of visual sense, and the mouth, with its mobile mandible, tongue, and palate, the midface serves as a platform and roof. Central to the paired maxillary sinus-malar areas is the nose, the most anterior projection of the resting human body and the arbiter of the senses of smell and, to some degree, taste. Remove the midface and the organism appears nonhuman, the spatial relationships defined in this small area separate us from our primate relatives.

Deformity in the region of the midface has several etiologies. Congenital abnormalities, particularly cleft lip and palate, may result in lack of projection of the midface, although the structural components are all present; reorganization of the relationship between maxilla and mandible will usually restore normality. Lateral clefts, whether genetically determined or intrauterine accidents, create lack of bony and soft tissue continuity in this region and should be considered not only in their frontal planar appearance, but as a three-dimensional deformity. Whether congenital or acquired, hemifacial atrophy or Romberg's disease affects the soft tissues surrounding the midface, creating a noticeable disfigurement and a particularly morbid, nonhuman effect.

Malignancy and the treatment of malignancy of the orbit and its contents, the skin, bone and soft tissues of the malar area, the paranasal sinuses and nasal cavity, and the upper oral cavity are the most common causes of major deformities in the midface. Skull base or occasionally intracranial tumors, either benign, malignant, or vascular, may extend inferiorly into the midface, affecting its structures and requiring en bloc resection as part of the effective therapy. Naturally, the characteristics of the deformity depend on the number of structures resected and thus dictate the needs for reconstruction.

The extent of resection in this complex area depends on tumor type and stage. Squamous cell carcinoma or adenocarcinoma from minor salivary glands of the respiratory epithelium of the paranasal sinuses is the most common reason for major resections, but esthesioneuroblastoma, sarcomas, and adenoid cystic carcinoma are also seen. The standard of surgical oncology, en bloc resection with a margin of normal tissue surrounding the tumor, remains the guideline for therapy, although the extent of the tumor may be modified by preoperative adjuvant radiotherapy. The bony walls of the sinuses may retard growth into the orbit or skin, but erosion of these bones and involvement of the periorbita or soft tissues outside the confines of the sinuses require resection of those tissues as well as orbital exenteration or inclusion of adjacent soft tissues. Similarly, encroachment on the cribriform plate or cephalad margins of the sphenoid sinus demands resection of the base of the skull. Combined intracranial and extracranial exposure, introduced in the 1960s by Ketcham and others and promulgated by numerous groups since then, allows safe exposure and improves the likelihood of obtaining a clear margin around the tumor.[8] Such resections, however, result in communication of the central nervous system and upper aerodigestive tract. Improvements in reconstruction that allow secure separation of the central nervous system from the sinus and pharynx have improved survival in these patients.

Radiotherapy as an adjuvant treatment may compound the effect of the extirpative surgery, causing chronic ischemia and soft tissue contraction or loss of bone and cartilage by osteoradionecrosis or chondronecrosis. Even when structures are left intact and radiotherapy or chemoradiotherapy is used as definitive treatment, considerable deformity may result. Treatment of orbital or maxillary rhabdomyosarcoma in children and retinoblastoma usually results in marked retardation of bone growth in the midface and atrophy of the skin and soft tissue structures, which greatly impair appearance and function, causing relative proptosis of the globe, trismus, abnormal texture and color of the skin, dental problems, and acute and chronic mucositis.

Trauma, both blunt and penetrating, regularly affects the midface, with troublesome sequelae. The relative anterior projection of the nose and malar areas and the juxtaposition of thick and thin bone put the midface at a high risk of deformity from deceleration injury. Nasoorbitoethmoid fractures disrupt the attachments of the periorbita and may destroy the foundation of the nose, allowing it to telescope into the sinus cavities and central airway. Lateralized blunt injury that is not adequately repaired may result in enophthalmos, facial flatness, and dental occlusal problems. A devastating and relatively common midface injury is the self-inflicted gunshot or shotgun wound, which may destroy most of the midfacial structures while leaving the brain intact. Placement of the gun in the mouth or beneath the chin in an anterosuperior aim will destroy the mandible, palate, nasal structures, and medial orbits with or without the eyes themselves. In addition to the loss of tissue, this deformity is compounded by impaction of small pieces of devascularized bone and sinus mucosa in the adjacent soft tissues. These nests of contaminated devitalized tissue subsequently create small abscesses and may impair local wound healing and infect nonvascularized bone grafts or synthetic implants. Reconstruction of this complex defect requires careful debridement and introduction of well-vascularized tissue.

Infection, either acute or chronic, may create significant deformity of the midface. Before the advent of antibiotics, dental infections and sinusitis, if uncontrolled, extended into the adjacent soft tissues, creating tissue loss, sinus tracks, or scar contractures. Similarly, cephalad or rostral extension could cause meningitis or brain abscess. Although still seen occasionally, bacterial infection is an uncommon source of major tissue loss in patients who are not immunocompromised. The success of organ transplantation, the epidemic of acquired immunodeficiency syndrome (AIDS), and better chronic treatment of diabetes mellitus have produced a large population of patients with impaired immune systems that are susceptible to invasive infection by resident organisms of the nasal passages, sinuses, and pharynx. Synergistic bacterial infection or fungal infection with aspergillus, mucormycosis, blastomycosis, and other organisms may create significant midfacial deformities if arrested before they invade the central nervous system, causing death. Noma and lethal midline granuloma, nonspecific names for a number of diseases including lymphoma and Wegener's granulomatosis, specifically affect the nasal cavity and sinuses; if controlled before causing death, they may leave subsequent deformity.

DESCRIPTIVE AND FUNCTIONAL ANATOMY OF THE MIDFACE

The anatomy of the midface, both descriptive and functional, is complex. The stationary mucosa-lined cavities of the nose, paranasal sinuses, and nasopharynx provide ingress to inspired air and humidify, warm, and clean it. These cavities separate the mucosa-lined oral cavity, with its numerous mobile structures that facilitate speech and swallowing, from the

relatively immobile anterior extension of the central nervous system, the eye and its protective and motor-surrounding tissues, the orbit, and the periorbita. One can consider each of these units a functional matrix or "a tissue or group of tissues performing a function."[15] Thus the eye and the orbital structures present visual information to the brain for processing; the nose, nasopharynx, and paranasal sinuses present and modify air to the lungs for smell, respiration, and speech; and the oral cavity presents and modifies the air to the lungs and food to the stomach for respiration, speech, taste, and alimentation. Three of the five senses—taste, smell, and sight—reside wholly in these functional matrices, and hearing is greatly influenced by changes in the area. Naturally, disruption of the normal anatomy and function may create a devastating problem.

A simplistic, conceptual model of midfacial anatomy can be constructed by considering each midface functional matrix to be a cube or a collection of cubes or parallelograms; those cubes are juxtaposed and surrounded and lined by their characteristic soft tissues (Figure 86-1). There are then the paired cubic structures, the orbits, the maxillary sinuses, the ethmoid sinuses, the frontal sinuses, and the single (although split by the septum and vomer) midline structure of the nose. The confluent cubic structure, the oral cavity, lies beneath these structures, and the confluent nasopharynx and sphenoid sinuses posterior to them. These units are modified by their intrinsic mucosal lining, soft tissues, nerves, and muscles to create the functional matrices. Pathology, tumor, trauma, and infection may destroy one or more of these cubic structures or whole functional matrices. Reconstruction should then be addressed at restoring whatever structure or function possible without damaging residual structural function. The intricate cavernous structure of the sinuses, with its ethmoid air cells,

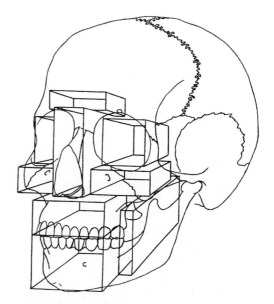

Figure 86-1. Conceptualization of the facial skeleton as a series of boxes juxtaposed. Each box serves a separate, usually unique function, and thus can be considered a separate functional matrix, which, when combined with adjacent matrices, defines the entire function of the face.

small draining passageways or foramina, and turbinates that greatly increase the surface area of this functional matrix when exposed to the inspired air, can obviously never be fully reconstructed, and neither can the precise motion and light-collecting ability of the eye or the amazing synergy of the oral and pharyngeal muscles, nerves, glands, and internal lining. Optimal reconstruction must then be limited to the restoration and facilitation of remaining function.

Another characteristic of the midface is its support of the calvarium—with its delicate contents, the brain, brain stem, and appendages—in the otherwise fairly mobile environment. (The mandible and oral cavity have constant purposeful and vegetative motion, and the neck and vertebral column allows the wide arc of motion with respect to the trunk.) Such support is provided by the structural framework of thick bone continuous through the bony suture lines between the calvarium and oral cavity. These midface buttresses are the foundation of the midface anatomy; in addition to protecting and providing support for the calvarium and orbits, they determine the characteristic appearance of the human face. The normal proportions of the facial structures as represented in Leonardo's square and other approximations of normal facial height and width depend on preservation or reconstitution of these buttresses. These vertical midface buttresses are, from medial to lateral, the nasofrontal, zygomatic, and pterygomaxillary buttresses, and the horizontal is the maxillary alveolar buttress.[7,9] Normal ocular and dental occlusive function, as well as appearance, depends on preservation of the anatomic relationships set by these buttresses. The concept of facial aesthetic units is the surface anatomy projection of the underlying functional matrices. The skin and soft tissues are draped over the bony framework, which maintains their shape, curvature, and anterior projection. Removal or destruction of the underlying framework results in collapse of the overlying tissues and contraction toward the center of the volume described by the missing buttresses (Figure 86-2).

ANALYSIS OF THE DEFECT

Three essential observations and a number of corollary judgments make up the appropriate analysis of a midface defect. Correct application of the analysis is the first step toward a successful reconstruction. Obviously, the *enumeration of missing structures* is paramount. Second, the *etiology* of the problem bears heavily on the approach. Oncologic defects must be assessed for the presence of residual tumor or the likelihood of recurrence. Infectious defects must be evaluated for the presence of invasive infection or for the likelihood that the reconstruction will change the milieu so that the colonization is turned into invasive infection. Therefore each cause of a midface defect has its own associated issues that affect closure and execution of reconstruction. The third parameter is the *function* of those structures destroyed by the disease process and the potential for restoring function. The relationship of functions that reside in adjacent functional matrices must also be assessed (e.g., how a defect of the nose or sinuses affects speech, swallowing, or ocular function). Other aspects of the defect or disease process include history of previous surgery or radiotherapy, the likelihood of subsequent surgery or radiotherapy, mobility, sensory capabilities, and secretory function.

Although the general functions of the area, including sight, respiration, and alimentation, have already been stated, a more

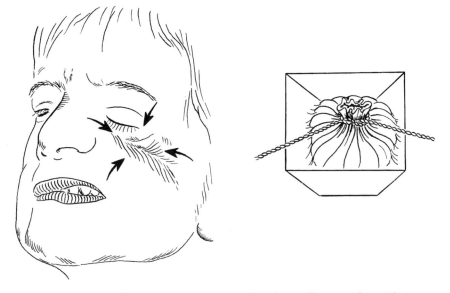

Figure 86-2. Diagram of patient previously treated with maxillectomy, hemipalatectomy, and adjuvant radiotherapy for adenoid cystic carcinoma arising in the maxilla. Loss of the midface buttresses allows collapse of the soft tissue structures toward the center of the defect, resulting in the displacement and derangement of the various functional matrices.

detailed examination is appropriate. Within the functional matrix of the orbit, the globe is the main processor of light-mediated visual information. The eyelids protect the globe from external trauma and facilitate lubrication and cleansing of the eye with the fluids secreted and drained by the lacrimal gland and lacrimal duct system. The eyelids also help the iris modulate the penetration of light into the globe.

The nose is the dominant aditus of air to the lungs. The circuitous route followed by the air is governed by the anatomy of the nose; its external and internal valves, the septum, the turbinates, and the choana protect the lungs from injury by large objects (e.g., insects) that might be inhaled. Respiratory epithelium contains secretory elements that provide mechanical and immunologic protection, and the high blood flow in the submucosal layers of the lining of the nasal cavity warms and humidifies the inspired air. These homeostatic mechanisms are so efficient that patients inhaling superheated air in a fire will not suffer thermal injury to the trachea or lungs. The orderly circulation of air through the nose allows chemical processing of inhaled substance by the olfactory apparatus and thus smell and, to some degree, taste. The paranasal sinuses contain the same lining as the nasal cavity and thus probably have served similar functions. Their progressive pneumatization during childhood growth probably indicates some function of cushioning or dispersion of energy between the mobile oral cavity and the neck and the fixed calvarium with its contents, the brain and brain stem. The multiple ciliated, mucosa-lined bony compartments suggest an effort to increase surface area, perhaps to allow greater contact between air and the heat-regulating processes or to modify expelled air, creating some resonance to speech. Linear nonturbulent bilateral flow of air is facilitated by the midline septum and perpendicular plate of the ethmoid bone, the vomer. The nasopharynx, with its connection to the ear via the eustachian tubes, helps equalize pressure internally and externally. The large amount of lymphoid tissue in the nasopharynx indicates its importance in immunologic processing. From front to back, the posterior wall of the frontal sinuses, the roof of the orbit, the cribriform plate, the superoposterior wall of the sphenoid sinus, and the roof of the nasopharynx form the inferior boundary of the cranial cavity, protecting the brain and keeping the cerebrospinal fluid contained.

The palate, the roof of the mouth, is the floor of the midface and separates the oral cavity from the nasal cavity. Its anterior extent, the rigid bony hard palate, is covered by a thick layer of keratinized, tightly adherent mucosa that is difficult to separate from the underlying periosteum. This masticatory mucosa extends partially into the dental sockets, creating a tight protective seal around the teeth. The maxillary alveolus or lateral and anterior extension of the palate forms the horizontal buttress of the midface, its thicker bone securely holding both primary and permanent teeth. The hard palate, with its mucosa lubricated by indigenous minor salivary glands, creates a rigid limit on which the tongue and mobile buccal area can manipulate the oral bolus to slide backward, ending the oral phase of swallowing and initiating the pharyngeal phase. Posterior to the hard palate, the velum or soft palate joins the tongue, oropharynx, and nasopharynx by the palatoglossus,

palatopharyngeus, tensor veli palatini, and levator palatini muscles and ascends and descends much like a trapeze to separate the oral cavity from the nasal cavity. This finely coordinated activity, combined with elevation and depression of the larynx and constriction and relaxation of the superior and middle constrictor and cricopharyngeus muscles, allows food to be propelled into the esophagus without going into the nose or larynx, routes inspired air from the nose into the lungs and not the stomach, and modifies the stream of air expelled from the lungs to pass through the mouth and nose, forming recognizable speech. Thus derangements of the palate cause many problems.

The interdependency of function and thus dysfunction in midface deformity can be illustrated by several relatively common clinical scenarios. Medial maxillectomy resection for squamous cell carcinoma of the medial wall of the maxillary sinus includes the nasofrontal buttress; the lateral nasal wall, including turbinates; and a portion of the anterior maxillary bone, with or without skin depending on the extent of the tumor. Although this is a relatively small amount of the total midface structure and two of the three vertical buttresses and the horizontal buttress remain intact, several problems might be seen. If the resection is carried high enough, the opening of the lacrimal drainage system into the nose might be damaged, causing possible obstruction and resulting in epiphora, ascending infection (dacryocystitis), or abscess. The normal airflow pattern in the ipsilateral nasal cavity will be altered, and the ensuing turbulence may result in drying, crusting and chronic inflammation, nosebleeds, or subtle voice changes. The classical maxillectomy for tumors involving the maxillary sinus or part of the palate includes resection of the oral and nasal surfaces of the hemipalate, including the alveolus; the nasofrontal, zygomatic, and pterygomaxillary buttresses; the lateral nasal wall and turbinate; and sometimes the infraorbital rim and floor of the orbit, depending on the extent of the tumor. The cavity created by such a unilateral resection in an adult man approximates a cube with the dimensions of $6 \times 6 \times 6$ cm or a volume of 216 cm^3. Since the bony framework has been removed, all of the boundary structures, the malar skin on the attached upper lip, the globe, the periorbita (if the orbital floor has been resected), the lateral facial skin and remaining pterygoid muscles and soft tissue and the remaining soft palate are pulled to the geometric center of that 216 cubic cm defect. Thus the upper lip will be pulled back, causing oral incompetence that affects speech and swallowing, while the malar skin will be pulled inward, decreasing the height and width of that side of the face. The pterygoid musculature and lateral soft tissues of the face will be pulled toward the center, decreasing their excursion and causing trismus or difficulty opening the mouth. The globe and orbital contents will be pulled down and inward, limiting the sphincteric actions of the orbicularis oculi and thus the elevation of the lower lid; this results in ectropion, lowers the visual axis of the globe, and restricts other extraocular movements, resulting in diplopia and other restrictions of the visual field (Figure 86-2 and 86-3). The wide open communication of the oral cavity, former maxillary sinus area, and nose creates disorders of oral

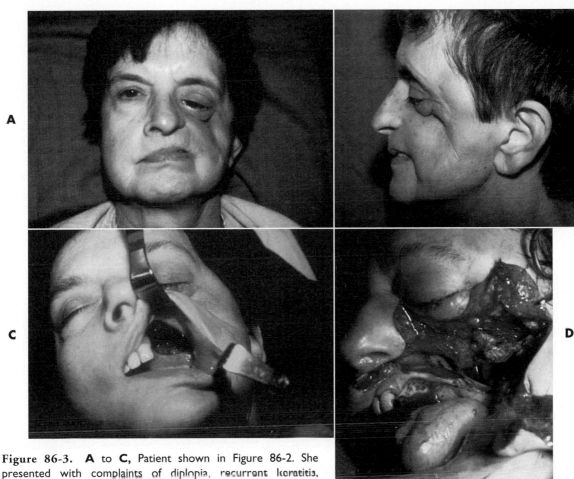

Figure 86-3. **A** to **C,** Patient shown in Figure 86-2. She presented with complaints of diplopia, recurrent keratitis, trismus, and inability to completely close the mouth, with the resultant oral incompetence and effect on speech and difficulty eating, because of poorly fitting prosthesis. **D,** Re-creation of the defect shows the extensive hemipalatectomy, hemimaxillectomy tissue loss with subsequent scarring and fibrosis from radiation and chronic infection. *Continued*

and nasal airway pressure and flow, disrupting the normal route of food and air. Contraction of the free margin of the soft palate may impair its normal motion and prevent obturation of the nasopharynx, resulting in velopharyngeal insufficiency. In addition to the obvious effects this would have on speech and swallowing, the turbulence of the air and the lack of normal warming and humidification create a surface environment of crusting, serum and mucus subject to superinfection, inflammation, and bleeding. The addition of radiotherapy as an adjunct to treatment makes the situation even worse, since damage to adjacent minor salivary glands creates xerostomia and decreases the ability of the airway to cleanse itself normally.

The goal of anatomic and functional assessment of the midfacial deformity is to suggest an appropriate method of reconstruction. Obviously, we are greatly limited in our abilities to recreate such complex functions as the eye's processing of light to stimulate a recognizable pattern by the brain. The intricate lattice of sinus surfaces with secretory function would be impossible to reconstruct. A more reason-

able approach for the present is to attempt to rebuild the damaged architecture to a form that will allow it to facilitate remaining function. A general principle to guide reconstruction would be to rebuild the missing surfaces that characterize the roughly cubic structure or if each surface cannot be exactly rebuilt, to restore those with the most functional importance and obliterate the remaining missing volume with well-vascularized soft tissue or some substitute such as a synthetic prosthesis. Although not addressing secretory, humidifying, olfactory, or other various functions, this conceptual approach satisfies the barrier and buttress characteristics of the midface and provides structure and separation of the oronasal and orbital cavities, and thus the complementary functions of respiration and alimentation. A simple iteration of this concept would describe the reconstructed midface as a solid cube with each of its surfaces having some functional importance: the palate, the lateral nasal wall, the posterior nasopharyngeal wall, malar buccal skin, the orbital floor, and the lateral pterygoid area (Figure 86-4). The following reconstructive procedures can be conceived of as addressing some or all of these

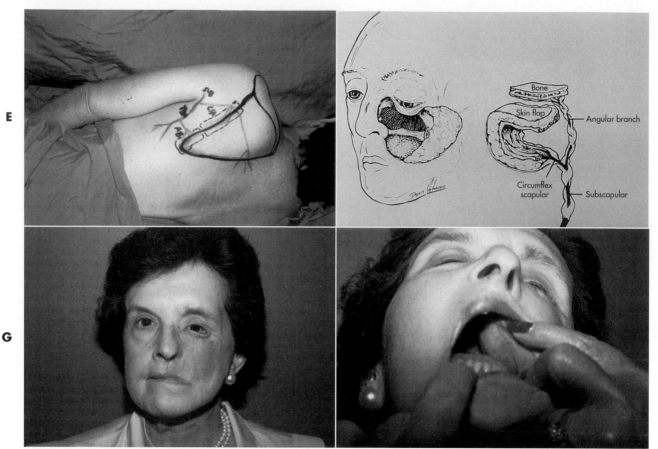

E   F

G   H

Figure 86-3, cont'd. **E** and **F,** A bipedicle scapula osteocutaneous flap was used to reconstruct the defect, with the skin based on the horizontal branch of the circumflex scapular vessels and the bone based on the angular branch of the thoracodorsal vessels. Thus the bone used to reconstruct the orbital floor has a widely independent arc of rotation from the skin. **G** and **H,** Postoperative results. Except for the ectropion, which was rectified with a skin graft at a subsequent minor operation, her functional problems were resolved by this single-stage reconstruction.

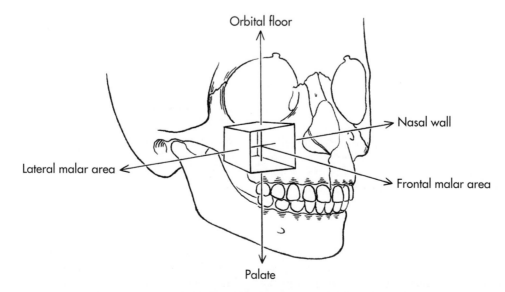

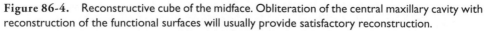

Figure 86-4. Reconstructive cube of the midface. Obliteration of the central maxillary cavity with reconstruction of the functional surfaces will usually provide satisfactory reconstruction.

considerations and can thus be judged on how many they satisfy.[5]

Radiographic analysis of the defect may make metachronous reconstruction more accurate and also plays a role in preoperative planning. Software programs combined with three-dimensional reformatting of computerized tomography allow definition of the defect and estimates of affected surfaces and remaining bony structures. Although reconstruction is limited by the availability of tissues and configuration of the tissues necessary to satisfy the defect, computerized tomography and plain radiographs may be used to identify bony structures left after the resection to which the reconstructed tissues may be fixed. Magnetic resonance imaging with or without contrast can be useful in followup of tumor patients, since recurrent tumor has different imaging characteristics from soft tissue used for reconstruction.

OPERATIONS

One of the tenets of craniofacial surgery is that orientation of the facial skeleton into its proper relationships will result in normal or improved soft tissue relationships. Although this may be true in growing children, it is not necessarily relevant in adult patients with problems secondary to malignancy, trauma, or infection. Provision of bone and soft tissue is optimal, but sometimes less than complete replacement of one structure may provide adequate reconstruction either by substitution or facilitation of complementary methods that combine to provide an acceptable whole.

The development of methods of midface reconstruction has been, to some degree, hampered by the widely held belief that maxillofacial prosthetics could resolve many of the problems created by such defects. Although clever and artistic constructs have been created, these are rarely sufficient unless the defect is limited. Even the simplest prosthetic reconstruction, the denture, is used successfully for chewing in a surprisingly small percentage of wearers. Larger prostheses that fill the maxillary sinus, nasal cavity, orbit, and other components of the midface require more daily care for cleansing and fitting, cause more discomfort, and are frequently rejected by even well-motivated patients after a short period of use (Figure 86-5). A combination of autologous tissue reconstruction, maxillofacial prosthodontics, and osseointegration of implants will likely produce the optimal functional and aesthetic result in the future. Preoperative analysis of the patient and projection of the expected defect by a multidisciplinary team, including surgeon, prosthetist, and others, are important steps in obtaining acceptable outcomes.[1,16]

The simplest and probably still most common method of reconstruction of midfacial deformities is skin grafting the raw surfaces or allowing reepithelialization and placement of a prosthesis after removal of temporary packing. Thus for the hemimaxillectomy defect, the malar skin that previously lay over the anterior wall of the maxilla is resurfaced with a skin graft. The lateral muscles and velar margin contract and epithelialize, leaving a cubic defect lined by skin graft and scar; this defect is to some extent obturated by a prosthesis consisting of a bulb to fill some of the cavity and to suspend the denture in the oral cavity. Such a reconstruction is unlikely to halt the progressive contraction of the skin graft toward the upper center of the defect and may be troublesome to care for daily, but if the defect is small, it may be satisfactory.

The midface is farther from the neck and thorax than the oral cavity and thus less amenable to single-stage reconstructions from thoracic musculocutaneous flaps. Because of the need for multiple-stage reconstructions, many surgically created defects of the recent past were left unreconstructed or cumbersome prostheses were fashioned to address some components of the problem. Prior to the elucidation of the musculocutaneous concept, tubed skin grafts were the most commonly attempted method of reconstruction and the goal was usually uniplanar reconstruction of one of the surfaces of the defect (malar skin or palate). Skin flaps from the posterior neck such as the Mutter or Zovickian flaps, or Tagliacotian flaps from the arm were the mainstay when such reconstructive attempts were made. The deltopectoral flap described in the mid-sixties was a more reliable axial-supplied skin flap; however, because of the distance of the resection from the chest wall, it required delay procedures prior to raising and inset. All of these skin flaps were based on the principle that a distant flap inset to the affected area would develop its intrinsic blood supply from the adjacent tissues, allowing the origin of the flap to be divided and the remaining tissue used for reconstruction. This process of parasitizing the blood supply is hindered by previous radiotherapy to the area, scar from previous surgery, high bacterial colonization or invasive infection, and the constant passage of air, mucus, and saliva around the wound. Again, these pitfalls discouraged the use of such techniques, and many patients were left with complex and morbid defects.

Bakamjian described the reconstruction of a palatal defect with a combined paddle of skin and sternocleidomastoid muscle and with the deltopectoral flap in the early sixties, well before the general appreciation of the musculocutaneous concept.[3] With the recognition that subjacent muscle can carry overlying skin, a number of other methods have been described. The pectoralis major musculocutaneous,[2] trapezius,[12] and latissimus dorsi[11] flaps may all, with some manipulation, include the midface within their arc of rotation. Their usefulness, however, is somewhat limited because most complex defects are at the very limit of their arc of rotation, subjecting the distal (most important) parts of the flap to relative ischemia. Unlike reconstruction of the lower oral cavity where the pedicle can be placed in the neck, reconstruction of the midface requires passage of the pedicle through the oral cavity or beneath the skin of the face,

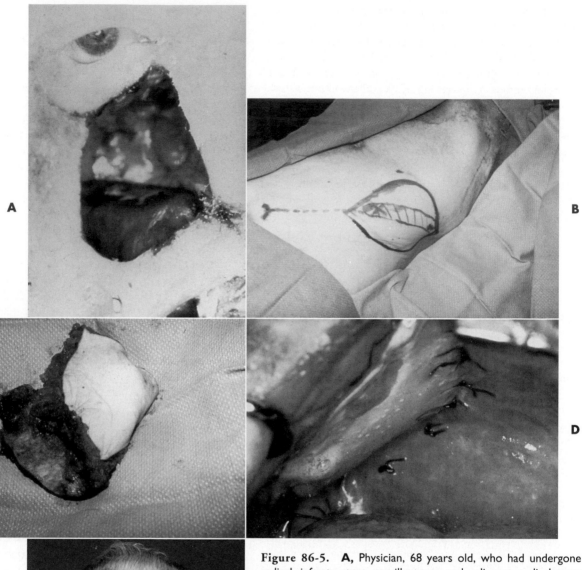

Figure 86-5. A, Physician, 68 years old, who had undergone radical infrastructure maxillectomy and adjuvant radiotherapy for squamous cell carcinoma invading through the skin. He was unable to function with a prosthesis despite multiple efforts. **B** and **C,** Left-sided deep circumflex iliac artery flap (DCIA) designed to carry skin for palate and malar surface and bone for the orbital floor. **D,** Postoperative appearance of reconstructed palate. **E,** Appearance 2 months after initial surgery. His malar skin area was debulked and replaced with a skin graft from the neck.

creating a significant secondary deformity. Staged operations involving removal of the bulky pedicle make such procedures similar to the earlier ones that relied on the local defect to supply the nutrient blood flow to the flap. Although a larger volume of tissue can be transported, the mechanics are not favorable. Initial enthusiasm for the sternocleidomastoid musculocutaneous flap has been dampened by recognition of a limited arc of rotation and poor blood supply to the skin island, with a high risk of subsequent necrosis. MacGregor described the forehead axial pattern skin flap, based on the superficial temporal vessels and transposed down into the palate, malar skin, or buccal area with a good blood supply but an unattractive donor site.

The temporalis muscle flap is useful for reconstruction of small-to moderate-sized defects of the palate and midface. Supplied by the internal maxillary artery, which enters the muscle on the deep surface, it can be mobilized from the temporal bone and zygoma and passed through the lateral buccal soft tissues to reach the contralateral buccal mucosa. It is also useful for resurfacing the orbit, reaching the medial orbital wall (Figure 86-6). Temporoparietal fascia based on the superficial temporal artery and vein can similarly be transposed into the orbital cavity midface or upper oral cavity. Vascularized calvarial bone can also be moved with the temporoparietal fascia to reconstruct orbital or midface bony defects.

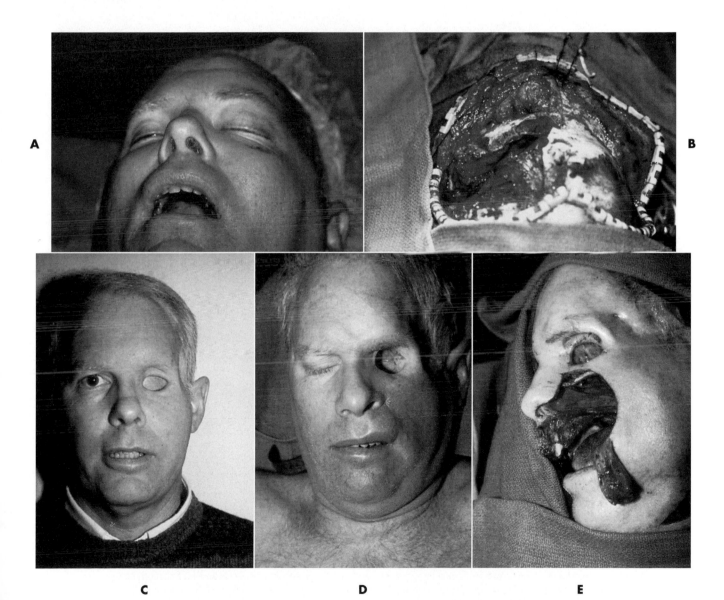

Figure 86-6. **A** and **B**, Patient with ethmoid tumor invading orbit who required orbitectomy with ethmoid and cribriform plate resection. **C**, The base of the skull and superoposterior orbital defects were reconstructed with a temporalis muscle flap resurfaced with a split-thickness skin graft. **D** and **E**, Massive recurrence in the maxilla and overlying skin necessitated radical resection including palate, lateral nasal wall, posterior orbital floor, and malar skin. *Continued*

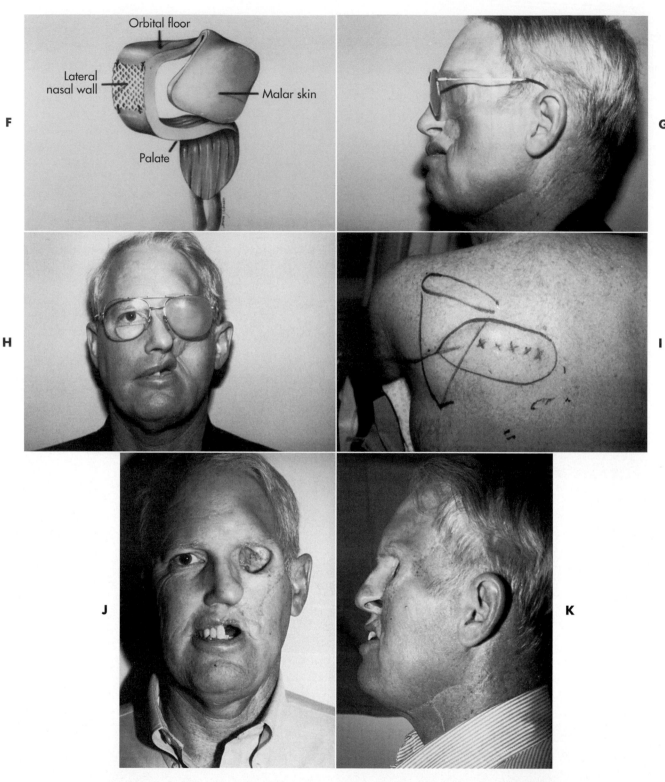

Figure 86-6, cont'd. **F,** Reconstruction was carried out with a rectus abdominis muscle flap and split-thickness skin grafts with excellent contour and functional result initially. **G** and **H,** Subsequent atrophy of the denervated rectus muscle led to unsatisfactory appearance and considerable lip retraction. The amount of atrophy of muscle flaps is unpredictable, so they are inferior to skin or musculocutaneous flaps for reconstruction in this area. **I** to **K,** A scapula skin free autograft was used to restore more normal contour and to lower the lip.

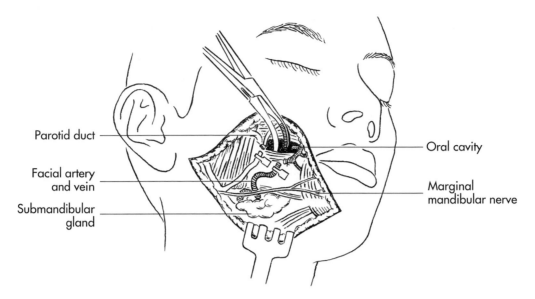

Figure 86-7. Dissection of a skin flap from the upper neck into the cheek in the subcutaneous plane will allow exposure of the facial vessels in the face. These are dissected out from beneath the marginal mandibular nerve. An incision through the buccinator muscle or buccal fat pad and mucosa allows entry into the oral cavity where the flap is placed to resurface the missing surfaces (palate, lateral nasal wall, orbit, base of skull).

In the mid 1980s it was recognized that the most efficient way of providing well-vascularized tissue to the midface and thus resolving the complex reconstructive issues was by free tissue transfer.[5] Unlike the situation with tumors of the oral cavity or laryngopharynx, the neck is rarely involved by regional metastases when defects are created in the palate, orbit, or maxillary area. The facial and occipital vessels or other branches of the external carotid and their venae comitantes or branches of the jugular vein are usually readily apparent, and the short distance between the upper neck where they reside and the palate or midface—even the orbit—is amenable to passing the vascular pedicle in a subcutaneous tunnel, thus minimizing secondary deformity (Figure 86-7). Muscle, skin, bone, or combinations of these tissues can be moved to satisfy various components of the midface defect at a single-stage operation or with one major operation and subsequent minor revisions. The obvious advantages of free tissue transfer are provision of tissue, with its independent blood supply, and an ample supply of tissue that can be manipulated to the defect in a single stage or used to overcorrect the deformity with subsequent refinement. These two characteristics obviate the previous problem of trying to resolve a large three-dimensional defect in multiple stages with a small amount of poorly vascularized tissue where each stage of such a reconstruction is likely to have complications undermining the ultimate result.

Since ample tissue is available with the latissimus dorsi, scapula, rectus abdominis, and other free tissue transfers, the unidimensional reconstruction is no longer the necessary approach. By folding the free flap on itself, the functionally important surfaces, the palate, lateral nasal wall, floor of the orbit, buccal malar soft tissue or skin, and base of skull, can all be satisfied with a single operation. The critical space bounded by these functional surfaces is obturated by the muscle or soft tissue, decreasing the likelihood of subsequent contraction and deformity and minimizing infection. Denervated muscle alone as a free tissue transfer may atrophy up to 70% of its volume, so care must be taken to suspend it adequately or to include skin or other soft tissue that is not as susceptible to shrinkage (see Figure 86-6). Composite flaps of bone and skin such as the fibula and scapula are also useful. The bipedicle osteocutaneous scapula free flap[6] is particularly useful for combined orbital and palatal reconstruction, since the arcs of rotation of the skin paddle and bone are widely independent. Although vascularized bone may be useful for reconstructing previous bony surfaces such as the orbital floor and hard palate, dermis, or skin, grafted muscle is frequently an adequate substitute. The suspension of the flap from remaining bony structures such as the palatal margin, frontal bone, zygoma, lacrimal bone, and sphenoid will create a semirigid surface that mimics bone and allows reasonable function (Figure 86-8).[4,14] When a well-vascularized soft tissue milieu has been created to close the defect, primary or secondary nonvascularized bone graft is more likely to be successful than without such surrounding tissue (Figure 86-9). This is particularly useful in the correction of ocular dystopia and its resulting diplopia. By using such techniques with free tissue transfer, lateral defects of large dimension can be reconstructed in a single stage.

A particularly difficult reconstructive challenge is the median midface defect. Although occasionally seen as a result

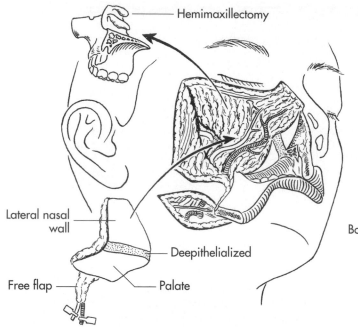

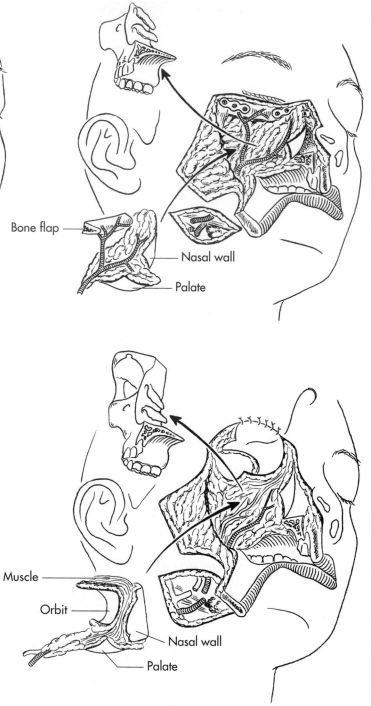

Figure 86-8. Reconstruction of various midface defects with microvascular free autografts with anastomosis in the neck and passage of the vessels through a subcutaneous tunnel in the cheek. **A,** When hemimaxillectomy and palatectomy are performed, the palate and lateral nasal wall may be reconstructed with a radial forearm, scapula, or rectus abdominis flap that is deepithelialized, sewn to the margin of the palate resection and the medial orbital wall, and folded back in and deepithelialized to fill the dead space. In younger patients, the alveolus may be reconstructed using radial forearm fibula or scapula osteocutaneous flaps, with the bone sandwiched between two layers of skin. **B,** When maxillectomy includes the orbital floor, but the globe and periorbita remain intact, the orbital contents should be supported with bone. Primary reconstruction is well performed with bipedicle scapula osteocutaneous flap, although the fibula and radial forearm flaps are also useful (see Figure 86-3). **C,** When orbital exenteration is part of the procedure, a larger muscle, musculocutaneous, or skin flap is used to reconstruct palate, lateral nasal wall, and orbit. In general, the orbit is lined with vascularized soft tissue, decreasing its volume, but leaving enough space to retain a silicone prosthesis. If the ultimate reconstructive goal includes an osseointegrated implant, a scapula or fibula free flap should be used to recreate the bony orbit.

of tumor resection, it is more frequently the result of self-inflicted trauma. Initial management consists of control of the airway, stabilization of remaining bony structures and their anatomic position to prevent contraction and secondary deformity, and debridement of the devitalized tissue. A single free flap fibula osteocutaneous or scapula osteocutaneous flap has been shown to be able to reconstruct both missing mandible and maxilla with bone or with bone and soft tissue.[13] Initial separation of the oral cavity and nasal airway and

restoration of as many of the midface buttresses as possible will provide a template upon which further reconstruction of the nose and midface soft tissues can be carried out. Maintenance of a central nasal airway facilitates rehabilitation. Multiple free tissue transfers may be necessary to provide enough tissue in cases of massive injury.

When adequate bone and soft tissue have been introduced to satisfy the functional disorders caused by the defect, local advancement flaps of remaining normal cheek and neck skin

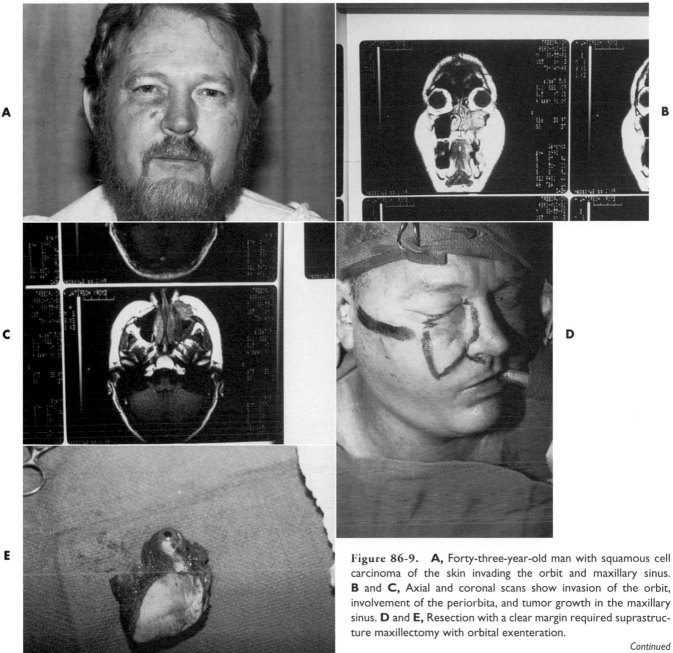

Figure 86-9. **A,** Forty-three-year-old man with squamous cell carcinoma of the skin invading the orbit and maxillary sinus. **B** and **C,** Axial and coronal scans show invasion of the orbit, involvement of the periorbita, and tumor growth in the maxillary sinus. **D** and **E,** Resection with a clear margin required suprastructure maxillectomy with orbital exenteration.

Continued

may improve appearance with time. Mustardé flaps or skin advancement flaps in a reverse facelift style are useful to disguise the distant tissue used for reconstruction (see Figure 86-9, *J* and *K*). Tissue expansion of adjacent normal skin may also provide an increased amount of more normal-appearing external coverage.

Although maxillofacial prosthetics are unlikely to resolve major problems by themselves, a combination of surgery and prosthetics may provide superior rehabilitation. Posi-

tioning of the free tissue transfer to allow purchase by an intraoral denture may improve appearance and function. Intranasal implants such as transantral Kirschner wires may also be useful, as are osseointegrated implants into the reconstructed bone, particularly the fibula.[10] Placement of intraosseous implants for fixation of a denture has been done as a secondary procedure after revision of the reconstruction, as part of the initial reconstruction, or as part of a prefabricated flap.

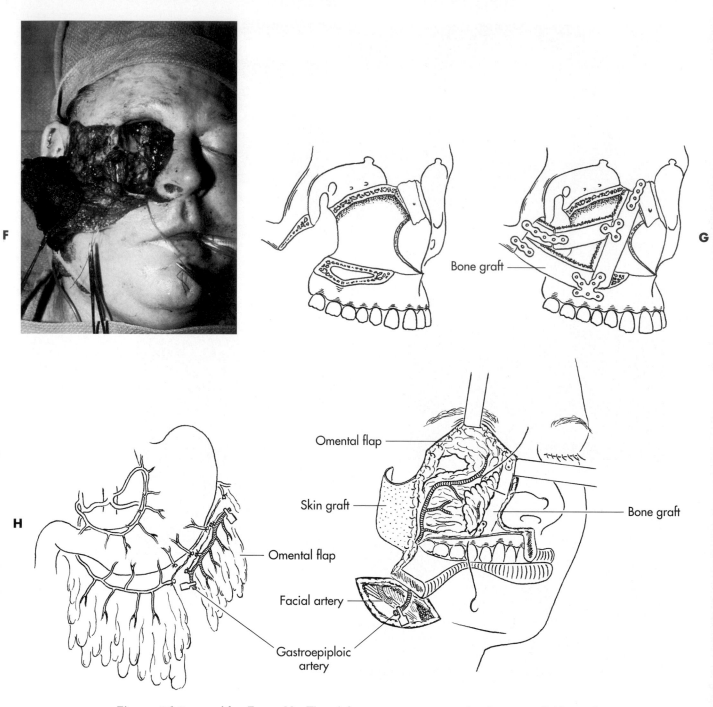

Figure 86-9, cont'd. F to H, The defect was reconstructed using a scaffolding of nonvascularized rib grafts that was then enveloped in an omental free flap. The palate was left intact. The external and nasal surfaces were skin grafted. *Continued*

OUTCOMES

There is a hierarchy of priorities for any therapy, operative or nonoperative. Survival from the underlying ailment is of primary importance, followed by restoration of normal function and appearance. The efficiency of the therapy or the ability to restore the patient to relative normality in a single state or in a short period of time, particularly in diseases where

recurrence or death may supervene, becomes a crucial parameter. A corollary to efficiency is obviously the cost of delivering the therapy, both in real dollars and in lost income and productivity.

In the United States, cancer and trauma are the leading causes of midface deformity. The multidisciplinary approach to resection of paranasal sinus tumors that includes surgery and radiotherapy, with or without chemotherapy, has improved survival from between 5% and 15% to between 40% and 60%

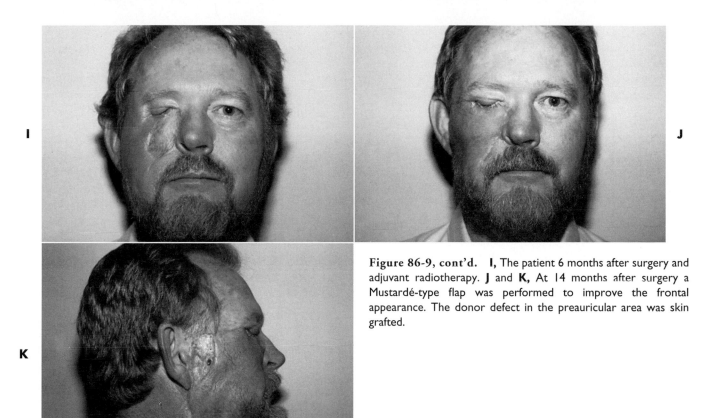

Figure 86-9, cont'd. **I**, The patient 6 months after surgery and adjuvant radiotherapy. **J** and **K**, At 14 months after surgery a Mustardé-type flap was performed to improve the frontal appearance. The donor defect in the preauricular area was skin grafted.

in recent years. Combined intracranial/extracranial resection, particularly with subsequent reconstruction using well-vascularized muscle flaps, has improved 5-year survival of such extensive paranasal and skull base tumors and decreased the occurrence of cerebrospinal fluid leaks to a much more manageable level. One potential drawback of immediate reconstruction of major midfacial cancer defects is the loss of the ability to inspect the resection site for tumor recurrence. Although this issue has not been satisfactorily addressed in the literature, there is considerable support for immediate reconstruction because of the late stage in which most of these tumors are diagnosed, the desperate functional state, and the hideous appearance that the unreconstructed patient presents. When self-inflicted trauma is the etiology of the injury, the underlying mental disorder must be addressed to prevent subsequent suicide attempts.

Functional goals have become more attainable with the recent ability to transfer large amounts of tissue to the midface. In most lateralized resections, a competent oral cavity separate from the nasal airway, with and without oronasal or oroantral fistula, may be successfully attained at the initial operation. A transnasal airway is usually possible even in the more extensive central midface trauma. Although restoration of vision is presently impossible, reconstruction of an orbital cavity will facilitate subsequent use of a prosthesis.

A reasonable appearance, the ability to breathe through the nose, and a competent oral cavity to produce speech and allow swallowing will speed the entry of the patient back into society and improve patient satisfaction with resection and reconstruction. Single-stage procedures, although costly, are more economical in terms of time and, ultimately, money than multiple-stage procedures. Creation of a soft tissue and bony matrix for the attachment of prostheses will further improve ultimate function and appearance.

REFERENCES

1. Anthony JA, Foster RD, Sharma A, et al: Reconstruction of a complex midfacial defect with the folded fibular free flap and osseointegrated implants, *Ann Plast Surg* 37:204-209, 1996.

2. Ariyan S: The pectoralis major for single stage reconstruction of the difficult wounds of the orbit and pharyngoesophagus, *Plast Reconstr Surg* 72:468-477, 1983.

3. Bakamjian V, Poole M: Maxillofacial and palatal reconstruction with the deltopectoral flap, *Br J Plast Surg* 30:17-33, 1977.

4. Coleman JJ: Osseous reconstruction of the midface and orbits, *Clin Plast Surg* 21(I):113-114, 1994.

5. Coleman JJ: Microvascular approach to function and appearance of large orbitomaxillary defects, *Am J Surg* 158:337-341, 1989.

6. Coleman JJ, Sultan MR: The bipedicle osteocutaneous scapula flap: a new subscapular system free flap, *Plast Reconstr Surg* 87:682-692, 1991.

7. Kayamoto HK: Correction of established traumatic defects of the facial skeleton. In Schultz RC, editor: *Facial injuries,* St Louis, 1988, Mosby.

8. Ketcham AS, Wilkins RH, Van Buren JM, et al: A combined intracranial facial approach to the paranasal sinuses, *Am J Surg* 106:698, 1963.

9. Manson PN, Hoopes JE, Su CT: Structural pillars of the facial skeleton: an approach to the management of Le Fort fractures, *Plast Reconstr Surg* 66:815-820, 1980.

10. Panje D, Hetherington H, LaVelle W: Bilateral maxillectomy and midfacial reconstruction, *Ann Otol Rhinol Laryngol* 104: 845-848, 1995.

11. Quillen CG: Latissimus dorsi myocutaneous flap in head and neck reconstruction, *Plast Reconstr Surg* 63:664-670, 1979.

12. Rosen HM: The extended trapezius musculocutaneous flap for cranio-orbital facial reconstruction, *Plast Reconstr Surg* 75:318-324, 1985.

13. Sadove RC, Powell LA: Simultaneous maxillary and mandibular reconstruction with an osteocutaneous free flap, *Plast Reconstr Surg* 92:141-146, 1993.

14. Schusterman MA, Reece GP, Miller MJ: Osseous free flaps for orbit and midface reconstruction, *Am J Surg* 166:341-345, 1993.

15. Tatum SA: Concepts in midface reconstruction. *Otolaryngol Clin North Am* 1997; 30:563-591, 1997.

16. Vinzenz KG, Holle J, Wuringer E, et al: Prefabrication of combined scapula flaps for microsurgical reconstruction in oromaxillofacial defects: a new method, *J Craniomaxillofac Surg* 24:214-223, 1996.

Reconstruction of the Eyelids and Orbit

Mark A. Codner

EYELID ANATOMY

The fundamental goals of any reconstructive procedure of the periorbital region are to restore the functional relationship between the orbit, globe, and eyelids and to ensure protection of the eye with preservation of vision. Although the eyelids represent less than a fraction of 1% of the total body surface area, the anatomy of this area is highly complex and requires detailed consideration. Appreciation of the highly specialized anatomic structures and function of the eyelids is helpful when managing reconstruction of acquired deformities.

The skin surface anatomy represents the topography of the eyelid region and is made up of the brow, upper eyelid, lower eyelid, and midface (Figure 87-1). The palpebral fissure has a vertical height of 10 to 12 mm and a horizontal width of 28 to 30 mm in the adult. The upper eyelid rests 2 mm below the upper corneoscleral limbus on forward gaze, its contour consisting of a gentle arch with the highest point medial to the pupil. The upper eyelid crease is formed by the insertion of the levator palpebrae aponeurosis into the pretarsal orbicularis and dermis. The distance from the lash margin to the apex of the crease in the Occidental male eyelid is 8 mm, 10 mm in the female. This distance is only 2 to 3 mm in the Asian upper lid due to the low fusion of the orbital septum and levator aponeurosis allowing inferior extension of the preaponeurotic fat into the pretarsal space.

The anatomic relationship between the upper eyelid and the eyebrow must be appreciated, since changes in brow position influence the appearance and function of the upper lid. The superior eyelid sulcus is the concavity between the upper eyelid and the superior orbital rim. Fullness in the central and medial superior sulcus generally represents herniation of periorbital fat. Prolapse of the orbital lobe of the lacrimal gland below the lateral orbital rim may create a lateral fullness in the sulcus. Instability of the support attachments of the eyebrow and prominence of the brow fat pad also contribute to obliteration of the superior sulcus. Deepening of the superior sulcus occurs with loss of orbital volume following fat atrophy, orbital fracture, and enucleation.

The lower lid normally rests at the lower corneoscleral limbus, with the eye in primary position. The lower lid contour consists of a gentle S-shaped curve, with the lowest position lateral to the pupil. The lower lid crease is formed by the insertion of the capsulopalpebral fascia with the lower lid orbicularis and dermis. The crease is formed 4 mm below the lash margin and angles inferotemporally, becoming less apparent with age. Anatomic contour changes that become more pronounced with age include formation of the malar crescent, nasojugal groove, and nasolabial fold (Figure 87-2). The orbitomalar ligament weakens along with the retaining ligaments of the face, resulting in descent of facial fat.[17,36] The malar crescent represents the junction between the orbicularis oculi muscle and the superior border of the malar fat pad.[22,66] A distinct transition exists between the thin eyelid skin, which lacks subdermal fat on histologic examination, and the thicker cheek skin, which has significant subcutaneous fat. The vertical distance between the lower lid and cheek junction increases with age as lower eyelid skin descends below the inferior orbital rim. The nasolabial fold deepens as the inferior portion of the malar fat pad descends and overlaps the nasolabial crease.

The layers of the eyelids can be divided into anterior and posterior lamellae. The anterior lamella primarily consists of skin and muscle, while the posterior lamella is made of the tarsal plates and conjunctiva (Figure 87-3). The orbicularis oculi muscle makes up the support layer of the anterior lamella and consists of three separate divisions based on the underlying anatomic structures: pretarsal, preseptal, and orbital. The pretarsal orbicularis is divided into a superficial and deep head and is primarily responsible for the involuntary eyelid blink. The preseptal orbicularis also has a superficial and deep component and functions as the lacrimal pump for tear drainage as well as voluntary eyelid closure (Figure 87-4). The orbital orbicularis has the widest distribution over the upper and lower orbital region and functions as a medial brow depressor and performs protective forced eyelid closure.

The orbital orbicularis has an insertion along the anterior lateral palpebral raphe. The medial insertion is into the frontal bone in the superior orbital region, and into the maxilla along the lower orbit converging on the anterior reflection of the

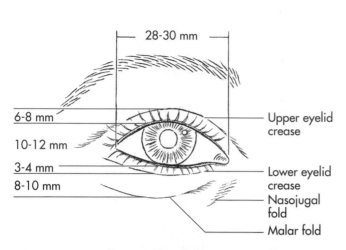

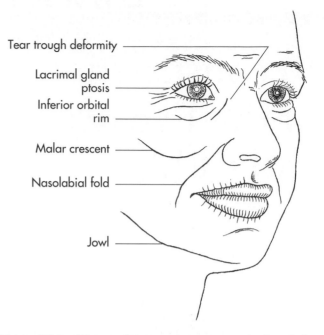

Figure 87-1. Anatomy demonstrating the topography of the periorbital region. The average distances in the youthful eyelid demonstrate the horizontal and vertical dimensions of the palpebral aperture and the relationships of the upper lid margin to the lid crease and lower lid margin to the malar fold.

Figure 87-2. Diagram demonstrating the anatomic changes that occur with aging. In the upper lid, ptosis of periorbital fat and the orbital lobe of the lacrimal gland obliterates the upper lid crease. The lower lid and midfacial region develop infraorbital hollowing with descent of the malar fat pad and increase in the distance from the lower lid to the cheek junction. Deepening of the nasojugal groove and nasolabial fold occurs.

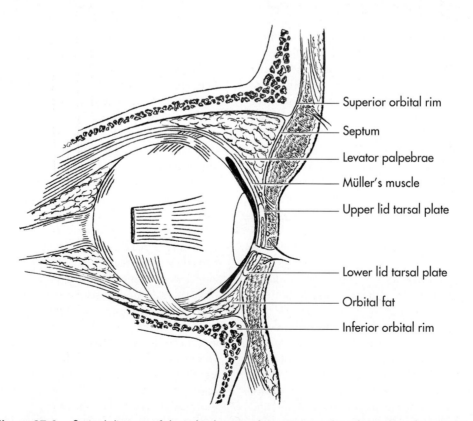

Figure 87-3. Sagittal diagram of the orbital region demonstrating the relationship of the eyelids to the orbit.

medial canthal tendon (Figure 87-5). The deep preseptal lateral orbicularis insertion forms the lateral palpebral raphe. The superficial preseptal fibers insert on the anterior crus of the medial canthal tendon. The deep preseptal fibers coalesce to form Jones' muscle, which inserts on the lacrimal fascia and functions as part of the lacrimal pump mechanism (Table 87-1). With eyelid closure, contraction of Jones' muscle creates negative pressure in the tear sac, which drains the canalicular system.[31] Pretarsal muscle surrounds the ampulla and canaliculi, causing compression and shortening with each blink. When the eye reopens, negative pressure is created in the ampullary system, causing the canaliculi to drain the tear lake from the fornix.

The pretarsal orbicularis fibers have a dense attachment to the upper and lower lid tarsal plates. The superficial fibers insert into the lateral palpebral raphe and the anterior crus of the medial canthal tendon along with the preseptal and orbital orbicularis. The deep head of the pretarsal orbicularis inserts on Whitnall's tubercle laterally within the lateral orbital rim. Riolan's muscle is a thin strip of pretarsal orbicularis that forms the subcutaneous component of the gray line along the lid margin (Figure 87-6). This provides an important anatomic landmark that is useful in reconstruction of the lid margin. The deep head of the pretarsal orbicularis joins the deep head of the preseptal fibers medially to form Horner's muscle, which passes deep to the canalicular system and lacrimal sac and inserts on the posterior lacrimal crest and deep lacrimal fascia. This deep medial insertion allows the eyelid to follow the curve of the globe and must be reconstructed following disinsertion of the medial canthal tendon following trauma or tumor resection.

The medial canthus is a complex structure that forms the fixation point of the medial commissure and consists of an anterior and posterior reflection of the medial canthal tendon

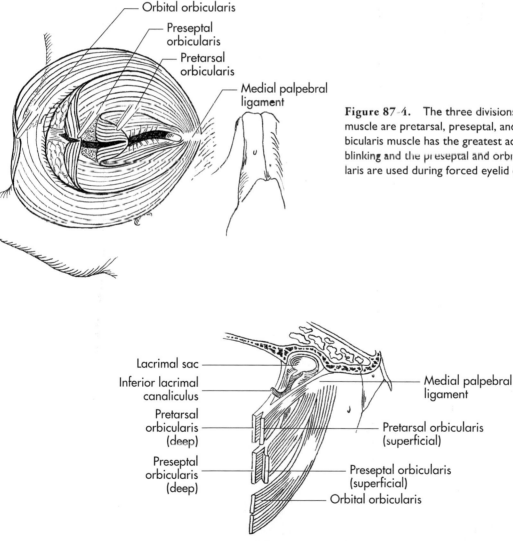

Figure 87-4. The three divisions of the orbicularis oculi muscle are pretarsal, preseptal, and orbital. The pretarsal orbicularis muscle has the greatest activity during involuntary blinking and the preseptal and orbital portions of the orbicularis are used during forced eyelid contraction.

Figure 87-5. Medial canthal insertion of the three divisions of the orbicularis oculi onto the medial canthal tendon. The pretarsal and preseptal muscles are divided into a deep and superficial component. The deep portions insert posterior to the lacrimal sac and the superficial muscles insert onto the anterior reflection of the medial canthal tendon.

Table 87-1.
Orbicularis Oculi Insertion

MUSCLE	MEDIAL INSERTION	LATERAL INSERTION
PRETARSAL		
Superficial	Anterior reflection medial canthal tendon	Whitnall's tubercle
Deep (Horner's)	Posterior lacrimal crest	Whitnall's tubercle
PRESEPTAL		
Superficial	Anterior reflection medial canthal tendon	Palpebral raphe
Deep (Jones')	Lacrimal fascia	Palpebral raphe
ORBITAL		
Upper lid	Frontal bone	Anterior raphe
Lower lid	Maxilla	Anterior raphe

and the medial retinaculum. The anterior reflection of the medial canthal tendon inserts on the anterior lacrimal crest formed by the frontal process of the maxilla and passes anterior to the lacrimal sac. The posterior reflection of the medial canthal tendon passes deep to the lacrimal fascia and inserts on the posterior lacrimal crest. The medial retinaculum is formed by the deep head of the pretarsal orbicularis, the orbital septum, the medial extent of Lockwood's ligament, the medial horn of the levator aponeurosis, medial rectus check ligaments, and Whitnall's ligament (Figure 87-7). The medial retinaculum is a relatively fixed fulcrum point for eyelid closure compared with the lateral retinaculum, which allows lateral canthal mobility with lateral gaze and voluntary blink.

The lateral canthus consists of a complex connective tissue framework that functions as an integral part of the suspension system of the lower lid. The lateral canthal tendon, 5 to 7 mm in length, is formed by the fibrous crura that connect the tarsal plates to Whitnall's lateral orbital tubercle within the lateral orbital rim. Ligamentous structures from the lateral horn of the levator aponeurosis, lateral check ligaments, Whitnall's superior suspensory ligament, and Lockwood's inferior suspensory ligament converge with the lateral canthal tendon to form the lateral retinaculum.[14]

The tarsal plates constitute the connective tissue support of the eyelids. The tarsoligamentous sling is the primary component of the posterior lamella. The upper lid tarsal plate is

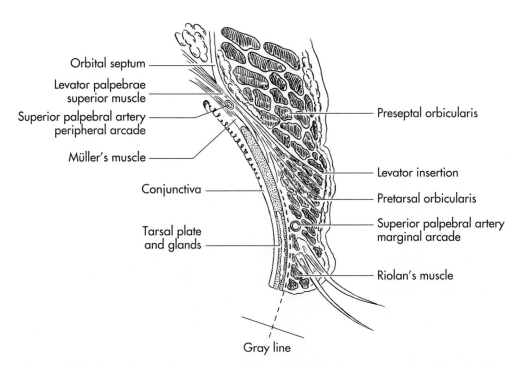

Orbital septum
Levator palpebrae superior muscle
Superior palpebral artery peripheral arcade
Müller's muscle
Conjunctiva
Tarsal plate and glands
Preseptal orbicularis
Levator insertion
Pretarsal orbicularis
Superior palpebral artery marginal arcade
Riolan's muscle
Gray line

Figure 87-6. Sagittal view of the upper eyelid demonstrating the anterior and posterior lamella. The anterior lamella consists of skin and orbicularis oculi muscle. The upper lid crease is formed by the dermal insertion of the levator aponeurosis and septum. The posterior lamella consists of tarsus and conjunctiva. The anatomic gray line of the lash margin is made of Riolan's pretarsal muscle.

30 mm in horizontal length and 10 mm at the point of maximal vertical height (Figure 87-8). Although the tarsal plate is positioned centrally over the midpupillary line in childhood, weakening of ligamentous support structures with age causes a shift over the lateral limbus in the adult. The attachments of the upper lid tarsal plate include the pretarsal orbicularis and levator aponeurosis on the anterior surface, Müller's muscle on the superior border, and conjunctiva on the posterior surface. The lower lid tarsal plate is 27 mm in horizontal width and 4 mm in vertical height. Attachments include the pretarsal orbicularis, capsulopalpebral fascia, and conjunctiva. The upper and lower tarsal plates have medial and lateral periosteal attachments to the orbital rim consisting of the canthal tendon, ligaments, and retinaculum. The canthal ligaments are the fibrous extensions of the tarsal plates, while the canthal tendons represent the insertions of the deep heads of the orbicularis muscle.[14]

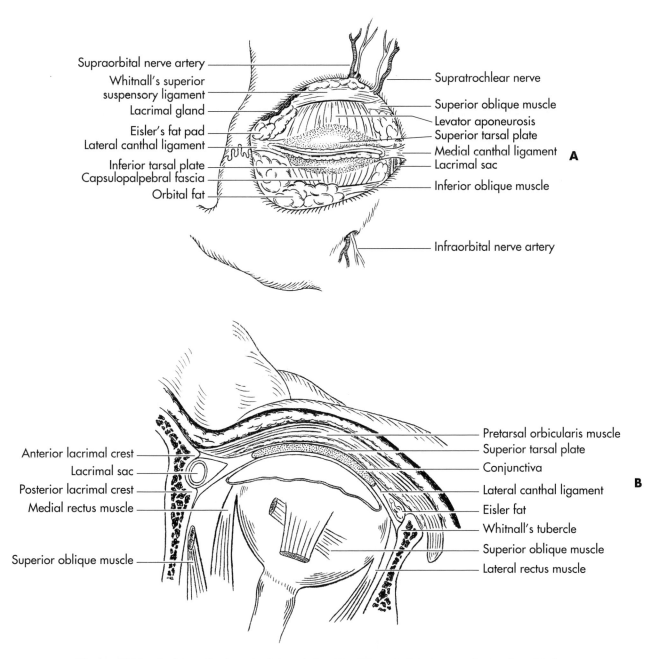

Figure 87-7.   A, Anatomic diagram of the relationship of the tarsoligamentous sling to the orbital rim. Eisler's fat pad is shown, which is an important landmark for canthoplasty suture placement above Whitnall's tubercle. **B,** Axial diagram demonstrating the medial and lateral insertion of the canthal tendons. The normal lateral canthus inserts on Whitnall's tubercle deep to the lateral orbital rim. The medial canthus has an anterior and posterior reflection divided by the lacrimal sac.

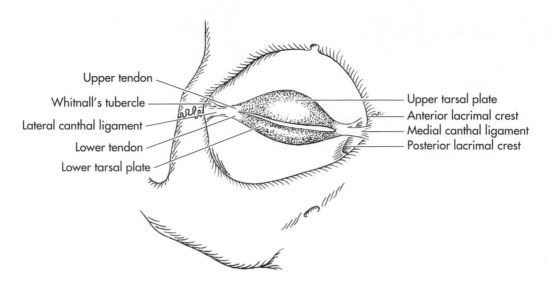

Figure 87-8. Diagram of the relationship of the tarsal plates to the medial and lateral canthal tendons and the orbit.

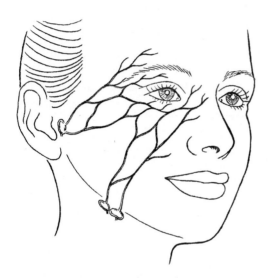

Figure 87-9. Lymphatic drainage of the upper eyelid and lateral canthus by the preauricular lymph nodes and the lower lid and medial canthus by the submandibular lymph nodes.

The lymphatic drainage of the upper and lower eyelids should be considered when evaluating a patient with a malignant neoplasm involving the periorbital region. The upper eyelid, lateral canthal region, and lateral half of the lower lid have lymphatic drainage to the preauricular lymph nodes (Figure 87-9). Metastatic spread from these areas will require a superficial parotidectomy along with management of cervical lymphatic spread with neck dissection. The medial canthus and medial half of the lower lid have lymphatic drainage through channels that travel with the facial vein inferiorly to the submandibular lymph nodes.[49] The distinct anatomic division of lymphatic drainage in the periorbital region may influence the detection of regional metastasis as well as attempts at curative surgical resection.

BENIGN EYELID TUMORS

INDICATIONS

Benign surface epithelial tumors, classified according to the histologic structures of origin such as epidermis, dermis, and adenexa, represent 37% of eyelid tumors taken from a large center registry[12] and can usually be diagnosed on the basis of their clinical appearance and behavior. In order to confirm the diagnosis, biopsy should be performed. Although smaller lesions can be completely removed with excisional biopsy including minimal margins, larger lesions may require incisional biopsy. All biopsies should include adjacent normal tissue and subcutaneous tissue deep to the tumor, particularly for all pigmented neoplasms. Superficial shave biopsy is only indicated for suspected epidermal or upper dermal lesions such as seborrheic keratosis.

Seborrheic keratoses represent common eyelid tumors found most frequently in the elderly population. Although the clinical appearance is often a waxy, "stuck-on" lesion, they may be confused with nevi, pigmented basal cell cancers, or melanomas. Biopsy confirms the diagnosis demonstrating hyperkeratosis limited to the epidermal layer with occasional extension into the dermis. The lesions are classified into three groups, depending on the histologic features: hyperkeratosis, adenosis, and acanthosis. In addition to excluding malignancy, large lesions may require excision from the eyelids if causing functional impairment of eyelid closure.

Benign pigmented lesions are another common group of eyelid tumors. These neoplasms arise from nevus cells, dermal and epidermal melanocytes. Nevocellular nevi commonly occur on the eyelid margin with varying degrees of pigmentation and have the benign appearance of lashes growing through the lesion (Figure 87-10). Junctional nevi arise from the deep layer of the epidermis and appear as flat, pigmented macular lesions. Compound nevi are more common with epidermal and dermal components of nevus cell nests. The most com-

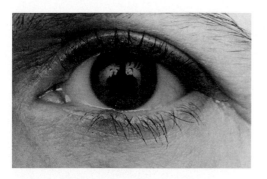

Figure 87-10. Benign appearance of a tumor of the lower lid margin with eyelashes that grow through the neoplasm.

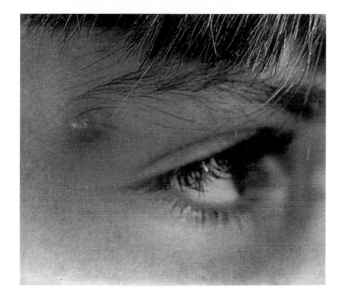

Figure 87-11. Typical location of a dermoid tumor at the lateral brow region near the frontozygomatic suture.

mon are the intradermal nevi, which have the morphologic appearance of dome-shaped lesions demonstrating nests of melanocytes within the dermis on histologic evaluation. Although junctional and compound nevi may undergo malignant degeneration into melanoma, this is rare in intradermal nevi. Morphologic changes including increase in size, change in the shape or color, and spontaneous bleeding are indications to proceed with biopsy.

Dermoid cysts are benign tumors that commonly present in infants and young children. The tumors often occur at the lateral brow near the frontozygomatic suture (Figure 87-11) and contain a sequestration of epidermal appendages at lines of embryonic closure.[6] Although dermoid cysts are present at birth, hair growth with sebaceous and eccrine secretions may cause a gradual increase in size. Large dermoids can cause mechanical ptosis or globe compression, which may result in astigmatism or amblyopia if not treated early. Occult orbital extension should be evaluated with a preoperative computed tomography (CT) scan or magnetic resonance imaging (MRI). Similarly, midline dermoid cysts may have an intracranial extension and should have preoperative radiographic evaluation. Complete surgical excision is therapeutic.

Benign tumors of the dermis are classified according to their cellular origin from blood vessels, nerves, lymphatics, and smooth muscle. Capillary hemangiomas are derived from vascular endothelial cell rests and represent the most common benign periorbital tumor of infancy. Although a small herald patch may be the only visible abnormality at birth, rapid increase in size occurs during the first year, which represents the proliferative growth phase. Spontaneous involution usually begins at 4 years of age and continues for several years. The clinical appearance changes from a raised bright red lesion to a lesion with a more spongy consistency, purple or pale in color and often surrounded by excess skin (Figure 87-12).

Treatment alternatives for hemangiomas in the periocular region depend on the degree of orbital extension and visual axis obstruction. Since hemangiomas that obstruct visual input in infants can result in amblyopia and serious, permanent impairment of visual development, the standard approach of watchful waiting and parental reassurance generally does not apply to hemangiomas of the eyelids.[74] Intraorbital extension should be evaluated with MRI prior to treatment.[19,29] Systemic steroids may be required if an incomplete response to intralesional injections occurs. Large hemangiomas or hemangiomas with a poor response to steroids require surgical resection. Postoperative patching of the uninvolved eye may decrease the risk of amblyopia by promoting increased use of the impaired eye. Parents should understand that despite these treatment efforts, the risk of astigmatism or decreased visual acuity remains significant.

Neurofibromas are tumors of Schwann cell origin that may arise as solitary benign tumors or may represent the cutaneous manifestation of von Recklinghausen's neurofibromatosis. Single neurofibromas occur more commonly in adults, whereas neurofibromatosis often presents during childhood. Histologic evaluation of the tumor demonstrates poorly circumscribed spindle-shaped Schwann cells embedded in an endoneurial myxoid stroma. Plexiform neurofibromas in the periorbital region appear as large flesh-colored tumors, diffuse in nature, and invading the supporting structures of the eyelids, causing mechanical ptosis (Figure 87-13). Indications for early surgery include visual obstruction, which may interfere with normal cortical visual development. Since complete resection is usually not possible due to the diffuse infiltrative morphology of the tumor, surgical debulking along with correction of ptosis is required to restore appropriate visual input. Parents should be made aware that these tumors will recur and often require multiple operations, sometimes including enucleation.[28]

OPERATIONS

Resection of benign eyelid tumors often results in superficial defects that may be closed primarily or, in the case of shave biopsies, allowed to reepithelialize. However, a subset of benign lesions may require more extensive resection, resulting in full-thickness defects that require immediate reconstruction. Several reconstructive procedures are available to the surgeon depending on the location of the defect, age of the patient,

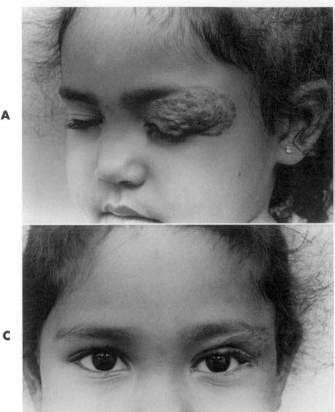

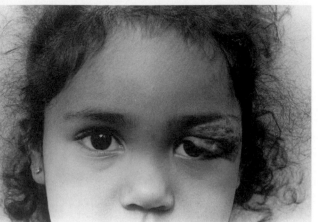

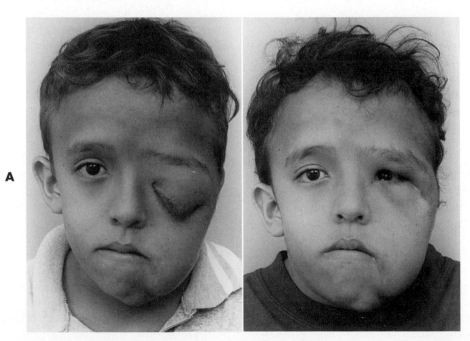

Figure 87-12. **A,** Periorbital hemangioma involving the upper lid causing mechanical ptosis in a 4-year-old child. **B,** Following involution of the hemangioma, excess skin is apparent. **C,** Reconstruction of the upper lid following excision of the hemangioma with tarsolevator advancement and posterior auricular skin grafting.

Figure 87-13. **A,** Neurofibromatosis involving the left upper eyelid and periorbital region in a 7-year-old child with near complete visual obstruction. **B,** Left eyelid reconstruction following excision of the eyelids with frontalis suspension and lower lid fascial support.

degree of tissue redundancy, and overall functional and aesthetic goals.

Direct Closure

Benign tumors of the lid margin requiring resection usually result in eyelid defects that are less than one third of the lid. In younger patients, defects as large as 30% of the upper lid margin can be closed with direct layered repair. Since tissue laxity generally increases with age, older patients can often undergo direct closure of upper eyelid defects of 40%. The suggested technique for full-thickness resection of upper eyelid lesions incorporates two parallel incisions with 1-mm margins on either side of the tumor beginning at the lid margin and extending to the upper border of the tarsal plate at the lid crease (Figure 87-14). Parallel excision of the tarsal plate should be performed to avoid notching of the lid margin. If a triangular wedge excision of the tarsal plate is performed, a notch of the upper lid with a peaked abnormal contour will result from tenting of the underlying tarsal plate.

Following tumor resection, the perpendicular edges should be grasped to assess the mobility of the lid margin. If there is too much tension for direct closure, the upper lid repair may result in postoperative mechanical ptosis. This can be avoided by

lateral cantholysis to allow relaxation of the upper limb of the lateral canthal tendon. A traction 7-0 silk suture is passed through the gray line to evaluate horizontal lid tension and eyelid position relative to the upper corneoscleral limbus. Once the lid margin is precisely reapproximated, the parallel cut edges of the tarsal plate are aligned and directly repaired with 7-0 silk sutures, which are passed through the tarsal plate in an interrupted fashion while avoiding penetration through the conjunctiva to prevent corneal irritation (Figure 87-15). The lash line is then precisely repaired with eversion of the lid margin to avoid postoperative notching. Following reconstruction of the posterior lamella, the anterior lamella should be repaired.

The skin and tightly adherent pretarsal orbicularis is approximated with 7-0 silk sutures beginning at the lash margin. Redundant skin above the upper lid crease may form a dog-ear, which is best managed by removal of two Burow's triangles keeping the incision within the upper lid crease as a T-shaped incision (Figure 87-16). Postoperative management includes ophthalmic antibiotic ointment with suture removal at 7 days. Early low lid position should be anticipated due to tension and swelling; however, postoperative ptosis should not occur if lid tension was not excessive. Relaxation of the tissue several weeks after surgery allows the lid to assume a normal position relative to the pupil.

As in the upper lid, reconstruction of full-thickness defects following resection of benign tumors of the lower lid margin can often be performed with direct closure. This should be considered for central eyelid defects of 30% in younger patients and up to 40% in older patients with increased tissue redundancy. When resecting lower lid neoplasms, the incision in the lower lid should be perpendicular to the lid margin, performing full-thickness resection of the tarsal plate with parallel edges. The incision in the skin and muscle below the lid margin, however, should be angled in a lateral direction in order to reduce the dog-ear formed by redundancy of the anterior lamella (Figure 87-17). This will shorten the length of the incision and place the scar parallel to the lines of tension in the lower lid region.

Reconstruction of the lower lid defect begins with a 6-0 silk

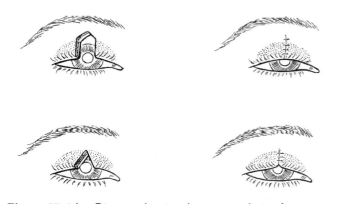

Figure 87-14. Diagram showing the correct design for resection of upper eyelid neoplasms including parallel full-thickness excision of the tarsal plate to avoid upper lid notching.

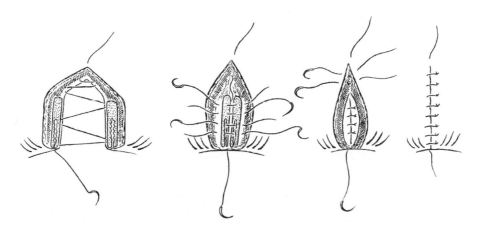

Figure 87-15. Repair of the posterior lamella of the upper lid following excision utilizes a stay suture reapproximating the gray line followed by repair of the tarsal plate.

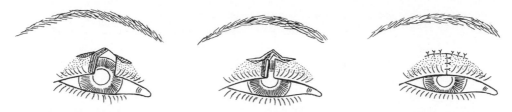

Figure 87-16. Repair of the anterior lamella of the upper lid begins at the lid margin with repair of pretarsal skin and muscle. Dog-ear resection can be hidden in the upper lid crease.

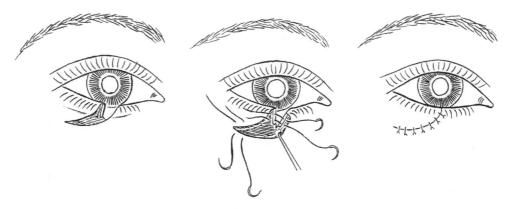

Figure 87-17. Lower lid neoplasms should be removed with full-thickness parallel excision of the tarsal plate. The skin incision is tapered laterally following the normal skin tension lines.

traction suture placed in the gray line to align the lid margin and evaluate tension on the repair. Excessive horizontal tension of the lower lid, particularly when combined with the presence of a prominent eye, may cause clotheslining of the lid below the globe, creating lower lid malposition with scleral show. Moderate tension can be reduced by lateral cantholysis of the inferior limb of the lateral canthal tendon and positioning the lid at the inferior limbus. The cut edges of the lower tarsal plate are repaired with interrupted 7-0 silk sutures. Accurate reapproximation of the tarsal plate is an integral part of lid repair to avoid postoperative dehiscence or notching. At this point, the musculocutaneous incision is repaired beginning at the lash margin. Redundant skin is excised within the lateral oblique incision and closed with 7-0 silk sutures. Postoperative ointment is applied to the incision, and the sutures are removed 1 week after surgery.

Excision of Dermoid Cysts

Treatment of lateral eyebrow dermoid cysts requires complete surgical excision. Surgery should not be delayed past 6 months to a year in infants to avoid significant increase in size, drainage, or infection. General anesthesia is required and a lateral brow incision provides direct exposure of the cyst. An alternative approach utilizes a remote incision in the temporal hairline with endoscopic visualization.[5] Midline dermoid cysts that show radiographic intracranial extension require a combined neurosurgical approach.

Skin Graft

Free tissue grafting techniques are often used to reconstruct large, superficial deformities of the anterior lamella. Grafts should match the reconstructed anatomic area as close as

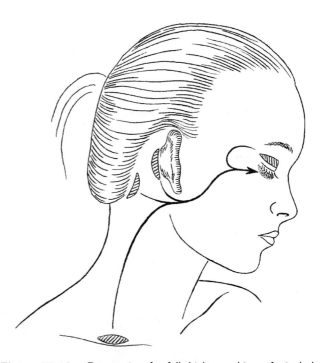

Figure 87-18. Donor sites for full-thickness skin grafts include the upper eyelid, the posterior auricular sulcus, and the supraclavicular region.

possible with respect to thickness and color in order to provide a good functional and cosmetic result. For eyelid reconstruction, a full-thickness graft is usually superior to split-thickness grafts. The upper eyelid is the ideal donor site with the best skin match for eyelid reconstruction. An elliptical incision is made in the excess skin in the lateral aspect of the upper eyelid. The skin is separated from the muscle by spreading with

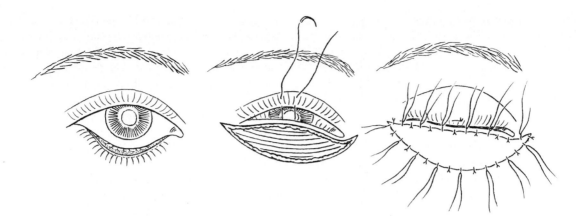

Figure 87-19. Placement of a skin graft to correct vertical skin shortage after lower blepharoplasty combined with lateral canthoplasty to restore lower lid position and Frost sutures for lid support during the early postoperative period.

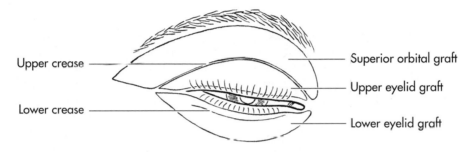

Figure 87-20. Diagram of design for extensive contracture release and full-thickness skin grafts for the correction of ectropion following burns to the periorbital region.

straight Iris scissors just beneath the dermis. Equal amounts of skin are removed from both eyes for postoperative symmetry. The nasal eyelid skin should not be used due to the risk of lagophthalmos. The donor site is closed directly following removal of the underlying orbicularis muscle.

Since the upper eyelid donor site can only provide a limited amount of skin graft, other donor areas used include posterior auricular skin, lateral cervical skin, and supraclavicular skin (Figure 87-18). A template of the defect can be created by placing steri-strips over the defect and tracing the underlying deformity. The posterior auricular sulcus should bisect the template, and an elliptical incision should be made around the outline of the graft. Since the dermis in the posterior auricular region is thicker than in the eyelid region, it should be thinned prior to grafting. For larger eyelid defects such as burn ectropion, the lateral cervical area just below the hairline and the supraclavicular area represent donor sites that provide large amounts of skin with an acceptable color match.

The edges of the eyelid deformity are freshened and the skin graft is sutured around the perimeter of the deformity with 6-0 silk bolster sutures (Figure 87-19). After the graft has been sutured into place, an 11-blade scalpel is used to incise the graft for drainage to avoid hematoma formation, which could reduce graft survival. A variety of bolster dressings such as moist cotton and a petroleum-coated gauze or dental wax or eyepads can be used to conform the graft to the defect. The eyelid margins are often sutured closed and the dressings are kept dry. The dressing and sutures are completely removed in 5 to 7 days.

Split-Thickness Skin Graft

Split-thickness skin grafts are reserved for large deformities of the upper and lower lids that may require multiple operations such as reconstruction of full-thickness burns to the eyelids and periorbital region.

A dermatome is used to harvest the skin graft from the upper thigh or buttock region. Following tangential excision of the burned eyelid skin or release of burn scar contracture, the eyelids should be sutured closed with a 5-0 nylon placed through the gray line, including the upper and lower tarsal plates. The skin can be protected with a padded bolster made from a 5-mm segment of red rubber catheter. Separate grafts should be placed from the lid margin to the upper lid crease and from the lid crease to the inferior border of the eyebrow. The grafts should extend several centimeters lateral to the canthus and parallel to the lines that would fall in the natural skin crease (Figure 87-20). Overcorrection by 50% to 75% should be performed to account for postoperative contraction of the skin grafts. Postoperative management includes a bolster dressing for 5 days. Since the eyelids should remain sutured closed for 4 to 6 weeks, unilateral staged reconstruction is recommended when both eyes are involved, if possible.

OUTCOMES

Since the general size of the deformity associated with benign eyelid neoplasms is usually less than one third of the lid margin, the complications associated with reconstruction are not as frequent as with malignant eyelid tumors. Preoperative clinical evaluation should include history of hypertension, use of aspirin, or any other factor that may contribute to postoperative bleeding. Hypertension should be medically controlled and aspirin products stopped 2 weeks prior to surgery involving the eyelids. The liberal use of ice and elevation for the first 48 hours after surgery is recommended.

Hematoma following eyelid reconstruction can have serious consequences with respect to both vision and flap failure. Early recognition is important with immediate evacuation to reduce the chance of compression of the optic nerve, which can lead to central retinal artery occlusion and blindness. All sutures should be removed with wide decompression of the orbital septum and lateral canthotomy to reduce the retrobulbar pressure. Hematoma formation under a flap or skin graft may result in necrosis and flap loss, which can further complicate the reconstruction.

Direct repair of eyelid margin deformities may be associated with a number of postoperative problems. When excessive tension is placed on the upper eyelid, mechanical ptosis may occur. A 3-month period of postoperative observation and temporizing treatment including lid massage is recommended prior to surgical intervention. Early edema may cause pseudoptosis of the upper eyelid, which resolves once the edema has improved. Ptosis that is present after the 3-month period may be due to tension on the repair, which generally requires surgical treatment. A lateral canthotomy will reduce the tension and allow the lid to assume a normal position.

Tension on the lid margin following direct repair can also contribute to the formation of notching or dehiscence. Early dehiscence with minimal separation of the lid margin should be managed in a conservative fashion with topical antibiotic ophthalmic ointment. The lid margin will generally heal satisfactorily by secondary intention without visible notching. If notching persists after a 3-month period, parallel excision of the tarsal plate with tension-free direct repair should be performed.

Multiple procedures should be anticipated following reconstruction of the eyelids for burn scar contracture. The acute management of burns to the periorbital region should focus on protection of the cornea from exposure keratitis due to dryness along with early excision and skin grafting. Full-thickness grafts provide the best initial attempt at reconstruction. Recurrent contraction of the grafts with lid malposition and lagophthalmos may be prevented by large interposition skin grafts. Careful slit lamp examination will provide continuous surveillance of the cornea.

MALIGNANT EYELID TUMORS

INDICATIONS

Effective recognition and management of malignant eyelid tumors require an understanding of the clinical and pathologic features of each subtype. There are a wide variety of rare malignancies that may involve the eyelid such as lymphoma, mucoepidermoid carcinoma, metastatic carcinoma, fibrosarcoma, sweat gland tumor, Merkel cell tumor, Kaposi's sarcoma, and others. The clinician should be familiar with these rare disease processes; however, the scope of this chapter will focus on the more common malignant eyelid tumors including basal cell carcinoma, squamous cell carcinoma, sebaceous carcinoma, and melanoma.

Basal Cell Carcinoma

Basal cell carcinoma was found to make up 12.4% of all eyelid tumors taken from a large registry of 5,392 tumors at the Wilmer Eye Institute of the Johns Hopkins Hospital over a 58-year period. Basal cell carcinoma was the most common malignancy, representing 90% of this series.[11,13] Clinically, basal cell cancers are more prevalent in fair-skinned individuals who have had significant exposure to sunlight. Since the effects of sun exposure on the skin are cumulative, skin cancers begin to manifest in middle-aged and older patients. Younger patients who present with multiple or repeated basal cell carcinomas should be evaluated for associated conditions with a predisposition to cutaneous malignancy such as xeroderma pigmentosum or Gorlin's basal cell nevus syndrome.[54,60]

Basal cell cancers occur more often on the lower eyelid and medial canthus than on the upper eyelid and lateral canthus. Lund originally described the morphologic patterns of basal cell carcinoma as nodular, ulcerative, morpheaform, and superficial spreading,[41] the most common being nodular with its appearance as a solid pearly lesion. With prolonged growth, spontaneous bleeding and central ulceration may occur. The histology of the nodular pattern consists of basaloid proliferation with no infiltration into the underlying tissues.

Ulcerative basal cell cancers may arise from untreated nodular tumors. Spontaneous bleeding often occurs from the friable telangiectatic vessels in the ischemic ulcer crater surrounded by a raised pearly edge. This is a more aggressive pattern of basal cell than the pure nodular form.

Morpheaform basal cell cancers represent the group of skin cancers that have the most aggressive tendency for diffuse infiltration into surrounding tissue. Although the surface epithelium of the tumor may appear relatively contained, cords of widespread basaloid cell proliferation occur through a dense connective tissue framework. Morpheaform cancer may present as a superficial nonhealing lesion of the lower eyelid with localized destruction of lashes (Figure 87-21). Due to the significant microscopic spread, Mohs' micrographic excision may require near total resection of the lower lid including tarsal plate and forniceal conjunctiva.

Studies have shown that recurrence rates for positive microscopic margins following excision of most basal cell carcinomas is approximately 50%.[59] Although this may be clinically acceptable in certain areas that can be closely followed and readily reexcised, definitive resection in the eyelid region should be performed with negative margins on intraoperative frozen section. Mohs' micrographic surgery has a reported success rate of 98% and is recommended for skin cancers in the eyelid region.[65] Clinical situations when Mohs' surgery should be used

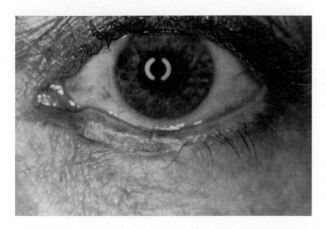

Figure 87-21. Basal cell carcinoma of the lower lid margin demonstrating malignant features of eyelash destruction.

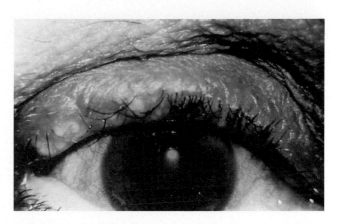

Figure 87-23. Sebaceous cell carcinoma of the nasal aspect of the upper lid margin.

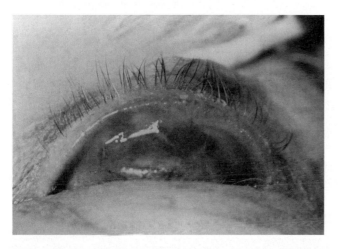

Figure 87-22. Squamous cell carcinoma involving the inner aspect of the upper lid.

include eyelid basal cell cancers that have morpheaform characteristics, involvement of the medial canthus due to the risk of intracranial extension, direct spread into the lacrimal sac, extension along cranial nerves, and direct invasion of the forniceal conjunctiva or globe.

Squamous Cell Carcinoma

Squamous cell carcinoma is the second most common malignant skin tumor in the eyelid region, representing 4% of all malignant epithelial tumors.[12] Squamous cell cancers typically arise from sun-damaged skin and often appear as erythematous, raised lesions on the eyelid margin with destruction of normal architecture and loss of lashes. However, squamous cell cancers can also occur on the inner conjunctival surface of the eyelid and therefore have an etiology other than sun exposure (Figure 87-22). Squamous cell cancers are invasive tumors that originate from the surface epithelium. The hallmark histologic feature of malignancy is dermal invasion by abnormal squamous cells from the epidermal rests. Although all squamous cell cancers are locally invasive, the metastatic potential varies depending on the etiology of the malignancy. Cutaneous squamous cell cancers that appear to be related to sun exposure have

a metastatic potential of less than 1%.[42,75] Those, however, that arise in areas following radiotherapy for eczema, acne therapy, or treatment of malignancy have a metastatic rate of 20%, and Marjolin's ulcer from chronic osteomyelitis has a very high metastatic potential of 44%.[55]

Sebaceous Cell Carcinoma

Although sebaceous cell carcinoma is a rare cutaneous malignancy outside of the periorbital region, it is the third most common eyelid malignancy, representing 1% to 2% of malignant epithelial eyelid tumors.[12,49] Sebaceous gland carcinomas arise primarily from the meibomian glands, although malignant transformation of pilosebaceous glands outside the eyelid region can occur. They are usually slow growing and most frequently arise on the upper eyelid (Figure 87-23) in patients over 60 years of age who may have been misdiagnosed with recurrent chalazion or chronic blepharoconjunctivitis. A delay in treatment of sebaceous cell carcinoma greater than 6 months is associated with a significant increase in mortality.[68] Despite early and aggressive management, the prognosis is unfavorable, with a 5-year survival of 60% to 70%.[4]

Since a superficial shave biopsy of the lid margin may not include the deep meibomian glands, a full-thickness biopsy including the tarsal plate is required to adequately confirm the diagnosis. Management includes wide local excision with intraoperative histologic confirmation of negative margins on frozen section, since the tumor is often multifocal. Margins are generally determined by adjacent anatomic structures in the eyelid region, and orbital extension requires orbital exenteration.[40]

Preoperative evaluation includes radiographic determination of orbital extension by CT scan or MRI and workup for distant metastasis, which most commonly occurs to the lungs, liver, and brain. The preauricular, submandibular, and cervical lymph nodes are evaluated for evidence of regional metastasis. Since advanced sebaceous cell carcinoma of the orbit can cause significant reactive hyperplasia in the draining lymph nodes without actual metastasis, open biopsy with frozen section confirmation followed by immediate neck dissection is an acceptable alternative treatment plan. The role of radiation therapy for the management of sebaceous gland carcinoma remains controversial. Although the tumor is somewhat radio-sensitive, radiotherapy is generally not curative, with reports of unacceptably high rates of recurrence.[23] Radiation therapy for the management of sebaceous cell carcinoma is therefore currently reserved for patients who are not surgical candidates and represents a form of palliative therapy to reduce tumor bulk.

Melanoma

Melanoma of the eyelids may occur as a primary cutaneous malignancy or may arise adjacent to an area of primary acquired melanosis of the conjunctiva. Similarly, melanomas of the forehead or cheek may involve the eyelids through direct extension. Diagnosis is made by full-thickness biopsy including subcutaneous tissue on the deep margin for determination of thickness (Figure 87-24).

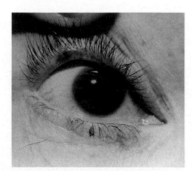

Figure 87-24. Nodular melanoma of the central aspect of the upper lid margin.

Management of eyelid melanoma should include preoperative staging for regional and distant metastasis. Clinical evaluation of involvement of the conjunctiva is crucial to determine if orbital exenteration is necessary for curative resection. Histologic evaluation of abnormal pigmented conjunctiva should be performed in order to make the distinction between melanosis and melanoma. Primary acquired melanosis of the conjunctiva may be managed with cryotherapy and preservation of the eye.[30] Melanoma of the conjunctiva requires enucleation or orbital exenteration. Cervical and preauricular lymphatic spread is treated with en bloc resection including superficial parotidectomy and neck dissection.

OPERATIONS

The initial evaluation of complex eyelid deformities should separate the component portions of the defect into deficiencies of the anterior and posterior lamella, upper and lower lid, and the support structures of the medial and lateral canthus (Box 87-1). Following this algorithm allows the surgeon to separate large deformities into multiple smaller deformities that require independent procedures to reconstruct each component part. The posterior lamella may require reconstruction of the tarso-ligamentous sling with shared tarsoconjunctival flaps from the opposite lid, free mucoperichondrium, or cartilage grafts. Similarly, defects of the anterior lamella may be closed with local rotation or transposition flaps, or may require free tissue grafting. Once adequate tissue replacements have been selected,

---

Box 87-1.
Decision Making in Eyelid Reconstruction

ANTERIOR LAMELLA
Skin muscle flap
Full-thickness skin graft
Split-thickness skin graft

POSTERIOR LAMELLA
Tarsoconjunctival flap
   free graft
   transposition flap
   lid sharing
Ear cartilage graft
Hard palate mucosa
Buccal mucosa
Septal mucoperichondrium

MEDIAL CANTHAL FIXATION
Direct repair posterior lacrimal crest
Nasal periosteal flap
Transnasal wiring
Miniplate fixation

LATERAL CANTHAL FIXATION
Direct repair Whitnall's tubercle
Lateral periosteal flap
Drill hole fixation
Miniplate fixation

ADJACENT TISSUE
Direct repair
Tenzel semicircular flap
McGregor temporal Z-plasty
Mustarde cheek rotation
Cervicofacial advancement flap
Subperiosteal cheek lift
Glabellar flap
Temporal forehead flap

OPPOSING EYELID TISSUE
Hughes tarsoconjunctival flap
Hewes transposition flap
Cutler-Beard bridge flap
Mustarde lid margin transposition
Tripier skin muscle flap
Fricke temporal brow flap

reconstruction of the medial and lateral canthal fulcrum points is required in order to restore the functional closure mechanism of the eyelids.

Posterior Lamellar Reconstruction

Although the most suitable tissue for reconstruction of the posterior lamella is replacement with nearly identical tissue, this may not be an option for large deformities and autogenous tissue substitutes are required.

SLIDING TARSOCONJUNCTIVAL FLAP. Reconstruction of isolated defects of the medial or lateral upper eyelid can be performed with a sliding tarsoconjunctival flap taken from the undersurface of the remaining upper eyelid.[47] The tarsal plate is designed to fit the defect, and a transposition flap is created based on the adjacent conjunctiva for blood supply and lining.

The upper eyelid is everted over a Desmarre retractor. The flap is designed 4 mm superior to the inferior edge of the remaining tarsal plate in order to maintain the integrity of the donor site and avoid problems with margin eversion (Figure 87-25). The incision is extended laterally corresponding to the width of the defect and angled superiorly to the border of the tarsal plate. Westcott scissors are used to dissect the tarsal plate and preserve the superiorly based conjunctival blood supply. The flap is transposed into the defect and sutured to the lateral orbital rim periosteum to create a new point of lateral canthal fixation. A 4-0 prolene is used to anchor the lateral edge of the

graft to the periosteum anterior to Whitnall's tubercle so that the lateral aspect of the reconstructed lower lid overlaps the lower lid margin. The medial edge of the tarsal plate is sutured to the remaining tarsus with 6-0 silk suture. The edges of the conjunctiva can be repaired using 6-0 plain catgut sutures with inverted knots to avoid corneal irritation.

The defect of the anterior lamella is reconstructed with an adjacent skin muscle flap or with a full-thickness skin graft taken from the lateral aspect of the opposite upper eyelid. The advantage of the sliding tarsoconjunctival flap is that the vascularized conjunctiva provides the blood supply for the overlying skin graft. Reapproximation of the skin graft is performed taking care to avoid overlapping skin at the lid margin, which could cause corneal irritation. The eyelids are sutured closed and a bolster dressing is placed to maintain gentle pressure on the skin graft for 1 week.

FREE TARSOCONJUNCTIVAL GRAFT. Shallow defects of the lower eyelid margin that include the tarsal plate can be reconstructed with a free tarsoconjunctival interposition graft from the upper eyelid. The upper lid is everted and a transverse incision is made through the conjunctiva and tarsal plate, preserving a 4-mm inferior lid margin. Vertical incisions are made corresponding to the length of the lower lid tarsal defect, and superior dissection continues to the upper edge of the tarsal plate, separating it from the overlying Müller's muscle (Figure 87-26). The conjunctiva is divided along the superior border

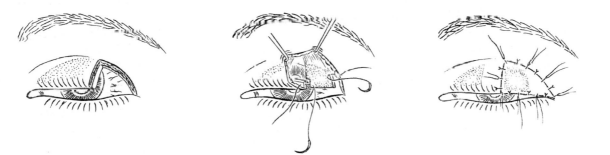

Figure 87-25. Sliding tarsoconjunctival graft used for posterior lamellar reconstruction of the lateral aspect of the upper lid. The tarsal flap is rotated laterally based on the conjunctival blood supply. The anterior lamella is reconstructed with a skin graft or skin muscle flap.

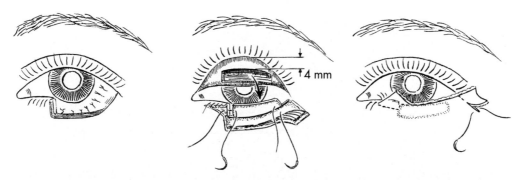

Figure 87-26. A free tarsoconjunctival graft taken from the upper lid can be used to reconstruct broad, shallow deformities of the lower lid. A 4-mm caudal margin of tarsus is preserved to avoid deformity of the lid margin. The graft is sutured in place and the skin muscle flap is advanced to provide blood supply to the flap.

and the free tarsoconjunctival graft is sutured in place in the lower lid using 7-0 silk to repair the cut edge of the graft to the edges of the lower lid tarsal plate. If the defect includes the medial or lateral canthal attachments, a 4-0 prolene is used to anchor the edge of the graft to the periosteum along the inner aspect of the lateral orbital rim or to the posterior reflection of the medial canthal tendon. The donor site heals rapidly with ophthalmic ointment without any change in normal upper lid position.[49]

EAR CARTILAGE GRAFT. The use of ear cartilage to reconstruct deficient posterior lamella is well described and represents the most commonly used autogenous tissue substitute.[2,3] Cartilage provides strong intrinsic support and can be used in larger defects. In addition to lid reconstruction, ear cartilage is used for correction of lower lid retraction as a spacer interposition graft following release of the capsulopalpebral fascia.[49] The exposed surface of the cartilage graft is generally well tolerated in the lower lid position and becomes epithelialized by adjacent conjunctiva over several weeks. Direct exposure to the cornea in upper lid reconstruction may cause irritation with blinking and should be avoided if possible.

Ear cartilage grafts are harvested from the scaphoid fossa rather than using conchal cartilage, which is too curved and thick. The scaphoid cartilage is flatter and similar in thickness to the tarsal plate. A curvilinear incision is made parallel to the helical rim on the posterior surface of the ear. The posterior perichondrium is undermined, exposing the posterior aspect of the scaphoid fossa. The elliptical graft is outlined and an incision is made 5 mm inside the helical rim through the cartilage to preserve the integrity of the helix and to avoid creating a visible contour deformity of the ear. The anterior perichondrium is bluntly elevated with a cotton applicator and the cartilage graft is harvested with Westcott scissors. The skin incision is repaired with 4-0 monocryl. The donor site is managed with cold compresses and ointment. The ear should be evaluated for hematoma formation postoperatively; however, morbidity associated with the donor site is uncommon.

HARD PALATE MUCOSAL GRAFT. The hard palate is a useful donor site for posterior lamellar reconstruction, offering the advantage of having both intrinsic support and mucosal lining.[1,9,35] Mucosal grafts may be used to reconstruct the posterior lamella of large deformities in the infraorbital area and lower eyelid including the lid margin. Additional uses include replacement of deficient tissue in severe cases of lid retraction associated with cicatricial ectropion, resection of malignant eyelid neoplasms, and Graves' ophthalmopathy. The mucosa of the hard palate is keratinized, stratified squamous epithelium that undergoes transformation to a nonkeratinized surface over several weeks following surgery. During this time, the keratinized surface may be irritating to the cornea and should be managed with liberal use of ophthalmic ointment. Mucosal hard palate grafts are too thick and irritating to the cornea to be used in upper eyelid reconstruction.

The graft is designed on the hard palate lateral to the midline, since the mucosa in the midline is thin and friable. A graft 10 mm wide is outlined from the alveolar ridge behind the canine tooth extending posteriorly to within 2 mm of the soft palatal junction (Figure 87-27). Following infiltration of local anesthetic with epinephrine, a partial-thickness incision is made with a 15-blade scalpel. The graft is elevated using Westcott scissors or a right-angled Beaver blade. The periosteum is left intact at the base of the palate to allow rapid granulation and decrease postoperative pain. Care is taken at the posterior extent of the incision to avoid the palatine artery, which exits the palatine foramen laterally and passes through the submucosal layer at the junction of the hard and soft palate. The graft can be thinned by excision of the residual submucosa and minor salivary glands. Hemostasis is achieved with liberal electrocautery, and Gelfoam is used to pack the donor site. Postoperative management of the donor site includes the use of topical Xylocaine jelly and dental paste to protect the palate. A soft diet is recommended after surgery until healing is complete.

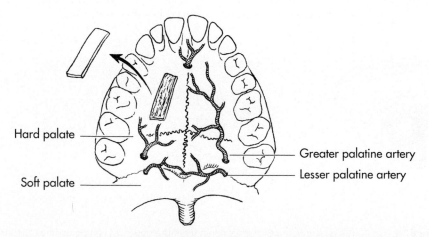

Figure 87-27. Diagram demonstrating the donor site for a graft of hard palate mucosa. The graft has intrinsic support and mucosal lining. Mucosa should be harvested from the paramedian location, avoiding the soft palate and palatine artery.

ORAL MUCOSAL GRAFT. When thin mucosal lining is required for eyelid reconstruction, full-thickness oral mucosal grafts can be harvested from the upper lip, lower lip, or buccal mucosa.[32,45] The primary uses include lining vascularized musculocutaneous flaps and reconstruction of the lid margin since the grafts are too thin to be used for tarsal support. Full-thickness mucosal grafts are preferred since there is less contraction. Split-thickness mucosal grafts are harvested with a mucotome and can be used for reconstruction of the conjunctiva of the fornix and episclera.

The lower lip is everted with skin hooks and the graft is outlined slightly larger than the defect, accounting for postoperative tissue contraction. The vermilion mucosa in the lip and Stensen's duct in the buccal recess are avoided. The mucosa is infiltrated using local anesthesia with epinephrine. An elliptical incision is made and the mucosa is undermined with straight Iris scissors. The graft is thinned by excising residual submucosa and minor salivary glands. Hemostasis can be obtained with Gelfoam, and large lip donor sites are allowed to heal by reepithelialization in order to avoid deformity of the lip contour. The buccal mucosa and small lip donor sites can be directly repaired with 4-0 monocryl.

SEPTAL CHONDROMUCOSAL GRAFTS. Eyelid deformities that require significant intrinsic support and mucosal lining may be reconstructed with chondromucosal grafts harvested from the nasal septum.[53] Septal chondromucosal grafts may be harvested up to a 25-mm square. Since this represents a significant amount of tissue to be used as a free graft, the indications generally include total upper and lower eyelid reconstruction or secondary reconstructive procedures when other donor sites may no longer be available. Furthermore, a well-vascularized musculocutaneous flap should be used for anterior lamellar reconstruction to provide the blood supply for neovascularization of the graft.

The nasal septum is blocked using local anesthetic with epinephrine and packed with 4% cocaine for maximal vasoconstriction. The graft is outlined on the nasal septum and an angled incision is made with a 15-blade scalpel parallel to the

dorsum and caudal septum, preserving 10 mm of septum as an L-strut for anterior support (Figure 87-28). A Freer elevator is used to separate the contralateral septal perichondrium from the cartilage graft, taking care to avoid perforation of the mucosa. The posterior septal mucosal and cartilage incisions are completed and the graft is removed. Any mucosal perforations must be repaired since a single layer of mucoperichondrium will make up the integrity of the septum while the donor site undergoes reepithelialization.

Following identification and harvesting of suitable grafts for replacement of deficient tissue of the posterior lamella, consideration must be given toward reconstruction of the lateral and medial canthal support structures prior to reconstruction of the anterior lamella.

Medial Canthal Reconstruction

Deformities of the medial canthus generally include loss of the medial support to the tarsoligamentous sling and a portion of the upper and lower eyelids. In order to restore the closure mechanism of the eyelids, the medial canthus requires reconstruction of the medial fulcrum point of the eyelids by reattaching the tarsoligamentous sling to bone. Direct fixation of the tarsal plate to the tendon can be performed if there is adequate residual medial canthal tendon. The point of medial canthal fixation should be posterior to the lacrimal sac corresponding to the normal posterior insertion point of the medial canthal tendon. The medial eyelid should approximate the posterior curve of the globe so that the inferior punctum is positioned for normal drainage of the tear lake.

The anterior lamella can be sutured to the anterior reflection of the medial canthal tendon in front of the lacrimal sac. If the tendinous portion of the medial canthus has been resected, a nasal periosteal flap can be elevated for reconstruction of the medial canthal tendon. The periosteum of the anterior lacrimal crest is divided as a rectangular flap 10 by 5 mm. The nasal periosteal flap is posteriorly based and can provide fixation for the upper and lower eyelids.[39]

When medial canthal deformities include loss of bone from tumor resection or trauma, a Y-shaped miniplate can be used to reconstruct a posterior fulcrum point for posterior lamellar support.[71] The plate is fixed to the thicker bone along the anterior lacrimal crest, and a 4-0 prolene is used to suture the tarsal plate to an empty hole in the miniplate, which corresponds to the posterior reflection of the medial canthal tendon. An alternative method for medial canthal support includes use of a Mitek anchor for bony fixation.[63] The anchor is made of a titanium alloy, which is placed in the medial orbital rim corresponding to the anterior reflection of the medial canthal tendon. The anterior lamella soft tissue can be sutured directly to the anchor.

Unilateral transnasal wiring can be used to reconstruct the medial canthus, particularly in cases of significant bony deficiency. Drill holes are placed posterior to the lacrimal sac fossa, and a 30-gauge stainless steel wire is used to tighten a 4-0 prolene suture placed through the medial canthal tendon remnant. As the wire is twisted, the medial canthal position is tightened by placing tension on the suture to avoid cutting through the soft tissue with the wire.[80]

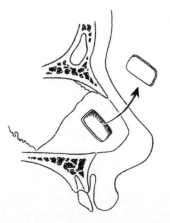

Figure 87-28. Graft of mucoperichondrium harvested from the nasal septum for reconstruction of larger eyelid deformities requiring lining and support.

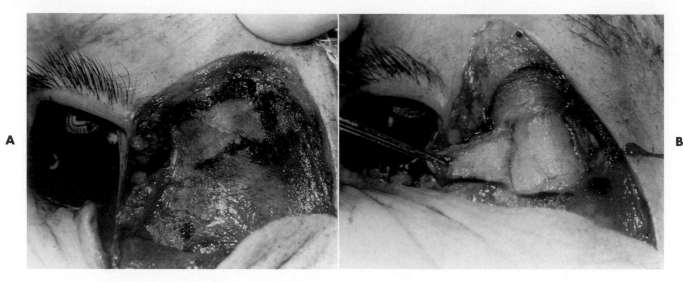

Figure 87-29. **A,** Lateral orbital rim exposed demonstrating outline of the lateral periosteal flap. **B,** The periosteal flap is elevated and rotated nasally, preserving the attachment at the lateral orbital rim superior to Whitnall's tubercle for lateral canthal reconstruction.

Lateral Canthal Reconstruction

The basic principles in lateral canthal reconstruction include separate points of fixation for the anterior and posterior lamella to the lateral orbital rim. The lower lid is fundamentally an adynamic structure and fixation is used primarily for lid support to prevent lower lid retraction. The upper lid is a more dynamic structure and the lateral canthus provides the lateral fulcrum point for functional movement of the upper lid. Without normal lateral fixation, upper lid closure may be impaired.

If resection includes the lateral canthal tendon, a lateral periosteal flap can be used to reconstruct the lateral canthal tendon. Following exposure of the lateral orbital rim, a rectangular flap of periosteum 10 by 5 mm is elevated. Parallel incisions are made through the periosteum and the flap is released from the junction of the deep temporal fascia (Figure 87-29). The flap is transposed medially and is based at the inner aspect of the lateral orbital rim above Whitnall's tubercle, thereby creating a neocanthal tendon. The tarsal plate is sutured to the periosteal flap with a 4-0 prolene.

Larger deformities that include the upper and lower limbs of the lateral canthal tendon can be reconstructed with crossed lateral periosteal flaps. Separate flaps are elevated, maintaining the periosteal attachments to the inner orbital rim superior to Whitnall's tubercle. The upper flap is transposed inferiorly to function as the tendon for the lower lid. The lower flap is transposed superiorly as the tendon for the upper lid, which should overlap the lower lid (Figure 87-30). When the periosteum of the orbital rim has been resected, drill holes through the lateral orbital rim can be used as an alternate method of fixation.

Lower lid and lateral canthal support may require the use of a fascia sling, which has medial and lateral points of fixation.

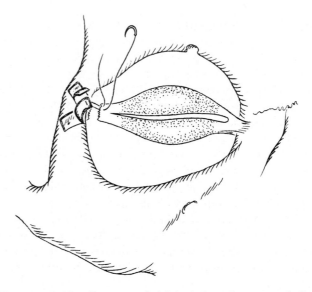

Figure 87-30. Diagram of bilobed lateral periosteal flap harvested from the lateral orbital rim for reconstruction of separate lateral canthal attachments for the upper and lower eyelids.

Although autogenous tensor fascia lata is preferred, preserved cadaveric fascia can also be used.[48] The anterior reflection of the medial canthal tendon is exposed through a small vertical incision. A hemostat is used to pass a fascial strip, which is sutured around the tendon with a 6-0 nylon. A Wright needle is used to thread the strip posterior to the pretarsal orbicularis. The strip is brought out a transverse incision made below the lid margin in the center of the lower lid. The fascia is passed back through the central incision to the lateral canthal incision. As the fascia is sutured to the periosteum of the lateral orbital rim, horizontal tightening of the tarsoligamentous sling is performed (Figure 87-31).

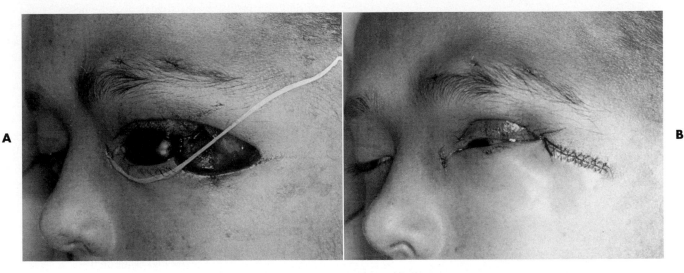

Figure 87-31.   A, Reconstruction of canthal support using autologous tensor fascia lata sling. The fascia is sutured around the anterior reflection of the medial canthal tendon. **B,** The fascia sling is passed through the pretarsal space and anchored to the periosteum of the lateral orbital rim. The anterior lamella is closed with advancement of the skin muscle flap.

Anterior Lamella Reconstruction

SEMICIRCULAR ROTATION FLAP. Although small defects of the eyelids following resection of malignant neoplasms can be closed by direct repair, larger deformities require the recruitment of adjacent tissue. One of the workhorse flaps used to reconstruct full-thickness defects of 40% to 60% of the central aspect of the upper or lower lid is the semicircular rotation skin-muscle flap described by Tenzel and Stewart.[77] For defects of the upper lid, the deformity is prepared by making sure the remaining cut edges of the tarsal plate are parallel similar to the principle used for direct repair. The semicircular flap is designed as a superiorly based musculocutaneous flap beginning at the lateral canthus and extending inferiorly as a semicircle, with a diameter of approximately 3 cm depending on the size of the defect (Figure 87-32). The flap is undermined deep to the orbicularis muscle until adequate mobilization is achieved for flap rotation. A lateral canthotomy is made in the upper limb of the lateral canthal tendon for release of the lateral aspect of the residual lid margin. The inferior limb of the lateral canthal tendon is preserved. Once the lid is detached from the lateral orbital rim, the full-thickness lid flap is advanced nasally. The lid margin is reapproximated with a 7-0 silk suture in the gray line.

Following nasal rotation of the flap, lateralization of the original central deformity occurs. The parallel edges of the tarsal plate are directly repaired with 7-0 silk suture with inverted knots. Lateralization creates a continuous lash margin over the nasal and central portion of the eyelid. For eye protection as well as aesthetic considerations, lash deficiency is better tolerated over the lateral aspect of the lid margin. Once the pretarsal skin and orbicularis have been reapproximated, lateral lid fixation is necessary to provide the lateral fulcrum for lid closure. The lateral canthus is recreated by suturing the edge of the semicircular flap to the periosteum with a 4-0 prolene suture at the point where the flap overlaps the lateral

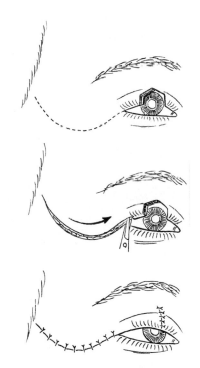

Figure 87-32. Tenzel semicircular rotation flap used for reconstruction of an upper eyelid deformity. Following elevation of the skin muscle flap, the lateral canthal tendon to the upper lid is divided and the flap margin is advanced nasally into the deformity. The Tenzel flap is sutured to the lateral orbital rim for lateral canthal support.

orbital rim. The posterior lamella is reconstructed by advancing the residual conjunctiva to the flap margin with a 6-0 plain catgut continuous suture. Following reconstruction of the lateral canthus, the semicircular skin-muscle flap donor site is closed with a continuous 6-0 nylon vertical mattress suture reapproximating the orbicularis and everting the skin edges.

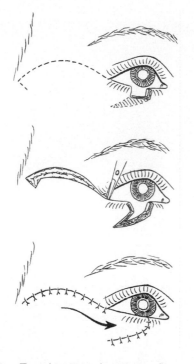

Figure 87-33. Tenzel semicircular rotation flap used for reconstruction of a lower eyelid deformity. The flap outline is shown and the lateral lid margin is released with canthotomy and advanced into the defect. The dog-ear is removed laterally along skin tension lines.

Excision of a small Burow's triangle may be necessary at the lateral aspect of the incision to prevent dog-ear formation. Antibiotic ophthalmic ointment, cold compresses, and head elevation make up the mainstay of postoperative management, with suture removal 1 week after surgery.

Lower lid defects that are too large for direct repair may be reconstructed with an inferiorly based, lateral semicircular skin-muscle rotation flap.[77] The lid deformity is prepared for reconstruction by creating full-thickness parallel edges of the tarsal plate. The rotation flap is designed beginning at the lateral canthus as a semicircle extending in a temporal direction just lateral to the eyebrow (Figure 87-33). The skin-muscle flap is undermined in the submuscular plane. A lateral canthotomy of the inferior limb of the canthal tendon is performed while preserving the superior limb for upper lid support. Large deformities of the periorbital region may also be reconstructed with a semicircular rotation flap in order to avoid downward tension on the lower lid (Figure 87-34).

Similar to the principle described for upper lid reconstruction, lateralization of the lower lid deformity occurs with nasal advancement of the remaining lateral lid flap. Excess skin and muscle in the lower lid region are removed with a laterally angled incision placing the scar parallel to the skin tension lines. Following closure of the lid deformity, the lateral canthus is reconstructed by suturing the muscle flap to the periosteum along the inner aspect of the orbital rim above Whitnall's

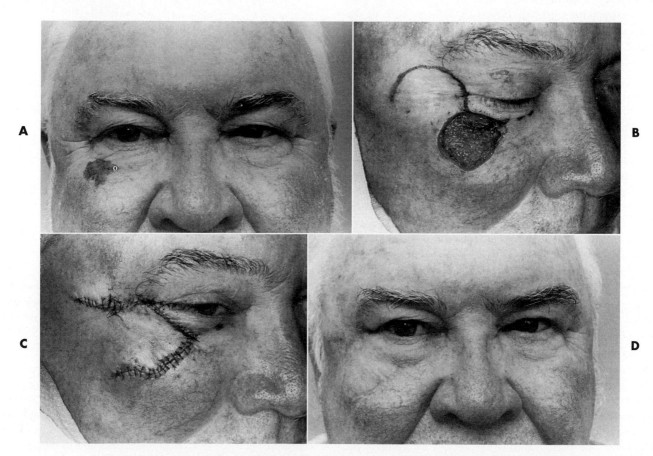

Figure 87-34. **A,** Lentigo maligna melanoma involving the right inferior periorbital region. **B,** Outline of Tenzel semicircular flap. **C,** Reconstruction following rotation of flap and lateral canthoplasty. **D,** Final result of reconstruction 6 months after surgery.

tubercle. The reconstructed lid margin should approximate the curved surface of the globe with superior overcorrection to account for postoperative lid descent. The conjunctiva is sutured to the flap margin and the skin and muscle are repaired.

TRANSPOSITION Z-PLASTY FLAP. Central lower lid deformities over 60% of the lid margin that include a large wedge resection below the eyelid may be reconstructed using a lateral orbital transposition flap. McGregor described a skin flap extending from the lateral canthal angle continuing laterally in a gentle upward curve to the lateral temporal hairline.[50] A prehairline incision is made inferiorly equal in length and parallel to the lateral edge of the lid deformity (Figure 87-35). A Z-plasty is made along the transverse incision to lengthen the lid margin corresponding to the width of the wedge resection from the lower lid. Following adequate mobilization of the skin flap, canthotomy is performed and the residual lateral lid margin is advanced medially. The tarsal plate and lid margin are reconstructed. The wedge resection is repaired following transposition of the skin flap nasally.

ROTATION CHEEK FLAP. Extensive full-thickness lower lid defects that extend inferiorly to the orbital rim and deformities of the infraorbital region may be repaired with a large rotation cheek flap, originally described by Mustarde[56,57] and described by Callahan and Callahan.[7] The flap is used to reconstruct defects with a significant vertical component. When the deformity involves the lid margin, the Mustarde flap is designed at the lateral canthus similar to the Tenzel flap, but extends into the cheek in the preauricular region following a

more gentle curve similar to the design of a facelift incision (Figure 87-36). The arc of rotation passes just below the lateral brow and can be extended into the neck with removal of a Burow's triangle from the lateral cervical region. This design allows tissue to be advanced superiorly in order to minimize retraction of the reconstructed lower lid. A wide base should be maintained to ensure adequate blood supply. The flap can be elevated in the subcutaneous plane or deep to the orbicularis oculi and superficial musculoaponeurotic system (SMAS) to maximize blood supply in high-risk patients such as cigarette smokers. Excess tissue may be excised as a dog ear with the incision placed in the nasolabial fold.

When total lower lid reconstruction is required, the posterior lamella is reconstructed with a mucous membrane graft harvested from the nasal septum, which includes a layer of septal cartilage for support. An alternative donor site is palatal mucoperichondrium, which has enough intrinsic support for posterior lamellar reconstruction. The graft is placed with the mucosa facing the surface of the eye to minimize corneal irritation. The length of the graft approximates the defect using approximately 25 mm for total lower lid reconstruction with a vertical width of 5 mm. The medial portion of the mucous membrane graft is sutured to the residual tarsal plate or to the posterior reflection of the medial canthal tendon using a 4-0 prolene. The lacrimal drainage system may require reconstruction and should be stented with placement of Crawford tubes. Following reconstruction of the medial tarsoligamentous support, the Mustarde flap is sutured to the anterior limb of the medial canthal tendon or to the periosteum of the medial orbital rim for anterior lamellar reconstruction.

After reconstruction of the medial portion of the deformity, the lateral canthus is reconstructed by suturing the mucous membrane graft to the lateral orbital rim periosteum with a

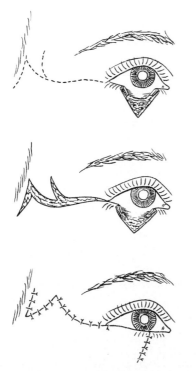

Figure 87-35. Repair of a V-shaped excision of the lower lid with lateral canthotomy and McGregor Z-plasty from the temporal region.

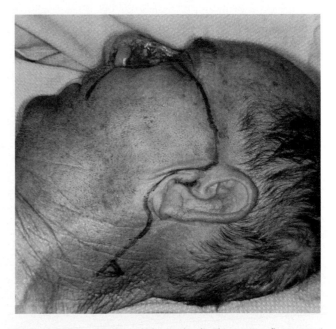

Figure 87-36. Outline of Mustarde cheek rotation flap extending in the preauricular region with removal of a Burow's triangle in the neck and medial dog-ear placed in the nasolabial fold.

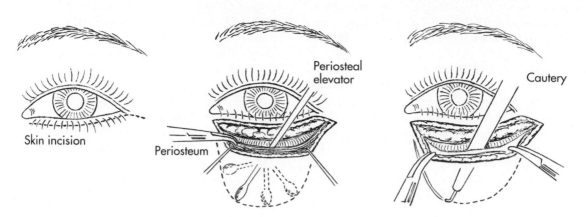

Figure 87-37. Diagram demonstrating the reconstructive cheek lift, which uses advancement of the midface following periosteal release for the reconstruction of lower lid deformities.

4-0 prolene above Whitnall's tubercle inside the orbital rim, with the graft positioned adjacent to the globe. A 6-0 plain catgut suture is used to suture the inferior edge of the graft to the residual conjunctiva in the fornix, completing the posterior lamellar reconstruction. Fixation of the cheek flap to the lateral orbital rim periosteum keeps the new lid margin positioned superior to the inferior corneoscleral limbus. The edge of the skin flap is sutured to the superior mucosal border with a continuous 6-0 plain catgut avoiding corneal exposure to the keratinized skin edge. Suspension of the cheek flap is completed with deep interrupted 4-0 monocryl sutures along the apex and preauricular portion of the lateral incision. The remainder of the skin incision is repaired with continuous 5-0 prolene.

SUBPERIOSTEAL CHEEK ADVANCEMENT. The lower lid skin and cheek tissue can be used as an advancement flap for reconstruction of deformities of the lower lid. Traditionally, these flaps have been elevated in the subcutaneous or submuscular plane for deformities of the medial canthus and nasolabial fold.[37] Subperiosteal dissection with periosteal release can be used to elevate the midfacial soft tissues for reconstruction of lower lid defects.[24] The cheeklift is particularly useful in patients with midfacial aging with increased tissue laxity. The cheek flap is anchored to the deep temporal fascia lateral to the orbital rim with a 4-0 prolene. Excess skin and muscle are recruited as a source of tissue for the reconstruction of defects with vertical inadequacy of the lower lid and infraorbital region. This technique can be used to correct deficient anterior lamella following resection of malignancy, reconstruction of burns to the eyelids, and repair of lower lid retraction following overresection of lower lid skin. The subperiosteal cheeklift can be used in order to avoid the need for a skin graft or staged lid-sharing procedure.

Prior to performing the subperiosteal cheek advancement, the degree of vertical inadequacy and tissue deficiency of the lower lid is evaluated. A lower lid subciliary incision is made with a slight lateral extension at the lateral cathal angle

following a prominent crow's foot line. The skin muscle flap is elevated anterior to the septum to the inferior orbital rim. The periosteum is divided along the inferior orbital rim from the medial canthus to the lateral canthus. A periosteal elevator is used to dissect the subperiosteal plane in a "U-shaped" area below the rim (Figure 87-37). Care is taken to divide the origin of the levator labii superioris preserving the infraorbital nerve, which exits the foramen just inferior to the levator of the upper lip. The infraorbital, zygomaticofacial, and zygomaticotemporal nerves are identified and preserved. Once the periosteum has been completely elevated, it is divided with a needle-tip bovie cautery along the inferior extent of the dissection at the piriform aperture of the maxilla. In order to elevate the cheek flap, the periosteal attachments must be completely released.

Depending on the extent of the lower lid deformity, a lateral canthoplasty may be necessary prior to the cheek flap elevation to control lower lid position with an independent point of fixation. The risk of ectropion has been significantly reduced when a lateral canthoplasty is performed with the cheeklift flap. The lateral canthoplasty is performed by suturing the cut edge of the tarsal plate to the periosteum of the lateral orbital rim with a 4-0 prolene. The point of suture fixation should be inside the orbital rim so that the lid follows the curve of the globe. The lid is positioned superior to Whitnall's tubercle with slight overcorrection in order to avoid postoperative lid retraction. Following completion of the canthoplasty, the cheek flap is elevated and sutured to the deep temporal fascia lateral to the orbital rim with multiple permanent sutures of 4-0 prolene. Elevation of the entire midfacial soft tissue complex allows a reliable framework on which to build the remainder of the lid reconstruction. The skin muscle flap is then inset into the deformity and a tension-free repair may be achieved (Figure 87-38).

LID-SHARING PROCEDURES. When adjacent eyelid tissue cannot provide suitable tissue for reconstruction, the best reconstructive option may be use of the opposing eyelid as the

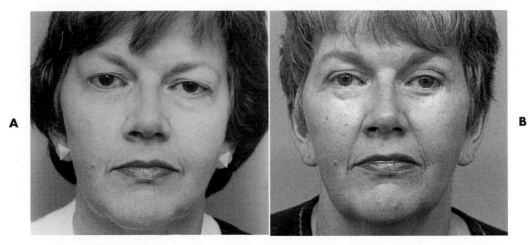

Figure 87-38. A, Patient with prominent eyes demonstrating lower lid retraction following lower blepharoplasty. **B,** Correction of lower lid malposition using cartilage grafts and subperiosteal cheeklift.

donor site. The advantage is use of identical components of the anterior and posterior lamella for reconstruction of complex deformities. The main disadvantage is that most of the lid-sharing procedures require multiple stages and temporarily obstruct vision of the involved eye.

TARSOCONJUNCTIVAL ADVANCEMENT FLAP. Reconstruction of full-thickness defects that involve greater than 50% of the lower lid margin without significant inferior extension can be reconstructed with a vascularized advancement flap of upper lid tarsal plate and conjunctiva. This procedure was originally described by Hughes [26,27] Use of a vascularized flap allows a free skin graft to be used if necessary for reconstruction of the anterior lamella and is safer for patients who have had previous radiation to the eyelids.

The horizontal width of the lower lid defect is measured under appropriate tension. The upper lid is everted over a Desmarre retractor and the advancement flap is designed preserving a 4-mm inferior margin of tarsal plate to avoid postoperative upper lid deformities (Figure 87-39). A 15-blade scalpel is used to make the transverse incision through the conjunctiva and tarsal plate. The vertical incisions are made corresponding to the width of the lower lid defect. Westcott scissors are used to dissect the tarsal plate and conjunctiva from the overlying Müller's muscle. Although Müller's muscle can be harvested with the flap, most surgeons prefer to harvest the tarsal plate based only on the conjunctiva.

Once the conjunctiva has been adequately mobilized above the upper border of the tarsal plate, the flap is advanced into the lower lid defect. The medial and lateral edges of the tarsal plate are repaired with interrupted 7-0 silk suture. The previous upper lid superior tarsal border is positioned as the newly reconstructed lower lid margin. The inferior tarsal margin is sutured to the conjunctiva in the lower lid fornix with continuous 6-0 plain catgut suture. The lower lid reconstruction is completed with placement of a skin graft or skin-muscle flap over the tarsoconjunctival flap.

Postoperative management primarily includes a light pressure dressing and use of ointment and eyedrops during the healing process. Traditional timing of flap division has been 6 weeks; however, earlier division at 2 weeks is usually safe in order to shorten the interval of visual impairment.[51] When the tarsoconjunctival flap is separated, a grooved instrument should be used to protect the cornea. The conjunctiva is divided along the superior aspect of the flap and is sutured to the cutaneous edge for lid margin reconstruction. In order to prevent superior retraction of the upper lid, the lid is everted and any fibrous attachments between Müller's muscle and the levator aponeurosis should be divided with Westcott scissors. This will release Müller's muscle back to its original level, avoiding the possibility of upper lid retraction similar to that performed by a Fasanella-Servat ptosis procedure.

TARSOCONJUNCTIVAL TRANSPOSITION FLAP. When the lower lid defect involves the lateral half of the lid margin including the inferior limb of the lateral canthal tendon, a laterally based transposition flap of tarsus and conjunctiva can be harvested from the upper lid. This flap was originally described by Hewes et al.[25] The advantage of this procedure is that it provides a one-stage vascularized tarsoconjunctival transposition.

The upper lid is everted over a Desmarre retractor. The flap is designed as an axial flap along the inner aspect of the superior border of the tarsal plate, which includes the superior arcade as the blood supply. The conjunctiva and superior edge of the tarsal plate are incised preserving the lateral base at the lateral canthal angle (Figure 87-40). The tarsoconjunctival flap is separated from the overlying Müller's muscle and transposed into the lower lid deformity, with the conjunctiva placed toward the globe. The edge of the tarsal plate is sutured to the remaining lower lid tarsus with 7-0 silk sutures. Lateral attachment of the flap to the periosteum is performed with a 4-0 prolene to avoid problems with lid retraction. The tarsoconjunctival flap may be covered with a skin graft or skin-muscle flap.

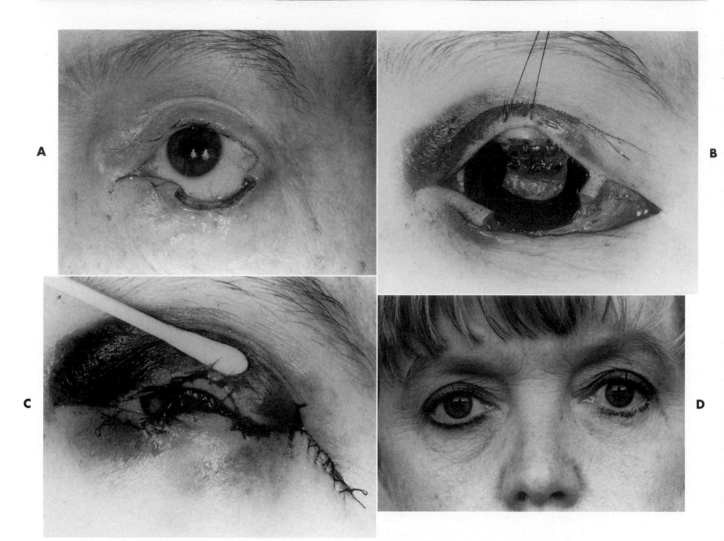

Figure 87-39. A, Lower lid defect following Mohs' excision of basal cell carcinoma. **B,** Reconstuction using lid sharing with a modified Hughes tarsoconjunctival flap from the upper lid. **C,** The flap is inset and the skin muscle flap advanced to the lid margin. **D,** Final reconstruction following division of the flap with make-up to simulate lower eyelashes.

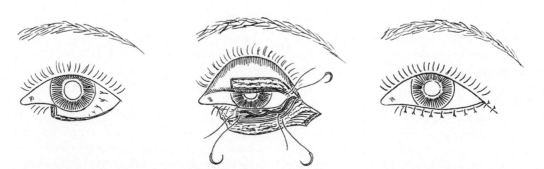

Figure 87-40. Reconstruction of lateral lower lid defect with a Hewes tarsoconjunctival transposition flap from the upper eyelid. The flap is based on the superior arcade. Following reconstruction of the posterior lamella, the skin muscle flap is advanced for anterior lamellar reconstruction.

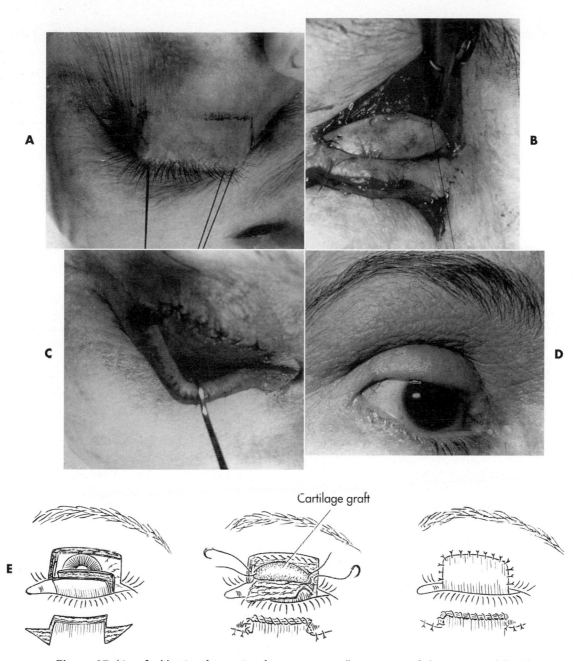

Figure 87-41. A, Margin of resection for squamous cell carcinoma of the upper eyelid with reconstruction using the Cutler-Beard lid-sharing bridge flap. **B,** Bipedicle bridge of lower lid margin with placement of ear cartilage graft in the upper lid position to reconstruct the tarsal plate. **C,** Retraction of lower lid bridge to show advancement of lower lid skin into the deformity. **D,** Final reconstruction of upper lid. **E,** Diagram of lower lid bridge flap. (Case courtesy of CD McCord.)

LOWER LID BRIDGE FLAP. Large full-thickness defects of the upper eyelid including total upper eyelid resection may be reconstructed with a full-thickness flap of skin, muscle, and conjunctiva harvested from the infraorbital region while preserving the lower lid margin as a bridge of tissue. This was originally described as the Cutler-Beard bridge flap.[10,72] The advantage is that a large amount of vascularized tissue can be harvested with little morbidity to the donor site. The flap can support a free cartilage graft used to reconstruct the upper lid tarsal plate. The primary disadvantages of the flap are that the

reconstructed eyelid is sutured closed for 6 weeks and eyelashes cannot be transferred with this technique.

The lower lid flap is designed as a rectangular advancement flap beginning 5 mm below the lower lid margin to preserve the inferior arcade, which will provide the blood supply to the bridge of the lower lid margin. The width of the transverse incision corresponds to the width of the upper lid defect. Parallel vertical incisions are made extending inferiorly to the fornix on the conjunctival side of the flap (Figure 87-41). The skin and muscle are divided down to the inferior orbital rim

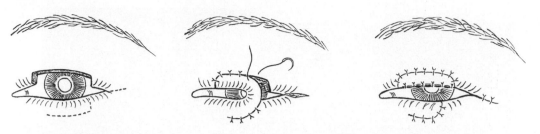

Figure 87-42. Reconstruction of shallow central upper lid defect with Mustarde lid-sharing flap from the lower lid margin. The lower lid flap is elevated as a full-thickness flap based on the medial arcade. The flap is divided and inset 6 weeks after the initial procedure.

and the flap is mobilized superiorly. Relaxing incisions may be necessary in the capsulopalpebral fascia in order for the flap to pass under the bridge of lower lid margin and into the upper eyelid defect with minimal tension.

The conjunctival layer of the flap is separated from the skin-muscle layer and sutured to the conjunctival defect of the upper lid with 6-0 plain catgut. A free ear cartilage graft is placed anterior to the conjunctiva and sutured to the remaining medial and lateral edges of the tarsal plate with 7-0 silk. If complete resection of the tarsal plate has been performed, the cartilage graft is sutured to the medial and lateral canthal tendons. In order to provide postoperative lid function, the superior edge of the cartilage graft must be sutured to the levator aponeurosis or to residual levator muscle. The skin-muscle flap is sutured to the cutaneous edges of the defect with interrupted 7-0 silk to complete reconstruction of the anterior lamella.

Postoperative management includes a light pressure dressing. Division and insetting of the flap are performed 6 weeks after the first stage. The cornea is protected, and the flap is divided 2 mm below the desired position of the upper lid margin to account for tissue contraction. A conjunctival flap is everted and sutured to the new lid margin to avoid problems with corneal irritation from the keratinized flap edge.

The lower lid donor site is repaired by insetting the lower lid margin. The bridge of tissue is deepithelialized and the remainder of the flap is replaced in the infraorbital region. The edges are reapproximated with 7-0 silk suture following excision of any excess tissue. The conjunctival surface is managed with ointment and allowed to reepithelialize.

PEDICLED LOWER LID SHARING. Broad, shallow defects of the central aspect of the upper lid can be reconstructed with a pedicled lid-sharing flap from the lower lid margin, which was originally described by Mustarde.[58] Although this technique requires a two-stage procedure with partial visual obstruction following the first stage, the primary advantage is reconstruction of the central lid margin with new eyelashes taken from the lower lid donor site.

The flap should be designed based on the central portion of the lower lid as the donor site for the lid margin. A full-thickness 5-mm vertical transection of the lid margin is made at the lateral limbus in order to preserve the lateral commissure. The inferior arcade provides the blood supply to the flap. The rectangular edge of the flap is elevated by extending the inferior incision parallel to the lid margin and inferior to

the marginal artery. The transverse incision continues medially until adequate mobilization of the pedicle lower lid flap has been achieved. The lateral edge of the lower lid tarsal plate is sutured to the medial edge of the upper lid tarsal plate (Figure 87-42). The gray line and lash margin are realigned with 7-0 silk sutures. Inspection for kinking of the blood supply should be performed. The inferior capsulopalpebral fascia can be released with Westcott scissors in order to reduce any tension on the flap.

The second stage of the procedure is performed 6 weeks after the initial reconstruction. The base of the lower lid flap is divided with an angled incision, and the remainder of the flap is rotated into the upper eyelid defect. The lateral upper lid margin is reconstructed by repairing the edges of the tarsal plate and the newly constructed lash margin. The lower lid donor site is repaired by medial advancement of the residual lateral lid margin. If tension is encountered, lateral canthotomy may be required to release the lateral lid margin to allow tension-free repair of the lower lid.

PEDICLED UPPER LID FLAP. Lateral deformities of the lower eyelid that are limited to the anterior lamella can be reconstructed with a pedicled musculocutaneous flap from the upper eyelid. This technique was originally described by Tripier.[78] The donor site requires excess tissue in the region of the upper eyelid crease. The flap can be designed as a unipedicle or bipedicle flap (Figure 87-43). The unipedicle flap is based laterally, with the inferior incision placed in the upper lid crease and the superior incision marked after utility forceps are used to evaluate tissue redundancy in the lateral aspect of the upper lid. The flap should have a lateral base of at least 10 mm and extend nasally to correspond to the length of the defect. Following undermining anterior to the septum, the flap is transposed into the lower lid defect and sutured in place with 7-0 silk sutures. The upper lid is closed similar to an upper lid blepharoplasty with continuous 6-0 nylon suture. The bipedicle flap is designed preserving a medial and lateral blood supply. Division of the pedicles and insetting the flap can be performed 2 weeks after the initial procedure.

Periorbital Donor Sites

When donor sites from adjacent eyelid skin are not available, periorbital sites can be used to provide large volumes of tissue for eyelid reconstruction. The primary disadvantages of the periorbital donor sites include the need for staged operations

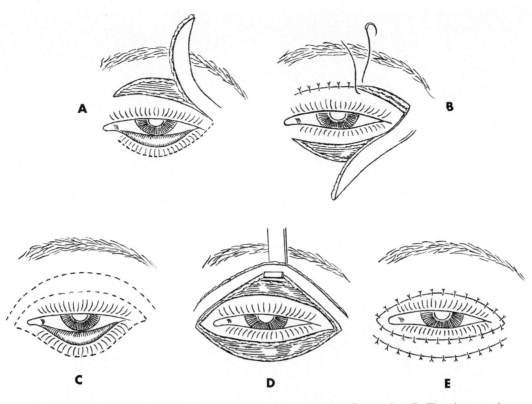

Figure 87-43. **A,** Donor site and flap outline of the unipedicle Tripier flap. **B,** The skin muscle flap is based laterally and transposed into the lower lid defect. **C,** Design of the bipedicle Tripier flap with dual blood supply. **D,** The skin muscle flap is transposed over the upper lid for reconstruction of wide lower lid defects. **E,** Diagram of lid-sharing flap.

and tissue that is significantly thicker and less pliable than eyelid skin. For these reasons, periorbital donor sites have limited use potential.

TEMPORAL FOREHEAD FLAP. The temporal forehead flap, described by Fricke,[16] uses tissue superior to the eyebrow as a transposition flap for defects of the upper eyelid and lateral canthal region. The scar is hidden in the superior brow margin and the brow is slightly elevated depending on the width of the flap. When used to reconstruct full thickness of the upper lid, the flap requires lining with a conjunctival flap or mucous membrane to avoid corneal irritation.

FOREHEAD FLAP. The forehead flap can be used for total upper and lower lid reconstruction. The flap, described by Kazanjian and Roopenian,[33] is based on the supratrochlear or supraorbital blood supply. The flap is elevated in the subgaleal plane with conservative thinning of the distal flap and is transposed into the deformity and undermining donor site laterally for forehead mobilization. The posterior lamella requires reconstruction with a conjunctival flap or mucous membrane graft. In order to give some function to the reconstructed upper lid, the flap should be reapproximated to the remaining levator aponeurosis. If the flap remains too thick, it can be thinned 2 weeks after the initial procedure while maintaining the blood supply from the pedicle. The pedicle can be divided and the flap inset after an additional 2 weeks.

GLABELLAR FLAP. Redundant tissue in the glabellar region can be used to reconstruct deformities of the medial canthal region. The glabellar flap is drawn as an inverted V-shaped flap extending superiorly between the eyebrows. The flap has a broad base and can therefore be safely thinned without compromising the blood supply (Figure 87-44). The flap is rotated into the medial canthal defect and the donor site closed primarily. Staged insetting may be required to complete the reconstruction depending on the contour of the flap.

OUTCOMES

The outcome of eyelid reconstruction following operations for curative resection of malignant neoplasms can be evaluated with respect to complications associated with the surgical procedures, functional outcomes including eyelid closure and protective mechanisms, and aesthetic result.

The most common complication following eyelid reconstruction is lower eyelid malposition. Lid retraction or ectropion may occur, from dynamic forces generated by a deficiency of skin in the anterior lamella or lack of stability of the tarso-ligamentous support structures of the posterior lamella from tumor resection. Despite appropriate reconstructive options and overcorrection of lower lid position, lower lid retraction may occur (Figure 87-45).

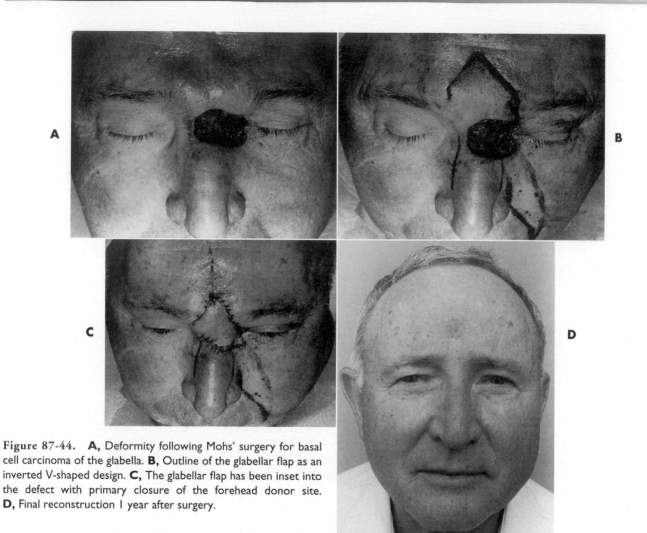

Figure 87-44. **A,** Deformity following Mohs' surgery for basal cell carcinoma of the glabella. **B,** Outline of the glabellar flap as an inverted V-shaped design. **C,** The glabellar flap has been inset into the defect with primary closure of the forehead donor site. **D,** Final reconstruction 1 year after surgery.

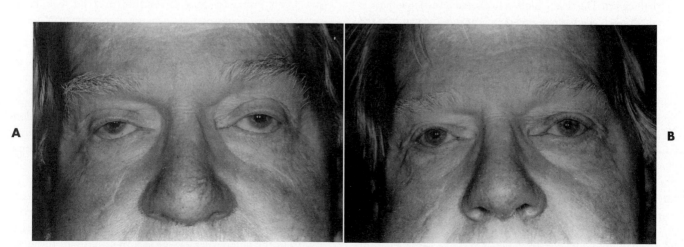

Figure 87-45. **A,** Bilateral lower lid senile ectropion and ptosis with prior right infraorbital reconstruction. **B,** Improved functional eyelid position following lateral canthoplasty and tarsolevator aponeurotic advancement.

Management of lower lid retraction is the most common indication for secondary surgical procedures following reconstruction of the lower eyelid and periorbital region. Treatment depends on the degree of corneal exposure and the timing after surgery. Early lid retraction may be due to edema of the reconstructive flap and should be managed conservatively with temporizing measures including massage and liberal use of eyedrops and ophthalmic ointment for corneal protection. Extreme cases of corneal exposure may be managed with bandage contact lens, moisture chamber, temporary Frost suture, or tarsorrhaphy. Lower lid malposition that is persistent 3 months after surgery will likely require surgical intervention.

Vertical inadequacy of the anterior lamella may occur with contraction of the flap or skin graft. Clinical evaluation reveals tightness in the lower lid region, with inability to elevate the lid margin above the inferior limbus with gentle upward pressure. Skin shortage may be managed with an interposition graft or readvancement of the reconstructive flap.

Once correction of anterior lamellar deficiency has been performed, the integrity of the tarsoligamentous sling should be evaluated by examining the fixation of the medial and lateral canthus as well as laxity of the lid margin. Spacer interposition grafts of ear cartilage or hard palate can be used to support the lid margin. Medial canthal fixation may require a periosteal flap, a fixation screw, or a fascia lata sling.

The most commonly performed procedure for the correction of lower lid malposition is the lateral canthoplasty. Selective canthotomy of the lateral canthal tendon to the lower lid is performed (Figure 87-46). After canthotomy, cantholysis of the lower lid should be performed by dividing the lower lid retractors parallel to the lid margin below the inferior arcade. Once the lower lid margin is fully mobile, the lid is tightened by overlapping the lid lateral to the orbital rim while elevating the lid margin above the inferior limbus. Full-thickness excision of the redundant lid is performed parallel to the lid margin.[8] The canthoplasty is performed with a 4-0 prolene suture placed in the exposed cut edge of the tarsal plate (Figure 87-47). The point of canthoplasty suture placement corresponds to the horizontal level of the pupil along the inner aspect of the lateral orbital rim (Figure 87-48). A mattress suture is tightened to correct any laxity and position the lower lid 2 mm above the inferior limbus.

In addition to lid malposition, blunting or webbing of the lateral canthal angle may occur after lid reconstruction. The lateral canthoplasty is also an effective method to correct these complications and restore a more normal lateral commissure. A 6-0 nylon alignment suture is placed in the gray line of the upper and lower lid to properly align the lateral commissure (Figure 87-49).

The functional outcome following reconstructive procedures of the eyelids is directly related to the extent of tumor resection. The goals of lower lid reconstruction include positioning the lower lid at the inferior limbus with apposition of the inferior punctum to the globe for functional drainage of the tear lake. Although the reconstructed lower lid functions adequately as an adynamic structure, the upper lid must maintain a dynamic relationship to the globe for normal eye protective mechanisms.

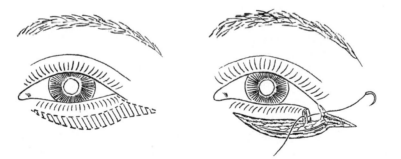

Figure 87-46. Lateral canthotomy is performed at the commissure with selective lysis of the inferior canthal tendon.

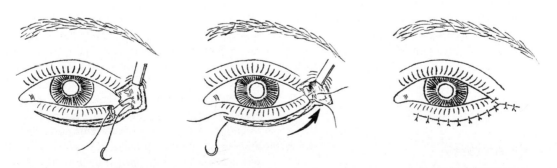

Figure 87-47. Diagram of lateral canthoplasty with suture placement through the tarsal plate to the inner aspect of the lateral orbital rim.

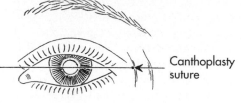

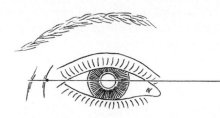

Canthoplasty suture

Figure 87-48. Point of canthoplasty suture placement at the horizontal midpupillary line on forward gaze.

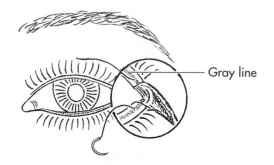

Gray line

Figure 87-49. Lateral canthal alignment technique to reconstruct the lateral canthal angle.

The levator palpebrae and orbicularis oculi muscles interact in order to coordinate functional opening and closing of the eyelids. Following partial resection of the levator, function can be maintained by fixation of the reconstructive flap to Whitnall's ligament or to the remaining orbital levator muscle. More extensive resection of the levator requires use of the frontalis muscle to elevate the reconstructed eyelid. Frontalis suspension is performed to restore function to the reconstructed upper lid as a secondary procedure.

The aesthetic outcome following reconstructive procedures of the eyelids should be given an importance comparable with that of the functional outcome. The aesthetic appearance of the reconstruction is generally better when the tissue used is adjacent to the deformity. Reconstruction of small defects with adjacent tissue often has excellent aesthetic results with a single procedure. When lid-sharing techniques are used, staged procedures should be anticipated and the patient should be informed that multiple procedures will be necessary. Larger defects of the eyelids often require flaps harvested from the periorbital region. Although these flaps provide larger volumes of tissue for reconstruction, the aesthetic results are compromised by the use of thicker tissue with less pliability. Multiple procedures for insetting and thinning are required to maximize the aesthetic outcome.

ORBITAL ANATOMY

The bony orbit is pyramidal in shape and consists of a medial and lateral wall along with the roof and floor. The surrounding structures include the frontal sinus and anterior cranial fossa superiorly, the nasal cavity and ethmoid and sphenoid sinuses medially, and the maxillary sinus inferiorly. The orbit is formed by seven separate bones including the frontal, zygomatic, maxillary, lacrimal, sphenoid, ethmoid, and palatine.[43] Since the overall dimensions of the orbit are variable, one should perform posterior orbital dissection with caution rather than relying solely on distances from the infraorbital rim to locate the optic canal. The optic foramen lies in the superior medial aspect of the posterior orbit (Figure 87-50).

The anteromedial portion of the orbital roof consists of the supraorbital extension of the frontal sinus. The remainder of the roof of the orbit is made of the thin orbital plate of the frontal bone and the lesser wing of the sphenoid posteriorly. The orbital roof is triangular in shape with a concavity in the superomedial rim, which is the periosteal insertion of the trochlea, and a superolateral concavity behind the edge of the rim, which is the location of the orbital lobe of the lacrimal gland. The orbital roof is very thin and extreme caution should be used during dissection to avoid fracture. The optic canal is located in the orbital apex, which is the posterior extent of the orbital roof. The optic canal is made up of the sphenoid body medially, the lesser sphenoid wing superiorly, and the optic strut, which separates the canal from the superior orbital fissure[15] (see Figure 87-50). The optic canal is 8 to 12 mm in length and 5 to 6 mm in diameter. The shape of the canal changes from a vertically oriented oval at the orbital side to a circular-shaped central canal, which enters the cranium as a horizontally oriented oval.[20] The optic nerve and ophthalmic artery pass through the optic canal.

The floor of the orbit is triangular in shape, extending from the inferior orbital rim to the posterior wall of the maxillary sinus. The majority of the orbital floor is made up of the orbital plate of the maxillary bone, which also forms the roof of the maxillary sinus. The palatine bone lies in the posterior aspect of the floor in the orbital apex. The zygomatic bone makes up the inferolateral orbital rim with a small contribution to the orbital floor. The medial aspect of the anterior orbital floor is the maxilloethmoid suture and the lateral boundary is the zygomaticomaxillary suture. The posterior lateral orbital floor extends to the inferior orbital fissure ending at the pterygopalatine fossa, and the orbital apex should not be considered part of the floor. The floor ends at the posterior antral wall, which is 35 to 40 mm from the inferior orbital rim.[15] The contents of the infraorbital fissure include the maxillary division of the trigeminal nerve, the zygomatic nerve, branches of the sphenopalatine ganglion, the infraorbital artery, and branches

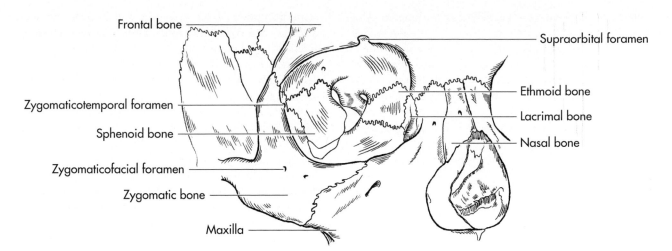

Figure 87-50.   Frontal view of the orbital bones

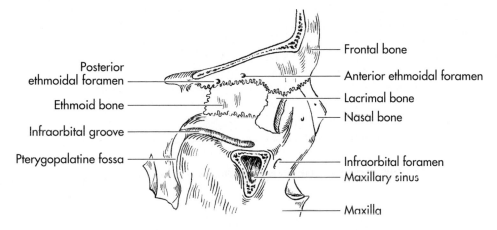

Figure 87-51.   Sagittal view of the medial orbital wall.

of the ophthalmic vein. The infraorbital canal continues as part of the central aspect of the orbital floor and appears as a slightly elevated bony ridge. The canal exits the maxilla as the infraorbital foramen.

The lateral wall of the orbit is made up of the frontal process of the zygomatic bone and the orbital plate of the greater wing of the sphenoid posteriorly. The lateral orbital wall has an oblique orientation at 45 degrees to the midsagittal plane. The thinnest part of the lateral orbital wall is 1 cm posterior to the lateral orbital rim, which facilitates surgical outfracture of the orbit. The lateral wall is separated from the floor by the inferior orbital fissure and the roof by the superior orbital fissure. The superior orbital fissure lies between the greater and lesser wings of the sphenoid. The annulus of Zinn creates the oculomotor foramen, which is an anatomic division of the superior orbital fissure that contains the structures that pass into the intraconal space. The nerves that pass through the oculomotor foramen include the superior and inferior divisions of the oculomotor nerve, the abducens nerve, and the nasociliary nerve. The remaining neurovascular structures exit the superior orbital fissure outside the oculomotor foramen into the extraconal space and include the trochlear nerve, the ophthalmic frontal and lacrimal branches of the trigeminal

nerve, and the ophthalmic veins. Two additional neurovascular structures pass through the lateral wall as the zygomaticotemporal and zygomaticofacial bundles, which represent terminal branches of the lacrimal artery and zygomatic nerves.

The medial orbital wall is parallel to the midsagittal plane and extends from the medial orbital rim to the orbital apex. The four bones that make up the medial wall include the maxillary, lacrimal, sphenoid, and ethmoid bones. The frontal process of the maxilla forms the anterior lacrimal crest and the anterior part of the lacrimal sac fossa (Figure 87-51). The lacrimal bone forms the posterior portion of the lacrimal sac fossa and the posterior lacrimal crest. The lamina papyracea forms the thin medial orbital wall separating the orbit from the ethmoid sinus. Care must be taken during dissection of this area to avoid penetration into the ethmoid sinus. The superior extent of the medial orbital wall is the frontoethmoid suture, which approximates the roof of the ethmoid sinus and the floor of the anterior cranial fossa. The cribriform plate may extend 5 to 10 mm inferior to the floor of the anterior cranial fossa. The anterior and posterior ethmoidal foramina represent important anatomic landmarks by approximating the level of the cribriform plate. During medial wall surgery, dissection should remain inferior to the ethmoidal foramina in the posterior orbit and inferior to the medial canthal tendon in the anterior orbit to avoid injury to the cribriform plate or anterior cranial fossa.[38] The anterior ethmoidal artery and the anterior ethmoidal branch of the nasociliary nerve exit the anterior ethmoidal foramen. The posterior ethmoidal artery and the sphenoethmoidal branch of the nasociliary nerve exit the posterior foramen. The posterior foramen lies 5 to 10 mm anterior to the optic canal. The posterior medial wall is formed by a small portion of the sphenoid bone, which overlies the sphenoid sinus and contributes to the medial portion of the optic canal.

INDICATIONS

The indications for orbital surgery can be broadly divided into the correction of acquired deformities including enophthalmos, exophthalmos, and anophthalmos. The position of the globe relative to the orbital rim is based on a volumetric relationship dependent on the soft tissue volume of the orbital contents and the bony dimensions of the orbit. The bony volume of the adult orbit is approximately 30 cubic cm.[69] Studies have shown that a 3-mm outward displacement of the floor or medial orbital wall associated with a "blow-out" fracture results in a 1.5 cubic cm or 5% increase in orbital volume, which causes 1 to 1.5 mm of enophthalmos.[67] More significant "blow-out" fractures result in greater degrees of enophthalmos. In addition, enophthalmos may occur after trauma or orbital tumor resection due to atrophy of orbital fat.

Similarly, enophthalmos can occur after enucleation. The normal adult globe occupies 7.5 cubic cm of the orbital contents.[69] Following enucleation, reconstruction is commonly performed with a sphere-shaped implant 18 to 20 mm in diameter, which represents 3 to 4 cubic cm. Following placement of the ocular prosthesis, there is generally a deficiency of 5% to 10% of the normal orbital volume, which contributes to enophthalmos and a superior sulcus deformity.

Enophthalmos that measures greater than 5 mm causes significant deformity of the orbit. Enophthalmos is measured by the relative position of the anterior globe to the lateral orbital margin. Although the position of the globe can be evaluated by CT scan with accurate comparison to the contralateral orbit, the most practical measurement is made clinically with a Hertel exophthalmometer. The device uses a prism to view the eye from the lateral position, measuring the distance from the lateral orbital rim to the anterior aspect of the globe. Normal measurements are dependent on the age, sex, and race of the patient and range from 16 to 20 mm. The relative difference between the normal eye is more useful than the absolute value of the involved eye.

The most common cause of enophthalmos is traumatic injury to the orbit. The etiology relates to displacement of a relatively constant volume of orbital soft tissue into an expanded bony orbit from a "blow-out" fracture or from a "tripod" fracture of the zygomatic-maxillary complex.[67] Trau-

matic disruption of the periorbita and ligamentous support structures also contributes to enophthalmos by decreasing the anterior conical projection of the orbital contents. Enophthalmos is often a late finding after orbital trauma and can occur despite early appropriate management of the acute traumatic injury. Additional clinical findings may include diplopia, upper eyelid ptosis, deepening of the superior and inferior orbital sulcus, and depression of the zygomatic prominence (Figure 87-52). Ptosis of the upper eyelid should be evaluated to determine if it is secondary to loss of orbital volume and downward displacement of the globe. This form of pseudoptosis will be corrected along with the correction of the enophthalmos. True ptosis caused by loss of function of the levator from direct trauma or injury to the third cranial nerve will require additional procedures for correction.

Exophthalmos is usually caused by an increase in the soft tissue volume of the orbital contents, which causes the globe to protrude from the bony orbit. The most common causes of exophthalmos are Graves' ophthalmopathy, orbital tumors, and vascular malformations including aneurysms. Pulsatile exophthalmos may be associated with neurofibromatosis causing sphenoid wing erosion and transmission of intracranial pulsations to the orbit.

The most common cause of exophthalmos is secondary to thyroid orbitopathy. Graves' disease often presents in middle-aged women with ophthalmic findings of exophthalmos, lid retraction, and in some patients the gradual onset of diplopia. Patients who present in the acute inflammatory phase should be managed medically with thyroid ablation and at least a 6-month interval for stabilization of orbital and eyelid changes. Indications for surgery during the acute phase are limited to compressive optic neuropathy with impending visual loss that does not respond to medical treatment. The goal of surgery for patients with compressive optic neuropathy is posterior apical orbital decompression in order to relieve pressure on the optic nerve and restore vision. For patients with significant exophthalmos that otherwise have good motility and normal vision, the goal of surgery is to cause retroplacement of the globe in order to restore the eye to a more normal position without causing motility imbalance of the extraocular muscles.[76] Additional indications for early surgery include severe exophthalmos with corneal exposure, entrapment of the eyelids behind the globe, and significant unilateral asymmetry (Figure 87-53). Otherwise, patients with exophthalmos should undergo elective surgery once the acute inflammatory phase has subsided with stabilization of eyelid changes. The sequence of surgery begins with orbital decompression to reduce the degree of exophthalmos. Once adequate globe position has been achieved, the patient should be evaluated for soft tissue surgery. Prior to performing eyelid surgery, clinically significant diplopia may require surgical correction. Patients require a 3-to 6-month healing period following orbital or extraocular muscle surgery before undergoing surgery of the eyelids. The most commonly performed procedures to improve the appearance of the eyelids include tarsolevator recession for the correction of upper lid retraction, and lateral canthoplasty with ear cartilage graft to correct lower lid retraction.

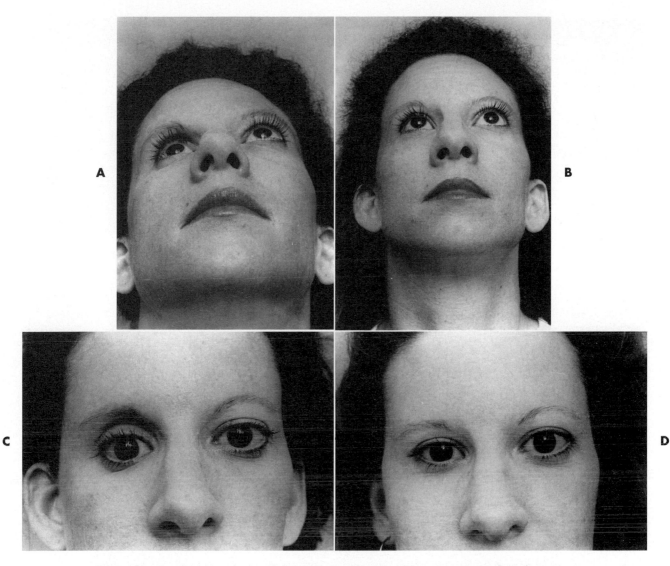

Figure 87-52. **A,** Late right enophthalmos 1 year after tripod fracture with significant bony loss. **B,** Reconstruction required grafting to the orbital floor for correction of the enophthalmos and onlay grafting to the maxilla and zygomatic arch for reconstruction of the midface. **C,** Soft tissue deformity includes deepening of the superior and inferior sulcus. **D,** Eyelid correction was performed with dermis fat graft to the deep superior sulcus and left canthoplasty to reduce the apparent prominence of the opposite eye.

Management of the anophthalmic socket requires both functional and aesthetic considerations. Following surgical removal of the eye, the acquired deformity of the orbit that follows includes enophthalmos, superior sulcus depression, upper lid ptosis, and lower lid laxity with secondary malposition.[52] This constellation of findings has been termed the *anophthalmic orbit syndrome*.[61] Enucleation changes the functional and structural relationship of the orbital soft tissues including the extraocular muscles and levator, Tenon's capsule, orbital fat, and connective tissue. The principles involved in reconstruction of the anophthalmic socket include replacement of the globe with an orbital implant of sufficient volume, preservation and reinsertion of the extraocular muscles for mobility of the prosthesis, adequate mucosal lining of the socket and fornix to accommo-

date a suitable prosthesis, and eyelids with proper anatomic position.

The indications for enucleation include a blind painful eye; a malignant intraocular tumor; trauma to the globe with risk of sympathetic ophthalmia and visual loss to the second eye; phthisis, which carries a risk of malignant degeneration; and congenital microphthalmos or anophthalmos (Figure 87-54).[62] True congenital anophthalmos is rare since there is generally a vestigial ocular remnant. The abnormality involves the orbit, which is underdeveloped, as well as the eyelids, which have severe lid hypoplasia with shallow fornices, contracted palpebral fissure, and poor levator function. Reconstruction of congenital anophthalmos requires multiple-stage procedures aimed at progressive orbital expansion and eyelid reconstruction in order to accommodate a prosthetic eye.

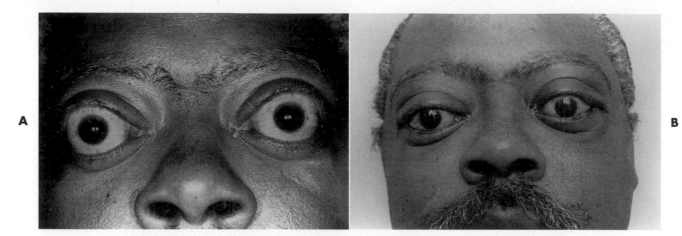

Figure 87-53. **A,** Significant exophthalmos due to Graves' disease with impaired eyelid closure and signs of corneal exposure. **B,** Early postoperative result following bilateral transorbital antroethmoidal decompression with lower lid lateral canthoplasty and no upper lid surgery.

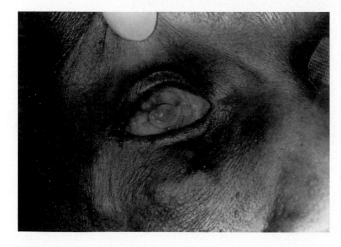

Figure 87-54. Chronic blind painful eye with clinical evidence of sympathetic ophthalmia.

Surgical management of the orbital socket following enucleation in an adult requires an orbital implant of sufficient volume. Central positioning of the implant will maximize the volume replacement within the orbit. Following completion of the final prosthesis, lower lid laxity, superior sulcus deformities, and upper lid ptosis should be corrected as secondary procedures.

OPERATIONS

Late enophthalmos that develops after traumatic injury to the orbit should be evaluated with preoperative CT scan with three-dimensional reconstruction to evaluate the bony volume of the orbit. Patients who had inadequate initial reduction of complex zygomaticomaxillary fractures should be considered

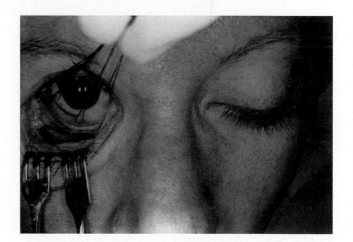

Figure 87-55. Exposure of the orbital floor through a fornix incision with lateral canthotomy using traction sutures in the extraocular muscles for anterior and superior positioning of the globe prior to grafting the orbital floor.

for osteotomies and readvancement with proper reduction of the fracture. Enophthalmos that has occurred despite proper reduction can be managed by building up the orbital floor with an implant to augment the orbital volume. Alloplastic material, hydroxyapatite, and bone grafts can be used.

An inferior fornix incision is preferred with lateral canthotomy to expose the entire orbital floor. Subperiosteal dissection of the orbital floor is performed with complete release of the periorbita. Traction sutures are placed through the tendinous insertions of the extraocular muscles with 4-0 silk in order to retract the globe anteriorly (Figure 87-55). The dead space between the periorbita and the globe represents the soft tissue volume deficiency contributing to the enophthalmos. This can be corrected with a cranial bone graft harvested to the corresponding volume and shaping the graft to rest posterior to the globe for maximal anterior projection. Methylmethacrylate alloplastic material has also been used, which can be easily molded into the posterior orbit to correct the orbital volume deficiency.[21] Care must be taken to irrigate the material during the exothermic reaction, which occurs with hardening, to avoid injury to the eye. Following completion of the infraorbital reconstruction, the stay sutures are used to make sure there is normal ocular motility without restriction from the graft. The reconstruction is completed with closure of the conjunctiva in the fornix with 6-0 plain catgut sutures and lateral canthoplasty to correct lower lid laxity and maintain normal lid position.

A number of surgical approaches exist for surgical decompression of the orbit, ranging from aggressive fat removal to reduce orbital volume to four-wall orbital decompression with a combined neurosurgical approach.[34,64] Each case should be individualized based on the anatomic problem, the degree of compliance of the orbital tissues, ocular motility, and presence of diplopia. Patients with exophthalmos who have good ocular motility, demonstrated by full extraocular range of motion without symptoms of diplopia, and who have easy retroplacement of the globe with gentle pressure generally have the best results following surgical decompression. Two-wall antroethmoidal decompression performed either through the orbit or maxillary antrum is the procedure of choice. This approach appears to have fewer adverse effects on ocular motility and eyelid function than procedures that decompress the posterior lateral orbital wall.

The transorbital approach to surgical decompression of the orbital floor and medial orbital wall is the most commonly performed technique for orbital decompression. Exposure to the inferior orbit is achieved by a transconjunctival inferior fornix incision combined with a lateral canthotomy. Lidocaine with epinephrine is used to infiltrate the fornix, orbital floor, and lateral canthal region. The ethmoid sinus is also blocked, and the nasal cavity is packed with Neo-Synephrine or cocaine. A lateral canthal incision is made, followed by canthotomy and inferior cantholysis. The conjunctiva of the inferior fornix is divided with a needle-tip cautery followed by division of the lower lid retractors. The septum should not be entered unless excessive prolapsing orbital fat requires removal. The periosteum along the inferior orbital rim is divided and the periorbita is elevated, exposing the orbital floor and medial ethmoidal area. Dissection along the medial orbital wall should remain inferior to the frontoethmoidal bony suture line to avoid injury to the cribriform plate.

The thinnest part of the orbital floor lies medial to the infraorbital canal and can easily be fractured with an osteotome. Once a window into the maxillary antrum has been created, Kerrison rongeurs can be used to remove the orbital floor up to the infraorbital neurovascular canal (Figure 87-56). For mild cases of exophthalmos with good motility, decompression of the orbital floor lateral to the infraorbital canal is not necessary. When more aggressive decompression is required, the orbital floor lateral to the canal can be removed with preservation of the neurovascular bundle. The junction between the medial orbital floor and the ethmoid sinus must be resected in order to

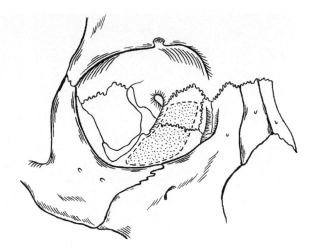

Figure 87-56. Schematic diagram demonstrating the extent of orbital floor decompression using the transorbital antroethmoid approach with preservation of the infraorbital neurovascular bundle.

decompress the medial orbital wall and ethmoidal air cells. The Kerrison or pituitary forceps is used to complete the ethmoidectomy. Hemostasis is achieved with electrocautery and use of surgical packing.

The periorbita is opened in order to complete decompression of the soft tissue orbital contents. Parallel relaxing incisions are made in the periorbita along the medial and lateral extent of the dissection. The window of periorbita is then removed and gentle pressure on the globe causes the orbital fat to prolapse into the osteotomies. This technique can generally achieve 4 to 6 mm of globe retroplacement. In cases of bilateral decompression, retroplacement of the globe can be judged on the first side in order to achieve similar decompression on the opposite side to maintain symmetry (Figure 87-57). The periosteal or periorbital openings can be enlarged if necessary.

Once the decompression is complete, the conjunctiva is closed with a 6-0 plain catgut suture. Lateral canthoplasty is performed with a 4-0 prolene suture with supraplacement of the lateral lid margin to correct any preoperative scleral show. Care should be taken to avoid making the canthoplasty suture tight, which may "clothesline" the lid inferiorly. Postoperative management includes elevation, cool compresses for 48 hours, and liberal use of ophthalmic ointment. Intraoperative and postoperative steroids are recommended to reduce edema.

Alternate approaches for correction of exophthalmos include the transantral antroethmoidal decompression, the transorbital approach to three-wall decompression, and combined transorbital neurosurgical four-wall orbital decompression. The transantral approach utilizes a Caldwell-Luc maxillary antrostomy to expose the orbital apex and posterior ethmoid sinus. This approach is primarily recommended for patients with compressive optic neuropathy because there is better exposure for posterior orbital decompression. Although posterior apical decompression reduces pressure on the optic nerve, it is associated with increased risk of ocular motility disturbances, resulting in postoperative diplopia.[46]

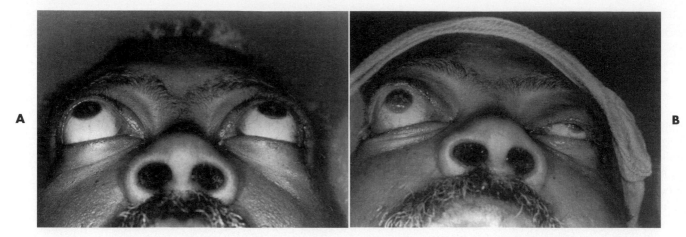

Figure 87-57. **A,** Intraoperative view demonstrating basal view prior to bilateral decompression. **B,** The degree of globe retroplacement can be appreciated following left orbital decompression when compared with the contralateral eye.

The transorbital three-wall decompression combines the standard antroethmoidal two-wall decompression with lateral orbitotomy performed by outfracturing the lateral orbital rim. In addition to increasing the orbital volume, the lateral orbitotomy increases the exposure of the posterior medial orbital wall for apical decompression by allowing the orbital contents to be retracted laterally.[44] The lateral orbital rim can be advanced anteriorly for orbital expansion and fixed with titanium miniplates.[18] Lateral canthoplasty is performed to achieve proper position of the eyelids.

The four-wall decompression has been described for patients with severe exophthalmos and requires a combined orbital and neurosurgical approach.[34] Following the standard lateral orbitotomy and antroethmoidal decompression, a bone cutting drill is used to remove the superolateral portion of the sphenoid wing down to the level of the dura, which overlies the temporal lobe. After completion of the decompression with removal of the orbital roof, the lateral orbital rim is advanced and rigid fixation is achieved with miniplates.

For patients with poorly compliant orbital tissue due to fibrosis who have severe exophthalmos or have failed antroethmoidal decompression, orbital expansion using craniofacial techniques can be used to manage the exophthalmos.[81] Orbital and midfacial expansion are performed by osteotomies, which are used to advance the lateral orbital wall or expand the entire orbital bar with decompression of the medial orbital wall and orbital floor. This approach is generally reserved for more difficult secondary cases.

Surgical management of congenital anophthalmos includes initial treatment with expansion of the socket within the infant's first month. Conformers are placed in the socket with progressive increase in size. A lateral canthotomy may be performed to allow insertion of maximal-sized conformers. Intraorbital dermis fat grafts have been used with gradual increase in the size of the graft concomitant with the child's growth,

resulting in effective orbital expansion.[70] Osteotomies of the orbit with orbital expansion are generally required to achieve the final reconstructive result. Reconstruction of the fornix with mucosal grafts and surgical correction of the hypoplastic lids are performed once adequate orbital expansion has been achieved.

Management of acquired anophthalmos begins with proper enucleation technique with placement of an orbital implant. Following induction of regional or general anesthesia, a self-retaining eyelid speculum is inserted. A 360-degree incision is made in the conjunctiva around the limbus, and Tenon's capsule is undermined to facilitate exposure of the extraocular muscles. Each of the four recti muscles is mobilized with a muscle hook, secured with a double-armed 6-0 Vicryl, and detached from the globe. The tendinous insertions of the oblique muscles are divided from the globe and allowed to retract. The globe and optic nerve are isolated from the extraocular muscles and a tonsil snare is used to divide the optic nerve within the posterior orbit. Once the optic nerve is divided, the central retinal vessels are cauterized to reduce the risk of bleeding.

The orbit can be measured with sizers, and a 20-mm implant is usually used for reconstruction (Figure 87-58). Although there are several options for ocular implants, porous hydroxyapatite spheres are most commonly used. The implant is soaked in gentamicin and placed in a shell of donor sclera. Four rectangular openings are made in the sclera for insertion of the four recti muscles. Following placement of the implant into the intraconal space and reinsertion of the extraocular muscles to the sclera with the Vicryl sutures, the reconstruction is completed with closure of the Tenon's layer and the conjunctiva. A conformer is placed and the lid margins are sutured together for 1 week after surgery. The patient is later referred for placement of an ocular prosthesis and evaluated for peg placement to increase ocular motility.

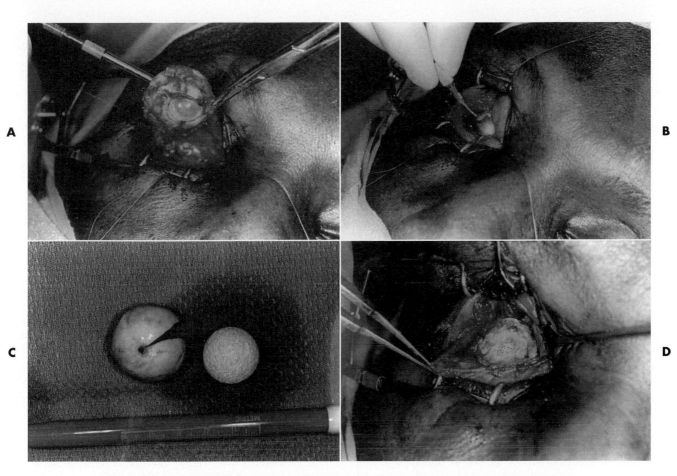

Figure 87-58. **A,** Right enucleation performed using the tonsil snare to divide the optic nerve. **B,** Orbital sizer placed to determine the maximal implant size. **C,** Scleral shell prepared for covering the hydroxyapatite implant. **D,** Placement of the implant into the intraconal space with reinsertion of the extraocular muscles into the scleral shell.

OUTCOMES

Late correction of enophthalmos is difficult to achieve due to fibrosis and contraction of the extraocular muscles. Patients often require multiple procedures aimed at the restoration of normal bony orbital volume and correction of soft tissue and eyelid deformities. Complications include resorption of bone grafts with recurrent enophthalmos, extraocular muscle imbalance, lower lid malposition, and superior sulcus deformity.[43] Recurrent enophthalmos may occur following the use of autogenous cranial bone, iliac bone, or rib grafts because of resorption of the graft material, and slight overcorrection at the time of the initial procedure may prevent this. Although use of alloplastic material prevents loss of volume due to resorption, there is an additional associated risk of infection.

Extraocular muscle imbalance with diplopia is not uncommon after orbital trauma because of direct injury to the extraocular muscles with late fibrosis and ptosis of the globe from increase in orbital volume. Muscle surgery may be required and should be performed 6 months following completion of surgery aimed at orbital reconstruction. The aim of extraocular muscle surgery is to achieve binocular vision in primary gaze and downgaze. Lower lid malposition may include ectropion or scleral show from scar contracture secondary to previous reconstructive procedures. Deformity of the lateral canthus may occur from downward displacement of the lateral orbital segment. After completion of bony reconstruction, secondary procedures including lateral canthoplasty may be necessary to correct lid malposition and canthal deformities. The superior sulcus deformity, which commonly occurs after orbital trauma or following enucleation, is secondary to the loss of orbital soft tissue volume and results from contraction of the superior rectus and levator muscles. This is managed by placement of a dermis fat graft. An elliptical graft is taken from the hip and placed in the preaponeurotic space. The deepithelialized side of the graft is oriented anteriorly and the fat is positioned posteriorly with overcorrection of the sulcus to account for postoperative fat resorption.

Complications after orbital decompression for exophthalmos include extraocular muscle imbalance with diplopia, residual proptosis, and hypoglobus. Early postoperative complications include edema, bleeding, and infection. Posterior decompression of the orbital apex is associated with risk of optic nerve injury. Examination of the patient's vision should be performed at regular intervals. Hematoma may occur from the anterior or posterior ethmoidal arteries as well as from the mucosal or bony surfaces, and immediate evacuation is necessary. Signs of sinusitis may develop after orbital decompression and should be treated with antibiotics and decongestants. Sinus drainage and placement of a nasoantral window may be necessary for persistent problems.

Patients frequently require multiple procedures including orbital surgery followed by extraocular muscle surgery for the correction of diplopia. Complications that are frequently seen after muscle surgery include orbital edema, which may result in a degree of recurrent exophthalmos. Eyelid surgery is performed to minimize the appearance of residual proptosis and reduce the risk of corneal exposure. Lateral canthoplasty with release of the lower lid retractors and ear cartilage graft may be required to correct residual lower lid retraction. Upper lid retraction may appear to worsen after orbital decompression due to the relative hypoglobus that occurs. This is managed by tarsolevator recession once the globe position has stabilized. Multiple surgical procedures for correction of eyelid position following orbital decompression should be anticipated.

Complications that occur following enucleation include enophthalmos, lower lid malposition, ptosis, and implant complications. Management of the sulcus deformity can be performed with dermis fat grafting techniques. Moreover, the ocularist can use the prosthetic eye to fill the sulcus and areas of soft tissue deficiency. With time, however, the prosthesis puts pressure on the lower lid, resulting in lower lid laxity and malposition[79] and requiring lateral canthoplasty to correct lower lid laxity and reinforce the lower lid for support of the prosthesis. Instability of the medial canthus will result in displacement of the inferior punctum with lateral canthoplasty and therefore requires a fascia sling to provide medial and lateral support.

Correction of upper lid ptosis should be performed after deformities of the superior sulcus and lower lid have been corrected. Although evaluation of the levator may reveal normal function, ptosis is caused by functional lengthening of the levator from laxity due to lack of support from the spherical implant compared with the more vertically shaped ocular globe. Additionally, dehiscence of the levator aponeurosis is common after trauma or following enucleation. An external tarsolevator aponeurotic advancement is performed if adequate levator function is present, or frontalis suspension when levator function is poor or absent.

Complications related to the orbital implant include migration or extrusion of the implant. Studies have found that up to two thirds of implants placed within Tenon's capsule migrate out of position.[73] Superior migration of the implant causes inferior displacement of the prosthesis, which may contribute to lower lid malposition. Inferior implant migration will interfere with the ability of the fornix to retain the prosthesis. Early extrusion is due to acute infection or surgical dehiscence from an implant that may be too large, late extrusion to chronic infection or erosion by a poorly fitting prosthesis. Both mandate removal of the implant with a course of intravenous antibiotics. Once the infection has been adequately treated, reconstruction can proceed with a smaller implant or replacement with a dermis fat graft. Dermis fat grafts provide significant orbital volume replacement and rarely undergo migration or extrusion.

REFERENCES

1. Bartley GB, Kay PP: Posterior lamellar eyelid reconstruction with a hard palate mucosal graft, *Am J Ophthalmol* 107:609-612, 1989.
2. Baylis HI, Pernam KI, Fee DR, et al: Autogenous auricular cartilage grafting for lower eyelid retraction, *Ophthal Plast Reconstr Surg* 1:23-27, 1985.
3. Baylis HI, Rosen N, Neuhaus RW: Obtaining auricular cartilage for reconstructive surgery, *Am J Ophthalmol* 93:709-712, 1982.
4. Boniuk M, Zimmerman LE: Sebaceous carcinoma of the eyelid, eyebrow, caruncle, and orbit, *Trans Am Acad Ophthalmol Otolaryngol* 72:619-642, 1968.
5. Bostwick J, Eaves FF, Nahai F: *Endoscopic plastic surgery,* St Louis, 1995, Quality Medical Publishing.
6. Brownstein MH, Helwig EB: Subcutaneous dermoid cysts, *Arch Dermatol* 107:237-239, 1973.
7. Callahan MA, Callahan A: Mustarde flap lower eyelid reconstruction after malignancy, *Ophthalmology* 87:279, 1980.
8. Codner MA, McCord CD, Hester TR: The lateral canthoplasty, *Op Tech Plast Surg* 5:90-98, 1998.
9. Cohen MS, Shoit N: Eyelid reconstruction with hard palate mucosa grafts, *Ophthal Plast Reconstr Surg* 8:183-195, 1992.
10. Cutler N, Beard C: A method for partial and total upper lid reconstruction, *Am J Ophthalmol* 39:1-7, 1955.
11. Doxanas MT, Green WR: Sebaceous gland carcinoma: review of 40 cases, *Arch Ophthalmol* 102:245-249, 1984.
12. Doxanas MT, Green WR, Iliff CE: Factors in the successful surgical management of basal cell carcinoma of the eyelids, *Am J Ophthalmol* 91:726, 1981.
13. Doxanas MT, Iliff WJ, Iliff NT, et al: Squamous cell carcinoma of the eyelids, *Ophthalmology* 94:538-544, 1987.
14. Dutton JJ: *Clinical and surgical orbital anatomy,* Philadelphia, 1994, WB Saunders.
15. Dutton JJ: Osteology of the orbit. In Dutton JJ, editor: *Clinical and surgical orbital anatomy,* Philadelphia, 1994, WB Saunders.
16. Fricke JCG: *Die bildung neuer augenlider (Blepharoplastik) nach zerstorungen und dadurch hervorgebrachten auswartswendungen derselben,* Hamburg, 1829, Perthes and Bessler.
17. Furnas DW: The retaining ligaments of the cheek, *Plast Reconstr Surg* 83:11-16, 1989.
18. Glassman RD, Manson PN, Vanderkolk CA, et al: Rigid fixation of internal orbital fractures, *Plast Reconstr Surg* 86:1103-1109, 1990.

19. Glatt HJ, Putterman AM, Van Aalst JJ, et al: Adrenal suppression and growth retardation after injection of periocular capillary hemangioma with corticosteroids, *Ophthalmic Surg* 22(2):95-97, 1991.

20. Goalwin HA: One thousand optic canals: clinical, anatomic, and roentgenologic study, *JAMA* 89:1745, 1922.

21. Gossman MD, Pollock RA: Acute orbital trauma: diagnosis and treatment. In McCord CD, Tanenbaum M, Nunery WR, editors: *Oculoplastic surgery,* New York, 1995, Raven.

22. Hamra ST: Arcus marginalis release and orbital fat preservation in mid-face rejuvenation, *Plast Reconstr Surg* 96:354-362, 1995.

23. Hendley RL, Rieser JC, Cavanagh HD, et al: Primary radiation therapy for meibomian gland carcinoma, *Am J Ophthalmol* 87:206-209, 1979.

24. Hester TR, Codner MA, McCord CD: Subperiosteal malar cheek lift with lower blepharoplasty. In McCord CD, Codner MA, editors: *Eyelid surgery: principles and techniques,* Philadelphia, 1995, Lippincott-Raven.

25. Hewes EH, Sullivan JH, Beard C: Lower eyelid reconstruction by tarsal transposition, *Am J Ophthalmol* 81:512-514, 1976.

26. Hughes WH: A new method for rebuilding a lower lid: report of a case, *Arch Ophthalmol* 17:1008-1017, 1937.

27. Hughes WH: Reconstruction of the lids, *Am J Ophthalmol* 28:1203-1211, 1945.

28. Jackson IT, Carbonnel A, Potparic Z, et al: Orbitotemporal neurofibromatosis: classification and treatment, *Plast Reconstr Surg* 92:1-11, 1993.

29. Jackson IT, Carreno R, Potparic Z, et al: Hemangiomas, vascular malformations, and lymphovenous malformations: classification and methods of treatment, *Plast Reconstr Surg* 91:1216-1230, 1993.

30. Jakobiec FA, Brownstein S: Cryotherapy for conjunctival melanotic neoplasms. In Jakobiec FA, Sigelman J, editors: *Advanced techniques in ocular surgery,* Philadelphia, 1984, WB Saunders.

31. Jones LT, Reeh M, Wirtschafter JD: *Ophthalmic anatomy,* Rochester, Minn, 1976, American Academy of Ophthalmology and Otolaryngology.

32. Jordan DR: Reconstruction of the upper eyelid. In Bosniak S, editor: *Ophthalmic plastic and reconstructive surgery,* Philadelphia, 1996, WB Saunders.

33. Kazanjian VH, Roopenian A: Median forehead flaps in the repair of defects of the nose and surrounding areas, *Trans Am Acad Ophthalmol Otolaryngol* 60:557-566, 1956.

34. Kennerdell JS, Maroon JC: An orbital decompression for severe dysthyroid exophthalmos, *Ophthalmology* 89:467-472, 1982.

35. Kersten RC, Kulwin DR, Levartovsky S, et al: Management of lower-lid retraction with hard palate grafting, *Arch Ophthalmol* 108:1339-1343, 1990.

36. Kikkawa DO, Lemke BN, Dortzbach RK: Relations of the superficial musculoaponeurotic system to the orbit and characterization of the orbitomalar ligament, *Ophthal Plast Reconstr Surg* 12:77-78, 1996.

37. Kroll SS, Reece GP, Robb G, et al: Deep plane cervicofacial rotation-advancement flap for reconstruction of large cheek defects, *Plast Reconstr Surg* 94:88-93, 1994.

38. Kurihashi K, Yamashita A: Anatomical consideration for dacryocystorhinostomy, *Ophthalmologica* 203:1, 1991.

39. Leibsohn JM, Hahn F: Medial canthal reconstruction with nasal periosteum, *Ophthal Plast Reconstr Surg* 8:35-40, 1992.

40. Lisman RD, Jakobiec FA, Small P: Sebaceous carcinoma of the eyelids, *Ophthalmology* 96:1021-1026, 1989.

41. Lund HZ, Tumors of the skin. In *Armed Forces Institute of Pathology, section 1, fascicle 2,* Washington, DC, 1957, Armed Forces Institute of Pathology, pp 205-234.

42. Lund HZ: How often does squamous cell carcinoma of the skin metastasize? *Arch Dermatol* 92:635-637, 1965.

43. McCarthy JG, Jelks GW, Valauri AJ, et al: The orbit and zygoma. In McCarthy JG, editor: *Plastic surgery,* Philadelphia, 1990, WB Saunders.

44. McCord CD: A combined medial and lateral orbitotomy for exposure of the optic nerve and orbital apex, *Ophthalmic Surg* 9:58-66, 1978.

45. McCord CD, Chen WP: Tarsal polishing and mucous membrane grafting for cicatricial entropion, trichiasis, and epidermalization, *Ophth Surg* 14:1021-1025, 1983.

46. McCord CD: Current trends in orbital decompression, *Ophthalmology* 92:21-33, 1985.

47. McCord CD, Wesley R: Reconstruction of upper eyelid and medial canthus. In McCord CD, Tannenbaum M, editors: *Oculoplastic surgery,* New York, 1987, Raven.

48. McCord CD, Ellis DS: The correction of lower lid malposition following lower blepharoplasty, *Plast Reconstr Surg* 92:1068-1072, 1993.

49. McCord CD, Codner MA: *Eyelid surgery,* Philadelphia, 1995, Lippincott-Raven.

50. McGregor IA: *Fundamental techniques of plastic surgery,* New York, 1989, Churchill Livingstone.

51. McNab AA: Early division of the conjunctival pedicle in modified Hughes repair of the lower eyelid, *Ophthalmic Surg Lasers* 27:422-424, 1996.

52. Migliori ME: Evaluation and management of the anophthalmic socket. In Bosniak S, editor: *Ophthalmic plastic and reconstructive surgery,* Philadelphia, 1996, WB Saunders.

53. Millard DR Jr: Eyelid repairs with a chondromucosal graft, *Ophthal Plast Reconstr Surg* 30:267-272, 1962.

54. Milstone EB, Helwig EB: Basal cell carcinoma in children, *Arch Dermatol* 108:523-527, 1973.

55. Moller R, Reymann F, Hou-Jensen K: Metastasis in dermatological patients with squamous cell carcinoma, *Arch Dermatol* 115:703-705, 1979.

56. Mustarde JC: *Repair and reconstruction in the orbital region,* Edinburgh, 1971, Churchill Livingstone.

57. Mustarde JC: *Repair and reconstruction of the orbital region: a practical guide,* Edinburgh, 1980, Churchill Livingstone.

58. Mustarde JC: Eyelid reconstruction, *Orbit* 1:33-43, 1982.

59. Nelson BR, Railan D, Cohen S: Mohs' micrographic surgery for nonmelanoma skin cancers, *Clin Plast Surg* 24:705-718, 1997.

60. Nerad JA, Whitaker DC: Periocular basal cell carcinoma in adults 35 years of age and younger, *Am J Ophthalmol* 106:723-729, 1988.

61. Nolan WB, Vistnes LM: Correction of lower eyelid ptosis in the anophthalmic orbit: a long-term follow-up, *Plast Reconstr Surg* 72:289-292, 1983.

62. Nunery WR, Chen WP: Enucleation and evisceration. In Bosniak S, editor: *Ophthalmic plastic and reconstructive surgery,* Philadelphia, 1996, WB Saunders.

63. Okazaki M, Haramoto U, Akizuki T, et al: Avoiding ectropion by using the Mitek anchor system for flap fixation to the facial bones, *Ann Plast Surg* 40:169-173, 1998.

64. Olivari N: Transpalpebral decompression of endocrine ophthalmopathy (Graves' disease) by removal of intraorbital fat: experience with 147 operations over 5 years, *Plast Reconstr Surg* 87:627-641, 1991.

65. Orengo IF, Salasche SJ, Fewkes J, et al: Correlation of histologic subtypes of primary basal cell carcinoma and number of Mohs' stages required to achieve a tumor free plane, *L Am Acad Dermatol* 37:395-397, 1997.

66. Owsley J: Lifting the malar fat pad for correction of prominent nasolabial folds, *Plast Reconstr Surg* 91:463-476, 1993.

67. Parsons GS, Mathog RH: Orbital wall and volume relationships. *Arch Otolaryngol Head Neck Surg* 114:743, 1988.

68. Rao NA, Hidayat AA, McLean LW, et al: Sebaceous carcinomas of the ocular adnexa: a clinicopathologic study of 104 cases, with five year follow-up data, *Human Pathol* 13:113-122, 1982.

69. Rizen AJ, Nikolic V, Banovic B: The role of orbital wall morphologic properties and their supporting structures in the etiology of "blow out" fractures, *Surg Radiol Anat* 11:241, 1989.

70. Shore JW, McCord CD, Bergin DJ, et al: Management of complications following dermis-fat grafting for anophthalmic socket reconstruction, *Ophthalmology* 92:1342-1350, 1985.

71. Shore JW, Rubin PAD, Bilyk J: Repair of telecanthus by anterior fixation of cantilevered miniplates, *Ophthalmology* 99:1133-1138, 1992.

72. Smith B, Obear MF: Bridge flap technique for reconstruction of large upper lid defects, *Plast Reconstr Surg* 38:45-48, 1966.

73. Soll DB: Evolution and current concepts in the surgical treatment of the anophthalmic orbit, *Ophthalmic Plast Reconstr Surg* 2:163-171, 1986.

74. Stigmar G, Crawford JS, Ward CM, et al: Ophthalmic sequelae of infantile hemangiomas of the eyelids and orbit, *Am J Ophthalmol* 85:806-813, 1978.

75. Szymanski FJ: Keratoacanthoma. In Graham JH, Johnson WC, Helwig EG, editors: *Dermal pathology,* Hagerstown, MD, 1972, Harper & Row, pp 625-635.

76. Tanenbaum M: Orbital decompression for Graves' orbitopathy. In Bosniak S, editor: *Ophthalmic plastic and reconstructive surgery,* Philadelphia, 1996, WB Saunders.

77. Tenzel RR, Stewart WB: Eyelid reconstruction by semi-circular flap technique, *Trans Am Soc Ophthalmol Otolaryngol* 85:1164-1169, 1978.

78. Tripier L: Du lambeau musculocutane en forme de pont applique a la restauration des paupieres, *Rev Chir,* 4, 1890.

79. Vistnes LM, Iverson RE, Laub DR: The anophthalmic orbit: surgical correction of lower eyelid ptosis, *Plast Reconstr Surg* 52:346-351, 1973.

80. Wesley RE: Medial canthal fixation in transnasal wiring. In McCord CD, Tannenbaum M, editors: *Oculoplastic surgery,* New York, 1987, Raven.

81. Wolfe SA: Modified three-wall orbital expansion to correct persistent exophthalmos or exorbitism, *Plast Reconstr Surg* 64:448-455, 1979.

CHAPTER 88

The Nose

Frederick J. Menick

INDICATIONS

Anatomically, the nose is made of thin, pliable, vascular lining; sculptured alar tip cartilages and bone and cartilage braces that buttress the dorsum and sidewalls; and a thin vascular canopy of skin that matches the face in color, texture, and hair-bearing quality. If all or part of the nose is missing, the requirements for reconstruction will depend on the extent of cover, support, and lining loss. The goals of restoration are, ideally, restoration of function and a normal and attractive nasal appearance, while also avoiding obstruction due to soft tissue collapse or excess bulk or a constricting scar.

Nasal defects that follow the surgical excision of skin cancer require the replacement of external skin and varying amounts of deeper tissues, depending on tumor extension. Basal cell carcinoma is the most common problem, growing slowly and locally and sometimes leading to severe deformity and death with orbital and central nervous system extension. Squamous cell carcinoma is less common but associated with more aggressive local growth and lymph node metastasis. Melanoma is even less common but more frequently associated with lymph node and systemic spread. Electrodesiccation and cryotherapy are destructive techniques frequently employed by dermatologists for small, superficial, primary basal cell carcinomas with well-defined borders. All other skin cancers are treated with surgical excision. Prior to removal, an incisional biopsy is performed to verify the histologic diagnosis of basal cell and squamous cell carcinoma. An excisional biopsy is used for all but large melanomas. Radiation therapy may be a safe, noninvasive treatment for selected basal cell and squamous cell carcinomas, but is usually limited to elderly patients who are poor surgical candidates due to the risk of postradiation osteitis and chondritis or other late radiation sequelae, including carcinogenesis. The cosmetic effects of radiation therapy can be good but vary with site, extent of disease, and expertise of the treating radiotherapist. Because head and neck surgery is associated with minimal systemic morbidity, surgical excision and reconstruction are the usually preferred therapy for significant skin cancers.

Skin cancers will recur unless adequately excised.[2] Surgical excision with examination of the specimen margin by permanent or frozen sections is adequate for small primary tumors with visible clinical margins, but may be inadequate in other circumstances. Certainly, all peripheral and deep margins must be examined for tumor extension and reexcised until clear. Mohs' micrographic surgery uses a technique of microscopically guided cold knife excision, which is particularly valuable for nasal lesions. All clinically visible tumor is excised in saucerlike layers, marking the exact size and shape of the tumor. Horizontal frozen sections from the undersurface of the excised specimen are examined microscopically, reexcising all tumor extensions as required. Mohs' surgical excision may be indicated for basal cell and squamous cell carcinomas that are large (greater than 2 cm), are recurrent, have poorly defined clinical borders, are morphea or sclerosing histology, or arise in "difficult" locations such as the nose, eye, or ear. The cure rate for a primary basal cell carcinoma by Mohs' excision is 99%, and for squamous cell carcinoma 95%. Recurrent tumors have cure rates of 95% and 90%, respectively. Because the cure rates of Mohs' frozen section excision are so high, delayed primary reconstruction can yield excellent results. Melanomas are excised with 1-, 2-, or 3-cm margins, depending on whether the tumor has a depth of less than 1 mm, 1 to 4 mm, or greater than 4 mm, respectively, verified by permanent section examination. Facial avulsion, human bites, and burns also present as skin losses with variable cartilage support and lining deficits.

Destruction or loss of nasal support alone may be an isolated sequela of facial fracture, but septal cartilage destruction without external cover loss more often follows intranasal lining necrosis due to the infectious complications of syphilis, leprosy or noma, or the illicit intranasal use of cocaine.[24] Inflammation and destruction of nasal mucosal lining exposes and devascularizes septal cartilage. Progressive nasal collapse due to loss of support and contraction of the lining follows. Except for full-thickness injuries due to noma or meningococcemia, the nasal skin cover may be relatively uninjured yet difficult to reexpand. Although not common, the multiply-operated cosmetic rhinoplasty cripple can present with scarred, contracted or excised nasal lining; absent or distorted nasal bone and cartilage framework; and avascular scarred and contracted external skin covering, which may require replacement of all three layers.

PREOPERATIVE ANALYSIS

The first step in nasal reconstruction is to make the diagnosis and formulate a plan.[1,3,7,8] The surgeon may have the opportunity to examine the patient prior to surgical excision of a skin cancer. A rough estimate of the tumor size and spread, as well as a visual determination of the wound likely to be present after excision, can be made. In other cases, the patient will present with an acute or old nasal defect following Mohs' surgery, trauma, or infection. It must be remembered that the apparent defect may not reflect what is actually missing. In acute wounds, edema, local anesthesia, gravity, and skin tension distort the tissues, usually enlarging the defect. In old wounds, secondary healing will draw the wound edges inward by contraction, decreasing the size. A previous repair that has simply patched the defect may further distort the original problem, wasting valuable donor materials or destroying the blood supply to useful flaps. The apparent defect may not be the true defect.

A clinical examination combined with an evaluation of medical photographs and if possible preinjury photographs will usually supply adequate information to make a surgical plan. Occasionally radiologic evaluation of large, complex defects involving bone or extensive soft tissue lesions by computed tomography (CT) scan or magnetic resonance imaging (MRI) is helpful. The surgeon must examine the defect in his or her mind's eye, repositioning the normal to its premorbid position to determine the three-dimensional character of actual anatomic loss.

The reconstructive surgeon, while evaluating the "hole," must also understand facial aesthetics and know the "normal."[29,31-34] Too frequently a facial defect is seen simply as an absence, a "hole to be filled." The surgeon becomes absorbed in examining the crater rather than in visualizing the three-dimensional facial feature that is absent. The emphasis may be placed only on anatomy or blood supply (flaps or grafts), looking to an encyclopedia of flaps or the reconstructive ladder to provide answers. Without an aesthetic goal clearly in mind, the operative planning is vague, nonspecific, unguided, inexact, and poorly staged.

It is frequently taught that a flap should be made smaller than the defect to conserve the donor site, or the flap made larger than the defect for safety's sake. If, however, such directions are followed, too much or too little tissue will be supplied and landmark symmetry distorted. Similarly, distortion caused by swelling or wound contraction may render an exact pattern of a defect inadequate. Even when enough bulk is successfully brought to a nasal defect, revisions may be poorly conceived and not integrated into an overall plan to restore the facial feature. The "hole" may be filled or the wound healed, but a normal appearance not restored.

Patients must be given choice and appropriate preoperative counseling. The defect can be allowed to heal by secondary intention or closed primarily by skin graft or flap. The number of surgical stages, donor morbidity, anesthesia requirements, and cost must be discussed; however, most patients are fastidious and wish the missing part to be restored to its original color, texture, contour, and function.

Reconstructive rhinoplasty may impair nasal function. After nasal amputation, the airways are patent unless clogged by bulky tissue or the contracted scars of failed attempts at surgical repair. Only by the judicious choice of pliable donor materials and the primary replacement of nasal support to anticipate the force of myofibroblast contraction can airway patency be maintained.

AESTHETIC NASAL RECONSTRUCTION

The external surface of the nose is crossed by ridges and valleys that separate it into slightly convex or concave surfaces—the tip, dorsum, paired sidewalls, alar lobules, and soft triangles. The nose is an aesthetic unit of the face, and the smaller parts are called regional or topographic subunits (Figure 88-1). Each regional unit is an adjacent topographic area with characteristic skin quality, outline, and contour.[3,6,8,28] The nose is a central facial unit seen in primary gaze with fixed outlines and landmarks. Reconstruction must be accurate because the opposite or contralateral side of each subunit (e.g., ala, hemitip) is available for immediate visual comparison. If part or all of the

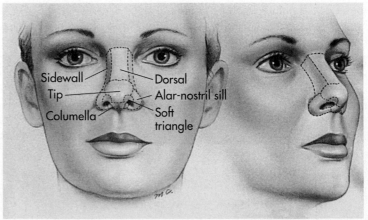

Figure 88-1. The nasal subunits: the dorsum, tip, columella and paired sidewalls, alae, and soft triangles. (From Burget G, Menick F: *Aesthetic reconstruction of the nose*, St Louis, 1994, Mosby.)

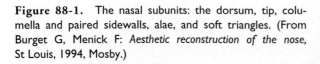

nose is missing, the basic elements that make a nose must be provided, deficiencies minimized, and the jarring abnormality mitigated so the repair does not draw attention to itself. To achieve the appearance of normal, the goal must be to restore the expected regional skin quality, subunit outline, and three-dimensional contour as it was before injury.

THE RESTORATION OF NASAL SKIN QUALITY

To look normal, the nose must be resurfaced with skin that matches the face in color and texture. The skin of the nose varies in texture and thickness over the nasal surface. The upper two thirds of the nose is covered by thin, smooth, mobile skin, whereas most of the lower third is thick and pitted, except along the alar rim and columella (Figure 88-2). These thick and thin skin zones do not correspond to subunit contour or outline, and are distinct from regional units.

Traditionally, the choice of the method of tissue transfer has been based on wound vascularity and defect depth. Skin grafts resurface well-vascularized superficial defects when only skin and a small amount of subcutaneous tissue are missing. Skin flaps resupply bulk to deep defects and cover a poorly vascularized recipient site or a wound with vital or support structures exposed or missing. Donor sites above the clavicle seem best suited for facial repair because cervicofacial skin has a better color and texture match than distant tissue.

Equally important to successful reconstruction is the effect of wound healing on grafts and flaps. Although a skin graft donor site may be chosen preoperatively because it matches in color and texture, the transient ischemia associated with skin graft take causes unpredictable color and texture changes after transfer. Postoperatively, skin grafts are typically shiny, atrophic, and hypopigmented or hyperpigmented. Also, a skin graft may shrink but rarely pincushions. Thus a shiny skin graft may be a good choice when used to resurface a superficial defect within the shiny, nonpitted skin of the nasal sidewall, but will stand out as a mismatched patch if used within the pitted, sebaceous tip where a flap would be a better choice. Skin flaps, in contrast, maintain their donor characteristics but have a tendency to pincushion and elevate above the surface of the defect, appearing as a bulge above adjacent normal skin. For these reasons, a flap is best employed to repair convex subunits within the rough, textured ala or tip.

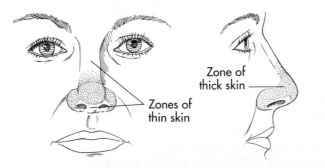

Figure 88-2. Zones of skin thickness. (From Burget G, Menick F: *Aesthetic reconstruction of the nose,* St Louis, 1994, Mosby.)

CREATING A SUBUNIT OUTLINE

If a normal nose is defined by its regional unit, then the surgeon must recreate the character of these subunits and not simply heal the wound or fill the defect. The presence or absence of scars is of much lesser importance.

If a graft or flap is designed from a pattern of a defect without regard to subunits, the repair may look like a distracting patch within the unit; however, if the defect is resurfaced so that the entire subunit is recovered, the quality of the nasal unit surface will be maintained. When practical, grafts and flaps should be designed to replace entire topographic units. When skin is replaced as a subunit rather than simply patching the defect, the scar is positioned in the joints between adjacent units, and the contractile force of the myofibroblast, which lies in the bed of scar under all transposed skin, is harnessed to simulate the surface contour of convex units. This means that the surgeon should take charge of the defect and not let the requirements of skin cancer excision or a traumatic injury dictate the extent of reconstruction required to achieve the best result.

The wound must be manipulated so that the reconstruction conforms to subunit principles,[9,18] which may demand changing position, size, outline, and depth. The defect may be enlarged, discarding adjacent normal skin so that an entire unit is resurfaced rather than part of it. As a general rule, if a defect encompasses more than 50% of a subunit, then residual normal skin is excised, enlarging the defect and permitting the replacement of subunit skin as a unit. If the defect encompasses more than one unit and extends into another, the wound margins may be advanced inward, positioning the scar along the border of adjacent units and allowing reconstruction of a single unit. Another approach is to enlarge the defect and resurface both units with a single flap, two separate flaps, or a flap and skin graft, depending on the wound and aesthetic requirements.

Tissue must be replaced in the exact amount necessary to restore a normal facial appearance. Exact three-dimensional foil templates should be made of the unit defect requiring reconstruction. If too much skin is supplied, it will contract postoperatively and obscure the detail created by an underlying support framework. If too little is supplied, it will be too tight, causing underlying cartilage grafts to collapse. The contralateral normal unit or subunit, or the ideal, can be used as a guide to create a template that exactly replaces the missing surface skin in size and outline. The defect, distorted by edema, wound tension, or late contraction, does not reflect the true dimensions of tissue loss.

Composite defects are those that overlap two or more facial contour units. Often a nasal defect will extend into the adjacent lip or cheek, producing a large three-dimensional wound that encompasses several facial units. The simplest solution is to fill the hole and replace missing bulk. This satisfies the basic objective of obtaining a healed wound but fails to position resultant scars so that they are hidden in normal contour lines. It is also difficult to reproduce the delicate three-dimensional character of multiple units with one flap. The inevitable force of wound contraction, the trapdoor effect, draws the flap into a domelike mass. Late attempts to divide and shape the single large flap and individual convex and concave surface contours are rarely successful. Also, if a defect encompasses parts of the cheek, lip, and nose, the cheek

and lip should be reconstructed at an initial operation. Once the platform is healed and the wound stable, the nose is rebuilt at a later operation. Cheek is used to restore the cheek unit; lip for lip[4,38,44]; and a forehead or nasolabial flap for the nose (Figure 88-3).

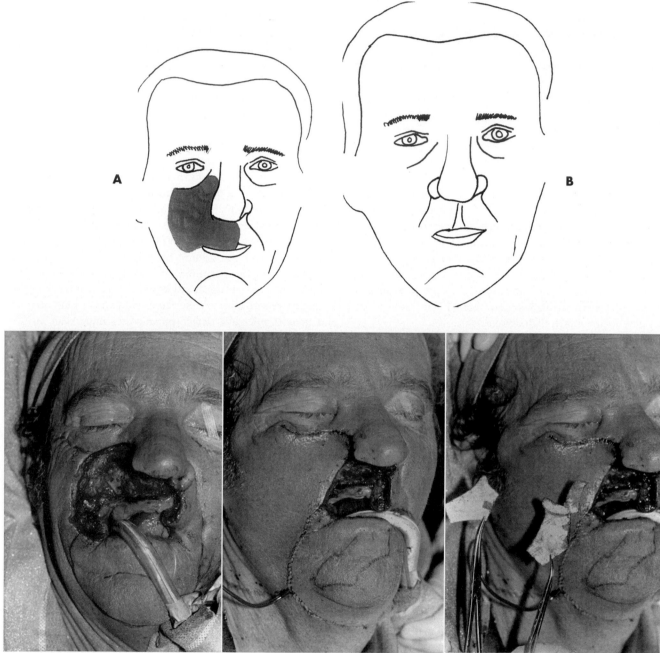

Figure 88-3. **A,** Composite defects overlap two or more facial units. As with any defect, they must be analyzed in terms of both anatomic (cover, lining, and support) and subunit visual unit loss. **B,** To restore the normal, the surgeon must visualize the skin quality, unit outline, and contour that determine the visual normal. **C,** This patient's composite defect includes a major loss of the medial cheek, two thirds of the upper lip, columella, and full-thickness right ala. **D,** First, a laterally based cheek flap, whose scar follows the nasolabial crease, is rotated to resurface the cheek unit. **E,** A pattern is made of the missing right lateral lip unit as well as an extended pattern to include the nostril sill and columella. This is used to design a cross-lip subunit midline Abbe flap to replace the missing one half of the upper lip, nasal sill, and columella. (**A** to **C** and **E** to **N,** From Menick F, Burget G: *Advan Plast Surg* 6:193, 1990.)

Continued

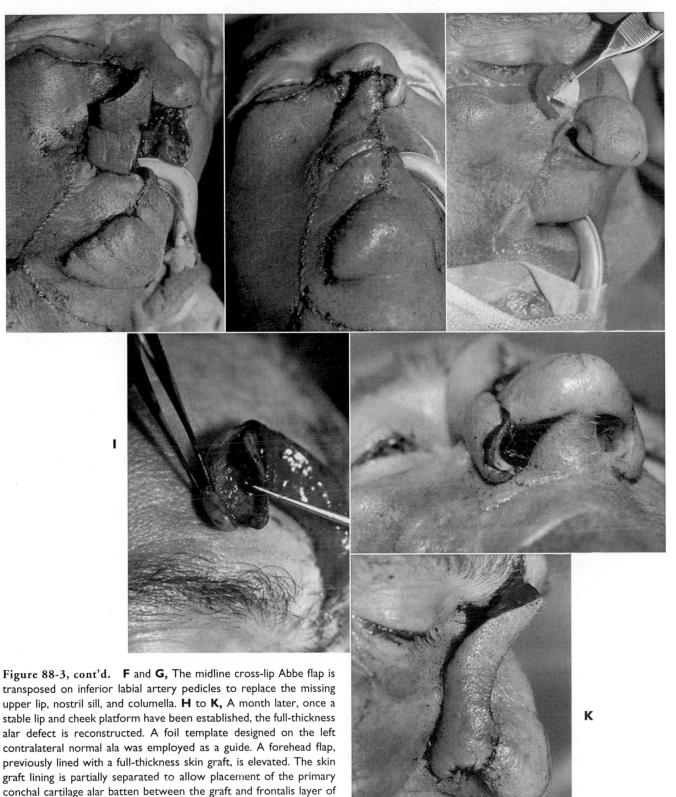

Figure 88-3, cont'd.   F and **G,** The midline cross-lip Abbe flap is transposed on inferior labial artery pedicles to replace the missing upper lip, nostril sill, and columella. **H** to **K,** A month later, once a stable lip and cheek platform have been established, the full-thickness alar defect is reconstructed. A foil template designed on the left contralateral normal ala was employed as a guide. A forehead flap, previously lined with a full-thickness skin graft, is elevated. The skin graft lining is partially separated to allow placement of the primary conchal cartilage alar batten between the graft and frontalis layer of the forehead flap. The forehead flap is positioned to reconstruct the right alar unit.   *Continued*

RECREATING A NASAL CONTOUR

The lighted ridges and shadow valleys of normal nasal contour reflect the underlying configuration of hard and soft tissue.[8] An ideal contour must be the primary reconstructive objective and its attainment integrated into the initial and all subsequent stages. This three-dimensional character of the nose is not restored by cover and lining alone. Flimsy, soft tissue must be positioned, made rigid, and shaped so that a nasal contour is recreated. A nasal framework provides support, projection, airway patency, and the expected shape. An underlying framework must be present or assembled to reestablish the correct external nasal shape. Primary cartilage grafts must be used to recreate a surface contour and to brace the soft tissues of cover and lining against collapse and contraction. The normal bony and cartilaginous framework of the dorsum, tip, columella, and sidewall must be restored if missing. Cartilage should also be placed along a new nostril margin, even if the alar lobule normally contains little cartilage. A cartilage graft will support the alar rim and prevent contraction upward and constriction inward, while recreating a bulging, convex alar contour.

A nasal support framework should be in place prior to completion of wound healing. In the past, bony and cartilaginous grafts have been placed secondarily months after the initial nasal reconstruction. Unfortunately, once the soft tissues have healed in place, they are fibrotic and edematous and can rarely be reshaped by secondary cartilage grafts.

PRINCIPLES OF SUBUNIT NASAL RECONSTRUCTION

Tenets of facial reconstruction have traditionally allowed the wound to determine the method of repair. The size, depth, and vascularity of the recipient bed and available local tissue determined whether a skin graft, local flap, or distant flap was used. Function was emphasized over form, perhaps forgetting that one of the most important functions of a face is to look normal. An aesthetic subunit approach to facial reconstruction divides the face visually into adjacent three-dimensional areas of characteristic skin quality, outline, and contour. The secret to success lies in visualizing, not the defect, but the ideal end result. A logical, thoughtful plan is formulated prior to the reconstruction to employ subunit principles to create the desired normal appearance. The subunit principles of facial reconstruction are[3]:

1. Patients wish to look normal.
2. The normal is defined by regional units—adjacent three-dimensional topographic areas of characteristic skin quality, surface outline, and contour.
3. The surgeon must restore regional units, not fill defects, if the normal is the goal.
4. The wound should often be altered in site, size, depth, and outline to allow unit replacement.
5. Adjacent normal tissue should be discarded, if it will improve the result.

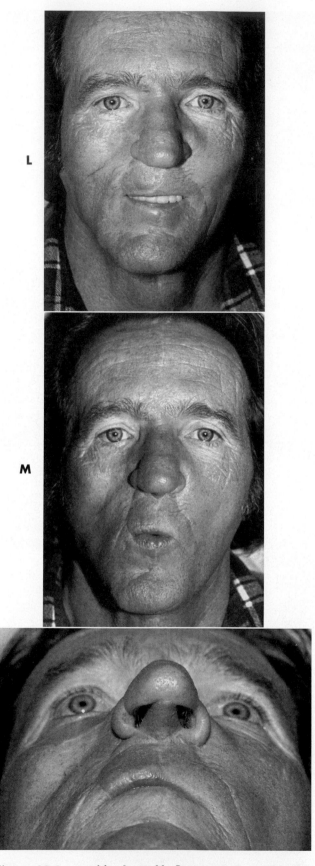

Figure 88-3, cont'd. L to N, Postoperative results after pedicle division. The units of the cheek, lip, columella, and right ala have been reestablished. The reconstructed upper lip is reinnervated and functions normally. (**A** to **C** and **E** to **N**, From Menick F, Burget G: *Advan Plast Surg* 6:193, 1990.)

6. Scars are best positioned in the borders between units where they will be less apparent.

7. Ideal donor materials and methods of tissue transfer should be chosen to allow the restoration of expected quality and contour.

8. Missing tissues must be replaced exactly in quantity.

9. The contralateral normal or ideal should be used for a template.

10. Contour should be integrated at each and every stage. A nasal support framework should be positioned prior to the completion of wound healing. Soft tissue sculpturing is employed prior to pedicle division.

OPERATIONS

For success in nasal reconstruction, the surgeon must analyze the clinical problem, define the desired end result, and set a plan, often in stages, with the goal in mind. The site, size, and depth of a nasal defect will determine the appropriate method of reconstruction.

COVER

It is useful to classify nasal deformities into small, superficial defects and large, deep defects. A small defect measures less than 1.5 cm. If a defect is larger than 1.5 cm, the nasal skin that remains around the defect will not provide enough surface area or mobility to be redistributed over the existing nasal skeleton. A local flap is unsuitable. If the best skin quality is desired, a regional flap will be required. When cartilage is lost and in defects greater than 1.5 cm, local flaps will collapse the delicate reconstructive framework because of the tension of local skin rearrangement. Thus a regional flap must be employed for cover.

RESURFACING THE SMALL, SUPERFICIAL DEFECT

Secondary Healing

Almost all wounds will heal by secondary intention by epithelialization and contraction with minimal pain and risk of infection simply by daily cleaning with soap and water and dressing with antibiotic ointment and a semi-occlusive dressing. A flat or depressed, pale, atrophic scar is the usual result. A superficial defect less than or equal to 0.5 cm and located on a concave or planar surface (i.e., the ala crease, medial canthal, or nasal sidewall) will heal satisfactorily and blend well, especially if it is away from mobile landmarks and the adjacent normal skin is smooth but irregularly pigmented or actinically damaged. In contrast, a similarly depressed, shiny scar in convex sebaceous tip skin will be extremely noticeable.

Skin Grafts

Split-thickness skin grafts are used only as a temporary wound dressing because of their poor color and texture match. Full-thickness skin grafts are used to resurface even large superficial defects of skin and fat in the thin skin zone of the upper two thirds of the nose, but not on the tip or ala. The hairless preauricular area is the best donor site. A strip of hairless skin 2 to 2.5 cm wide can be harvested, even in men. The donor skin is excised as an ellipse with the posterior incision placed in the preauricular crease. A layer closure is performed after superficial cheek undermining. Skin grafts must remain immobile and be placed on a well-vascularized bed. Temporary quilting stitches and a stent dressing for 48 to 72 hours prevent shearing and enhance skin graft take. Postauricular skin and supraclavicular skin are also potential donor sites, but often appear more red or brown, respectively.

Because skin quality and contour have priority, the subunit principle of excision of adjacent normal skin within a subunit may be disregarded when using a skin graft or a small local flap for reconstruction of small superficial defects, encompassing less than 50% of a subunit. Border scars, however, may be more visible if they do not lie between subunits.

Composite auricular grafts may be employed to repair losses of the ala margin. Most often a two-layer sandwich of skin containing cartilage or fat is taken from the helical root, rim, or lobule. The scar surrounding the defect can be excised or hinged over to create small lining flaps that diminish the area of full-thickness repair. The bed must be well vascularized and the graft less than 1.5 cm in diameter if successful revascularization is to occur. With time, however, composite grafts usually look shiny and irregularly pigmented, no longer matching the color and texture of the adjacent normal nose. Contour is rarely symmetric to the opposite side (Figure 88-4).

Local Flaps

Single lobe transposition flaps (Banner, Rhomboid) give a slightly better result than a skin graft in the thin and lax skin of the upper two-thirds.[13] For defects less than 1.5 cm they are an alternative to skin grafts; however, their 90-degree arc of rotation makes them unreliable for small defects within the thick and rigid skin of the tip and ala because of dog-ear and vascularity problems.

The larger dorsal nasal flap of Reiger transfers skin from an area of glabellar excess to the tip and can be used to resurface the tip or ala with skin of similar kind.[50,51] The results are fairly good but are jeopardized by the movement of thick pitted glabella skin into the thin nasal sidewall near the medial canthus, which creates an iatrogenic canthal fold. Such flaps are also of non-subunit design. The bilobed flap for smaller defects[56] or a regional forehead flap for larger defects usually creates a more normal result.

The geometric bilobed flap is the flap of choice for repair of defects between 0.5 and 1.5 cm in the thick skin zones of the tip and ala (Figure 88-5). Rules for design of the geometric bilobed flap apply[27,53,56,57]:

1. Allow no more than 50-degree rotation for each lobe, a total of 100 degrees for the whole design to prevent dog-ears.

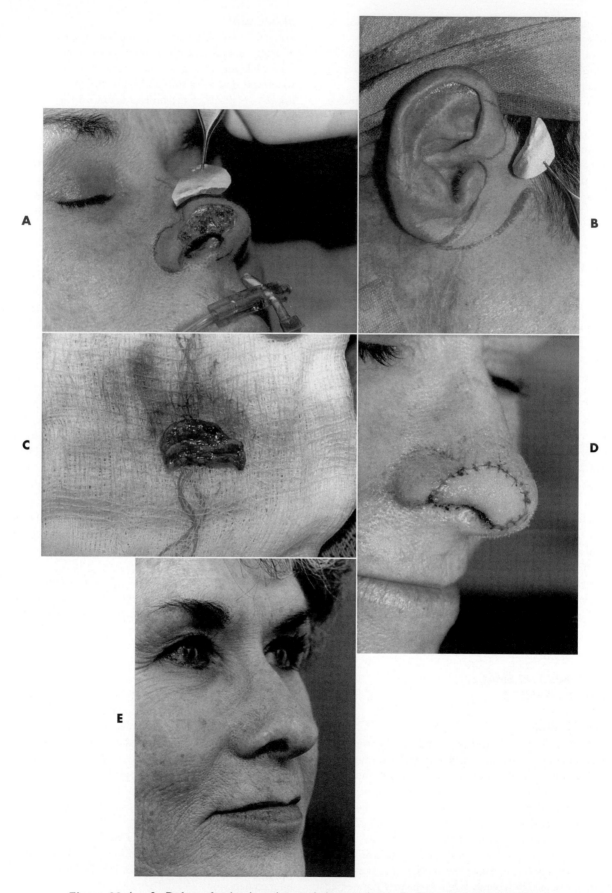

Figure 88-4. **A,** Defect of right ala and tip including rim lining. **B,** Foil template designed and positioned over the left helix. **C,** Composite skin cartilage containing ear cartilage for nasal lining and cover. **D,** Graft replaces the defect. **E,** Postoperative result. Composite graft somewhat shiny and atrophic.

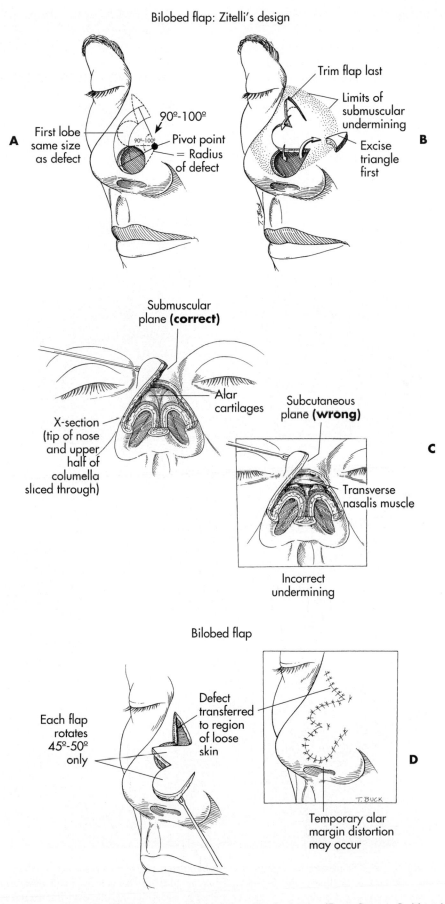

Bilobed flap: Zitelli's design

A First lobe same size as defect   90°-100°   Pivot point = Radius of defect

B Trim flap last   Limits of submuscular undermining   Excise triangle first

Submuscular plane (**correct**)   Alar cartilages   X-section (tip of nose and upper half of columella sliced through)

Subcutaneous plane (**wrong**)   Transverse nasalis muscle   **C**

Incorrect undermining

Bilobed flap

Each flap rotates 45°-50° only   Defect transferred to region of loose skin   **D**

Temporary alar margin distortion may occur

Figure 88-5.   A to **D,** The geometric bilobed flap: Zitelli design. (From Burget G, Menick F: *Aesthetic reconstruction of the nose,* St Louis, 1994, Mosby.)

2. Excise a triangle of dog-ear between the defect and flap pivot point before the flap is rotated.

3. Undermine widely above the periosteum and perichondrium on both sides of the incision to diminish later trapdoor formation. Include well-vascularized muscle with the overlying skin.

4. Make the diameter of the first lobe equal to the defect. The second lobe can be reduced in width to ease donor closure.

5. Use the bilobed flap for defects less than or equal to

1.5 cm. A larger flap design will not fit onto the nasal surface (Figure 88-6).

RESURFACING LARGE, DEEP NASAL DEFECTS

The Nasolabial Flap[19,21,22]

A moderate amount of excess skin is available within the nasolabial fold for flap transfer in one or two stages to resurface the ala. However, a nasolabial flap is inadequate in size and arc

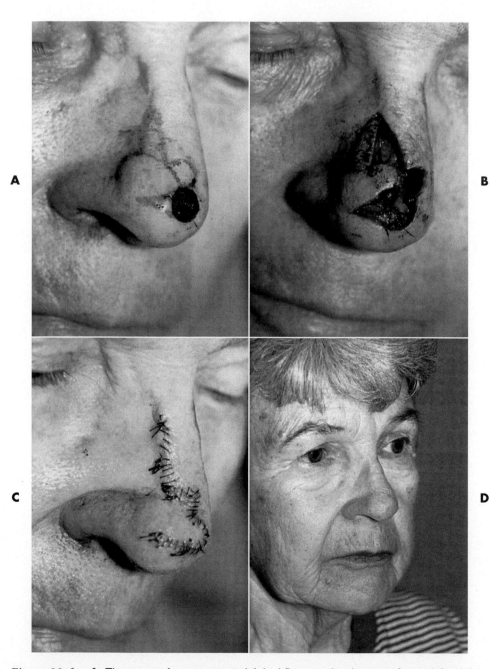

Figure 88-6. **A,** The pattern for a geometric bilobed flap is outlined to resurface a defect of the nasal tip within the thick cheek zone. **B** and **C,** The revascularized flap is incised and elevated over the periosteum and perichondrium. The defect is filled by redistributing skin over the nasal surface. **D,** Postoperative result. Skin quality and contour have been restored. Nasal scars usually heal well.

of rotation to resurface the tip, dorsum, or hemi-nose. The soft, fatty flap also has a propensity to contract into a hemisphere, standing up above the surface of residual skin and disrupting contour; therefore it is best used to resurface the entire alar convex subunit, not to patch a partial defect of the alar lobule or to repair the premaxillary platform on which the alar base normally sits. A two-stage nasolabial flap permits a delicate re-creation of the alar crease, base, and sill. When transferred in one stage as an extension of an advancing cheek flap, these

nasal contour details are not reestablished.[59] However, it is a very useful technique when employed for smaller defects up to 2.5 cm in size that include both the sidewall and ala and do not involve the alar base inset. The forehead flap with its superior color, texture, pliability, and size is donor site of choice for all other nasal repairs.

Under local anesthesia or general anesthesia as an outpatient, the two-stage nasolabial flap is designed as follows:

First, an exact three-dimensional template of the contralateral normal ala is cut, shaped, inverted, and positioned just on the ipsilateral nasolabial crease at, or slightly below, the oral commissure to ensure an adequate arc of rotation. The pattern is marked with ink 1 mm larger to allow for expected soft tissue contraction. The superior subcutaneous base is richly perfused by underlying perforators of the facial and angular arteries passing through the levator labii muscle (Figure 88-7). The pedicle is tapered to a point at the upper nasolabial crease. Distally a triangular dog-ear excision is designed with its medial border following the nasolabial line exactly (Figure 88-8). When so designed, the donor site can be closed exactly in the line of the lazy-S nasolabial crease and will not extend onto the nasal sidewall. The defect is enlarged so that the entire alar subunit is resurfaced, positioning border scars in the joins between subunits (Figure 88-9). Expected flap contraction will enhance the result. Even though no cartilage is normally present in the ala lobule, a septal or ear cartilage graft must be fixed to the remaining or repaired lining to support and shape the soft tissues. The flap is elevated from distal to proximal. The distal one-half of the inset is thinned, leaving 2 to 3 mm of subcutaneous fat. Then the dissection passes more deeply over the underlying proximal facial muscles. The proximal broad subcutaneous

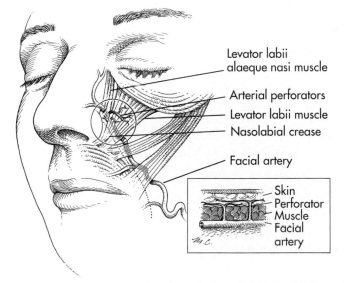

Figure 88-7. Anatomy of the medial cheek. (From Burget G, Menick F: *Aesthetic reconstruction of the nose,* St Louis, 1994, Mosby.)

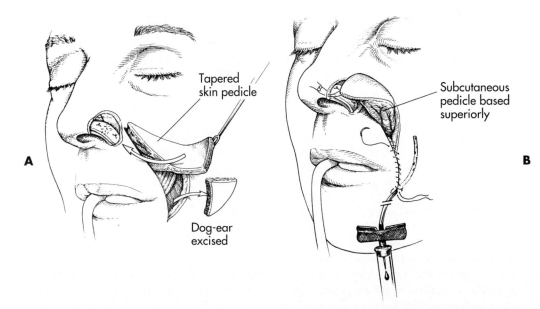

Figure 88-8. A and **B,** Design for the two-stage nasolabial flap. (From Burget G, Menick F: *Aesthetic reconstruction of the nose,* St Louis, 1994, Mosby.)

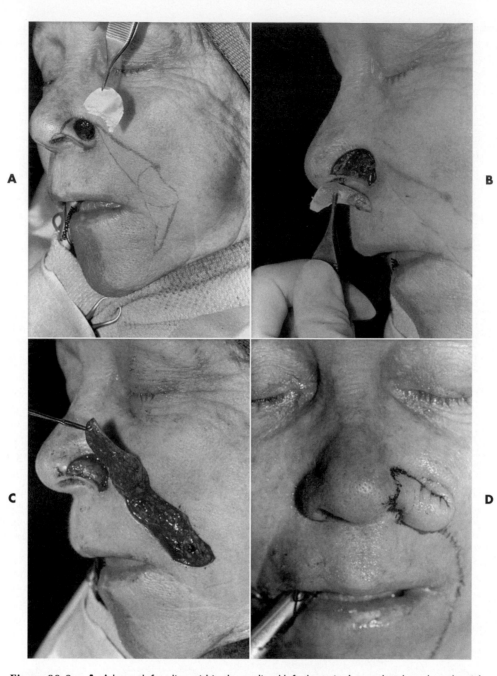

Figure 88-9. **A,** A large defect lies within the outlined left alar unit. A template based on the right contralateral normal ala is positioned to abut the left nasolabial fold and used to design a nasolabial flap tapered both proximally and distally. **B,** A primary cartilage conchal graft is positioned to support the left alar rim lining after excision of residual normal surface skin within the alar unit. **C,** The nasolabial flap is elevated from distal to proximal. Distally, it is raised with only 1-2 mm of fat. The underlying axial vessels near the alar base supply its proximal base. **D,** The flap is transposed to resurface the entire left alar unit. Residual normal skin within the unit has been excised. The donor site is closed, leaving a scar that lies exactly within the left nasolabial crease. (From Menick F. In *Surgical reconstruction of the face: the nose, midface and anterior skull base,* Philadelphia, 1997, WB Saunders.)

base is mobilized by dividing fibrous bands while preserving the blood supply and is released enough to allow rotation. The proximal skin paddle is narrow or nonexistent. The donor site is closed by advancement over a suction drain after cheek undermining. Three weeks later the pedicle is divided at the level of the cheek, partially elevated off its inset, thinned, and shaped. It is wrapped inferomedially to form the

alar base. The proximal donor site is excised as a pointed ellipse and closed so that the final scar lies exactly in the nasolabial crease (Figure 88-10).

The Forehead Flap

Well vascularized and lying adjacent to the nose, the forehead is acknowledged as the best donor site for nasal reconstruction

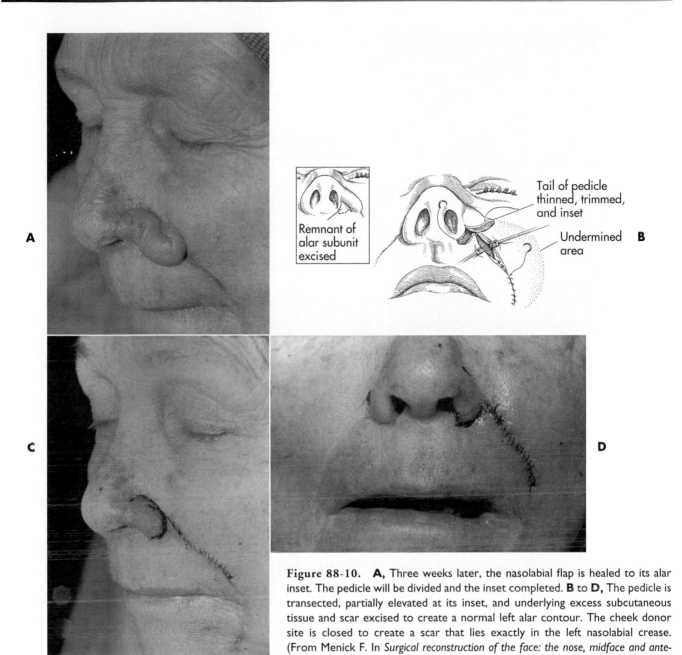

Figure 88-10. A, Three weeks later, the nasolabial flap is healed to its alar inset. The pedicle will be divided and the inset completed. **B** to **D,** The pedicle is transected, partially elevated at its inset, and underlying excess subcutaneous tissue and scar excised to create a normal left alar contour. The cheek donor site is closed to create a scar that lies exactly in the left nasolabial crease. (From Menick F. In *Surgical reconstruction of the face: the nose, midface and anterior skull base,* Philadelphia, 1997, WB Saunders.) *Continued*

because of its superb color and texture match.* The classic median Indian forehead flap carried midline tissue on paired supraorbital and supratrochlear vessels.[5,12,35,49,54] Its 180-degree arc of rotation and high pivot point limit its reach. However, bilateral pedicles are not essential for flap viability, and a paramedian forehead flap centered over the medial canthus and eyebrow of one side permits transfer of midforehead skin to resurface part or all of the nose. Forehead skin, however, should only be used for nasal losses. Restoration of the three-dimensional contour of the alar base, lip, and cheek requires that non-nasal units not be rebuilt with a single flap of forehead skin but by other methods such as cheek advancement or cross-lip flaps. Other regional flaps based on the superficial temporal artery transfer forehead skin (New's sickle flap[49] or Converse scalping flap[12]) or postauricular skin (the Washio

flap).[55] These operations are of greater magnitude than the paramedian forehead flap, require a skin graft for donor site closure, and create a heavy hanging pedicle that stretches across the orbital region during transfer. They are inherently less well vascularized and may require a delay. They are poor second choices.

Tissue expansion is a mechanical technique used to increase the amount of local tissue available for transfer to a recipient site, hopefully diminishing the detrimental consequences of tissue loss at the donor area. It is useful because it can enlarge the skin surface in two dimensions, increasing both length and width of available excess. The expanded skin may, however, become thin and atrophic, distorting donor subcutaneous tissues and the underlying frontal bone at the donor site. The fibrous rind that forms about the expander surface decreases the pliability of the transferred skin and adds unpredictable contraction to the final result. Skin expansion is ideally

*References 12, 16, 17, 25, 47, 48, 55.

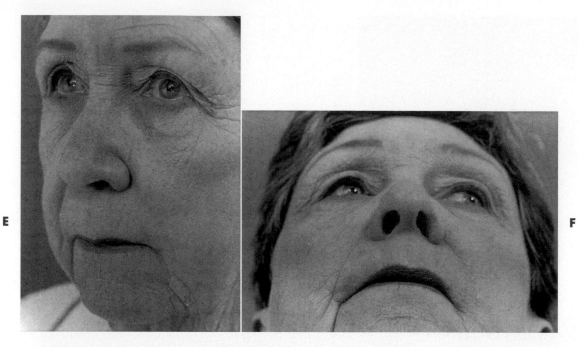

E and **F**

Figure 88-10, cont'd. **E** and **F,** Postoperative results. Scars lie hidden in the junction between the ala, soft triangle, tip, sidewall, and cheek units. Because the nasolabial donor site lies within the nasolabial crease, it is not apparent. (From Menick F. In *Surgical reconstruction of the face: the nose, midface and anterior skull base,* Philadelphia, 1997, WB Saunders.)

Figure 88-11. The forehead is richly perfused by vertically and axially oriented vessels arising from the angular, supratrochlear, and supraorbital arteries and veins. (From Burget G, Menick F: *Aesthetic reconstruction of the nose,* St Louis, 1994, Mosby.)

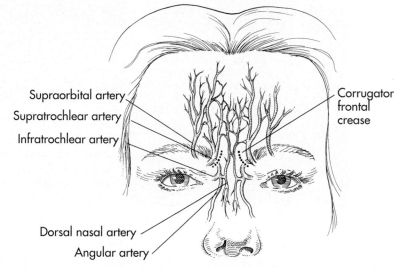

Supraorbital artery
Supratrochlear artery
Infratrochlear artery
Corrugator frontal crease
Dorsal nasal artery
Angular artery

suited to supply skin to a flat surface by simple advancement (cheek, forehead) rather than to the complex and variable shape and texture of the nose. Tissue expansion of the forehead is rarely necessary in nasal reconstruction. Forehead skin is available in adequate excess to resurface the entire nasal unit. In those rare instances when expansion of the forehead would be appropriate, it is probably best to first rebuild the nose with nonexpanded skin, and then use an expander secondarily to improve the donor deformity.

The use of nonfacial tissue for nasal skin resurfacing has a long history.[24] Tagliacozzi pedicled upper arm skin.[48] More recently, freed from the constraints of a short pedicle, distant tissue from the back, forearm, or dorsum of the foot has been transferred by microvascular surgery. In all instances, however,

distant tissue moved to the face has a poor color and texture match and should be used for what it does well—revascularize a wound, fill dead space, create a platform, or provide invisible lining—rather than as a covering for the nose. If any forehead skin is available for transfer, it should be moved on whatever pedicle is available and be employed to resurface the external nose.

Under general anesthesia with a short-stay hospitalization, a paramedian forehead flap is designed as follows:

The forehead is supplied by an arcade of vessels from the supraorbital, supratrochlear, infratrochlear, and dorsal, nasal, and angular vessels (Figure 88-11). They ascend from the brow vertically passing over the periosteum inferiorly, then through the frontalis muscle until they are subcutaneous in the midfore-

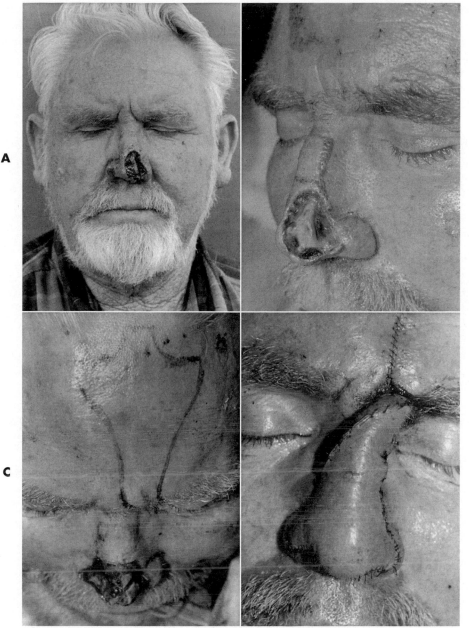

Figure 88-12. A and **B,** Extensive defect of the nasal tip and dorsum with absence of the left lateral crus after Mohs' excision. The nasal subunits are marked with ink. Adjacent normal tissue will be excised within the tip and part of the dorsal unit. **C,** The missing left lateral crus is repaired with a conchal cartilage graft. Adjacent normal tissue within the tip and dorsal unit has been discarded. A three-dimensional foil template is employed to create an exact pattern of the missing nasal skin of the tip, part of the dorsum, and medial aspects of each alar unit. The template design is drawn over the left supratrochlear vessels. **D,** The forehead flap is elevated and transferred to the nose without thinning. A split-thickness skin graft is placed on the raw surface of the proximal pedicle. The forehead donor site was undermined but could not be completely closed. A 2.5-cm defect in the midforehead was allowed to close by secondary intention. (**A** to **D,** From Menick F. In Evans G, Shusterman M, editors: *Operative plastic surgery,* Stanford, 1998, Appleton & Lang.) *Continued*

head or superior forehead, almost adherent to the dermis. A vertically designed paramedian forehead flap is an axial flap. The distal flap can be thinned of frontalis and some subcutaneous tissue. The proximal flap is elevated over the periosteum. Arc of rotation is increased 1.5 cm by extending the flap design into the scalp (clipping off hair bulbs from the deep surface of the flap at the time of transfer to diminish late hair growth), and

further lengthened 1.5 cm by lowering the pivot point inferiorly across the orbital rim toward the medial canthus, dividing corrugator fibers and preserving blood vessels with care.

The nasal defect is evaluated and recreated, if necessary, by the excision of granulation tissue or contracted scar. Subunit outlines are marked in ink and adjacent normal skin within subunits excised, if appropriate (Figure 88-12, *A* and *B*).

Missing lining and support are restored. The contralateral normal, or ideal, is then used to fashion an exact three-dimensional template of the missing surface skin. This pattern is flattened and placed on the forehead over the supratrochlear vessels identified by Doppler (Figure 88-12, *C*) lying just lateral to the medial frown crease. If the defect is unilateral, the flap is designed on the same side as the defect to decrease the arc of rotation. If the defect is located in the midline, the side with the best quality skin is chosen. The pattern is oriented vertically to maintain the axial blood supply and is placed to abut or extend slightly over the hairline. The proximal pedicle is narrowed to approximately 1.2 cm to allow easy rotation of the flap and tensionless closure of the inferior donor defect. Elevating from distal to proximal, the flap can be thinned to

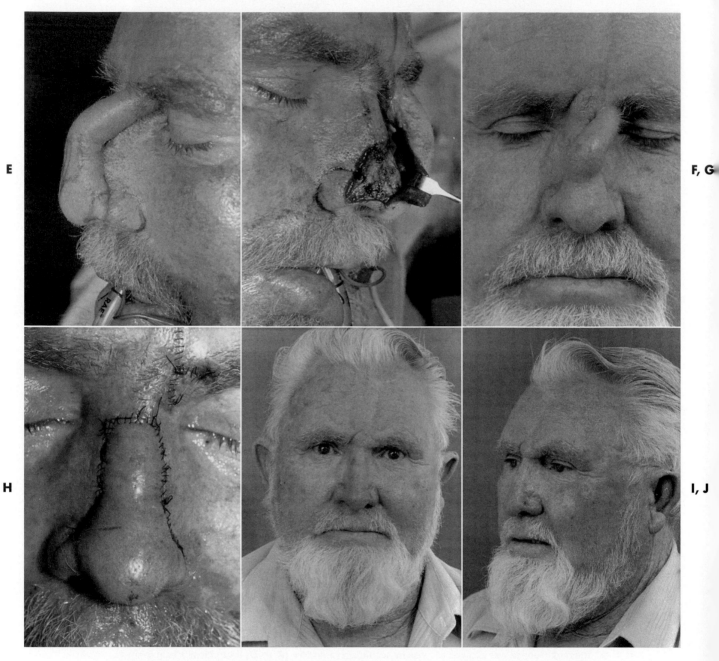

Figure 88-12, cont'd. **E to G,** Three weeks after the initial operation, the forehead flap appears bulky. The nasal subunits are drawn on the flap's surface as a guide. Leaving it attached proximally to its pedicle and distally along the alar margin and columella, the forehead flap is elevated and underlying soft tissues aggressively thinned to sculpt the wound bed into a nasal shape. The flap is then repositioned on the nose. **H,** Three weeks later (6 weeks after the initial operation), the pedicle is divided and inset proximally as a small inverted "V" in the medial brow and along the dorsal subunit lines on the nose. **I and J,** Postoperative result. The nose has a nasal shape, and the scars lay largely invisible within the junction of normal contour units. The forehead has healed secondarily, with minimal distortion. (**A to D,** From Menick F. In Evans G, Shusterman M, editors: *Operative plastic surgery,* Stanford, 1998, Appleton & Lang.)

include only a small amount of subcutaneous tissue for the distal 1.5 cm, if desired. Be cautious in smokers. Dissection is then deepened to the loose areolar plane over the periosteum, lifting the frontalis to the brow. The flap is transposed 180 degrees to the nose and sutured with a single layer of fine interrupted stitches (Figure 88-12, D). Necrosis of a forehead flap is rare. Aggressive thinning should be avoided, especially in any random transverse limbs that have been designed to cover the ala. Any interrupted suture that causes blanching should be released.

The forehead is undermined over the periosteum into both temples, advanced, and closed under moderate tension inferiorly. Layered closure is performed after the placement of 2 to 3 key tension sutures. Any residual defect in the superior forehead is dressed with petrolatum gauze and allowed to heal secondarily. Skin grafts, local flaps, or expanders to assist forehead closure are not required.

Although the pedicle can be divided at 3 weeks, it is helpful, especially in smokers or in major defects, to plan an intermediate operation between the initial operation and sectioning of the pedicle. Three weeks after the first operation, the flap is elevated off its bed at a superficial subcutaneous level over most of the nasal surface, leaving it attached proximally to its pedicle and distally along the alar margin and columella. With a bipedicle blood supply, the flap is aggressively thinned and soft tissue and scar sculpted from the underlying wound bed. Further support grafts may also be placed. The flap is then re-inset with quilting sutures to eliminate dead space (Figure 88-12, E to G).

At 6 weeks (3 weeks after the intermediate operation) the pedicle is divided (Figure 88-12, H to J). Proximally frontalis muscle, fat, and scar are excised and the donor site of the inferior forehead partially opened to allow the pedicle skin stump to be replaced as a small inverted "V," which will visually appear to be a frown crease. Distally the forehead flap is reelevated from its inset for several centimeters, underlying soft tissue sculpted, and the cephalic aspect of the defect pared to a subunit design. The forehead flap is then thinned and inset to complete coverage of the nasal skin surface defect.

ESTABLISHING NASAL SUPPORT

Primary bone and cartilage grafts taken from the ear, nasal septum, ribs, ilium, or cranium (1) provide support against gravity and external physical forces; (2) act to create nasal tip projection and nasal length; (3) form a subcutaneous sheet of hard tissue that braces nasal covering and lining against centripetal trapdoor contraction. Support must extend from the nasal bone superiorly down to the alar margin inferiorly and from the nasal tip anteriorly to the maxilla posteriorly; and (4) are individually carved to resemble in slight miniature a surface subunit of the nose. This framework of grafts will impart a normal surface contour to the nose when seen through thin covering tissues.

Although most often the entire subunit of skin will be replaced, only partial subunit reconstruction with cartilage grafts is required. Residual intranasal support, combined with a fabricated replacement of those areas of framework that are missing, is covered by a thin skin flap to resist postoperative wound contraction and allow the underlying framework to show through. Because the external skin that covers these grafts is thicker than normal, the nasal framework must have not only a precise normal nasal shape, but also must be reduced in all its external dimensions by 2 to 3 mm.

The most useful graft materials are cartilage and bone of the nasal septum, the cartilage of the floor and walls of the auricular concha, the costal cartilages (especially the eighth costal cartilage), and occasional cranium or iliac bone grafts. An 8-mm-wide L-shaped dorsum and caudal strut must be maintained to support the nose after harvesting septal cartilage. Costal cartilage is an ideal replacement for the nasal dorsum and can be shaped into thin slices to repair the nasal sidewall, alar lobule, or even the alar cartilage. The cartilage of the concha may be removed through a posterior or anterior incision. All these cartilage grafts have the great advantage that they are seldom resorbed over time. In patients less than 35 years of age, however, costal cartilage may warp postoperatively despite following Gibson's rules of balanced carving.[15] Although surgeons may staunchly defend the cranium, ilium, septum, or concha as the ideal donor site for a nasal framework, the material chosen is not of great importance. It is a subtle and exact shape that creates an ideal or normal nasal framework.

Requirements for nasal framework include (Figure 88-13):

1. A 4-mm-wide strut of septal or conchal cartilage is scored and bent to form a replacement for one or both alar cartilages. These alar cartilage replicas are sutured to the stumps of the residual medial crura, the projecting ends scored and bent laterally, and then sutured to intact or reconstructed lining of the vestibule. Further tip projection can be achieved by adding a one- or two-layered Peck-style tip graft 4×9 mm wide at the top of the newly reconstructed alar cartilage domes.

2. A brace of ethmoid perpendicular plate and attached cartilage or rib graft can be trimmed to a trapezoidal shape and positioned on the nasal sidewall as replacement for the missing upper lateral cartilage and bone. It supports the middle vault against collapse and provides a platform for eyeglasses. Such a graft also braces the nasal sidewall against upward contraction.

3. A 4- to 6-mm-wide batten of conchal or septal cartilage can be fastened along the caudal edge of the lining sleeve from the alar base to the nostril apex. This fixes the new alar rim in position and gives a normal bulging contour to the ala even though the ala does not normally contain cartilage.

4. An architectural flying buttress of layered septal grafts, conchal cartilage, or rib graft can be installed along the dorsum to prevent upper contraction and postoperative shortening of the nose. It also gives shape to the nasal bridge and recreates the form of the dorsal subunit.

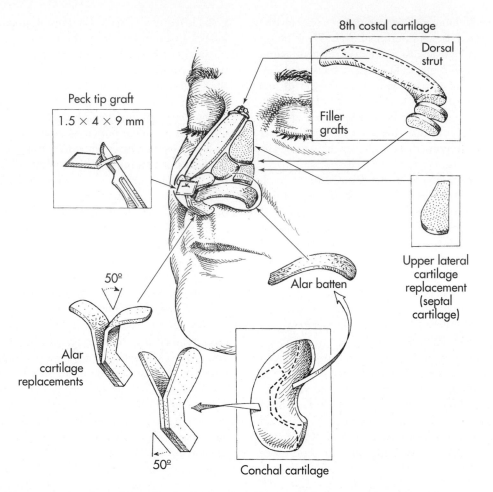

Figure 88-13. A nasal framework of primary cartilage grafts restores nasal support and contour, and braces the reconstruction against the forces of wound healing. A dorsal strut, a sidewall brace, alar batten, and alar cartilage replacements. (From Burget G, Menick F. In *Aesthetic reconstruction of the nose,* St Louis, 1994, Mosby.)

NASAL LINING

A forehead flap can resurface the nose with vascularized skin of matching quality. Support and contour are supplied by a skeletal framework. However, most often a failure in reconstruction results from a shortage of lining. The lining chosen for replacement must be vascular enough to support primary cartilage grafts, supple enough to conform to the proper shape, and thin enough that it neither obstructs the airways nor distorts the external shape.

Unraveling Contracted Lining

If the lining loss is minimal along the alar margin, residual vestibular skin can often be freed from its attachment superiorly and pulled inferiorly like the hem of a skirt until it reaches the level of the proposed nostril margin. An advancement of 2 to 3 mm can be obtained but must be fixed into position by a bolster of primary cartilage graft to prevent its retraction.

In a patient who has undergone previous surgery, the alar rim may be distorted and retracted. If a true lining deficit exists, it must be replaced. However, after excision of scar and replacement of tissues in their normal position, ample lining may remain, having been folded on itself by scar contraction. When released, the alar margin is repositioned and the lining buttressed with cartilage grafts.

Local Hinge-over Flaps

Thin, stiff, lining flaps can be created by turning over the skin and scar adjacent to a healed nasal defect. Uninjured adjacent skin, previously placed skin grafts surrounding a defect, or areas of scar may be hinged over. The main disadvantage is the unreliability of their blood supply.[40-43,45] Because of their relative avascularity, such turnover flaps must be kept short, 1 to 1.5 cm. Primary cartilage grafts can be placed but cartilage infection and necrosis occur more often. It should also be remembered that skin damaged by sun or radiation, if placed inside the nose as a lining flap, may later develop a skin cancer within the hidden recesses of the nose. Turnover flaps also preclude immediate reconstruction, since the wound edges must first be allowed to heal (Figure 88-14, *A* to *E*).

In the past the rolling over of bilateral nasolabial flaps to line both the ala and the columella was a popular method. When the blood supply from the angular and facial arteries is

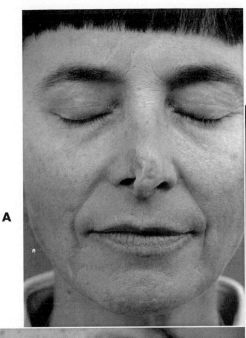

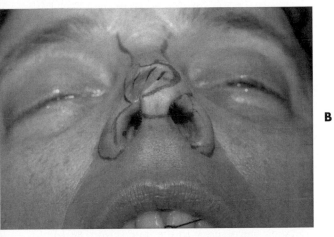

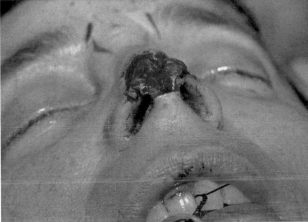

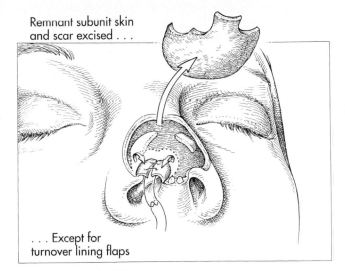

Remnant subunit skin and scar excised . . .

. . . Except for turnover lining flaps

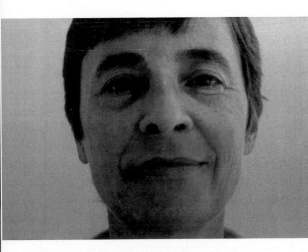

Figure 88-14. **A,** Healed Mohs' nasal defect with missing skin of the tip and ala, alar tip cartilages, and right nasal rim lining. **B** to **D,** The tip unit is outlined. Residual normal skin is excised and hinged over at the healed periphery of the defect to line the vestibule. **E,** Conchal cartilage grafts are positioned to recreate columella support and lateral crural replicas. Additional tip graft is placed. **F,** Postoperative result after pedicle division. (From Menick FJ. In *Operative techniques in plastic and reconstructive surgery: facial and nasal reconstruction,* Philadelphia, 1998, WB Saunders.)

respected, these flaps will remain viable; however, they are always too thick and cannot be thinned at the initial stage without jeopardizing their blood supply. This thick and shapeless lining must then be covered with an inappropriately large forehead flap. With the borderline vascularity of such lining flaps, primary cartilage grafts are precluded because of the significant risk of necrosis and liquefaction of support structures. The shape of the new nose is totally controlled by the bulk and contour of the lining flap, crowding the vestibule and bloating the external shape. They are rarely useful.

Prefabricated Skin Graft and Cartilage Lining of a Forehead Flap ("Building the Nose on the Forehead")

During preliminary operations, composite grafts from the ear or septum or separate pieces of skin and cartilage graft may be placed under the distal edge of a forehead flap at donor site before elevation and transfer to the nose (Figure 88-14, F). When they survive, these preinstalled lining grafts can create a delicate nostril margin.[11,39,46] Unfortunately such grafts retain the cartilage shape of their donor concha or septum and are fixed by the scar that formed about them during healing on the forehead. The shape is not correct and cannot be modified when all the pieces are finally assembled, hurting their usefulness.[35-37]

Folding a Forehead Flap or Nasolabial Flap for Both Cover and Lining

In general, the folding of a cover flap for lining is to be condemned. Doubling a cover flap on itself magnifies donor morbidity due to excessive flap length; diminishes the distal blood supply, increasing the risk of necrosis; and necessitates the creation of thick, shapeless, and unsupported alar margins.

Intranasal Lining Flaps

Although not apparent, significant amounts of lining normally remain within the residual nose and the piriform aperture. Lining flaps from intranasal donor sites (the vestibule, the middle vault, and the septum) are thin. They neither distort the shape of overlying cartilage grafts and covering skin nor bulge into the airway, obstructing breathing. Such lining flaps are vascular enough to nourish primary cartilage grafts without the risk of necrosis and are soft enough to conform to the shape of a cartilage framework.[11,30,47]

The arterial supply of the nasal septum arrives posteriorly through the septal branches of the sphenopalatine artery and anteriorly superiorly from the ethmoidal arteries (Figure 88-15). The major anterior inferior arterial supply enters from the upper lip. Arising from the facial artery, the superior labial artery winds medially through the orbicularis oris muscle at the level of the skin vermilion junction. Lateral to the philtral column, the septal branch of the superior labial artery passes almost vertically upward and enters the nasal septum lateral to the nasal spine. Thus a flap of septal mucoperichondrium,

either unilateral or bilateral, and with or without a bone or cartilage component, will survive if based on a 1- to 1.2-cm pedicle located in the zone between the anterior plane of the upper lip and the lower edge of the piriform aperture—the zone containing the septal branches of the superior labial artery. Such flaps of septal mucoperichondrium, cartilage, and bone may extend from the nasal floor below to the level of the medial canthal above and posteriorly onto the ethmoid perpendicular plate.

Unilateral mucoperichondrial flaps[3] based either on the right or left superior labial artery can be transposed laterally to replace the missing lining of the vestibule or the lateral sidewall. A unilateral leaf of septal mucous membrane can be used in combination with a bipedicle of vestibular skin based medially on the anterior septum and laterally on the nasal floor, supplied by branches of the facial artery at the alar base. It may also be used in combination with a contralateral mucoperichondrial flap based on the dorsum of the septum that is hinged laterally to line the sidewalls of the middle and upper vault as originally described by deQuervain and later by Kazanjian,[23] Converse, and Millard. In total nasal reconstruction, a bilateral flap of mucoperichondrium and septal hard tissue can be pivoted anteriorly on an inferior base to supply support and lining for the vestibules and columella, the middle and upper vaults, or the entire nasal dorsum. Millard has also described a proximally based septal L-shaped chondromucosal flap that is advanced up and out of the vestibule, fixing the inferior limb on the nasal spine, creating a cantilever. This full-thickness septal flap is pivoted out of the nose and does provide septal support, although it does not supply lining for other areas of the nose, unlike the inferior-based septal composite flap. These various intranasal flaps can be used in any combination (Figure 88-16, A to G).

In a unilateral alar defect, residual vestibular skin that lies above the defect may be incised in the area of the intercartilaginous line, creating a bipedicle flap approximately 6 mm wide and based medially on the septum and laterally on the nasal floor. The bipedicle vestibular flap is advanced inferiorly to the level of the proposed alar rim, and the defect that remains above is filled with an ipsilateral septal mucoperichondrial flap based anteriorly and inferiorly on the superior labial artery branches. Exposed septal bone and cartilage are removed and employed later for cartilage support, leaving the raw surface of the contralateral septum intact to heal secondarily. Alternatively the residual defect above the vestibular flap can be filled by a dorsally based contralateral mucoperichondrial flap passed through a slit in the ipsilateral septal mucoperichondrium (Figure 88-16, H).

In larger heminasal defects when the size of the lining loss precludes the use of residual vestibular skin, an ipsilateral septal flap may be hinged and transposed laterally across the nasal airway to line the lower vestibule and alar margin, with a second contralateral mucoperichondrial flap based on the dorsum of the septum and receiving branches of the anterior ethmoidal artery hinged laterally to line the upper vault

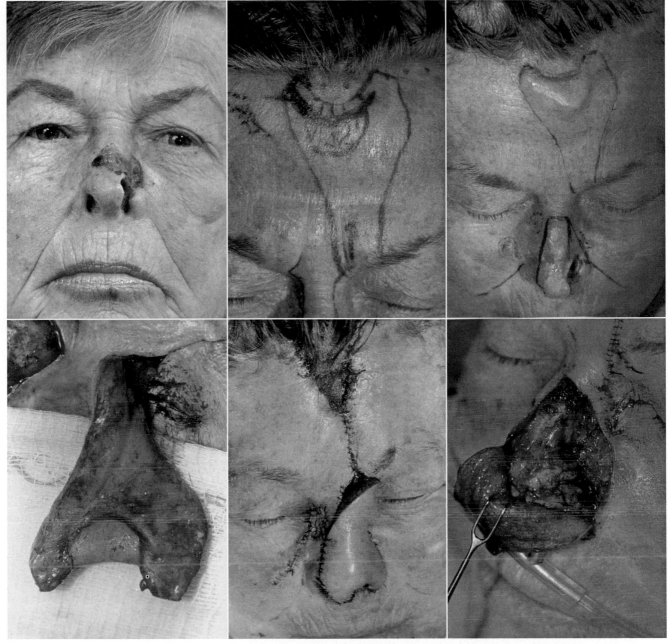

Figure 88-15. **A,** Partially healed Mohs' defect with the tip, dorsum, left ala, and sidewall. This elderly patient was a respiratory cripple on constant nasal oxygen. Intranasal manipulation should be minimized. Forehead flap reconstruction was planned under local sedation anesthesia. The patient had a high aesthetic standard and was insistent on reconstruction. **B** and **C,** At the first stage, a paramedian forehead flap was designed utilizing a three-dimensional foil template and positioned over the supratrochlear vessels. The peripheral outline was incised to delay the flap. It was partially elevated distally, and the deep frontalis surface skin grafted. Within a subcutaneous tunnel between the forehead skin and frontalis layer, a conchal cartilage alar batten is positioned. **D** and **E,** Three weeks later the forehead flap is elevated. The primary healing of the skin graft and cartilage graft is evident. The forehead flap is transferred to the nose. **F,** Three weeks later (6 weeks after the first stage), the forehead is divided and the flap elevated toward the tip and ala. An additional conchal cartilage tip graft is placed. (From Menick FJ. In *Operative techniques in plastic and reconstructive surgery: facial and nasal reconstruction,* Philadelphia, 1998, WB Saunders.)

Continued

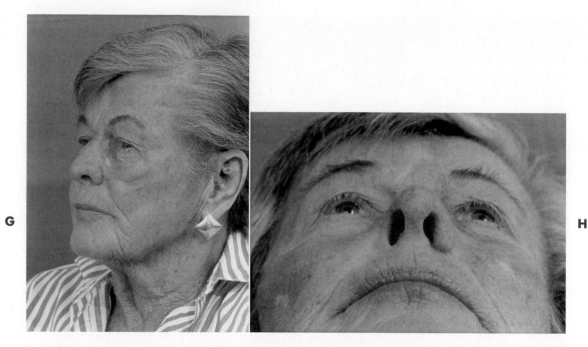

Figure 88-15, cont'd. G and **H,** Postoperative result after pedicle division. The nasal rim is supported, the airway is patent, and the aesthetic result good. (From Menick FJ. In *Operative techniques in plastic and reconstructive surgery: facial and nasal reconstruction,* Philadelphia, 1998, WB Saunders.)

(Figure 88-17). This second flap may be swung as a composite flap with its adherent septal bone and cartilage, but it is often more satisfactory to remove the exposed cartilage and bone of the septum as graft material prior to incising the dorsally based flap. After the lining is restored, cartilage grafts are replaced to support the sidewall. The large septal fistula that is created is usually asymptomatic.

When a large central nasal defect is present, but residual septum remains intact within the piriform aperture, a composite flap centered over both septal branches of the right and left superior labial artery can be utilized to move full-thickness septal tissue out of the nose to the level of the nasal bridge. As the flap pivots into position, its distal end pops over the exposed stump of the nasal or frontal bone and may be locked into position, maintaining bone-to-bone contact. It is best to design this flap overly wide, creating an intentional dorsal hump. At a subsequent operation when this hump is lowered, the extra lining can be folded laterally to line the dorsal nasal vaults. This technique provides a stable central nasal platform and ample lining for the middle and upper vault in the one stage. With this septal "I-beam" firmly healed to the nasal root and strong enough to resist wound contraction, other lining and cover flaps can be brought into position at a later operation (see Figure 88-16, *D* to *G*).

Staged Sequential Skin Grafts For Lining[3]

Although a full-thickness skin graft is soft and pliable, it has no intrinsic blood supply and must rest against a highly vascular bed for its survival. Primary cartilage grafts cannot be placed between a skin graft and its recipient bed because they would prevent skin graft revascularization. Without primary support at the time of reconstruction, uncontrollable skin contraction and soft tissue collapse invariably lead to postoperative shrinkage and external distortion; however, a paramedian forehead flap is bilaminar, composed of a superficial axial skin and subcutaneous layer (see Figure 88-15) and a deep musculofascial layer of galeofrontalis muscle and fascia, all of which are perfused by an axial blood supply based on the supratrochlear vessels. The superficial skin and subcutaneous component may be separated from the deeper galeofrontalis layer at the initial operation, placing one or more contoured cartilage grafts within tunnels developed between the two lamellae to provide a supporting contour for nasal reconstruction. These grafts remain completely surrounded by well-vascularized soft tissue and will survive, restoring support, projection, and contour and ensuring airway patency. A full-thickness skin graft, raw surface outward, is sutured to fill the lining defect and fixed to the well-vascularized frontalis surface of the forehead flap with quilting sutures. In small unilateral defects in which residual normal vestibular skin remains intact above the defect, a bipedicle flap of remnant vestibular skin based medially on the septum and laterally on the alar base may be incised and transposed inferiorly to the proposed level of the new alar margin (Figure 88-18), repairing the secondary lining defect above the vestibular flap with a full-thickness skin graft sutured to the frontalis muscle of the forehead flap. Primary cartilage grafts can be sutured to the raw surface of the vascularized alar margin bipedicle flap during the first stage. Tip and rim support is applied primarily, although the superior aspect of the nasal defect remains temporarily

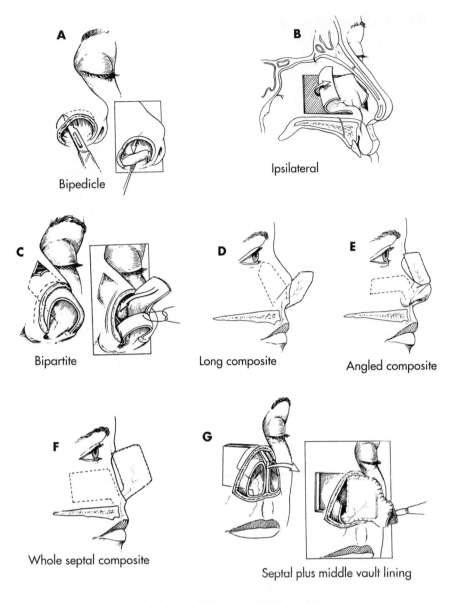

A
Bipedicle

B
Ipsilateral

C
Bipartite

D
Long composite

E
Angled composite

F
Whole septal composite

G
Septal plus middle vault lining

Variations of the septal pivot flap

Figure 88-16. **A** to **H,** The nasal septum has a rich vascular supply based anteroinferiorly on the septal branches of the superior labial arteries and superiorly on the anterior ethmoid vessels. Septal mucosal flaps can be elevated for lining, which will vascularize primary cartilage grafts. (From Burget G, Menick F. In *Aesthetic reconstruction of the nose,* St Louis, 1994, Mosby.)

Continued

unsupported. Three weeks later, once skin graft take is ensured and before flap contraction can occur, the forehead flap can be reelevated; excessive subcutaneous tissue and scar excised, both from the overlying flap and its underlying bed; and cartilage support positioned for the nasal sidewall. In this way, a complete nasal framework is restored. Depending on the specifications of both the defect and its inset, the forehead flap can be divided at this stage or at a third stage. Regardless, an unbroken sheet of hard tissues lies throughout the defect and braces the reconstruction against retraction or collapse (Figures 88-19 and 88-20).

Distant Tissue for Lining

Although distant tissue matches the face poorly when used for nasal cover, it can provide useful lining for difficult cases. The radial forearm flap, anastomosed to vessels in the neck, is placed with the skin side facing inward and is folded on itself for cover or temporarily skin grafted. Once survival is ensured and the flap healed to its inset, the superficial surface of the flap is thinned, primary cartilage grafts positioned, and the reconstruction covered with the ideal skin of a forehead flap, thus creating a nasal framework and providing covering skin that matches the face. *Text continued on p. 1492*

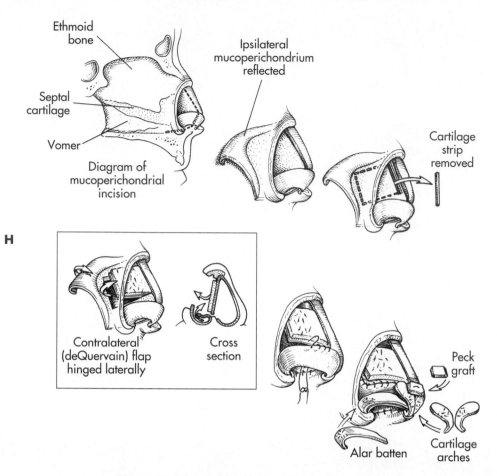

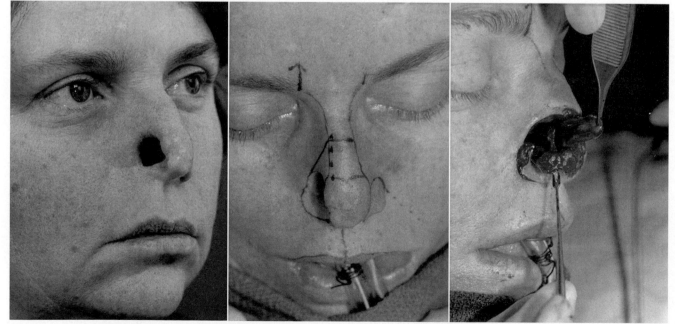

Figure 88-16, cont'd. For legend see previous page.

Figure 88-17. A, Full-thickness defect of right tip, ala, sidewall. Previous right nasolabial flap resurfaces the nasal base and sill. **B,** Nasal units outlined and nasal base inset, positioned, marked based on a left hemi-upper lip template. Residual normal skin of tip, dorsum, and sidewall will be excised. **C,** A bipedicle flap of residual vestibular skin alone. The defect based on the septum medially and alar base laterally is incised and positioned inferiorly to line the new alar rim. A contralateral septal flap based dorsally is passed through a horizontal slit in the ipsilateral septum to line the sidewall defect alone.

Continued

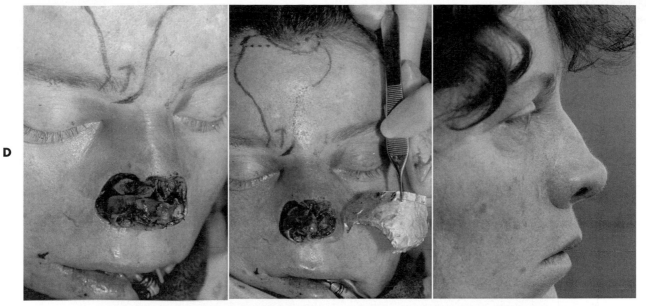

Figure 88-17, cont'd. **D,** Nasal skin subunits excised and cartilage grafts used to create structure. **E,** Template and forehead flap design for external cover. **F,** Postoperative result.

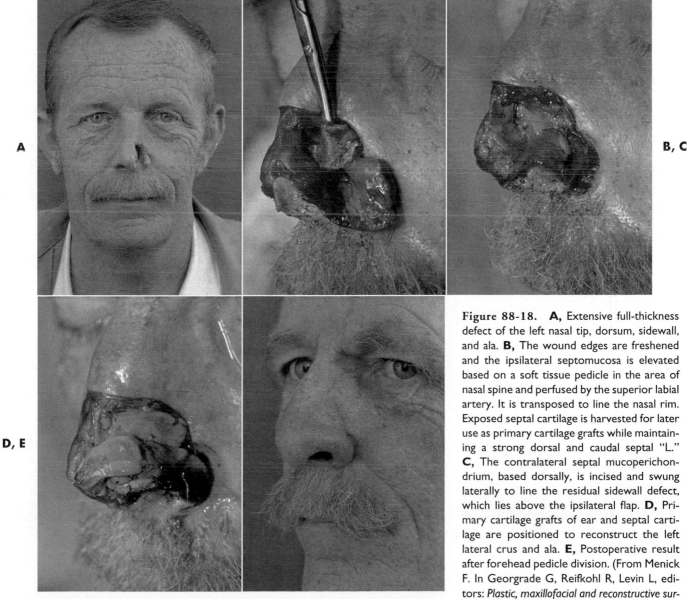

Figure 88-18. **A,** Extensive full-thickness defect of the left nasal tip, dorsum, sidewall, and ala. **B,** The wound edges are freshened and the ipsilateral septomucosa is elevated based on a soft tissue pedicle in the area of nasal spine and perfused by the superior labial artery. It is transposed to line the nasal rim. Exposed septal cartilage is harvested for later use as primary cartilage grafts while maintaining a strong dorsal and caudal septal "L." **C,** The contralateral septal mucoperichondrium, based dorsally, is incised and swung laterally to line the residual sidewall defect, which lies above the ipsilateral flap. **D,** Primary cartilage grafts of ear and septal cartilage are positioned to reconstruct the left lateral crus and ala. **E,** Postoperative result after forehead pedicle division. (From Menick F. In Georgrade G, Reifkohl R, Levin L, editors: *Plastic, maxillofacial and reconstructive surgery,* 1996, Baltimore, Williams & Wilkins.)

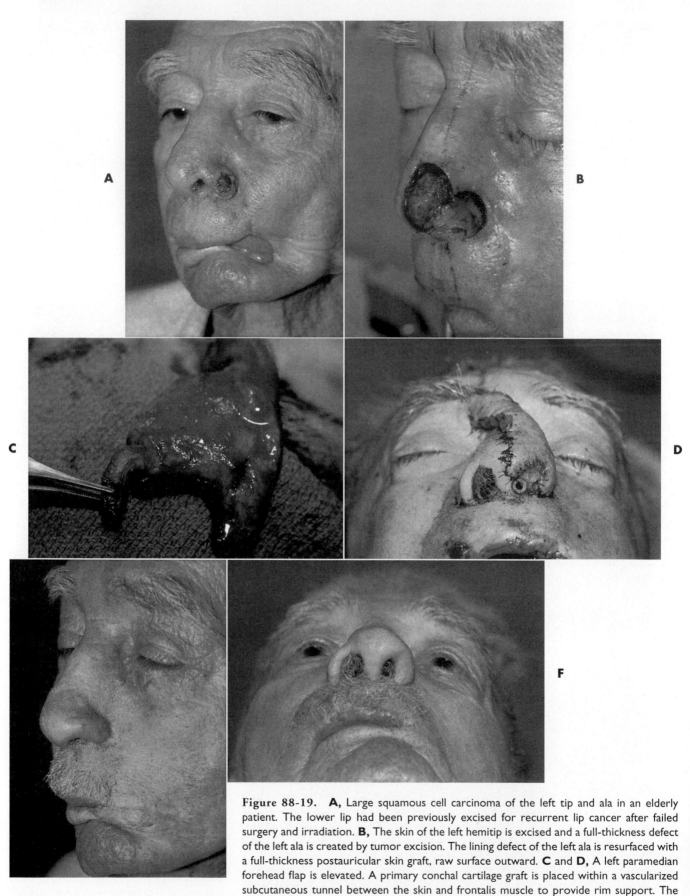

Figure 88-19. **A,** Large squamous cell carcinoma of the left tip and ala in an elderly patient. The lower lip had been previously excised for recurrent lip cancer after failed surgery and irradiation. **B,** The skin of the left hemitip is excised and a full-thickness defect of the left ala is created by tumor excision. The lining defect of the left ala is resurfaced with a full-thickness postauricular skin graft, raw surface outward. **C** and **D,** A left paramedian forehead flap is elevated. A primary conchal cartilage graft is placed within a vascularized subcutaneous tunnel between the skin and frontalis muscle to provide rim support. The forehead flap is then positioned over the skin graft lining, fixed with quilting sutures and a light nasal pack. **E** and **F,** Postoperative result after pedicle division.

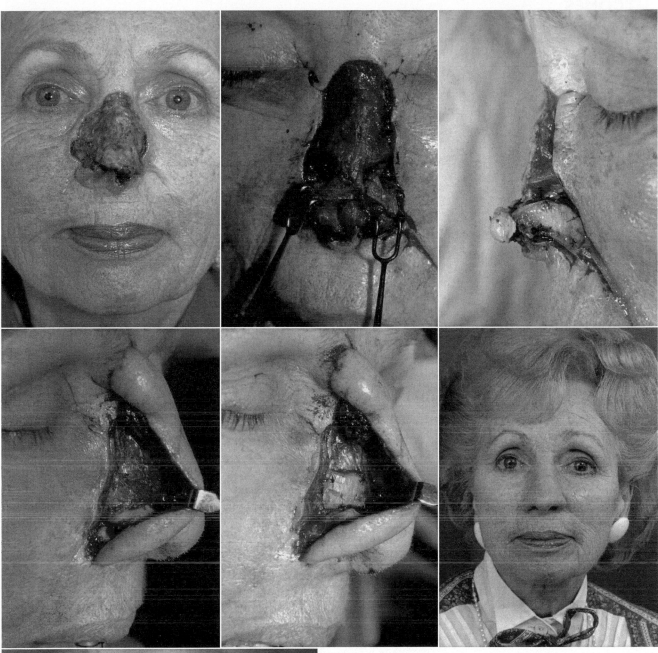

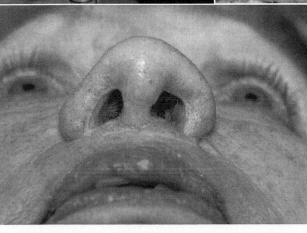

Figure 88-20. **A,** Mohs' defect of the nasal unit with extension onto the medial cheeks. Lining is absent medially along each alar rim. **B,** Bipedicle flaps placed medially on the septum and laterally on the alar base are incised at the intercartilaginous line and positioned inferiorly to recreate lining for the alar rims. The defect created above is filled with full-thickness postauricular skin grafts, raw surface outward. **C,** The highly vascular bipedicle flaps allow placement of conchal cartilage alar battens and tip grafts. No primary cartilage grafts are positioned over the skin graft. **D** and **E,** Three weeks later, at an intermediate operation the forehead flap is elevated, maintaining a proximal base and a distal inset. The skin grafts in the area of the sidewall are indistinguishable from normal nasal lining, and delayed primary cartilage grafts are positioned to support and contour the sidewalls. They will also brace the reconstruction against upward contraction. **F** and **G,** Postoperative result after pedicle division. Airways are patent. (From Menick FJ. In *Operative techniques in plastic and reconstructive surgery: facial and nasal reconstruction,* Philadelphia, 1998, WB Saunders.)

OUTCOMES

The most common indication for nasal reconstruction is destruction of the nose due to skin cancer.

Skin cancer will recur if the tumor is not completely destroyed or excised. This is best ensured by a complete pathologic examination of all lateral and deep margins. It can be accomplished with frozen sections, permanent sections, or by Mohs' histographic excision.

Zitelli,[58] a Mohs' surgeon, has analyzed comparative costs for treatment by destruction (electrodesiccation and curettage), simple office excision, ambulatory surgical facility excision, radiation therapy, and Mohs' micrographic surgery for small skin cancers between 1 and 2 cm in size. In each case the biopsy, standard pathology, anesthesia, facility, and laboratory costs were considered. Wounds were allowed to heal by second intention or closed by simple suture, depending on the technique employed. The cost for destruction of a 1- to 2-cm skin cancer was $653, with a 7.7% recurrence rate. Similar fees for office excision were $1,239, with a 10% recurrence rate. Ambulatory surgical facility excision was $2,112, with a 10% recurrence rate; radiation therapy was $2,573, with a 9% recurrence rate; and Mohs' surgery was $1,252, with a 1% recurrence rate.

Barton et al[2] have examined the reconstruction of difficult basal cell carcinomas. Lesions in critical anatomic areas (eye, nose, and ear), greater than 2 cm in size, recurrent, or with indistinguishable clinical margins (morphea) have a greater than 50% recurrence rate after standard electrodesiccation and curettage excision or radiation therapy. In their patient population of 281 patients with 359 basal cell carcinomas undergoing delayed primary reconstruction by primary closure, flaps, or grafts after Mohs' histographic excision, with a 64-month follow-up, there was only a 1.4% recurrence rate and a 1.9% infection rate, with less than one third causing failure of reconstruction.

Outcomes of tumor control must be differentiated from those of a successful reconstruction. It must be remembered that one of the most important functions of the face is to look normal. The face tells the world who we are and influences what we can become. A nose functions properly when it permits easy nasal breathing and appears normal. Before the birth of Christ, Sushruta[54] in the Hindu Book of Revelation exclaimed, "The love of life is next to the love of our own faces in the mutilated cry for help." In modern times, Freud[14] noted, "A terrible sensation took possession of the patient. No way out. No escape. There remained only one activity—to look constantly in his pocket mirror, attempting to establish the degree of his mutilation." Interestingly, Harris,[20] a British plastic surgeon, evaluated a series of cosmetic and reconstructive patients and noted that the psychogenesis of symptoms in patients who are treated for gross disfigurements, whether from congenital malformation, disease, or injury, is the same as in those patients treated for aesthetic surgery.

Few patients are happy with an artificial prosthesis. Facial reconstruction patients, just as breast reconstruction patients, have a constant fear of prosthetic displacement and their deformity being "found out."[26] Moreover, a prosthesis is never integrated into the body's self image. Although a temporary prosthesis may be employed for a period between tumor excision and the beginning of a complex reconstruction, unless indicated by poor health or a high risk of recurrence requiring continued visual observation, most patients prefer that their nose be rebuilt with their own tissues. The costs of artificial prostheses are high. Medicare reimburses $2,000 for a full or partial nasal prosthesis in Arizona. Prosthesis color and integrity deteriorate with time, requiring prosthesis replacement every 1 to 2 years, although Medicare will replace it only every 4 to 5 years. Required adhesives cost about $100 a year. Osseointegrated implants fixed to the maxilla or glabella can also be employed using two to three titanium implants at $1,000 to $1,400 an implant. The retention clips and bar required to fix the prosthesis to the implants add another $1,400 independent of the prosthesis itself.

Importantly and ironically, prosthetists are recommending removal of the residual normal septum even if not involved with malignancy to simplify prosthetic retention. Loss of vascularized septal lining significantly complicates and may even preclude later surgical reconstruction.

Radiation therapy is used to treat skin cancer, aiming to avoid the deformity associated with excision and the need for reconstruction. It claims an overall cure rate of 92% in the treatment of skin malignancies, but the technique requires specialized personnel and equipment, and is normally reserved for older individuals who are not surgical candidates. It may be recommended for larger lesions to preserve tissue, but the resultant scar tends to worsen over time and may even ulcerate, with a finite risk of radiation osteitis and chondritis or late radiation-induced cancer. Radiation also complicates a future reconstruction. Utilizing an electron beam linear accelerator, 20 to 30 fractions would normally be given to larger skin cancers over 4 to 6 weeks at approximately $125 per treatment, a cost of $4,000 to $6,000. Although obtaining satisfactory cure rates, radiation therapy has generally not been found to provide as good a cosmetic result as surgical modalities.[52]

Plastic surgical reconstruction of a defect following surgical excision can create the appearance of normal in one, two, or three stages, which will not deteriorate over time. The total Medicare reimbursement for the surgeon, anesthesiologist, and all hospital charges, including overnight stay if needed, for a one-stage reconstruction with a nasolabial flap and ear cartilage graft is approximately $2,280. For a two-stage reconstruction with nasolabial flap and ear cartilage graft it is $3,260. A two-stage forehead flap and cartilage graft reimbursement is $6,670. A three-stage forehead flap and cartilage graft reimbursement is $7,000, and with multiple septal mucosal lining flap it is $11,500.

Complications after properly executed nasal reconstruction are relatively infrequent. They are often associated with a failure to identify preexisting risk factors such as smoking or a prior history of facial surgery or injury that interferes with tissue blood supply. Technical misadventures, such as excessive thinning of flaps or closure under tension at initial stages, or a failure to stage procedures properly must be avoided. These are often errors of judgment. Flap necrosis can be avoided by careful design, maintaining axial vasculature, and utilizing staged reconstructions. Cartilage graft loss and infection are unusual, and present as an acute, purulent infection or as a slowly progressive chondritis with overlying inflammation and prolonged drainage. They usually follow loss of lining or covering skin. Prophylactic antibiotics are appropriate. If a nasolabial or forehead flap is found to be necrotic at its tip, rather than waiting for spontaneous separation of the necrotic wound, aggressive surgical excision prior to development of infection is vital, coupled with immediate resurfacing with healthy tissue. Although minor loss of the tip of a forehead flap may seem insignificant, it may lead to exposure of the underlying cartilage framework, lingering infection, and shrinking of the overlying covering flap, which can rarely be expanded secondarily.

Burget et al[10] have reviewed their 5-year experience with unipedicle and contralateral septal flaps for full-thickness heminasal losses of the tip, ala, and sidewall. Forty percent of patients also had associated cheek or lip defects. All patients had high aesthetic standards and wished to look normal. Reconstructions were completed in two to six procedures, utilizing cheek flaps, forehead flaps, septal and ear cartilage grafts, and contralateral superior based septal mucoperichondrial flaps or inferior-based ipsilateral septal flaps, with an average follow-up of more than a year. All patients were satisfied with the aesthetic result. There were no losses of flap, soft tissue, or cartilage grafts. Nasal fistula that followed the use of septal flaps was asymptomatic.

REFERENCES

1. Barton FE Jr: Aesthetic aspects of nasal reconstruction, *Clin Plast Surg* 15:155-166, 1988.

2. Barton F, Cottell W, Walker B: The principle of chemosurgery and delayed primary reconstruction in the management of different basal cell carcinomas, *Plast Reconstr Surg* 68:746, 1981.

3. Burget GC, Menick F: *Aesthetic reconstruction of the nose,* St Louis, 1994, Mosby.

4. Burget GC, Menick F: Aesthetic reconstruction of one-half of the upper lip, *Plast Reconstr Surg* 78:583, 1986.

5. Burget GC, Menick FJ: Nasal reconstruction: seeking a fourth dimension, *Plast Reconstr Surg* 78:145, 1986.

6. Burget GC, Menick FJ: Nasal support and lining: the marriage of beauty and blood supply, *Plast Reconstr Surg* 84:189, 1989.

7. Burget GC, Menick FJ: Restoration of nasal defects—an aesthetic viewpoint. In Jurkiewicz M, Krizek T, editors: *Plastic surgery—principles and practice,* St Louis, 1988, Mosby.

8. Burget GC, Menick FJ. In Reilly T, editor: *Restoration of the nose after skin cancer. Plastic Surgery Educational Foundation: Instructional Courses, Vol 1,* St Louis, 1988, Mosby.

9. Burget GC, Menick FJ: Subunit principle in nasal reconstruction, *Plast Reconstr Surg* 76:239, 1985.

10. Burget G, Murrel G, Toriumi D: Most current technique for aesthetic reconstruction of the confluence of the nose, lip and cheek. In *Operative techniques in plastic and reconstructive surgery,* Philadelphia, 1997, WB Saunders.

11. Converse JM: Composite graft from the septum in nasal reconstruction, *Trans Lat Am Congr Plast Surg* 8:281, 1956.

12. Converse JM: Reconstruction of the nose by the scalping flap technique, *Surg Clin North Am* 39:335, 1959.

13. Elliot RA Jr: Rotation flaps of the nose, *Plast Reconstr Surg* 44:1A47, 1969.

14. Freud S: *The ego and id,* London, 1927, Hogarth.

15. Gibson T, Davis WB: The distortion of autogenous grafts: its cause and prevention, *Br J Plast Surg* 10:257, 1958.

16. Gillies HD, Millard DR: *The principles and art of plastic surgery,* Boston, 1957, Little Brown.

17. Gillies HD: *Plastic surgery of the face,* London, 1920, Oxford Medical.

18. Gonzalez-Ulloa M, Castillo A, Stevens E, et al: Preliminary study of the total restoration of the facial skin, *Plast Reconstr Surg* 13:151, 1954.

19. Guerrerosantos J, Dicksheet S: Nasolabial flap with simultaneous cartilage graft in nasal alar reconstruction, *Clin Plast Surg* 8:599, 1981.

20. Harris D: The symptomatology of abnormal appearance—an anecdotal survey, *Br J Plast Surg* 35:312, 1982.

21. Herbert DC, Harrison RG: Nasolabial subcutaneous pedicle flaps. 1. Observations on their blood supply, *Br J Plast Surg* 28:85, 1975.

22. Herbert DC: A subcutaneous pedicle cheek flap for reconstruction of ala defects, *Br J Plast Surg* 31:79, 1978.

23. Kazanjian VH: Reconstruction of the ala using septal flap, *Trans Am Acad Ophthalmol Otolaryngol* 42:338, 1937.

24. Mazzola RF, Marcus S: History of total nasal reconstruction with particular emphasis on the folded forehead flap technique, *Plast Reconstr Surg,* 72:408, 1983.

25. McCarthy JG, Lorenc PZ, Cutting C, et al: The median forehead flap revisited: the blood supply, *Plast Reconstr Surg* 76:866-869, 1985.

26. McGregor I, McGregor F: *Cancer of the face and mouth,* Edinborough, 1986, Churchill Livingstone.

27. McGregor JC, Soutar DS: A critical assessment of the bilobed flap, *Br J Plast Surg* 34:197, 1981.

28. Menick FJ: Aesthetic restoration of the face. In Cohen M, editor: *Problems in general surgery,* Philadelphia, 1989, JB Lippincott.

29. Menick F: Artistry in facial surgery: aesthetic perceptions and the subunit principle. In Furnas D, editor: *Clinics in plastic surgery, vol 14,* Philadelphia, 1987, WB Saunders.

30. Menick FJ: Principles of head and neck reconstruction. In Cohen M, editor: *Mastery in surgery: plastic and reconstructive surgery,* vol 3, Boston, 1994, Little Brown, pp 842-863.

31. Menick FJ: The aesthetic use of the forehead flap for nasal reconstruction—the paramedian forehead flaps. In Tobin G, editor: *Clinics in plastic surgery,* Philadelphia, 1990, WB Saunders.

32. Menick FJ, Burget GC: Reconstruction of the nose. In Cohen M, editor: *Mastery in surgery: plastic and reconstructive surgery*, vol 3, Boston, 1994, Little Brown, pp 883-905.

33. Menick FJ, Burget GC: Nasal reconstruction: creating a visual illusion. In Habal M, editor: *Advances in plastic surgery, vol 6*, St Louis, 1989, Mosby.

34. Menick FJ, Burget G: Regional units in aesthetic reconstruction of the face. In Coiffman F, editor: *Cirugia plastica, reconstructiva y estetica*, Barcelona, 1997, Sabat Editores.

35. Meyer R: Aesthetic aspects in reconstructive surgery of the nose, *Aesthetic Plast Surg* 12:195, 1988.

36. Millard DR: Congenital nasal tip retrusion and three little composite ear grafts: case report, *Plast Reconstr Surg* 48:501-504, 1971.

37. Millard DR: Secondary corrective rhinoplasty, *Plast Reconstr Surg* 44:545-557, 1969.

38. Millard DR: The fat flip flap: a method of blending a pedicle implant, *Plast Reconstr Surg* 44:202-204, 1969.

39. Millard DR: Three very short noses and how they were lengthened, *Plast Reconstr Surg* 65:10-15, 1980.

40. Millard DR: Aesthetic reconstructive rhinoplasty, *Clin Plast Surg* 8:169, 1981.

41. Millard DR: Reconstructive rhinoplasty for the lower half of the nose, *Plast Reconstr Surg* 53:133, 1974.

42. Millard DR: Reconstructive rhinoplasty for the lower two-thirds of the nose, *Plast Reconstr Surg* 57:722, 1976.

43. Millard DR: Hemirhinoplasty, *Plast Reconstr Surg* 40:440-445, 1967.

44. Millard DR: Alar margin sculpturing, *Plast Reconstr Surg* 40:342-347, 1967.

45. Millard DR: Total reconstructive rhinoplasty and a missing link, *Plast Reconstr Surg* 37:167, 1966.

46. Millard DR: *Principilization of plastic surgery*, Boston, 1986, Little Brown.

47. Millard DR: Versatility of the chondromucosal flap in the nasal vestibule, *Plast Reconstr Surg* 50:580-587, 1972.

48. Miller TA: The Tagliacozzi flap as a method of nasal and palatal reconstruction, *Plast Reconstr Surg* 76:870, 1985.

49. New GB: Sickle flaps for nasal reconstruction, *Surg Gynecol Obstet* 80:497, 1945.

50. Rieger RA: A local flap for repair of the nasal tip, *Plast Reconstr Surg* 40:147, 1967.

51. Rybka FJ: Reconstruction of the nasal tip using nasalis myocutaneous sliding flaps, *Plast Reconstr Surg* 71:40, 1983.

52. Silverman M, Kopf A, Gladstein A, et al: Recurrence rates of treated basal cell carcinoma, *Dermatol Surg Oncology*, 18:549, 1992.

53. Spear SL, Kroll SS, Romm S: A new twist to the nasolabial flap for reconstruction of lateral alar defects, *Plast Reconstr Surg* 79:915, 1987.

54. Sushruta S. In Bhishagratna KKL, editor: *Sushruta Samhita*, Calcutta, 1907-1916, Bose.

55. Washio H: Retroauricular temporal flap, *Plast Reconstr Surg* 43:162, 1969.

56. Zimany A: The bilobed flap, *Plast Reconstr Surg* 11:424, 1953.

57. Zitelli JA: The bilobed flap for nasal reconstruction, *Arch Dermatol* 125:957, 1989.

58. Zitelli JA: Personal communication.

59. Zitelli JA: The nasolabial flap as a single stage procedure, *Arch Dermatol* 126:1445, 1990.

CHAPTER

Reconstruction of Acquired Ear Deformities

Robert J. Havlik
Thomas S. Moore

INDICATIONS

The external ear derives both its importance and its vulnerability from its projection from the surface of the head. The primary importance of the external ear lies in its aesthetic characteristics. Although few would argue that the ear is beautiful, its absence, size discrepancy, or distortion is immediately apparent, almost always not attractive, and often subject to ridicule.[58] *Cartilaginous* in structure, aesthetically critical, and vulnerable to injury, the ear is similar to the only other structure that projects from the surface of the craniofacial skeleton—the nose. The ear's functional role, establishing the directional source of sound, is relatively insignificant, and unlike other animals, the muscles associated with the human ear are atavistic. The auricle's primary function in man may be its adapted role as support for eyeglass frames.[60,78]

The projection of the ear from the side of the head makes it susceptible to sun exposure, actinic damage, and ultimate degeneration into cutaneous malignancies, as well as to injury from direct trauma by contusion, abrasion, laceration, avulsion, and thermal injury. The most frequent indications for reconstruction of acquired ear deformities are tumor resection and direct trauma. In addition to the auricle itself, the condition of the surrounding tissues (e.g., scalp, temporal vessels, facial skin) will greatly impact on resective and reconstructive strategies.

CANCER OF THE EXTERNAL EAR

Each year more than 600,000 cases of cutaneous malignancies are reported in the United States, with over 90% involving the head and neck region and 5% to 10% the ear.[7,12,22,55,88] Predominantly a disease of elderly white males,[24,28,78,88] the average age for development of a cutaneous malignancy of the ear is in the sixth and seventh decades of life.[24,28,78,79,88]

The 9:1 ratio of men to women may be secondary to occupational hazards (e.g., farming, construction) and traditional differences in hairstyles.*

Unlike most other areas of the skin, where basal cell carcinoma predominates, on the external ear the incidence of squamous cell cancer may equal or actually exceed that of basal cell cancer,[28,88] with several of the larger series showing squamous cell cancer at 50% to 60%, basal cell carcinoma at 30% to 40%, and melanomas at approximately 5% to 10%.† Furthermore, 5% to 10% of all melanomas will be found on the ear, a disproportionately high risk area.[12] Ear lesions may have the clinical appearance of basal cell cancer, yet histology proves them to be squamous cell cancer with its much higher recurrence rate and invasive potential.[55,80,88] Squamous cell carcinoma has, in fact, a higher recurrence and metastatic rate in the ear (5% to 18%) than in any other site.[24,55,78,80,88] In children, the ear is also a common site for rhabdomyosarcoma, being second in frequency only to the orbit in the head and neck region.

As many as 60% of cancers will present with initial involvement of the helix,[24,79,88] with the remaining typically found on the antihelix, triangular fossa, concha, and posterior auricular skin.

Management of carcinomas of the auricle is surgical. Several large series of patients treated by radiation have demonstrated higher recurrence rates.[42,51] Moreover most patients are at continued risk of solar radiation exposure and thus have the potential for second and even third primary cancers of the ear.[24] In the lower half of the ear, there is more subcutaneous tissue between the skin and perichondrium, and it is often possible to perform an excisional biopsy of the lesion without removing the underlying cartilage. In the upper half, however, the skin is more adherent to the perichondrium, usually mandating excisional wedge biopsy for diagnosis. If the lesion is larger, various star-shaped patterns of excision may be necessary to prevent "buckling" of the cartilage as the wedge is closed (Figure 89-1).[80] Full-thickness resection of skin, perichondrium, and cartilage is appropriate.

---

*References 12, 24, 28, 42, 78-80.
†References 12, 24, 78, 80, 82, 88.

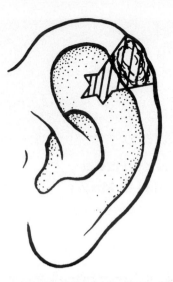

Figure 89-1. If a simple wedge excision creates buckling, the wedge can be converted to a star-shaped excision, which allows for reduction of the scapha, or if extended further medially, the conchal bowl, and allows approximation of the cartilage to minimize distortion.

If perichondrium and cartilage are involved, as they may be in up to one third of these lesions, a more aggressive resection is indicated, because of less predictable tumor extension along this plane.[33,82] Mohs' surgery may not confer any particular advantage over wide resection with frozen section control in lesions of the periauricular region.[55] Surgical therapy includes resection with a negative margin and appropriate treatment of the parotid, postauricular, and cervical regional nodal basins. The incidence of nodal involvement in primary squamous cell carcinomas of the ear ranges from 5% to 20%, and even small carcinomas (<2 cm) can have an appreciable incidence of metastatic disease,[24,33,55,78] leading to significant recurrence rates of 14% to 25%.[12,24,28,79] Concern regarding aesthetic appearance of the resulting ear is clearly secondary to adequate management of the malignancy. The choice of reconstructive technique for auricular defects after cancer excision is determined by the defect, the adjacent tissue available, the presence or absence of radiation injury, and considerations for clinical follow-up.

TRAUMA OF THE EXTERNAL EAR

The prominent unprotected position of the ear makes it susceptible to abrasion, laceration, contusion/hematoma, thermal injury, and avulsion. It is protected somewhat from physical injury by its resilient cartilage, which bends easily and recoils.[64] As a "prize" of political and physical conquest, it is subject to amputation in battle. Japanese samurai, having invaded and conquered Korea 400 years ago, hacked off the noses and ears of tens of thousands of Koreans and buried them at the Mimizuka, or "ear mound," a three-story-high hill outside the ancient Japanese capital of Kyoto. Few Japanese outside of Kyoto know of this ear mound, but most Koreans do, and this bizarre relic remains to Koreans a symbol of a Japanese aggression,[54] one of the world's most macabre war memorials. In Colonial America as an act of domination and demonstration of resolve, King Charles I nailed the ears of rebellious Puritans and other colonists to a post.[33] Therefore the ear, despite its natural resiliency, does not escape much.

Since head trauma accompanies three quarters of motor vehicle accidents, the auricle is frequently involved. After life-threatening problems have been addressed, methodical assessment of the external auricle, external auditory canal, tympanic membrane, hearing status, postauricular ecchymosis, otorrhea, and facial nerve function, as well as a complete neurologic evaluation, should be performed for every acute injury. The external auricle should be assessed for lacerations, abrasions, missing skin cover, missing cartilage, or hematoma formation.

Lacerations

Lacerations and abrasions are the most frequently seen ear injuries. Following the administration of local anesthesia, the fundamental principle is cleansing of tissue with minimal debridement (Figure 89-2) aimed at maximal preservation of tissue. Even tissue deemed "marginal" should be cleansed and used in the repair, since it can always be debrided if demarcation occurs.[62] The principle of working from "known to unknown" assumes increasing importance as the severity of the injury increases.[62,64] The surgeon will visualize the next step in the process of completing the repair, as the fragments "line-up" with traction.[62] Tissue approximation must be meticulous, taking care to align all discernible landmarks. If it is not possible to repair all sites, healing by secondary intention will often occur in small defects, since the ear has a remarkable ability for secondary epithelialization.[62] If the perichondrium is intact and epithelialization does not occur promptly, areas of exposed perichondrium should be grafted.[64] Abrasions should be cleansed extensively, debriding fragments of "road rash," lest they result in fixed "traumatic tattoos." The initial management is almost never the time for major reconstructive intervention, with the exception of those isolated cases in which the whole ear is amputated and there is the possibility of replantation. Postoperative support of the injured ear parts (including both dressings and wound care) is crucial to good outcome.[10]

Hematomas

Hematomas occur with blunt trauma to the ear when blood accumulates between the cartilage and the perichondrium, presenting as a fluctuance over the ear with bluish discoloration. These should be drained early and copiously irrigated through an incision designed so as to be hidden or camouflaged in the hollow of the scapha, concealed by the helical rim.[53] Following complete evacuation of the hematoma and irrigation of the potential space, the skin and perichondrium should be coapted to the underlying cartilage framework using a tie over bolster or dental roll to prevent recurrent fluid accumulation below the perichondrium, which may serve as a nidus for further cartilage formation, leading to a loss of

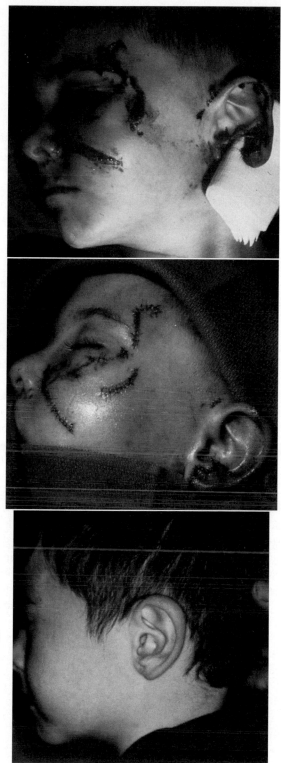

Figure 89-2. Lacerations of face and ear. **A,** The lower third of the ear is avulsed as a superiorly based flap. **B,** Meticulous cleansing and reapproximation lead to uneventful healing with a favorable aesthetic result **(C)**.

definition of the auricle's cartilage framework and creating a "cauliflower ear." This difficult problem requires contouring and shaving the excess cartilage to improve the definition of the underlying auricular framework and is better treated by prevention.

Thermal Injury

Thermal injury may occur from either frostbite or burns. Below 19E F, the sensibility of exposed tissues is diminished. Frostbite occurs when the exposed tissue has actual freezing of extracellular fluid with ice crystal formation. The key points in management are: (1) rapid rewarming of the tissue with sterile, water-soaked towels or cotton gauze at 100E to 108E F, (2) avoidance of further trauma or injury to tissue, and (3) use of topical antibiotics such as bacitracin, Silvadene, or Sulfamylon. The process of rewarming is painful, requiring analgesics. No tissue should be debrided initially, and none should be debrided at all unless clear demarcation has occurred.

The ears are involved in 90% of all facial burns.[41] Superficial and partial-thickness burns are cleansed and treated with topical antibiotics. Deep partial-thickness and full-thickness burns should be treated with Sulfamylon since it penetrates skin and cartilage well. Critical to the treatment of any thermal injury to the auricle is the prevention of further tissue injury by avoiding pressure and additional trauma and by minimizing the risk of infection. Because facial burns may necessitate ventilation and sedation, further injury from pressure on the auricle can convert partial-thickness injury to full-thickness injury. The head must be carefully positioned and turned frequently to prevent pressure related insults to the burned ear. The ear is usually allowed to heal following conservative treatment with topical antimicrobials, and reconstruction delayed. Early debridement, iontophoresis, and early skin grafting may, however, be important in the prevention of severe deformities.[75] Bacterial chondritis secondary to cartilage exposure occurs in up to one fourth of all patients with burns involving the ears[41] and requires that aggressive debridement be combined with the use of intravenous antibiotics, topical antibiotics, and possibly iontophoresis to prevent invasive tissue destruction.

OPERATIONS

The approach to reconstruction of the external ear is similar to reconstruction of any other area of the body. The reconstructive surgeon must adequately assess the defect, catalog the missing components, and delineate the tissues available for reconstruction. The tissue available after resection of a helical rim basal cell carcinoma differs markedly from that available after an episode of chondritis following a major burn. In those cases where there is the loss of skin only with an intact perichondrium, skin grafts can be applied. The favored donor sites include the posterior auricular area, the auriculocephalic sulcus, the retroauricular area, the upper inner arm, the scalp, and the buttock.[10] When there is also the loss of perichondrium, grafting is not possible, and flap coverage is necessary. There is, however, a readily available "reservoir" of tissue for flap reconstruction on the posterior aspect of the auricle, in the auriculocephalic sulcus, and in the retroauricular skin and soft tissue overlying the mastoid region. More extensive injury with loss of this reservoir may require the use of a superficial temporoparietal fascial flap or other tissue transfer. Cartilage is usually required for reconstruction of defects of the antihelix and helix, whereas cartilaginous defects of the scapha or concha can be adequately resurfaced with either skin flaps or grafts if the outer cartilage framework of the helix and antihelix persists. The presence of either the helical or antihelical cartilage struts is the key to reconstruction of a normal appearing ear.[15] Cartilage donor sites include the same ear, the contralateral ear, and rib cartilage from the costochondral junction. When conchal cartilage from the ipsilateral or contralateral ear is harvested, an intact antihelical strut will prevent collapse and further deformity.[15,16] Collapse and

deformity of the helical rim after tumor excision and primary closure or skin grafting can be prevented by use of a composite graft of skin with a small amount of auricular cartilage, although this seldom yields better results than a simple extension of the resection into the concha and wedge closure, or the use of a chondrocutaneous rotation advancement flap.

Unfortunately the complexity of ear reconstruction does not increase linearly with the amount of tissue loss, but rather exponentially. The problems encountered in acquired auricular deformity can be categorized according to the segmental site of loss, and techniques available for reconstruction can be tailored to each site. Special consideration is given to the total ear reconstruction and to the management of the burned ear.

CUTANEOUS DEFECTS

The presence of supple and well-vascularized skin is essential for success in ear reconstruction. Because the cutaneous cover of the ear is tightly adherent over most of its surface, there are relatively few instances following trauma (other than thermal injury) or tumor ablation in which the skin and subcutaneous tissue are lost and the perichondrium is intact and able to support skin grafting.[33] Partial-thickness losses of the ear can be treated by (1) wedge resection and closure; (2) local flaps; (3) excision of cartilage and skin grafting the deep surface of the opposite cutaneous surface (Figure 89-3); or (4) open treatment and healing by secondary intention.[62] Fortunately, the adjacent posterior aspect of the auricle, the auriculocephalic sulcus, and mastoid area can provide this hairless skin and subcutaneous tissue for flap coverage of the visible anterior surface of the ear.[50] Such flaps, either axial or random, can be based anteriorly, superior to the root of the helix, and transposed directly (Figure 89-4)[36] or if necessary elevated from the posterior surface to provide additional tissue in the area of the deficit (Figure 89-5, A to C), with or without a cartilage graft for additional support, covering the donor defect with a skin graft.[67] Alternatively, the flaps can be based

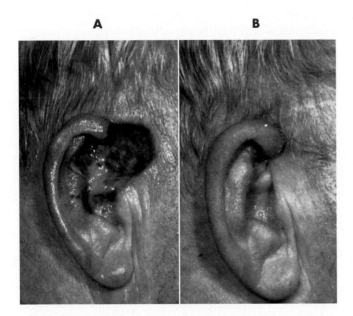

Figure 89-3. Defects of the concha and root of the helix can often be simply treated with grafting. **A,** Defect after Mohs' treatment of a squamous cell carcinoma. **B,** Several months following skin grafting.

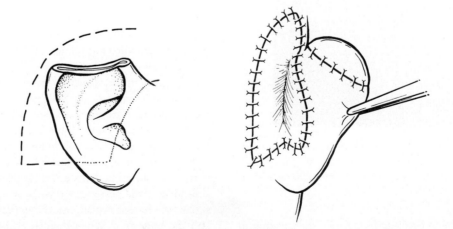

Figure 89-4. A superiorly based flap from auriculocephalic sulcus used for coverage of the helical rim and other more extensive defects. The donor site of the flap is closed by advancing the mastoid skin, or when the flap is relatively wide, skin grafted.

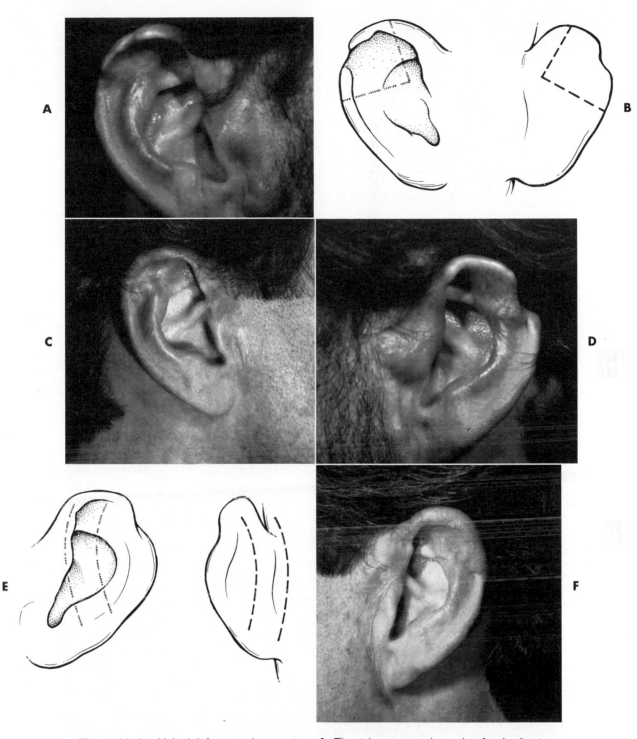

Figure 89-5. Helical defects in a burn patient. **A,** The right ear several months after healing in a firefighter who sustained multiple second-and third-degree burns of the face and ears. Most of the helical rim is intact, but markedly thinned. **B,** Design of V-to-Y flap on posterior auricular surface. The flap is laterally based (toward the helical rim), and is undermined onto the posterior surface of the ear with lateral advancement of the posterior auricular skin, which is rolled on itself, creating a new helix. **C,** Result after 6 months. **D,** The left helical rim in the same patient with loss of the helical margin in the upper two thirds of the ear. **E,** Design of a bipedicle flap of posterior auricular sulcus, measuring 2×5 cm. **F,** Following division and inset of the flap in several stages under local anesthesia.

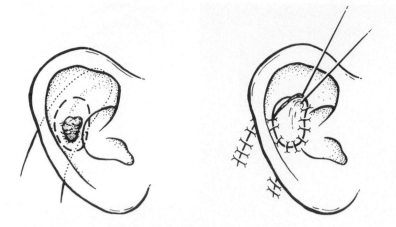

Figure 89-6. Defects of the anterior (or lateral) surface of the external ear are aesthetically important. They can be reconstructed by developing a flap in the mastoid region, and passing this flap through an incision in the cartilage to resurface the anterior ear and provide excellent results.

posterior on the skin overlying the mastoid, and draped over the helix for closure of the cutaneous defect, with subsequent division of the base of the flap and release of the ear (Figure 89-5, D to F).[33] A window created in the cartilage will allow passage of the flap to the anterior (lateral) surface of the ear for one-stage reconstruction (Figure 89-6). Such cutaneous flaps will provide an effective single-stage reconstruction for composite defects of the concha, with little need to replace the cartilage. The defect created by the flap can usually be closed primarily, or with the placement of a skin graft on the perichondrium or on the periosteum. The excellent blood supply of the cutaneous coverage in this area is responsible for the consistent reliability of "random flaps." A chondrocutaneous flap based on the middle branch of the posterior auricular vessels has been described for reconstruction of conchal defects.[27,71]

The "reservoir" of tissue on the posterior auricular surface, the auriculocephalic sulcus, and the retroauricular area of the mastoid can be a critical determinant of the end result following not only an isolated cutaneous loss, but also the loss of a composite portion of the ear. It is essential to recognize the importance of this tissue in successful ear reconstruction and carefully plan incisions to avoid limitation of staged or subsequent reconstructions.

RECONSTRUCTION OF THE HELIX

The helix is the most prominent part of the ear, and is visible when viewing the face from the front or on profile.[56] The helix is the area most susceptible to actinic damage and malignant degeneration[24,25,80] and to traumatic injury, particularly thermal injury. Because the skin is so thin and adherent in the anterior, or lateral, surfaces of the ear, these sites are most commonly burned (see Figure 89-5).[75] Rosenthal stresses the importance of maintaining the thin lateral helical lip, or outer edge, to avoid a flattened

"cartoonlike appearance," since reconstruction can be inordinately difficult.

Smaller defects of the helix can be closed by extending the defect centrally and closing this directly as a wedge or a modified star (see Figure 89-1). Wedge closure becomes less desirable in defects larger than 15 mm, since this results in a smaller auricle, buckling, and distortion of the remaining cartilage framework. To prevent distortion, the surgeon must reestablish the proper relationship between the available peripheral and central components—increase the former or decrease the latter.[60] This principle underlies the three main techniques for reconstruction of larger helical rim defects: the chondrocutaneous advancement flap (Antia-Buch), the "tunnel" procedure of Converse, and the tubed pedicle flap.

The chondrocutaneous advancement flap of Antia and Buch uses an incision of the anterior aspect of the ear in the concealed hollow of the scapha,[4] which extends through the anterior skin, perichondrium, and cartilage. The posterior skin of the auricle is elevated from the perichondrium in the area of the incision medially toward the skull (Figure 89-7). This leaves the existing helical rim mobile as a composite flap, with the posterior skin of the auricle as a pedicle. The root of the helix is incised and rotated posteriorly in a V-to-Y fashion, and the inferior aspect of the helix and lobule is elevated and rotated superiorly. Closure of moderate to large defects of the helix and scapha is achieved in a single stage without a secondary donor site, concealing the incision in the scapha within the "shadow" of the helix. Although the technique was originally described for reconstruction of defects of the upper third of the ear,[4] it works equally well in reconstruction of middle and lower third defects.[16] In a cadaver study, reconstruction of helical defects with helical rim advancement always led to closure with less wound tension than did wedge excision and primary closure.[26]

The Antia-Buch helical rim advancement techniques does, however, have limitations. In the cadaver study, closure of a 20-mm defect in the helical rim through the use of the helical

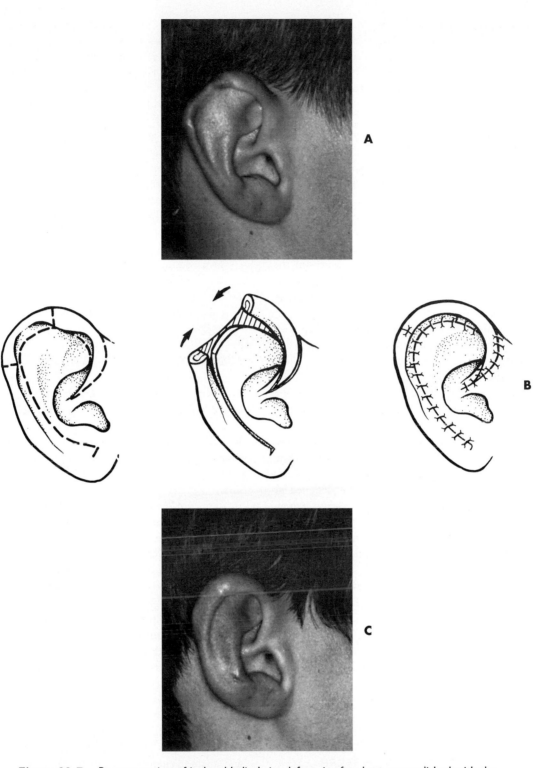

Figure 89-7. Reconstruction of isolated helical rim defects is often best accomplished with the use of the Antia-Buch chondrocutaneous flap technique. **A,** An 11-year-old boy has a 2-cm defect of the helical rim due to a horse bite. **B,** The principle of the chondrocutaneous flap is illustrated. Note that the helical rim is mobilized completely with the posterior auricular skin serving as the base of the flap. Also note that both the helical root and the helical rim can be mobilized if needed. In the case shown, only the posterior and inferior helix was used for rotation and advancement. **C,** The result 1 year after reconstruction.

rim advancement decreased ear height from 72 mm to 63.5 mm, an 11.8% decrease.[26] As the helical rim defect exceeds 25 to 30 mm, significant distortion occurs, limiting its use to defects less than 3 cm in length.[61,62] Although this technique has been largely limited to defects of the helical rim, several alternative procedures based on a similar principle of segmental advancement have been described for defects of the helix including the scapha and antihelix.[5,48]

For defects larger than 30 to 35 mm, a staged approach is necessary.[15] The tunnel procedure first advocated by Converse[30,31,33] involves suturing the margins of the helical defect to the retroauricular skin at the first stage. If wound conditions permit, a strut of cartilage, harvested from a second donor site (usually rib), is placed; if not, a second stage is required for placement of the cartilage (Figure 89-8). In the final stage, the cartilage strut is elevated with its envelope of skin from the retroauricular area. This technique allows reliable reconstruction of large defects of the helical rim and scapha and does not lead to a diminution in size of the auricle.

Reconstruction of the helix using a tubed pedicle flap is an excellent technique when adequate adjacent skin is available (see Figure 89-5, E).[6,33,43,74] For larger defects, two thin tubes of retroauricular skin are constructed sharing a common base. The free ends of these tubes are attached to the ends of the helical defect, with the shared central component remaining anchored in the retroauricular area. At the second stage, division and inset of the shared common central component complete the helical margin. Donor site problems are uncommon and the thin skin allows a favorable aesthetic result. Fine caliber tubed pedicle flaps can be designed at distant sites (e.g., cervical skin) but require more stages, which may compromise reliability. A similar procedure for helical reconstruction was described by Lewin and based on a postauricular mastoid flap transferred to the helical defect, leaving an exposed raw surface posteriorly.[56] The contour of the helical rim is then reconstituted as the raw surface of the flap heals, causing the flap to tube on itself. Like any pedicle flap, the second stage of the procedure requires division and inset of the flap. The theoretic advantage of this technique is that it creates a natural, thin helix, which is often difficult with tubed pedicle flaps. When using "skin-only" techniques, the surgeon must routinely consider whether the long-term results would be improved by the use of a cartilage component for structural support.[16]

RECONSTRUCTION OF THE UPPER THIRD OF THE EAR

Defects of the upper third of the ear can be partially concealed by hair; however, this area is functionally very important for supporting eyeglasses. Five main techniques have been identified for reconstruction of defects of the upper third of the ear.[16] Minor losses confined to the helical rim are amenable to a helical rim advancement flap as described above or a preauricular banner flap. Intermediate-sized loss is reconstructed with the anteriorly based flap of tissue from the

auriculocephalic sulcus described by Crikelair (see Figure 89-4).[36] Brent suggests that major losses in the upper third are most successfully reconstructed with a contralateral conchal cartilage graft, originally described by Adams.[1] He cautions, however, that if the recipient bed skin is unfavorable, this technique should not be used.[16] In fact, in major losses of the upper third of the ear, the skin is seldom adequate to support a large composite graft. In such cases, a fifth method, in which the entire concha is rotated upward as a chondrocutaneous composite flap on a small anterior pedicle of the crus helix, is useful (Figure 89-9).[38] Donelan has reported very favorable results in a series of 24 upper third ear reconstructions in burn patients with this method.[40] Although this technique restores the silhouette of the ear, the antihelical contour is absent, sometimes resulting in a "shell" appearance.

Two additional techniques for larger defects of the upper third of the ear include the tunnel procedure (see Figure 89-8)[33] and the fabrication of a cartilage framework and coverage with a temporoparietal fascial flap and skin graft.

MIDDLE THIRD DEFECTS

Loss of the middle third of the ear is very deforming. Because of the mobile tissue, both superior and inferior, most auricular tumors in this area can be excised and closed by wedge or helical advancement,[15,16] albeit with corresponding diminution in ear height. Larger defects may require the Converse tunnel procedure (Figure 89-10).[30,31,33] In this staged procedure, the margins of the defect are opened and parallel incisions are made in the retroauricular tissue overlying the mastoid. The marginal incisions allow elevation of a small rim of tissue on the posterior, or medial, aspect of the ear, which is sewn to the retroauricular incision. A tunnel is then created between the retroauricular incisions, and a carved costochondral graft is inserted beneath the tunnel and secured to the native ear cartilage superiorly and inferiorly. The anterior limb of the marginal incisions is then sewn to the flap of skin overlying the tunnel of retroauricular skin. At a second stage, two incisions are extended posteriorly from the tunnel and connected with an incision parallel to the costal cartilage. This flap of retroauricular skin is elevated with the cartilage graft, and is then folded over the cartilage graft to complete the ear reconstruction. The donor site is closed by either advancement or skin graft. This technique provides reliable reconstruction with the hairless posterior auricular skin, with excellent color and texture match.

LOWER THIRD DEFECTS

Because it is difficult to obtain a natural appearing result in this area, defects of the lower third of the ear involving more than the earlobe are particularly problematic. Most of the described reconstructive techniques for this area involve designing a local flap that can be elevated and doubled over on itself to provide soft, flexible tissue.[16] The exact

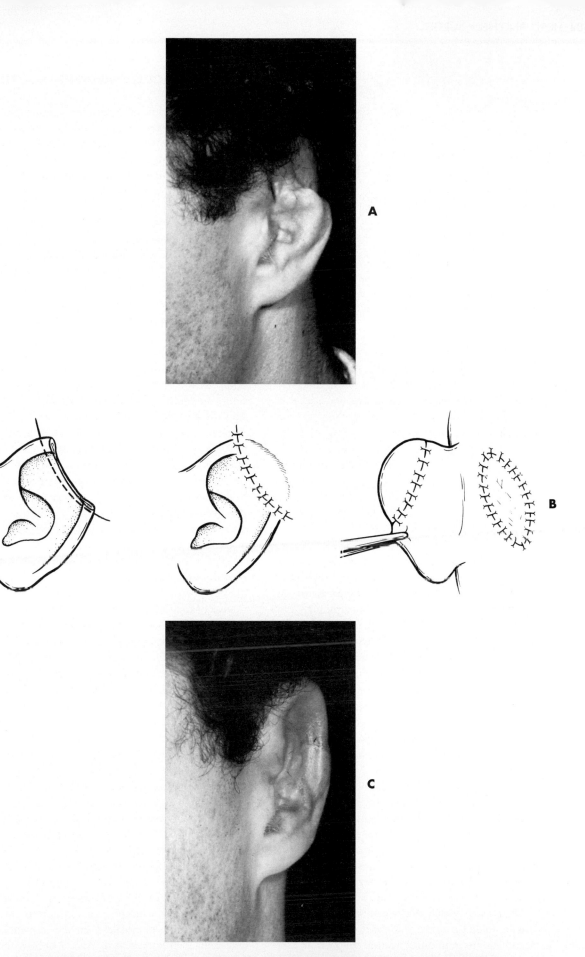

Figure 89-8. Defect of the upper third of the ear from an automobile accident. **A,** Appearance 1 year after injury. **B,** The upper third was reconstructed using a rib cartilage graft in a tunnel procedure. The cartilage graft is buried beneath the skin and secured to the cartilage framework. At a second stage, the flap is elevated. **C,** Result 6 months later.

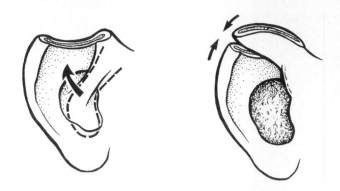

Figure 89-9. Reconstruction of upper third ear defects using the conchal cartilage as a pedicle flap based on the crus of the helix, as described by Davis. The entire conchal cartilage and its cutaneous cover may be elevated and transposed superiorly.

orientation of the flap design can be varied somewhat, and indeed may need to be altered, depending on the integrity of the skin in this area. Despite the need for soft and even floppy tissue in this area, Brent recommends the use of a contralateral conchal cartilage graft in order to enhance the reliability of reconstruction of this area.[16] The graft helps provide support during the wound contraction of the initial healing process, and also provides support to ensure long-term contour.[16]

ACQUIRED EARLOBE DEFORMITIES

Defects of the earlobe are largely related to ornamental piercing. Previously exclusively seen in females, they now appear with increasing frequency in males. The problems are either traumatic clefts from an earring pulling through the lobule, or the development of keloids following ear piercing. Cleft earlobes can be closed in many different ways, but it is important to offset the closure at the free border of the ear to prevent a notch from developing during healing. This can be done either with a Z-plasty or overlapping closure.

Keloids of the earlobe are common, and represent a particular challenge. Excision followed by steroid injection on a monthly basis with pressure provided by special clasp earrings as an adjunct in the postoperative course may decrease recurrence.[16]

Total reconstruction of a missing ear lobe is similar to reconstruction of lower third defects mentioned above. Converse described a bilobed flap folded on itself to create the lobule.[30] Alanis recommends reconstruction with a vertical banner type flap extending off of the inferior aspect of the ear, and folded back on itself.[2] Brent has also described a "reverse" helical rim advancement flap for earlobe reconstruction that extends posteriorly and inferiorly from the lower area of the helical rim.[14] These techniques basically rely on the creation of a flap that can be folded over on itself and closed to allow healing to occur and to minimize wound contraction and secondary deformation.

TOTAL AURICULAR RECONSTRUCTION

Major auricular loss usually occurs following traumatic injury or subtotal or total resection of the external ear for cancer. Essential components of total auricular reconstruction include the establishment of adequate and reliable cutaneous cover, the creation of an acceptable framework, and the provision of skin cover for the posteromedial aspect of the ear after elevation.[33]

Cutaneous Coverage
NATIVE SKIN COVERAGE. In major traumatic loss, coverage for the reconstructed ear can be provided by the native retroauricular skin, tissue expansion, or the temporoparietal fascial flap. Posttraumatic total or subtotal reconstruction differs from reconstruction of severe congenital microtia in several important ways. Since there is often scarring or adjacent tissue loss, the local cutaneous coverage may be unsatisfactory. No additional skin is available from unfurling the microtic ear remnant, and the presence of a fully developed external meatus limits the usefulness of an anterior incision and thus the facial skin. In such defects, the cutaneous pocket is best developed through a peripheral incision, avoiding a posterior incision, which may compromise both the local circulation and the total amount of available skin cover. These constraints on the development of the area and volume of the pocket may limit the size of the cartilage framework, and thus the definition of the reconstructed ear. For these reasons, the following alternatives for cutaneous coverage may need to be considered.

TISSUE EXPANSION. Tissue expansion has the potential to provide additional tissue for cutaneous coverage from the existing postauricular tissue. Neuman was the first to describe the use of tissue expansion in ear reconstruction.[68] Like tissue expansion elsewhere, this technique has the primary advantage of creating donor tissue that is virtually the same color, thickness, texture, and sensation as the recipient site (Figures 89-11 to 89-13). Expanded skin from the postauricular area is thin, pliable, well vascularized, and non–hair-bearing.[77] Tissue expansion can produce a sufficient amount of tissue to drape over framework without violation of the native hairline and allows delay of the major commitment of obtaining a rib cartilage graft until the second stage, when the integrity of the skin coverage has been established.[93]

Cases for tissue expansion should be carefully selected to exclude those with excessive scarring.[10] If significant scarring is present, an alternative method of reconstruction, such as the temporoparietal fascial flap, should be selected. At surgery the expander is placed through a remote incision, usually in the posterior scalp with its axis oriented radially to the site of tissue expansion. A remote valve expander is preferred.[11,77] The pocket is readily dissected in the subgaleal plane. Pre-placed galeal closure sutures prior to implant insertion preclude the use of needles near the implant, decreasing the risk of inadvertent puncture. After 2 or 3 weeks, the expander is inflated once or twice weekly. At the time of expander

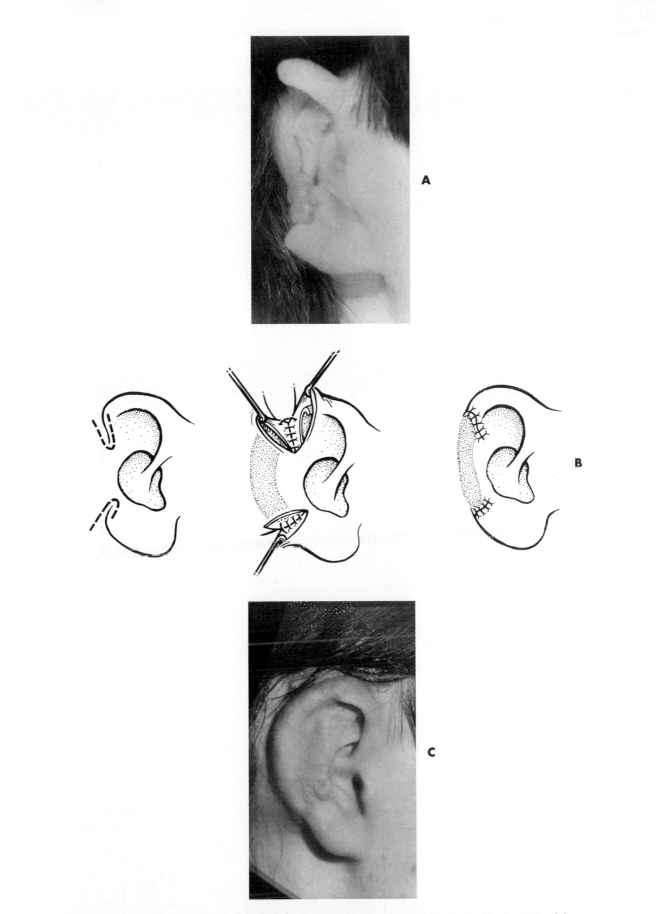

Figure 89-10. **A,** This large defect of the middle portion of the ear occurred in an automobile accident. **B,** The ear was reconstructed in a two-stage repair using the principles of the tunnel procedure. During the first stage a rib cartilage is contoured and inserted in the retroauricular skin. Several months later, the ear is elevated, using the skin over the mastoid to fold down over the rib cartilage graft. The mastoid area is then grafted. **C,** The result 6 months following the elevation of the framework.

A   **B**   **C**

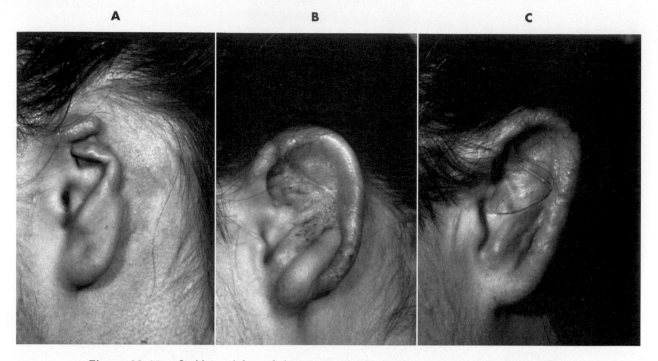

Figure 89-11. **A,** Major defect of the upper two thirds of the ear 6 months following an automobile accident. All that remains is the concha, the root of the helix, and the earlobe. **B,** A tissue expander was placed in the retroauricular skin overlying the mastoid, and a new ear framework fabricated from rib cartilage and inserted. **C,** Appearance of ear after rotation-transposition of lobule.

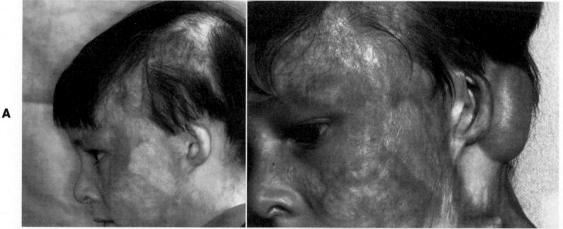

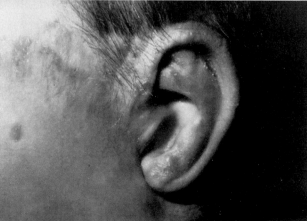

Figure 89-12. **A,** This patient sustained extensive third-degree burns of the body, face, and left ear. There is major loss of the ear except for the concha. **B** and **C,** The final result following a four-stage repair: during the first stage a tissue expander was placed in the retroauricular skin; a rib cartilage framework was fabricated and positioned during the second stage; the third stage consisted of a V-to-Y release of the earlobe; and finally, release of the auriculocephalic sulcus and skin graft of the postauricular space.

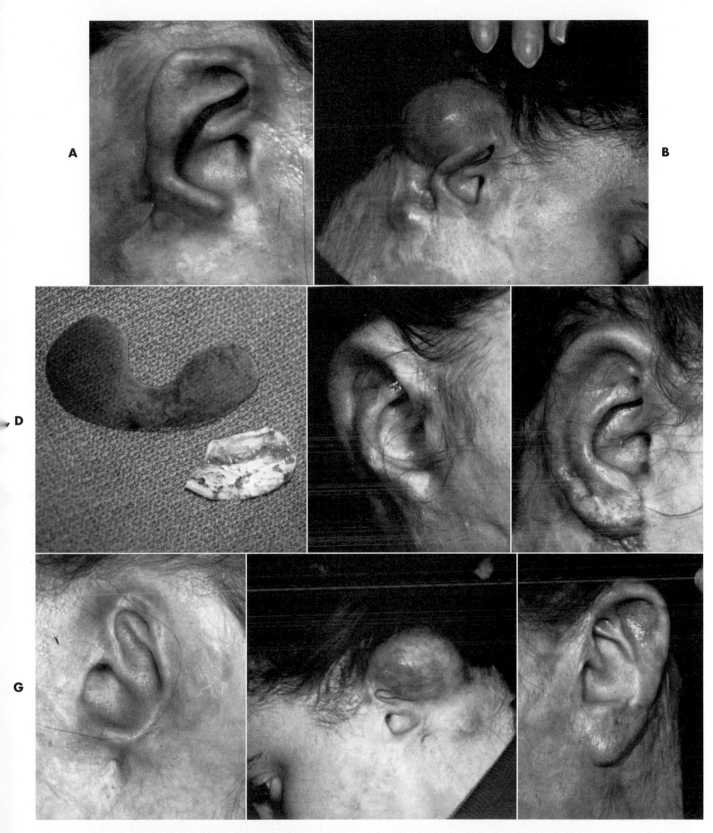

Figure 89-13. Near-total ear reconstruction in burn patient. **A,** The ear 1 year after extensive burn in a 26-year-old woman who ignited herself with gasoline. **B,** Tissue expansion was performed in the retroauricular skin in preparation for a rib cartilage graft. **C,** A pattern and rib graft to reconstruct the ear lobule. **D,** Several months following sculpting and insertion of a framework from rib cartilage. Unfortunately, the framework was not large enough to allow creation of the ear lobule. **E,** Final result after placement of the rib cartilage and the release and skin graft of the ear lobule in a subsequent stage. **F,** The opposite ear in the same patient prior to reconstruction. **G,** Appearance after placement of a tissue expander. **H,** Final result after sculpting a rib cartilage framework, and release and skin graft of the posterior auricular area.

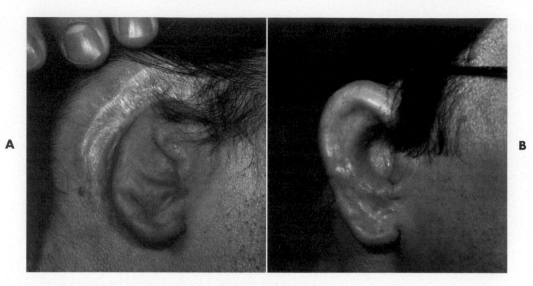

Figure 89-14. **A,** Failed Silastic implant ear reconstruction with prominent scarring and skin cover that is fibrotic and contracted. **B,** Following reconstruction with rib cartilage framework and temporoparietal fascial flap, a favorable aesthetic result is obtained.

removal, the fibrous capsule surrounding the tissue expander may be removed, if the skin cover is thick, to allow tight coaptation of the cutaneous coverage to the cartilage framework[10]; however, if the skin cover is thin in the expanded area, there is no need to remove the capsule and potentially jeopardize the quality of skin cover.

Despite many theoretic advantages, use of tissue expanders has not been uniformly successful in ear reconstruction. Sasaki has reported 12 patients, seven for helical defects and five for both helical and antihelical defects, noting that the most common minor complication was contraction of thin skin over carved cartilage framework.[77] Although not of sufficient degree to deform the framework, it did diminish the depth of the postauricular sulcus. He concludes that under favorable conditions, tissue expansion is an acceptable and reliable method for partial or total ear reconstruction[77]; however, several other authors have been disappointed with their results.[44,49] Citing inherent problems in the skin of this specific area of the scalp, Bauer cautions that even in the most experienced hands, complications of expansion of the ear have been more frequent than expected, and the risk of compromising the final reconstruction without significantly enhancing the final result must not be underestimated.[11] Potential problems of infection and exposure require meticulous attention to detail during both placement of expanders and the expansion process.[11] A critical issue is obviously case selection, since expansion in the face of scarring is futile.

"Instantaneous" tissue expansion has also been recommended for posttraumatic reconstruction. Unlike true tissue expansion, "instantaneous" expansion uses a Foley balloon at the time of surgery and relies on tissue creep, compression, dehydration, and circumferential migration of the skin.[13,75]

REGIONAL FLAPS. When adjacent tissue is scarred or not pliable, other sources for skin coverage must be considered.

Although several approaches to this problem have been recommended, including platysma flaps[6] and "superthin" skin and subcutaneous flaps,[81] the real workhorse for regional flap coverage in this area has become the temporoparietal fascial flap. Edgerton and Bachetta had described a "fan flap" in which the temporalis muscle and fascia were brought down to provide coverage over silicone frameworks.[45] A refinement of this technique also including temporalis muscle was presented by Ohmori.[69] Tegtmeier and Gooding were the first to describe the technique for dissection and elevation of the isolated temporoparietal fascial flap in auricular reconstruction with silicone frameworks, recognizing that inclusion of the temporalis muscle was not necessary for the successful and reliable use of this fascial flap.[87] Due to the requirement of thin coverage over any auricular framework, the temporoparietal fascial flap, or superficial temporal fascia as it has frequently been called, provides superior coverage characteristics (Figures 89-14 and 89-15). Erol et al adopted it for coverage of costochondral frameworks in reconstruction of the burned ear,[47] methods later refined by Brent and Byrd.[19]

The temporoparietal fascia is a thin, gossamer-like layer of tissue between the subcutaneous tissue of the scalp and the deep temporal fascia, extending approximately 12 cm by 14 cm from the zygomatic arch inferiorly to the area of the temporal crest of the skull superiorly, and from the lateral orbital rim anteriorly to the occipitoparietal area posteriorly. The anterior limit of flap elevation is generally the frontal branch of the facial nerve. About 2 to 3 mm thick in its native state, it is readily distinguished from the underlying deep temporal fascia, which has a dense white fibrous fascial appearance and directly overlies the temporalis muscle. The flap's main vascular pedicle is the superficial temporal artery and vein, which enters the base of the flap just anterior to the ear. The vessels are of sufficient size (2 mm) to allow transfer of the tissue as a free flap.[21] The anterior and posterior extent of

A　　　　　　　**B**　　　　　　　**C**

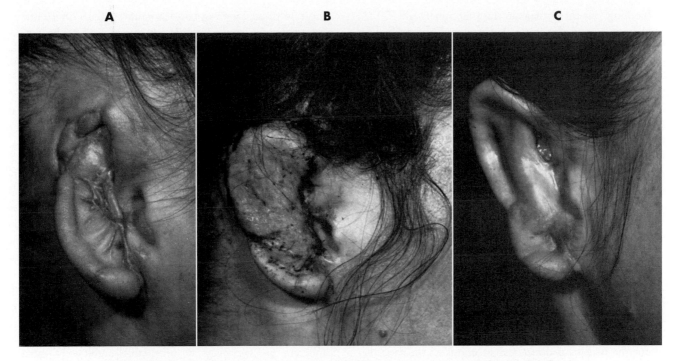

Figure 89-15. A, The ear several months following unsuccessful use of the Mladick-Baudet technique in a patient who sustained an auricular avulsion in an industrial accident. **B,** The ear early after rib graft reconstruction with coverage using a temporoparietal fascial flap and skin graft. **C,** The final result at 1 year without any additional surgery. Note the improved definition with this technique after enough time is allowed for edema and swelling to subside in the temporoparietal fascial flap.

the flap can be "back cut" to enhance the mobility of the flap without compromising its viability. When the flap is to be isolated completely on the superficial temporal pedicle, as in free tissue transfer, care must be taken to avoid injury to the vein, which lies superficial directly beneath the subcutaneous fat of the scalp. During elevation of the skin off the fascia in the subdermal layer there is risk of damage to the hair follicles, which may result in areas of alopecia. Otherwise, donor site morbidity is minimal. Variations of this flap may also be raised on the posterior auricular vessels or the occipital vessels if the superficial temporal vessels have been injured or if the area to be reconstructed is suitable for these posterior vessels.[10,19]

Because of its luxuriant vascularity, the flap can readily be skin grafted after it is draped over the cartilage framework or can wrap the entire cartilage framework for single-stage ear reconstruction. Following the use of the temporoparietal fascia for coverage of a cartilage framework, the highlights of the cartilage will be muted by edema, which resolves over 6 months to a year, leading to greater definition of the details of the cartilage framework. This prolonged resolution must be explained to the patient preoperatively to avoid unrealistic expectations (see Figure 89-15).

In secondary reconstruction of the ear after failed or unacceptable microtia reconstruction, Nagata reports that there are virtually identical constraints to those of other acquired ear deformities (see Figure 89-14). All necrotic skin and scar tissue from the primary reconstruction must be removed, limiting the available skin for secondary reconstruc-

tion. The presence of scar tissue and loss of tensile strength in the subdermal layer makes it difficult to construct a subcutaneous pocket for grafting of the three-dimensional framework, and in patients with full-thickness grafts over native periauricular skin, contraction of the skin grafts has been noted.[66] The temporoparietal fascia flap can serve as a lifeboat in these difficult secondary reconstructions.

Brent has also recommended the use of the temporoparietal fascial flap for acute coverage in the setting of auricular amputation when replantation is not possible.[19] In the few cases in which acute avulsive injuries have been reattached and covered with temporoparietal fascial flaps acutely, all have showed poor definition of the cartilage highlights.[3,52] The problem may lie not in the temporoparietal fascial flap, but rather in the inexorable impact of poorly controlled wound contraction on the thin and frail native auricular cartilage.

Ear Framework
SALVAGE OF AURICULAR CARTILAGE. The complex convolutions of the auricular cartilage have confounded countless surgeons. Surgical attempts to create a thin cartilage framework with cutaneous cover on both sides have consistently failed. Although these efforts may initially yield an acceptable result, the thin cartilage framework is unable to resist the powerful deforming forces of wound contraction during healing, placing a high priority on preservation of the traumatically amputated ear cartilage in the reconstruction and suggesting several salvage methods.[33]

"Banking" the ear cartilage in the abdominal wall[35,83,84,86] or the neck,[29] until the amputated site could be readied for transfer has been suggested by several authors. Mladick described the "pocket principle," in which the severed ear is dermabraded on both the anterior and posterior surfaces, sewn back in anatomic position, and covered with the retroauricular skin elevated off the mastoid region and advanced to cover the framework. After 2 weeks, the dermabraded ear is released and allowed to reepithelialize.[63] Mladick's single case report noted later problems with wound contraction. Baudet modified this technique, dermabrading the posterior surface and fenestrating the cartilage with relatively large holes to allow the soft tissue more surface area for neovascularization.[9,27]

Although all three of these "salvage" techniques have enjoyed a significant amount of discussion in the literature, there has been little documentation of their clinical utility. In 1967, Musgrave pointed out that only one of the cases published had a photograph.[64] Twenty years later, Bauer commented that there still were very few cases documented in the literature in which amputated parts, greater than 2 cm in their smallest dimension, had been successfully replanted without the benefit of direct reanastomosis of their vasculature.[10] Very few publications show acceptable photographs, and fewer still show any long-term documentation. Although these techniques (e.g., pocket principle, Baudet's fenestration technique) may show initial "success," long-term follow up frequently shows unacceptable deformity (see Figure 89-15).[10] The degradation with time may occur secondary to delay in revascularization[10] or as a result of the inexorable process of wound contraction, two processes that may be interlinked. Amputated ears reattached by microvascular surgery do not undergo the same process of degradation with time.

In the ear that cannot be reattached by microvascular surgery, an alternative would be to drape the temporoparietal fascial flap over the reattached and denuded auricular cartilage. The dense blood supply in this fascial flap may provide for effective revascularization, and thereby limit the ultimate loss of ear contour. However, reports using this technique for salvage of amputated auricular cartilage have shown ultimate poor definition of the auricular cartilage.[3,52] It is clear that the temporoparietal fascial flap can effectively cover costochondral grafts and yield a favorable result, but the costochondral framework is much stronger than the native auricular cartilage, and can more effectively counter the forces of wound contraction. At this point in time, nonmicrosurgical reattachment of a native auricular cartilage has not been proven consistently reliable by any method. The surgeon must carefully consider whether nonmicrosurgical or microsurgical (see below) reattachment is indicated and whether success or failure in this endeavor will jeopardize the more reliable technique of reconstruction with a temporoparietal fascial flap over a carved costochondral framework.

COSTOCHONDRAL FRAMEWORK. In most cases following total or near-total ear loss, the surgeon is ultimately faced with a total ear reconstruction, requiring fabrication of a costochondral framework. Pierce was the first to describe

creation of an ear from costochondral cartilage in 1930.[33,74] Several notable contributions and refinements have been made to the construction of the cartilage framework since then.* The successful grafting of a well-sculpted cartilage framework is the foundation for a sound ear repair.[18] The framework fabrication in the acquired auricular deformity is virtually identical to that in the congenital ear deformity (see Figures 89-11 to 89-15). The framework should not be sculpted to resemble a denuded auricular cartilage, but rather crafted with an exaggeration of the helical height and antihelix to compensate for the increased thickness of the covering skin.[18] The actual fabrication of the cartilage framework can also be more difficult in the acquired ear deformity than in the congenital ear deformity, since cartilage sculpting is more difficult in the adult patient. The rib cartilage is much firmer between 30 and 50 years of age, because of calcification and ossification. Adolescent cartilage, since it is undergoing a transition to its adult state, may be inhomogeneous, making sculpting problematic.[18]

ARTIFICIAL FRAMEWORK. Because of the complexities inherent in sculpting an acceptable autologous cartilage framework, there have been several attempts, largely unsuccessful, to develop an acceptable "off-the-shelf" artificial ear framework. Beginning with Cronin's initial use of a silicone ear framework, the complications of exposure, infection, and immediate or delayed extrusion have plagued synthetic frameworks (see Figure 89-14). Cronin suggested reserving its use for patients not prone to trauma, such as young girls and adults.[37] Ohmori reported a 10% extrusion rate with less than 2-year follow-up,[70] and complication rates in reported series are typically over 50%.[37,57] Success rates vary inversely with the length of follow-up.[57] In 1977, Brent and Converse remarked "that the bell tolls, in fact the knell has already sounded for the inorganic implant as a framework for auricular reconstruction."[33] Although some preliminary data suggest that porous polyethylene may behave more favorably than silicone with respect to tolerance of exposure and response to wound contraction,[91,92] there have been no long-term data published to suggest that artificial frameworks have anything but a limited role in ear reconstruction.

MICROSURGICAL REPLANTATION

Reattachment of the avulsed or amputated ear with a blood supply provides the best reconstruction of these devastating injuries. These replanted ears look essentially normal, and have not been subject to the loss of definition and wound contraction characteristic of other techniques.[39,90] Unfortunately, although it has now been over 30 years since Malt and McKhann's seminal report of arm reattachment,[59] and reattachment of digits, hands, and limbs is now relatively commonplace, the successful reattachment of ears is still a rarity.[65] Pennington et al were the first to report successful

---

*References 13, 17, 30, 32, 34, 85, 86.

replantation of the ear in 1980,[73] but in total there are fewer than 20 successful cases in the English literature.[39,76,90] Buncke notes that "without a doubt, the ear is one of the most difficult structures to replant because of the small size of the vessels in the pinna. I have tried and failed to replant two ears."[23] In addition to the small size of the vessels, several factors contribute to this relative infrequency. Although ears are frequently injured, they are less frequently completely amputated than avulsed. The occurrence of an avulsion, as opposed to a sharp amputation, decreases the success of finding a suitable vessel for vascular anastomosis. The vessels of the ear are extremely small and difficult to locate, being between 0.3 and 0.7 mm. All reported cases have had difficulty identifying suitable vessels, differentiating arteries from veins, and performing both inflow and particularly outflow anastomoses. A useful guide to the location of the vessels may be the small nerves that often accompany the vessels.[90] Use of the superficial temporal artery and vein or their branches almost always requires interpositional vein grafts from the dorsal foot for end-to-side anastomosis. Careful consideration of the probability of successful replantation must be weighed against the possibility of requiring further reconstruction with a temporoparietal fascial flap, since an end-to-end anastomosis to the superficial temporal vessels, or injury to these vessels, will result in the loss of the temporoparietal fascial flap as a salvage procedure should the microvascular replantation fail.[20] Whereas microvascular replantation provides the potential for exceptional results, the temporoparietal fascial flap provides the most reliable salvage for total auricular loss, and thus the preservation of the superficial temporal vessels is axiomatic.

Total auricular loss may also occur with a major scalp avulsion injury (Figure 89-16). In such cases, although the total amount of tissue avulsed is greater, replantation may be technically easier. The scalp has predictable sites of vascular supply, and the vessels are larger. The avulsed ear is reattached as a portion of the larger replantation with the potential for an excellent aesthetic result (see Figure 89-16).

BURNED EAR

The ears are frequently involved in thermal injury. In one series, over 60% of all admissions to the Brooke Army Medical Center Burn Unit had burns to the face, and 90% of these facial burns involved the ears.[41] The initial management is nonsurgical, but to obtain optimal results, management must be active, and the surgeon must not relegate the ear to secondary reconstruction after other higher priority issues have been addressed. The initial assessment after burn injury frequently reveals a pattern of regions of necrosis intermixed with areas of stasis and hyperemia. Unlike a classical traumatic tissue injury model, the complex convolutions of the ear often affect the proximity and amount of thermal injury sustained. Moreover, the amount of subcutaneous tissue between the skin and the cartilage framework varies from place to place on the ear, with the skin tightly adherent to the cartilage framework on the superior and lateral surfaces of the ear, and with the

amount of subcutaneous tissue progressively increasing toward the inferior aspect of the ear and lobule of the ear. Therefore a thermal injury that is less severe, such as a flash burn, may lead to an injury of the helix and antihelix of the ear, with preservation of the scaphal and conchal tissue; and also there may be valuable tissue preserved in the "shadow" of the ear in the postauricular and retroauricular areas, as well as the auriculocephalic sulcus (see Figures 89-5, 89-12, and 89-13).

Initial burn management must focus on preservation of viable cells by maintaining an internal milieu conducive to nutrition and repair.[75] Cartilage is extremely vulnerable to desiccation and must be rigorously protected. Initial treatment includes frequent washings, the application of Sulfamylon cream, and soft supportive head dressings to minimize pressure on the injured ear. In major burns, patients are frequently ventilator dependent and immobile. A potentially salvageable ear can be readily converted to a total loss if a pressure insult is added to the thermal injury. Similarly, the effect of desiccation or infection is additive to the initial thermal injury. Even when another agent is used elsewhere on the body, Sulfamylon has clear advantages for the ear.[41,46,75] The eschar should not be debrided initially, since it provides protection against desiccation and the Sulfamylon can penetrate effectively through this barrier.[75] The earliest signs of chondritis can be difficult to assess because of the swelling that occurs in the ear from the burn injury; however, any evidence of suppuration should be addressed promptly to minimize the spread of infection and limit structural damage. The usual pathogens are *Staphylococcus* and *Pseudomonas* species,[41,75] and debridement for chondritis may involve a helical rim incision and bilobing the ear,[41] which may result in a totally unusable ear.[46] Alternative approaches include prompt cartilage resections limited to the area of suppuration, leaving areas of viable cartilage with adherent perichondrium. Some centers also have reported the favorable use of iontophoresis for chondritis, where the polar molecules of the antibiotics penicillin and gentamicin are driven into the avascular cartilage by a direct current. These centers have found iontophoresis more effective than the intravenous delivery of antibiotics.[75]

The prime consideration in management of the burned ear is the salvage of the complex cartilaginous framework. An important step to understanding surgical management is that this salvage is not an all or none approach. Similar to major abrasions and lacerations, an attention to detail with a piecemeal use of major fragments and rebuilding of the ear may yield an aesthetically superior result. Exposed nonviable cartilage must be excised to prevent further loss. Narrowing the helix symmetrically or by the segmental removal of the antihelix, lobe, and tragal subunits will not unduly deform the ear if structural relationships are not obliterated.[75] If the cartilage is viable and perichondrium is intact, skin grafts may be applied. The need for a suitable bed and the potential for grafts to become irregular make this a secondary reconstructive choice. The granulation tissue over the ear can be sculpted to provide three-dimensional relief and enhance the aesthetic reconstruction.[75] A fundamental error is to try and cover the entire ear with a sheet graft as if it were an "aesthetic subunit"

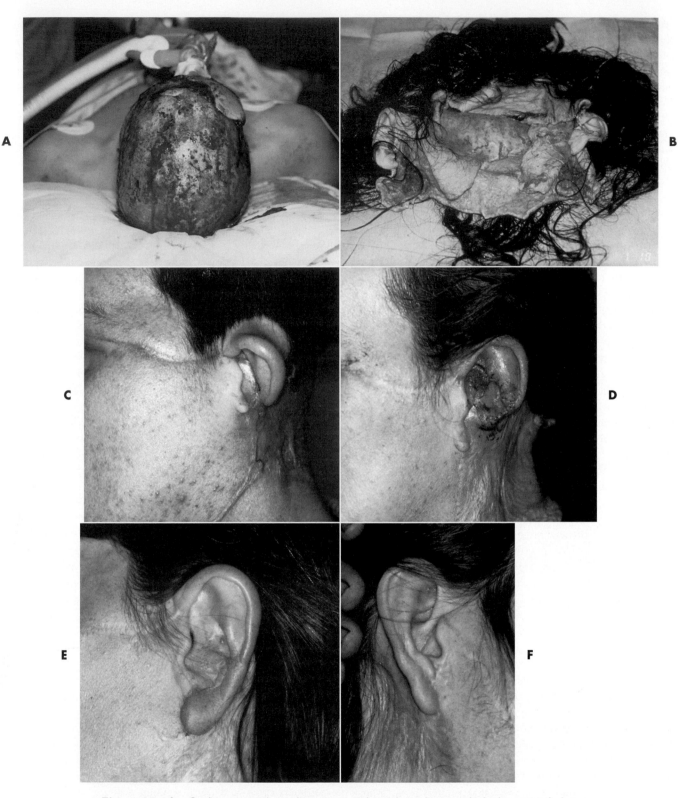

Figure 89-16. **A,** A major scalp avulsion in an industrial accident in which the patient's hair was drawn into a machine. **B,** The avulsed scalp. Note that both ears have been totally avulsed. **C,** The left ear after successful replantation of the entire scalp/ear complex. Unfortunately, there was loss of the lower and central portions of the ear. **D,** The ear shortly after a conchal chondrocutaneous flap from the upper portion of the concha used to lengthen the ear. The donor area was skin grafted. **E,** The ear following reconstruction of the lower third using a tubed pedicle cervical flap. **F,** The contralateral ear that survived replantation. (From *J Reconstr Microsurg* 6:3, 1990.)

of the face. Draping a sheet graft across the helix, scapha, and antihelix will predictably lead to a loss of definition of these areas. Better results are possible by preserving existing cutaneous cover in the scapha, which is generally less severely injured, and using grafts over the helix and antihelix.[75]

In the frequent case where perichondrium has been lost, local flap coverage may be necessary. Tissue can be imported from the posterior auricular surface, the auriculocephalic sulcus, or the retroauricular area. The plane of elevation of the flaps is the subcutaneous tissue directly over the perichondrium, and this elevation can be facilitated by hydrodissection with lidocaine.[75] Appropriate care must be taken since the entire field of tissue has been previously injured, and elevation of flaps within this field must be done judiciously.

The helical rim is frequently injured in burns, and its reconstruction depends on whether the loss is segmental or over one third of its length. Smaller losses can be corrected with an Antia-Buch chondrocutaneous flap. If the perichondrium is preserved or the tissue is granulating, the entire helical rim can be sheet grafted. If flap coverage is necessary, and the retroauricular skin is intact, the entire ear rim can be buried and elevated at a subsequent stage (see Figure 89-5).

The antihelix is also seldom spared in thermal injury. In addition to the flaps that have been noted in prior sections, Rosenthal has reported that the burned antihelix can be favorably reconstructed using the conchal tissue for flap coverage, with a more favorable result than grafting.[75]

Reconstruction of upper third and middle third segmental defects of the ear can be performed according to the principles outlined in previous sections. Specific to thermal injury is the innovative technique of Donelan using the Davis chondrocutaneous flap for upper third reconstruction (see Figure 89-9).[40] The upper third of the ear is frequently burned due to its prominence and its lack of protective subcutaneous tissue, and the burned ear conchal tissue is preserved because of its protected position, allowing its use in reconstruction of the upper third of the ear.

If ear loss is more substantial, reconstruction will require a more extensive approach and more complex surgery. In secondary reconstruction, the first step is the release of existing burn scar contractures, either through excision or Z-plasty or V-Y advancement techniques[46]; however, if the ear reconstruction will require fabrication of a rib cartilaginous framework, reliable skin cover is necessary to prevent distortion or exposure of the framework, and a temporoparietal fascial flap may be required, similar to other traumatic injury.

OSSEOINTEGRATED IMPLANTS

Occasionally because of medical or social issues, or simply because of the patients desire to pursue a prosthetic reconstruction, total ear reconstruction may not be desirable. Prosthetic ears present many challenges, including inadequate color match as the patient's skin tans or lightens with seasonal sun exposure and unreliable fixation. Presently available adhesives and glues may result in insecure fixation and dislodgment of the prosthesis at inopportune times, as well as chronic skin irritation secondary to sensitization to the adhesives.

Over the past 2 decades, osseointegrated implants have developed into a reliable alternative choice for prosthetic fixation. The advantages to the osseointegrated implants include shorter surgery, which often can be performed under local anesthesia requiring only two stages, and greater similarity of form and projection than autogenous reconstruction. However, significant disadvantages include the need for ongoing care and prosthetic support. The procedure should not be offered to individuals who have little understanding or commitment to the use of the prosthesis, or those with limited manual dexterity.[93] Unfortunately, these restrictions can often exclude those very patients with infirmities for which local anesthesia and a limited operative time would be most suitable.

In 1986, the combined U.S., Canadian, and Swedish experience with osseointegrated implants for nonoral maxillofacial prosthetic reconstruction totaled 1365 implants in 637 patients. In the patients who had not received radiation, the implant retention rate was 97.5%, whereas in radiated patients, the implant retention rate was 69%.[72] Since that time, the technique has been more widely applied. In 1995, it was estimated that over 250,000 patients have been treated with over 1 million Branemark implants, but the vast majority of that experience has been with dental implants.[89] Only 3000 patients have been treated with nonoral craniofacial prostheses or bone-anchored hearing aids, and bone-anchored hearing aids likely account for the majority of those patients.[89]

A recent analysis of time of treatment and cost was reported by Wilkes and Wolfaardt in the Canadian health system. Total treatment time from the initial surgery until the final delivery of the prosthesis was 4 to 5 months. For autogenous reconstruction of four stages, the total time was 9 months. The cost in the Canadian system was $9050 for the typical four stages of autogenous reconstruction, versus $6500 for reconstruction with a temporoparietal fascial flap. For prosthetic reconstruction, the cost was $8900. Ongoing costs with the prosthetic reconstruction include maintenance for the first year of $450, and $250 for each subsequent year,[93] making overall cost and treatment time of reconstruction with the two techniques comparable.

OUTCOMES

An assessment of the outcomes following ear reconstruction for acquired defects is an extremely difficult task. The defects are varied, the tissue available for reconstruction is not constant, and the damage to the adjacent tissue may vary from normal to mild contusion to extensive radiation or thermal injury. Therefore in this section, we will review the major complications that can occur, discuss patient satisfaction, and outline an approach to reconstruction of the ear based on our experience.

INFECTION

In all surgical procedures, infection is a consideration. Fortunately, except in burn cases, infection following delayed reconstruction of the ear for acquired auricular defects is rare. Infection may occur soon after cartilage grafting or may be a delayed phenomenon. If erythema or tenderness develops in the postoperative phase, it should be assumed that early chondritis is developing and it should be treated aggressively by hospitalization and intravenous antibiotics. Although there can be a variety of causative organisms, *Staphylococcus* and *Pseudomonas* species should be included in the initial antibiotic coverage regimen. We have been successful with intravenous antibiotic regimens alone and fortunately have not experienced failure of the reconstructive effort due to infection. The use of iontophoresis, advocated by others, may have a definite role in the treatment of postburn or other extensive cartilage infections.

FRAMEWORK EXPOSURE

In total ear reconstruction, exposure of the ear framework can occur, particularly with synthetic prosthetic frameworks, and may lead to loss of the entire implant. In autologous rib graft reconstruction, this problem occurs occasionally, usually soon after the cartilage grafting procedure and almost always along the helical rim. This may be secondary to the compromised vascularity of the overlying skin from a cartilage graft that is too large, from pressure by a tight bandage, or from the patient lying on the ear before protective sensation returns. This can usually be prevented by patient education and careful application of the protective bandage. If the area of skin necrosis is only a few millimeters in diameter, successful conservative treatment by the continuous application of a topical antibiotic ointment is possible. More commonly, however, this should be treated aggressively with early closure to prevent subsequent chondritis. A bipedicle flap from the retroauricular area is quite helpful in coverage of helical skin defects, but larger areas of skin loss may require a small temporoparietal fascial flap. We have found that this is seldom necessary. It is crucial that exposure of a cartilage graft or of native cartilage should be treated aggressively by early closure rather than risk the possibility of desiccation or chondritis.

SCAR CONTRACTURE

Scar contracture is an inexorable process that may negatively influence an otherwise favorable early postoperative result. In total ear reconstruction, this may occur following ear release and skin grafting. We have seen contracture of the auriculocephalic sulcus on several occasions and have had to repeat the release and grafting procedure. Our technique for ear release involves undermining and advancement of the remaining scalp into the retroauricular area. A thick split-thickness skin graft or full-thickness graft is applied to the postauricular area only and not to the retroauricular defect, since the obvious difference in texture and color match of a graft over the mastoid is unsightly. Although there is some tendency for the scalp skin to retract after advancement into the retroauricular space, we believe that the aesthetic results are far superior to that achieved with skin grafting the mastoid area. We have also seen scar contracture in reconstructed earlobes when soft tissue only is used. For this reason, some sort of cartilage graft is required to maintain form.

PATIENT SATISFACTION

We conducted a retrospective survey of patients with major acquired auricular deformities requiring rib cartilage graft reconstruction. A questionnaire was mailed, and over half of the patients responded. All patients reported that they were pleased with their results and would recommend the reconstructive ear surgery to others. None reported any deformity or functional disability at the donor area. All believed that their result was unchanged over the long term. There were no significant problems reported in caring for the reconstructed ear.

FUNCTIONAL OUTCOMES

As mentioned previously, the function of the external ear is to establish a directional source for sound and to perhaps amplify this sound; however, this does not appear to be an important function in modern man. Perhaps the main role of the auricle is to support eyeglasses, an important consideration in reconstruction of acquired deformities. Deformity of the ear with or without other areas of the face can inhibit comfortable social interaction as well. The goal of this surgery is to return the appearance of the ear to as normal as possible, clearly a reconstructive rather than cosmetic goal.

COST

In today's changing medical environment, reduction of cost of treatment without sacrificing the quality of the final result is of paramount importance. The majority of the procedures that have been described can be performed safely and effectively on an outpatient basis. What initially appears to be a more expensive or costly procedure may ultimately be less costly. An example of this is the use of a temporoparietal fascial flap and a skin graft to provide coverage for a cartilage graft in total or subtotal ear reconstruction. This reconstruction can frequently be accomplished in a single stage in contrast to the use of tissue expansion followed by cartilage grafting and eventual ear release, which may require multiple stages. In our practice, we have successfully performed all of the operations that have been discussed on an outpatient basis, except when a large graft or a temporoparietal fascial flap is performed. In these situations, a 1-or 2-day hospitalization is required. Cost of reconstruction also has to be measured in lost days from work or school. In the early postoperative period, we do not allow patients to return to occupations that are not in a clean environment or in which the ear may be subject to trauma. Each patient requires individual consideration regarding the time to return to full activity or work.

RECONSTRUCTIVE PREFERENCES

In this chapter, we have attempted to review many of the options that are available to the surgeon faced with the challenge of reconstructing an acquired auricular deformity. Innumerable possible traumatic injuries exist, and the experience of the individual plastic surgeon with any specific defect is often limited.[8] Because the tissue loss and circumstances following reconstruction for acquired defects are so variable, there are few published reports of series of patients with specific defects that were treated in the same way. Based on our experience in reconstruction of acquired auricular defects, we have developed our own preferences and philosophy of treatment. What follows is our opinion regarding these surgical options and the basis for our preference of technique.

Helical Defects

Helical rim defects are common problems in acquired deformities, since the helical rim is prone to malignant degeneration following actinic damage, and is also prone to thermal injury. By far, we favor the Antia-Buch chondrocutaneous flap for small-to-moderate-sized defects of the helix.[4] This technique produces a superior aesthetic result with an almost imperceptible donor site. We have closed defects over 2.5 cm using only the inferior pedicle. This results in a slight flattening of the earlobe, but no appreciable deformity. Fortunately, in most individuals, any diminution in height caused by the rotation advancement flap is not apparent, since both ears are rarely viewed simultaneously. The superior pedicle utilizing the root of the helix is used sparingly only for larger defects, since the flap does not advance as easily and the donor site scar is more visible. Both procedures, however, have the distinct advantage that they can be performed in an outpatient setting under local anesthesia.

Upper and Middle Third Defects

For larger defects of the upper or middle third involving the helical margin of the ear when the retroauricular skin is intact, we prefer the tunnel procedure utilizing rib cartilage. Frequently, the cartilage requirements are small and can be satisfied using the free-floating ninth rib, which is easily accessible under local anesthesia and/or regional block. We

prefer rib cartilage over conchal cartilage, since it is more rigid and maintains its contour better against the forces of wound contraction and, in our hands, can better simulate the gentle roll of the helix. A disadvantage is that because of its thickness, care must be taken to avoid "notching" at its junction with the native cartilage of the ear remnant by careful tailoring and inset of the graft.

Lower Third Defects

Defects of the lower third of the ear are often undermanaged. The randomly based skin flaps, or tubed pedicles mentioned previously, can be useful for partial or total loss of the earlobe. In our hands, the best result for total earlobe reconstruction involves using conchal or rib cartilage to provide structure for the reconstructed earlobe, with a second stage if necessary to release the flap from the mastoid area with a skin graft.

Major Traumatic Defects

For major traumatic defects in which cartilage grafts are required, the surgeon must decide whether there is enough native skin available or if additional skin coverage is needed. In burned ears there is usually unburned postauricular and retroauricular skin available because of protection from the thermal blast in the "shadow" of the ear itself. This may be sufficient to provide helical coverage, or coverage of a graft or cartilaginous framework after tissue expansion. The skin also may be expanded for delayed reconstruction or in acute salvage following burns, as described by Rosenthal.[75] We believe this postauricular and retroauricular skin is often underutilized following trauma and especially in burns. Of course, if the skin is scarred or unavailable, then coverage with a temporoparietal fascial flap will be required.

Ear Avulsion

Options for treatment of the avulsed ear when the amputated part is available vary in complexity from simply burying the framework in an adjacent or distant site to the microvascular replantation. We have had success with one case of microvascular replantation associated with a scalp avulsion. We have yet to attempt microvascular repair of an isolated ear avulsion. If presented with this situation, we believe that an attempt at microvascular replantation is worthwhile, since this has the potential to produce the best aesthetic result. The replantation plan, however, will preserve the integrity of the superficial temporal vessels, to allow the best salvage via the temporoparietal fascial flap should replantation not be successful.

We have not had good success with burying the amputated ear in distant sites or in the retroauricular area.[9,63] Although we have seen survival of the amputated cartilage, there has been significant distortion of the cartilage over time, leading to an inferior aesthetic result. Another major disadvantage is scarring of the postauricular skin. This experience has led us to abandon these techniques in favor of a delayed reconstruction with a rib cartilage framework. Cutaneous coverage for the rib cartilage framework can be provided either by expanded postauricular and retroauricular skin or by a temporoparietal fascial flap and skin graft.

SUMMARY

The exposed position and delicate anatomy of the ear make its structure especially susceptible to trauma and sun exposure and make its reconstruction especially challenging. Whenever possible, local tissue, because of simplicity and color match, should be the basis for reconstruction. Furthermore, meticulous preservation of the existing cartilage framework should be attempted. The one exception to this rule is in the totally avulsed ear that is not amenable to microvascular replantation. In this case, it is better to start with a rib cartilage framework that can resist the forces of wound contraction. Careful planning includes avoiding "burning any bridges" by sacrificing the superficial temporal vessels in a case where there may be later need for the temporoparietal fascial flap. Initial treatment is primarily directed at preservation of viable tissue. Major reconstruction is frequently delayed, especially in traumatic cases where contamination or poor vascularity is possible. There is a definite learning curve for dealing with these problems, and this is not an area for the inexperienced surgeon. Ear reconstruction following trauma or tumor ablation is one of the most challenging, yet potentially rewarding, procedures facing the plastic surgeon. Success depends on careful planning, proper execution, and patient cooperation.

REFERENCES

1. Adams WM: Construction of upper half of auricle using composite concha cartilage graft with perichondrium attached on both sides, *Plast Reconstr Surg* 88:88-96, 1955.
2. Alanis SZ: A new method for earlobe reconstruction, *Plast Reconstr Surg* 45:254-257, 1970.
3. Anous MM, Hallock GG: Immediate reconstruction of the auricle using amputated cartilage and the temporoparietal fascia, *Ann Plast Surg* 21:378-386, 1988.
4. Antia NH, Buch VI: Chondrocutaneous advancement flap for the marginal defect of the ear, *Plast Reconstr Surg* 39:472-477, 1967.
5. Argamaso RV, Lewin ML: Repair of partial ear loss with local composite flap, *Plast Reconstr Surg* 42:437-441, 1968.
6. Ariyan S, Chicarelli ZN: Replantation of a totally amputated ear by means of a platysma musculocutaneous "sandwich" flap, *Plast Reconstr Surg* 78:385-389, 1986.
7. Arons MS, Savin RC: Auricular cancer, *Am J Surg* 122:770-776, 1971.
8. Bardsley AF, Mercer DM: The injured ear: a review of 50 cases, *Br J Plast Surg* 36:466-469, 1983.

9. Baudet J, Tramond P, Goumain A: A propos d'un procede original de reimplantation d'un pavillon de l'oreille totalement separe, *Ann Chir Plast* 17:67, 1972.
10. Bauer BS: Reconstruction of major congenital and acquired auricular deformities. In Riley WB Jr, editor: *Plastic surgery educational foundation instructional courses,* St Louis, 1988, Mosby, pp 146-178.
11. Bauer BS: The role of tissue expansion in reconstruction of the ear, *Clin Plast Surg* 17:319-325, 1990.
12. Blake GB, Wilson JSP: Malignant tumours of the ear and their treatment, *Br J Plast Surg* 27:67-76, 1974.
13. Brent B: Ear reconstruction with an expansile framework of autogenous rib cartilage, *Plast Reconstr Surg* 53:619, 1974.
14. Brent B: Earlobe reconstruction with an auriculo-mastoid flap, *Plast Reconstr Surg* 57:389-391, 1976.
15. Brent B: The acquired auricular deformity, *Plast Reconstr Surg* 59:475-485, 1977.
16. Brent B: Reconstruction of traumatic ear deformities, *Clin Plast Surg* 5(3):437-445, 1978.
17. Brent B: The correction of microtia with autogenous cartilage grafts: I. The classic deformity, *Plast Reconstr Surg* 66:1-12, 1980.
18. Brent B: Auricular repair with autogenous rib cartilage grafts: two decades of experience with 600 cases, *Plast Reconstr Surg* 90:355-374, 1992.
19. Brent B, Byrd HS: Secondary ear reconstruction with cartilage grafts covered by axial, random, and free flaps of temporoparietal fascia, *Plast Reconstr Surg* 72:141-151, 1983.
20. Brent B, Furnas DW: Ear reconstruction complications, *Perspect Plast Surg* 3:47-68, 1989.
21. Brent B, Upton J, Acland RD, et al: Experience with the temporoparietal fascial free flap, *Plast Reconstr Surg* 76:177-188, 1985.
22. Broders AC: Epithelioma of the ear: a study of 63 cases, *Surg Clin North Am* 1(5):1401-1410, 1921.
23. Buncke HJ: Discussion: microsurgical reattachment of totally amputated ears, *Plast Reconstr Surg* 79:541, 1987.
24. Byers R, Kesler K, Redmon B, et al: Squamous carcinoma of the external ear, *Am J Surg* 146:447-450, 1983.
25. Byers RM, Smith JL, Russell N, et al: Malignant melanoma of the external ear: review of 102 cases, *Am J Surg* 140:518-522, 1980.
26. Calhoun KH, Slaughter D, Kassir R, et al: Biomechanics of the helical rim advancement flap, *Arch Otolaryngol Head Neck Surg* 122:1119-1123, 1996.
27. Cheney ML: Acquired deformities of the auricle. In Nadol JB Jr, Schuknecht HF, editors: *Surgery of the ear and temporal bone,* New York, 1993, Raven, pp 449-469.
28. Conley J, Schuller DE: Malignancies of the ear, *Laryngoscope* 86(8):1147-1163, 1976.
29. Conroy WC: Salvage of an amputated ear (Letter), *Plast Reconstr Surg* 49:464, 1972.
30. Converse JM: Reconstruction of the auricle—Part I, *Plast Reconstr Surg* 22:150-163, 1958.
31. Converse JM: Reconstruction of the auricle—part II, *Plast Reconstr Surg* 22:230-249, 1958.

32. Converse JM: Construction of the auricle in congenital microtia, *Plast Reconstr Surg* 32:425, 1963.

33. Converse JM, Brent B: In Converse JM, editor: *Deformities of the auricle: acquired deformities,* Philadelphia, 1977, WB Saunders, pp. 1724-1769.

34. Converse JM, Wood-Smith D: Corrective and reconstructive surgery in deformities of the auricle in children. In Mustarde JC, editor: *Plastic surgery in infancy and childhood,* Edinburgh, 1971, Churchill Livingstone.

35. Conway H, Neuman CG, Gelb J, et al: Reconstruction of the external ear, *Ann Surg* 128:226-239, 1948.

36. Crikelair GF: A method of partial ear reconstruction for avulsion of the upper portion of the ear, *Plast Reconstr Surg* 17:438-443, 1956.

37. Cronin TD: Use of a Silastic frame for total and subtotal reconstruction of the ear: preliminary report, *Plast Reconstr Surg* 37:399-405, 1966.

38. Davis JE: Auricle reconstruction. In Saad M, Lichtveld P, editors: *Reviews in plastic surgery,* Amsterdam, 1974, Elsevier and Excerpta Medica, p 129.

39. deChalain T, Jones G: Replantation of the avulsed pinna: 100 percent survival with a single arterial anastomosis and substitution of leeches for a venous anastomosis, *Plast Reconstr Surg* 95:1275-1279, 1995.

40. Donelan MB: Conchal transposition flap for post-burn deformities, *Plast Reconstr Surg* 83.641-652, 1989.

41. Dowling JA, Foley FD, Moncrief JA: Chondritis in the burned ear, *Plast Reconstr Surg* 42:115-122, 1968.

42. Driver JR, Cole HN: Treatment of epithelioma of skin of the ear, *AJR* 48:66-75, 1942.

43. Dujon DG, Bowditch M: The thin tube pedicle: a valuable technique in auricular reconstruction after trauma, *Br J Plast Surg* 48:35-38, 1995.

44. Edgerton MT: Discussion: secondary reconstruction for unfavorable microtia results utilizing temporoparietal and innominate fascia flaps, *Plast Reconstr Surg* 94:266-267, 1994.

45. Edgerton MT, Bachetta CA: Principles in the use and salvage of implants in ear reconstruction. In Tanzer RC, Edgerton MT, editors: *Symposium on the reconstruction of the auricle,* St Louis, 1974, Mosby, p 58.

46. Eriksson E, Vogt PM: Ear reconstruction, *Clin Plast Surg* 19:637-643, 1992.

47. Erol OO, Parsa FD, Spira M: The use of the secondary island graft-flap in reconstruction of the burned ear, *Br J Plast Surg* 34:417-421, 1981.

48. Fata JJ: Composite chondrocutaneous advancement flap: a technique for the reconstruction of marginal defects of the ear, *Plast Reconstr Surg* 99:1172-1175, 1997.

49. Firmin F: Microtie: reconstruction par la technique de Brent, *Ann Chir Plast Esthet* 37:119, 1992.

50. Gingrass RP, Pickrell KL: Techniques of closure for conchal and external auditory canal defects, *Plast Reconstr Surg* 41:568, 1968.

51. Hansen PB, Jensen MS: Late results following radiotherapy of skin cancer, *Acta Radiol (Therapy)* 7:307-319, 1968.

52. Jenkins AM, Finucan T: Primary nonmicrosurgical reconstruction following ear avulsion using the temporoparietal fascial flap, *Plast Reconstr Surg* 83:148-152, 1989.

53. Kelleher JC, Sullivan JG, Baibak GJ, et al: The wrestler's ear, *Plast Reconstr Surg* 40:540-546, 1967.

54. Kristof ND: *400th anniversary for grisly memorial in Japan,* New York, September 14, 1997, New York Times.

55. Lee D, Nash M, Har-El G: Regional spread of auricular and periauricular cutaneous malignancies, *Laryngoscope* 106:998-1001, 1996.

56. Lewin ML: Formation of a helix with a postauricular flap, *Plast Reconstr Surg* 5:432-440, 1950.

57. Lynch JB, Pousti A, Doyle JE, et al: Our experience with Silastic ear implants, *Plast Reconstr Surg* 49:283-285, 1972.

58. MacGregor FC: Ear deformities: social and psychological implications, *Clin Plast Surg* 5:347-350, 1978.

59. Malt RA, McKhann CF: Replantation of severed arms, *JAMA* 189:716, 1964.

60. Menick FJ: Reconstruction of the ear after tumor excision, *Clin Plast Surg* 17:405, 1990.

61. Millard DR: Reconstruction of one-third plus of the auricular circumference, *Plast Reconstr Surg* 90:475-478, 1992.

62. Mladick RA: Salvage of the ear in acute trauma, *Clin Plast Surg* 5(3):427-435, 1978.

63. Mladick RA, Horton CE, Adamson JE, et al: The pocket principle, *Plast Reconstr Surg* 48:219-223, 1971.

64. Musgrave RH, Garret WS: Management of avulsion injuries of the external ear, *Plast Reconstr Surg* 40:534-539, 1967.

65. Mutimer KL, Banis JC, Upton J: Microsurgical reattachment of totally amputated ears, *Plast Reconstr Surg* 79:535-540, 1987.

66. Nagata S: Secondary reconstruction for unfavorable microtia results utilizing temporoparietal and innominate fascia flaps, *Plast Reconstr Surg* 94:254-265, 1994.

67. Navabi A: One stage reconstruction of the partial defect of the auricle, *Plast Reconstr Surg* 33:77-79, 1964.

68. Neuman C: The expansion of skin by progressive distention of a subcutaneous balloon, *Plast Reconstr Surg* 19:124-130, 1957.

69. Ohmori S: Reconstruction of microtia using the Silastic frame, *Clin Plast Surg* 5:379, 1978.

70. Ohmori S, Matsumoto K, Nakai H: Follow-up study on reconstruction of microtia with a silicone framework, *Plast Reconstr Surg* 53:555-562, 1974.

71. Oshumi N, Iida N: Ear reconstruction with a chondrocutaneous postauricular island flap, *Plast Reconstr Surg* 96:718-720, 1995.

72. Parel SM, Branemark PI, Tjellstrom A, et al: Osseointegration in maxillofacial prosthetics: II. Extraoral applications, *J Prosth Dent* 55:600-606, 1986.

73. Pennington DG, Lai MF, Pelly AD: Successful replantation of a completely avulsed ear by microvascular anastomosis, *Plast Reconstr Surg* 65:820-823, 1980.

74. Pierce GW: Reconstruction of the external ear, *Surg Gynecol Obstet* 50:601-605, 1930.

75. Rosenthal JS: The thermally injured ear: a systematic approach to reconstruction, *Clin Plast Surg* 19:645-661, 1992.

76. Sadove RC: Successful replantation of a totally avulsed ear, *Ann Plast Surg* 24:366-370, 1990.

77. Sasaki GH: Tissue expansion in reconstruction of acquired auricular defects, *Clin Plast Surg* 17:327-338, 1990.

78. Schewe EJ, Pappalardo C: Cancer of the external ear, *Am J Surg* 104:753-756, 1962.

79. Shiffman NJ: Squamous cell cancer of the skin and pinna, *Can J Surg* 18:279-283, 1975.

80. Shockley WW, Stucker FJ: Squamous cell carcinoma of the external ear: a review of 75 cases, *Otolaryngol Head Neck Surg* 97(3):308-313, 1987.

81. Song Y, Song Y: An improved one stage total ear reconstruction procedure, *Plast Reconstr Surg* 71:615-622, 1983.

82. Songcharoen S, Smith RA, Jabaley ME: Tumors of the external ear and reconstruction of defects, *Clin Plast Surg* 5:447-457, 1978.

83. Spira M, Hardy SH: Management of the injured ear, *Am J Surg* 106:678-684, 1963.

84. Suraci AJ: Plastic reconstruction of acquired defects of the ear, *Am J Surg* 66:196, 1944.

85. Tanzer RC: Total reconstruction of the external ear, *Plast Reconstr Surg* 23:1-15, 1959.

86. Tanzer RC: The reconstruction of acquired defects of the ear, *Plast Reconstr Surg* 35:335, 1965.

87. Tegtmeier RE, Gooding RA: The use of a fascial flap in ear reconstruction, *Plast Reconstr Surg* 60:406-411, 1977.

88. Thomas SS, Matthews RN: Squamous cell carcinoma of the pinna: a 6-year study, *Br J Plast Surg* 47:81-85, 1994.

89. Tjellstrom A, Granstrom G: One-stage procedure to establish osseointegration: a zero to five years follow-up report, *J Laryngol Otol* 109:593-598, 1995.

90. Turpin IV: Microsurgical replantation of the ear, *Clin Plast Surg* 17:397-404, 1990.

91. Wellisz T: Reconstruction of the burned external ear using a Medpor porous polyethylene pivoting helix framework, *Plast Reconstr Surg* 91:811-818, 1993.

92. Wellisz T, Dougherty W: The role of alloplastic skeletal modification in the reconstruction of facial burns, *Ann Plast Surg* 30:531-536, 1993.

93. Wilkes GH, Wolfaardt JF: Osseointegrated versus autogenous ear reconstruction: criteria for treatment selection, *Plast Reconstr Surg* 93:967-979, 1994.

Scalp and Calvarial Reconstruction

Rajiv Sood
John J. Coleman III

INDICATIONS

The scalp is a highly specialized skin unit designed not only to cover the cranium but also, because of its unique arrangement of hair and accessory structures, to convey an aesthetic sense of the individual. Therefore loss of all or part of this specialized organ results in both a functional (i.e., exposure of the cranium) and an aesthetic problem.

The scalp is divided into five distinct layers (Figure 90-1): the skin (S), subcutaneous tissues (C), galea aponeurotica (A), loose subaponeurotic areola tissue (L), and the pericranium (P) (SCALP). Each of these layers has unique yet interdependent relationships to the forehead and facial tissue planes that must be understood by anyone who undertakes scalp repair or reconstruction. The skin of the scalp is 3 to 4 mm thick anteriorly and temporally and up to 8 mm thick posteriorly toward the occiput.[17,59] The thickness of the scalp skin and its ability to rapidly heal with hair-bearing skin make it ideal for the harvesting of partial-thickness skin grafts. This is particularly true in the pediatric patient with a large body-surface-area burn because other donor sites might be limited. The subcutaneous tissue layer contains the vasculature, lymphatics, and sensory nerves. This layer is somewhat unique because it is compartmentalized by fibrous septa extending from skin to galea, much like the hyponychium of the digits. This anatomic peculiarity is responsible for two clinical consequences: (1) a large amount of bleeding is encountered with scalp lacerations because blood vessels cannot retract secondary to their fibrous connections, and (2) the localization of infections in and around this layer by the septate compartments produces local pressure and subsequently pain and necrosis.[39]

The third layer, the galea aponeurotica, consists of the paired occipital muscles posteriorly, the frontalis muscles anteriorly, and their thick connective tissue facial connections across the vertex. This continuous layer is connected to the occipital protuberance and superior nuchal line posteriorly, the temporoparietal fascia laterally, and the supraorbital ridges and adjacent musculature anteriorly.[16,39] Clinically the galeal layer creates a thick barrier to infection of the underlying tissues and, because of its attachment to the skin and subcutaneous

tissues, facilitates approximation of these layers after laceration. The galea is believed to be continuous with the temporoparietal fascia laterally, which in itself is continuous with the superficial musculoaponeurotic system (SMAS) layer of the face and the platysmal layer of the neck representing a confluent embryonic fascial plane.[62,64]

The fourth layer is the subaponeurotic layer (loose areolar plane, subgalea fascia, innominate fascia).[16] This layer is continuous with the parotid masseteric fascia and is the layer that allows the scalp to slide on the skull. This areolar plane is clinically important since avulsions of the scalp from the skull typically occur in this layer. Recent advances in the understanding of scalp anatomy have allowed the use of this layer as locoregional pericranial flaps for coverage of exposed calvarium. The deepest layer of the scalp is the pericranium, which is tightly adherent to the underlying bone. Bone denuded of pericranium is unsuitable for skin grafting, since the periosteum has a very rich vascular supply.[15] The periosteum fuses with the deep temporal fascia above the superior temporal line[62,64] (See Figure 90-1, *B*).

The blood supply to the scalp is rich (Figures 90-2 and 90-3), arising from four major arteries and their venae comitantes, the superficial temporal arteries anteriorly, and the paired occipital arteries posteriorly. In addition, the posterior auricular artery, smaller branches of the external carotid artery, and the supraorbital and supratrochlear vessels also supply the lateral and anterior scalp. These vessels form an interconnecting vascular plexus in the subcutaneous layer, which is important clinically because the entire scalp can potentially survive on a single arterial anastomosis.[16,17] These vessels travel in the supragaleal plane and send communicating branches down through the galea to the cortex. The anterior portion of the scalp is supplied by the supratrochlear and supraorbital vessels, which, by midforehead, travel along the superficial surface of the frontalis muscle anastomosing freely with the superficial temporal vessels, which ascend laterally. The superficial temporal vessels, the terminal branches of the external carotid artery, supply the lateral aspect of the scalp. Anterior to the tragus of the ear, they arise from beneath the parotid and are frequently encountered during rhytidectomy procedures. The vessels then travel along the temporoparietal fascia and bifurcate into an

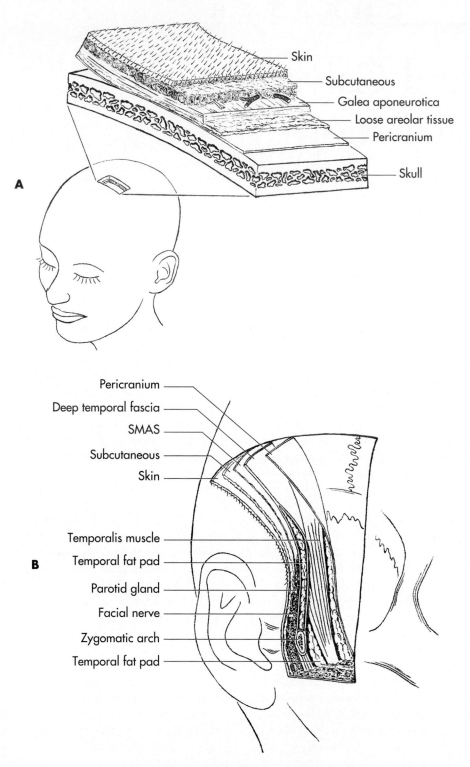

Figure 90-1. **A** and **B,** Cross section of scalp.

anterior and posterior branch approximately 2 cm above the zygomatic arch. Posteriorly, the occipital arteries enter the scalp just 2 cm lateral to the midline and divide into medial and lateral branches. A well-formed vascular arcade exists between these vessels, the postauricular vessels, and the posterior branch of the superficial temporal vessels.[17]

The nerve supply of the scalp is similarly multiple (see Figure 90-2). Sensation to the anteriormost portion of the scalp is supplied by branches of the fifth cranial nerve, the

supraorbital and supratrochlear nerves exiting the skull at the junction of the middle and medial one third of the superior orbital rim. The lesser occipital nerve (a branch of second or third cervical nerve) supplies the posterior scalp. Motor innervation to the lateral temporal scalp is supplied by the auriculotemporal nerve, a branch of the mandibular division of the trigeminal nerve. The frontal branch of the facial nerve supplies the lateral forehead and part of the lateral scalp (see Figure 90-2) and can potentially be injured with lateral

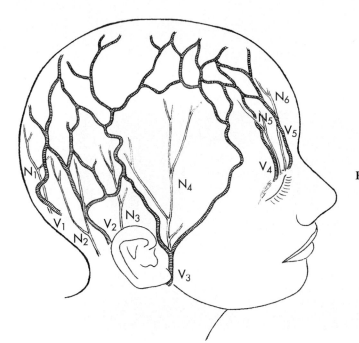

Figure 90-2. Blood supply and neural innervation of the scalp.

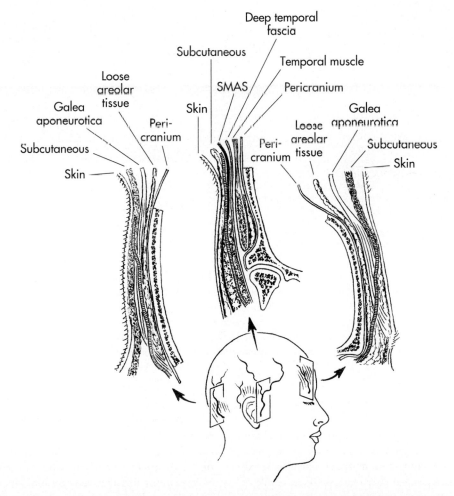

Figure 90-3. The blood supply to the frontal scalp exits from the supraorbital notch, travels for about a centimeter just above the periosteum, then ascends through the frontalis muscle and at about midforehead runs in the subcutaneous layer, where it remains throughout its course. The superficial temporal and occipital vessels follow a similar pattern, running from deep to superficial.

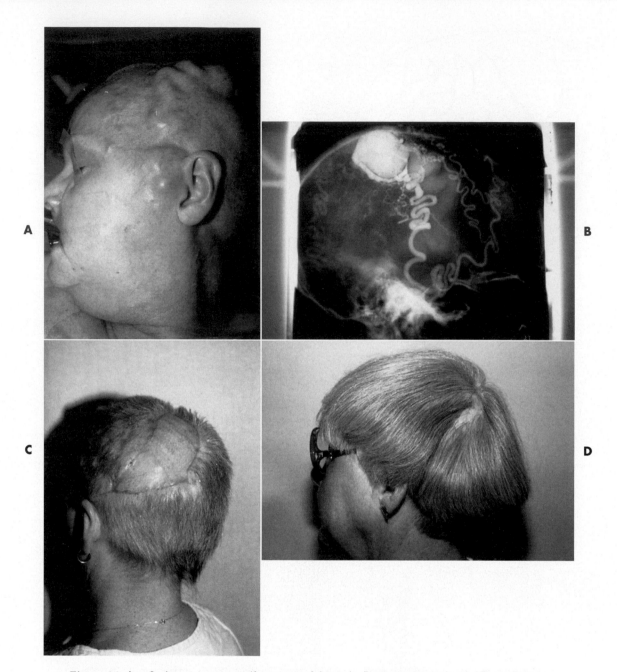

Figure 90-4. **A,** Arteriovenous malformation of the scalp. Patient presented with 17-year history of enlarging subcutaneous vessels, which presented 2 years after trauma to scalp. Symptoms included constant sound in left ear and shortness of breath. **B,** Arteriogram shows extensive lesion continued to the distribution of the external carotid artery and involved only the scalp. **C,** Wide excision of the lesion and scalp advancement allowed split-thickness skin grafting of periosteum. **D,** Several scalp advancements over a 3-year period resolved the alopecia.

approaches to the zygomatic arch from the scalp, such as the Gillies approach.

Congenital indications for scalp reconstruction include aplasia cutis congenita, hemangiomas and arterial venous malformations, extravasation injuries, and the rare syndrome of craniopagus. Aplasia cutis congenita is a rare, sporadic congenital deformity, most often seen in first-born female children. The cause seems to be a failure of differentiation of the skin early in embryonic life, with presentation that ranges from subtotal to total absence of the skin, fat, skull, dura, and occasionally the underlying brain. The scalp is involved in 60% of cases, especially in the vertex, and the ulcers may be multiple. Aplasia cutis ulcers present as sharply marginated ulcers with a reddish base[16,39] that usually heal rapidly by secondary intention with appropriate wound care.[3,66] Exposed structures must be kept moist and observed carefully, since the formation of an eschar and subsequent eschar separation may lead to infection and hemorrhage in the underlying subeschar space.[20]

Hemangiomas and vascular malformations may present on the scalp (Figures 90-4 and 90-5). These are described in detail

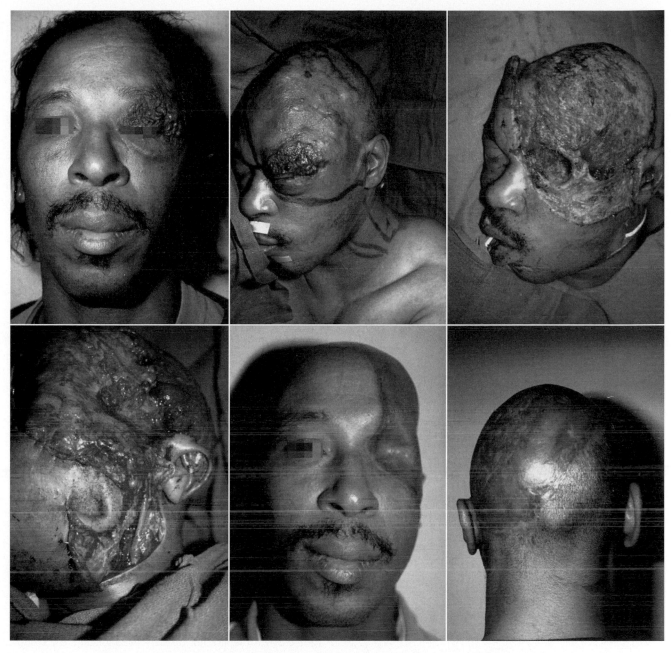

Figure 90-5. A and **B,** Congenital vascular malformation in a 42-year-old man. He had undergone eight previous surgical procedures. The lesion, which now had characteristics of a high flow arteriovenous malformation, gave symptoms of fatigue, obstructed visual field, decreased visual acuity, and constant sound. The orbital contents were involved, but the only connection to the intracranial circulation was the ophthalmic vessels and the emissary veins of the calvarium, and there was no intracranial lesion. **C,** Resection of the orbital contents and involved scalp and face was performed in the subperiosteal plane. **D,** Coverage of the scalp was achieved with a latissimus-serratus free muscle flap. The serratus vessels were brought through a preauricular incision and the thoracodorsal vessels through a postauricular incision, and vascular anastomosis was performed to the occipital artery and the posterior face vein. **E** and **F,** Split-thickness sheet grafts and the muscle flaps create an excellent simulation of the scalp.

in other chapters in this book. Management of these lesions has to take into account the layers involved and the ideal reconstruction. This may range from simple closure of the scalp after excision to preexcision tissue expansion to complex reconstruction with free tissue transfer for the larger arterial venous malformations. Involvement of the underlying skull

and/or brain needs to be assessed preoperatively by magnetic resonance imaging (MRI). Intravenous fluid extravasation, typically antibiotics, calcium agents, and hyperalimentation, is frequently seen in the neonatal population where scalp veins are a preferred route for fluid administration. Although full-thickness wounds may result, conservative treatment with

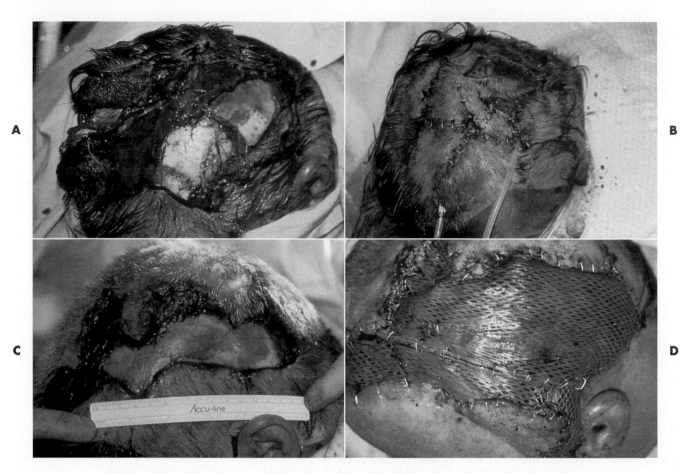

Figure 90-6. Clinical example of scalp laceration. **A,** Initial presentation. Scalp laceration due to blunt trauma. **B,** Following repair. **C,** Subsequent loss of portion of frontoparietal scalp. **D,** Definitive coverage with rectus free flap/skin graft.

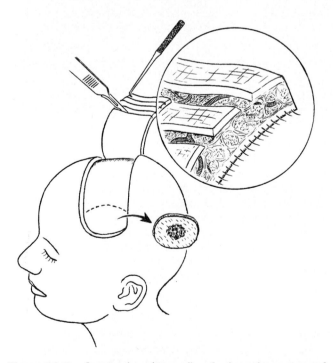

Figure 90-7. Scoring the galea to allow further advancement of the scalp. Care must be taken to avoid injury to the axial vessels in the subcutaneous layer.

moist dressing changes usually leads to secondary wound healing. Delayed reconstruction can certainly be carried out if necessary. Craniopagus is a rare anomaly seen in 1 in 600 twin births and 1 in 60,000 live births. It consists of symmetric twins who are joined at the skull, brain, and/or scalp. The deformity may be partial or total (brains are connected). Problems with separation of these twins include the complex sharing of the brain and particularly the venous drainage[22,46] of the brain. Separation of the skin has been facilitated by the use of tissue expansion.[60] Separation of conjoined twins is a potentially lethal surgical undertaking, and therefore careful and extensive discussion with the parents should occur preoperatively.

Traumatic defects of the scalp may range from simple lacerations to scalp avulsion to burns of indeterminate depth. The basic principles of management of scalp lacerations include a careful history and physical examination with identification of possible associated injuries (i.e., skull fractures or brain injury) and assessment of the layers of scalp involved with the laceration (Figure 90-6). Operative principles include irrigation and debridement; careful hemostasis, especially of the galeal vessels; and repair of the galeal layer to prevent a depressed scar. Galeal scoring may allow some additional advancement of the scalp with traumatic wounds (Figure 90-7).

Traumatic injuries may result in partial-or full-thickness loss of the scalp. Management of these wounds depends on the particular layers injured, the usual site being the plane of the loose areolar tissue; the amount of skull exposed; and concern over the long-term aesthetic outcome in terms of hair-bearing skin. The range of options for closure include simple skin grafting over intact pericranium, composite grafting of the injured part (which usually does not work well),[11] and local or distant flaps. Conservative treatment allowing healing by secondary intention and subsequent skin grafting is another option, albeit not ideal. Complex local flaps should not be performed at the acute stage when there is any question of the blood supply to the adjacent tissues. It is, however, important to remember that the grafted defect may be secondarily reconstructed with tissue expansion.

The treatment of full-thickness scalp avulsion, including total scalp avulsion, has improved significantly with the advent of microsurgery. Total scalp avulsion (Figure 90-8) frequently occurs in individuals with long hair while they work with machinery. The level of avulsion is at the plane between the galea and the periosteum, and typically includes the forehead, eyebrows, upper lids, and ears.[39] Miller et al reported the first successful total scalp replantation by microvascular anastomosis.[44] This is now the treatment of choice for total or near-total avulsions of the scalp.[2,33,41,55,70] The advantages of microsurgical replantation include the concept of replacing "like with like" tissue. A successful replantation usually results in return of scalp sensibility, hair growth, and restoration of the aesthetic units of the forehead and upper lid.[33] Failure to successfully replant the scalp results in a significant deformity. Acute management of these wounds includes debridement, coverage with temporary substitutes including pigskin or cadaveric allograft, and delayed skin grafting (see Figure 90-8). Unfortunately, the results of failed replantation are psychologically devastating to the patient.

Burns represent another indication for subtotal or total reconstruction of the scalp. Burns of the head and neck are seen in almost 25% of all burn unit admissions, especially in children. Scalp burns are frequently seen resulting from electrical injuries as well.[1] Because of the increased resistance to electric current offered by the scalp and skull, a great deal of local heat is produced, increasing the amount of local tissue damage. Although several classification systems exist,[26,27,53] Achauer has proposed a classification system that breaks these wounds into mild (less than 15% of the scalp), moderate, extensive without brain involvement, and those with full-thickness skull or brain involvement.[1] Another problem with burns of the scalp is that it is frequently difficult at initial evaluation, and even later, to make an accurate diagnosis of the extent and/or depth of involvement. The mechanism of injury in these cases is important, since grease, chemical, and electrical injuries result in much deeper burns than scald or thermal burns. The treatment options include conservative therapy consisting of early debridement of nonviable tissue and local wound therapy. This is preferred as long as invasive infection is prevented to help preserve hair-bearing skin. A second treatment option is tangential excision of the scalp if it becomes necessary to debride eschar. In this option there is an attempt to preserve hair follicles and deeper dermal structure if not burned. The diagnosis of a bony injury associated with a scalp burn can also be quite difficult. An outer cortical table burn may be treated either by conservative treatment with moist dressing changes to stimulate granulation tissue arising from the emissary veins in the skull or by lightly abrading the outer table to promote bleeding and the formation of granulation tissue. It is imperative in these patients with bony injury that an underlying brain injury be ruled out by computed tomography (CT) or MRI scan with or without electroencephalogram (EEG). Some authors have advocated bone biopsy and early coverage of suspected bony injury.[69] Scalp burn alopecia is seen in almost 30% of children with burns[10] (Figure 90-9). Treatment of this problem most often involves either serial excision of the alopecia area or the use of tissue expansion of the remaining hair-bearing skin. Loss of pericranium makes reconstruction slightly more challenging. It is well known that skin grafts will take well on pericranium, however, the resultant coverage may still be unstable and aesthetically displeasing. In the absence of pericranium, several pedicle flaps have been described.[50]

Tumors involving the scalp that are either benign or malignant, hemangiomas, vascular malformations, and congenital nevi may result in defects requiring reconstruction (Figure 90-10). Nevus sebaceus of Jadassohn presents as a hairless plaquelike lesion at birth, which eventually becomes nodular secondary to papillomatous hyperplasia of the epidermis.[35] The risk of malignant degeneration to epidermal appendage or basal cell tumors (10% to 40%) suggests excision of these lesions is wise. Larger nevi (giant congenital nevi) involving the scalp, back, and neck may also be associated with leptomeningeal melanosis, and an MRI scan of the brain should be obtained in these patients. Because of the increased risk of melanoma in these giant congenital nevi, excision is indicated. Our primary modality of therapy includes excision of these lesions and coverage with cultured epithelial autograft. Other tumors seen in the scalp include basal cell and squamous cell carcinomas (nonmelanoma skin cancers [NMSC]).[61] It is estimated that one in six Americans will develop NMSC in their lifetime,[21] 80% of which occur on the face and/or head and neck.[58] Because the scalp can easily be disguised by a cap or scarf, some patients—whether from fear or denial—will allow extensive growth and calvarial or even dural invasion before presenting to a physician. Routes of lymphatic spread from the scalp are twofold. The forehead and frontoparietal regions typically drain to the superficial parotid gland and to retromandibular nodes. Posteriorly located lesions will drain to the occipital nodes and occasionally to the posterior triangle cervical nodes.[16] We have seen many examples of basal cell carcinoma of the scalp, often ignored by the patient for many years, with subsequent deep invasion and destruction locally.

Metastatic tumors to the scalp include renal cell carcinoma and carcinoma of the breast. Meningiomas may also have direct extension through the bony cortex into the scalp, presenting as tumors of the scalp.

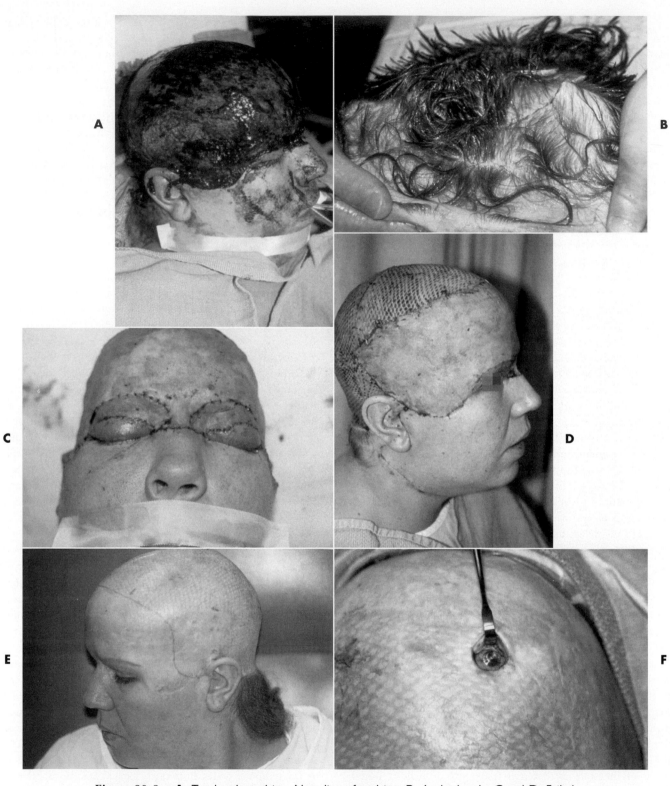

Figure 90-8. **A,** Total scalp avulsion. Note line of avulsion. **B,** Avulsed scalp. **C** and **D,** Failed replant—coverage with sheet graft of frontal area, full-thickness skin graft to upper eyelid, and meshed autograft to the rest of the scalp. **E,** Result at 1-year postinjury. **F,** Placement of osseointegrated implants for ease of placement of hairpiece.

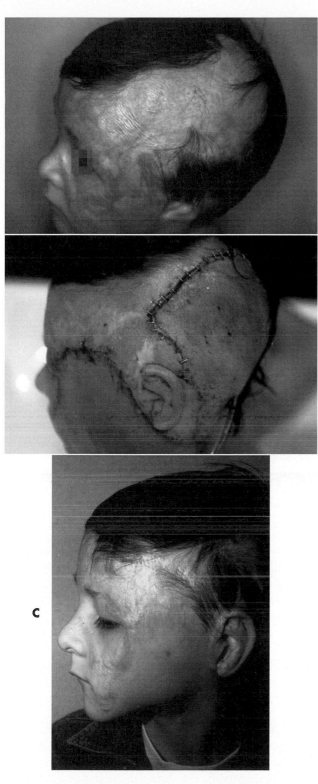

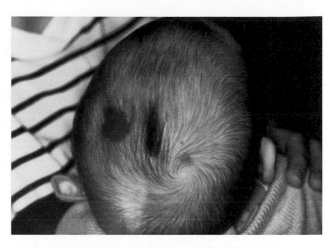

Figure 90-10. Congenital nevus of the scalp.

Figure 90-9. **A,** Burn alopecia in a child with a 45% total body surface burn treated with split-thickness skin grafts. **B,** Tissue expansion of the hair-bearing scalp allowed advancement flaps and excision of grafted areas. **C,** Appearance after first expansion. Subsequent advancements addressed the burned facial skin.

OPERATIONS

References to reconstruction of the scalp and cranial deformities appeared in the fourteenth and fifteenth centuries, when surgeons noted that in order to cover the exposed calvarium, one needed to expose the diploic space to enhance formation of granulation tissue. As is true for many reconstructive procedures in plastic surgery, the drive to develop these procedures was accelerated by current world events. Such events as the scalping injuries of the Native Americans, the Industrial Revolution, the era when women starting to work with heavy machinery, and the World Wars have all been instrumental in the evolution of these procedures.[16] Development of rotation flaps significantly increased the reconstructive options available to the plastic surgeon[19]; prior to this era, skin grafts were essentially the only option available, but now single-pedicle flaps could cover dura and exposed calvarium. Kazanjian devised a bipedicle flap, with relaxing incisions adjacent to the wound with skin grafting of the wake to cover scalp and calvarial wounds.[32]

Orticochea, in 1967, reported the entire scalp raised as either three or four pedicle flaps to cover defects up to 24 cm in diameter.[31,49,51] Radovan's principles of tissue expansion, used so extensively in breast reconstruction, were also applied to the scalp, making it possible to expand hair-bearing skin to cover large defects, particularly for burn alopecia.[36] The advent of microsurgery added two dimensions to scalp reconstruction: total scalp avulsions could now be replanted using microvascular techniques,[44] and, subsequently, microvascular transfer of muscle, skin, and/or bone allowed three-dimensional reconstruction of the scalp and calvarium.

One of the principal tenets of scalp reconstruction is that any reconstructive effort should optimally be based on a stable bony platform. Calvarial reconstruction has had a similarly interesting evolution. Initial reconstruction of the bony skull dates back to prehistoric Roman times, when a skull defect was reconstructed with gold plates.[39] In the late 1800s, osteoperiosteal bone grafts from the tibia were utilized to bridge bony defects of the calvarium.[14] The early 1900s heralded the use of rib or iliac crest grafts for bony reconstruction in addition to numerous metals including tantalum, Vitallium, and stainless steel.[39] Outcome analyses of these patients revealed a high incidence (10% to 12%) of complications, especially when the overlying soft tissue was not well vascularized.[67]

The advent of craniofacial surgical principles and techniques in the 1960s and 1970s heralded the use of split cranial bone graft, although this had initially been described in the late 1800s.[45] Herein, the outer table of the calvarium could be split from the inner and used as bone graft.[38,42,57] The advantages, according to Marchac, are that no foreign material is used, the donor site morbidity (if carefully done) is minimal, and—especially in children—the bone is able to be molded to fit the defect.[16] The parietal skull is the favored donor site considering factors including the absence of underlying venous sinuses and the thickness of the calvarium. Two techniques of bone graft harvest exist: the so-called *in-vivo technique,* wherein the outer table is split from the inner table, and the *ex-vivo technique,* wherein a true craniectomy is performed, the calvarial bone is split, the inner table is used as the bone graft, and the outer table is replaced in the donor site.[24]

Split rib cranioplasty (Figure 90-11) provides another alternative for bony reconstruction of the skull. Ribs will regenerate if periosteum is left intact. The donor deformity is acceptable if no more than two or three ribs are taken and care is used to avoid a pneumothorax. The disadvantage of rib cranioplasty is that ribs, particularly in adults, are somewhat more difficult to mold and may actually resorb over time, leading to contour irregularities.[16]

Alloplastic implants have had a wide usage in calvarial reconstruction. Methylmethacrylate is still most frequently chosen by "non-plastic surgeons," and infection and exposure continue to be problems—especially if the overlying soft tissues are not healthy or viable or if even minor wound infection supervenes. Although methylmethacrylate and other synthetic calvarial substitutes are simple, with no resultant donor deformity, they are contraindicated when there is exposure to either the sinuses or the nasal cavity, a history of previous infection at the site of reconstruction, and/or poor soft tissue coverage.[39]

Extensive research is underway to delineate the optimal synthetic bone graft substitute.[24] Bone substitutes that are currently being used include demineralized bone implants,[23] hydroxyapatites, and calcium phosphate and calcium sulfate[9] (Figure 90-12).

The indications for scalp reconstruction have been delineated in the previous section. When evaluating a patient for scalp reconstruction, important points to be obtained in the history include the etiology of the defect (i.e., a history of infection, trauma, or previous surgery). Evidence of underlying injury to the skull or brain must be assessed prior to undertaking reconstruction. Physical examination should identify the amount of scalp needing reconstruction, the hair pattern status of the underlying skull, and the nodal drainage basins, as well as the extent of tumor involvement in cancer cases. Radiographic

assessment is necessary mostly in trauma patients to rule out concomitant neck or skull injury and in those patients presenting with primary or secondary tumors of the scalp. CT scans, including three-dimensional CT scan reconstruction of the calvarial defect, are most effective for evaluation of bony defects, and MRI is useful for intracranial and/or extracranial soft tissue assessment. Both are important in helping to prioritize and plan reconstruction (see Figure 90-12).

Lacerations of the scalp are repaired using basic principles of wound debridement and closure in layers. Because of the luxuriant blood supply, hemorrhage can be significant and even life threatening. Careful repair of the galea layer will help prevent a depressed scar. Partial-thickness wounds, if quite small, can be observed and allowed to heal secondarily; this is sometimes preferable to split-thickness skin grafting, which leaves an unsuitable aesthetic result. Skin grafts, however, may be allowed to contract and can be excised with or without tissue expansion secondarily, particularly in children. Skin grafting may also be useful in grafting the failed scalp replant when pericranium is not injured. Finally, skin grafts may be placed on total or partial burns to the scalp in the anticipation that tissue expansion of the remaining hair-bearing scalp will be performed secondarily. Occasionally, burring the outer table of the skull to enhance granulation tissue is necessary prior to skin grafting, especially in children with total scalp burns. Basic principles of skin grafting include harvesting relatively thick (.012 to .015 inch) skin grafts, careful hemostasis, and fixation of the grafts (Figure 90-13).

Small full-thickness wounds of the scalp (i.e., less than 15%) can be treated with skin grafting if pericranium is available. In the absence of pericranium, local periosteal flaps may be rotated based on an axial blood supply.[63] These flaps have also been described as subgaleal-periosteal turnover flaps based on cortical blood supply.[34] Local hair-bearing flaps adjacent to the defect can also be rotated, keeping in mind standard angiosome concepts[25,56,68] (Figure 90-14). These subcutaneous flaps are excellent for very small defects only and may be transposed or rotated, depending on the geometry of the wound. A pinwheel-type rotation flap has also been described that is a variation of a Limberg-type flap.[65] Larger full-thickness wounds can be managed by skin grafting, coverage with local pedicle flaps, tissue expansion (better for secondary reconstruction), or free tissue transfer. Numerous options exist for local pedicle flaps. The most common and versatile options are the four-flap and, subsequently, three-flap scalp reconstruction techniques of Orticochea.[50,51] These axial flaps allow the entire remaining scalp to be elevated to cover large defects (Figure 90-15). The three-flap (banana peel) technique incorporates an anterior supraorbital and supratrochlear vessel pedicle, a lateral superficial temporal artery and posterior auricular vessel pedicle, and a posterior lateral and medial occipital vessel pedicle. To gain further length with these flaps, longitudinal galea incisions perpendicular to the long axis are recommended. It is imperative not to damage immediately adjacent vasculature when making these relaxing incisions.[48] These flaps are particularly useful for reconstruction of frontal and occipital areas of the scalp. Technical refinements to optimize results

Text continued on p. 1533

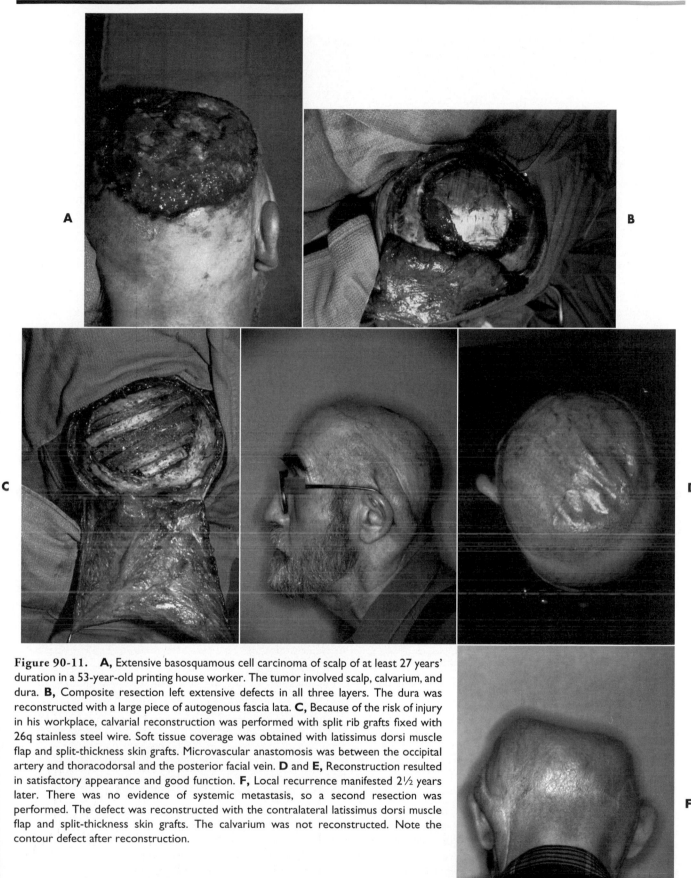

Figure 90-11. **A,** Extensive basosquamous cell carcinoma of scalp of at least 27 years' duration in a 53-year-old printing house worker. The tumor involved scalp, calvarium, and dura. **B,** Composite resection left extensive defects in all three layers. The dura was reconstructed with a large piece of autogenous fascia lata. **C,** Because of the risk of injury in his workplace, calvarial reconstruction was performed with split rib grafts fixed with 26q stainless steel wire. Soft tissue coverage was obtained with latissimus dorsi muscle flap and split-thickness skin grafts. Microvascular anastomosis was between the occipital artery and thoracodorsal and the posterior facial vein. **D and E,** Reconstruction resulted in satisfactory appearance and good function. **F,** Local recurrence manifested 2½ years later. There was no evidence of systemic metastasis, so a second resection was performed. The defect was reconstructed with the contralateral latissimus dorsi muscle flap and split-thickness skin grafts. The calvarium was not reconstructed. Note the contour defect after reconstruction.

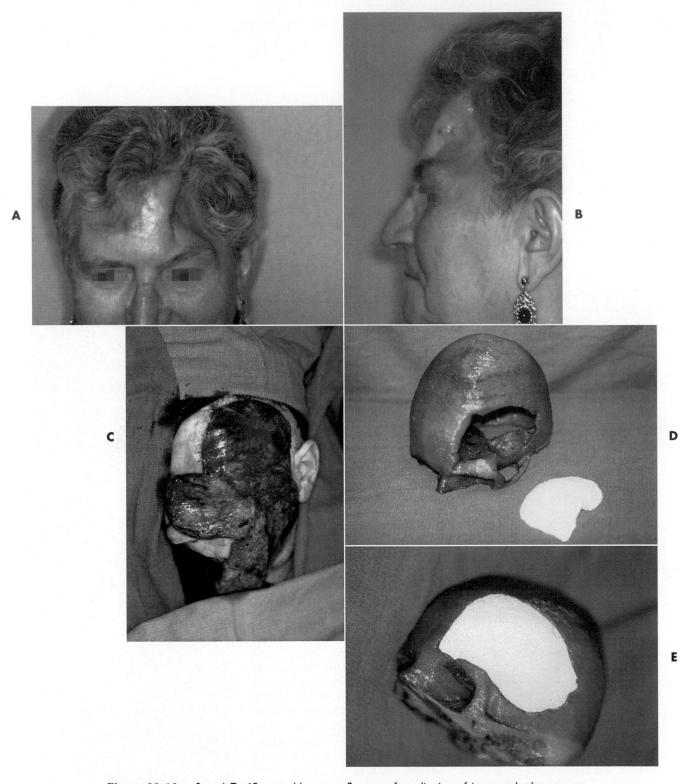

Figure 90-12. **A** and **B,** 65-year-old woman 2 years after clipping of intracerebral aneurysm complicated by wound infection with methicillin-resistant *Staphylococcus aureus* and loss of bone flap. At presentation, she had already undergone two attempts at calvarial reconstruction, both of which failed from postoperative infection. The skin covering of the dura was very atrophic, with several chronic draining sinuses. **C,** Her first operation included debridement of the bone edges and sinuses and interposition of a latissimus dorsi muscle free microvascular autograft between the skin and dura to provide stable soft tissue coverage. **D** and **E,** Using three-dimensional computed axial tomography, a customized porous acrylic composite was created for calvarial reconstruction.

Continued

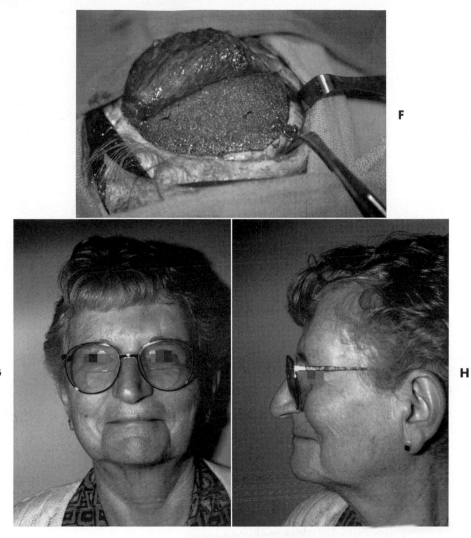

Figure 90-12, cont'd. F, Her second operation was planned for 6 months later, but this was delayed by Dilantin-induced thrombocytopenia. At 14 months, the composite was placed beneath the scalp and muscle flap. G and H, Four years after surgery she has remained well healed, with no episodes of infection.

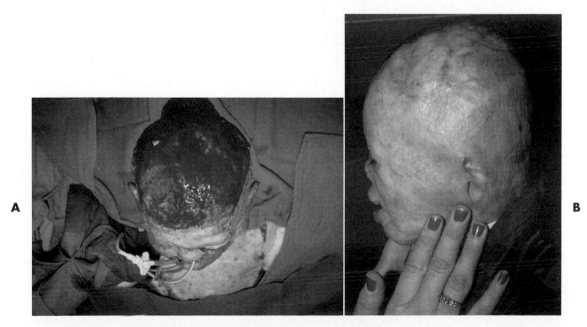

Figure 90-13. A, This 18-month-old child sustained an 80% total body surface area burn, including fourth-degree burn of the entire scalp and calvarium. The calvarium was treated by abrasion of the outer table and wet dressings, and over the course of several months, granulation tissue from the diploë and adjacent areas covered the entire cranium. B, Subsequent split-thickness skin grafting has provided coverage without breakdown for 3 years.

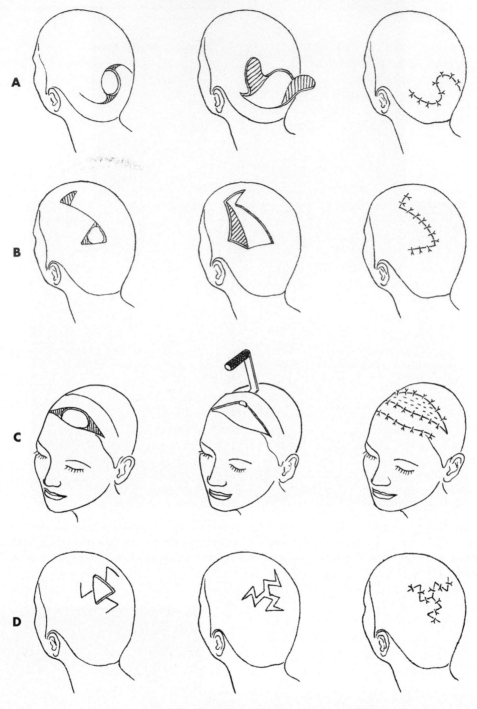

Figure 90-14. **A** to **D,** Local subcutaneous scalp flaps.

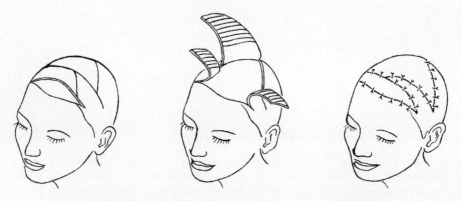

Figure 90-15. Diagrammatic representation of an Orticochea flap.

with the Orticochea flap include careful preoperative planning; basing each flap on its own axial blood supply; making the third flap very large with a wide pedicle, thereby enhancing its vascularity and using it to close the donor defects of the first and second flaps; and galeal scoring. Galeal scoring may, in fact, allow up to a 20% increase in coverage area. Disadvantages of these flaps include the possible need for delay with repeat procedures, donor defects that may subsequently require skin grafting, and the potential need for transfusion.[5,16] In the acute trauma or burn setting, extensive flap transposition is dangerous because damage to adjacent tissues may be present. If possible, conservative debridement and stabilization of the wound are more appropriate, with subsequent definitive reconstruction by flap transposition.

Juri has described several scalp flaps particularly useful for coverage of frontal or frontoparietal areas with hair-bearing skin.[30] The temporoparietal occipital and the temporoparietal occipitoparietal scalp flaps are based on the superficial temporal vessels. Again, these flaps are dissected in the subgaleal plane, taking care not to injure the vascular network that lies immediately above in the subcutaneous tissues. Intraoperative Doppler mapping is useful to identify the pedicle and allow proper marking of the flap. The temporoparietal occipital flap may be 30 to 32 cm long and 4 cm wide and is best performed with a delay procedure. It leaves a central area of alopecia in its wake. When recreating the anterior hairline, Juri recommends deepithelializing the anterior 2 mm of these flaps to produce an even suture line.[29] These flaps are best suited for the treatment of male pattern baldness; however, they can obviously be used for other reconstructive needs. Of the thoracic musculocutaneous flaps, the trapezius is the most useful and the latissimus dorsi a distant second (Figure 90-16). The trapezius is a large, flat, triangular-shaped, paned muscle with an origin of the occipital protuberance, ligamentum nuchae, and T1-T12 thoracic vertebrae. It inserts into the lateral third of the clavicle, spine of the scapula, and the acromion, and has a Type II pattern of circulation, with the transverse cervical artery and vein off the thyrocervical trunk as its dominant pedicle, and the dorsal scapular and lumbar vessels and branches of the occipital artery and vein as its minor pedicles. The trapezius serves to rotate and elevate the scapula during abduction and flexion of the arm and is innervated by the spinal accessory nerve. Loss of function results in a shoulder droop deformity, but this is prevented by leaving the superior muscle fibers attached to the spine of the scapula, making this the focal point for rotation. It is particularly useful for coverage of the occipital scalp with non-hair-bearing skin.

Tissue expansion represents a major advance in scalp reconstruction. For secondary reconstruction of the scalp it can be used alone or in concert with the above-described scalp flaps to either recruit additional tissue or help close resultant donor sites. It is especially useful in the management of burn alopecia and in providing hair-bearing tissue following excision of benign lesions (i.e., nevi, in the pediatric population). The principles of scalp tissue expansion have historically been extrapolated from breast tissue expansion by Argenta et al[4] and Manders,[36] suggesting that up to 50% of hair-bearing scalp can be replaced by expansion. Scalp tissue can be reexpanded as well and readvanced following initial expansion.[4] Crescentic-shaped expanders are positioned in multiple locations adjacent to the defect via incisions through the leading edge of the defect. The incision should be placed perpendicular to the axis of expansion. Expansion can begin at 10 to 14 days following placement of the expander and can be repeated weekly or biweekly. The port of the expander can be integrated, remote, or external. We prefer the integrated ports. In the child, expansion may require an operating room setting with mask anesthesia, but with EMLA cream, it is possible to perform expansion in an outpatient setting, especially for the older child. Estimating the amount of expansion necessary to cover a defect can be difficult. The available area is estimated by calculating the distance over the expander and subtracting the distance of the base. About 20% of the measured expanded skin is lost during advancement; therefore one should overexpand by 20% to 30%.[16] Once maximal volume and the desired expansion parameters are met, the expanders can be removed and the scalp flap(s) advanced. It has been shown that the capsule is important to the blood supply of the expanded tissue. We prefer to leave the capsule intact. Careful capsular scoring can be done, if needed, to further increase the length of the expanded flap. Previously expanded scalp tissue can be reexpanded, usually after 4 to 6 months. The gain in length using secondary reexpansion is often less than in primary expansion.

Microsurgical replantation of the scalp has been possible since its first description in 1976[44] and has now become the preferred treatment for near-total or total scalp avulsion injuries. The pattern of avulsion typically seen is described in the Indications section. The technique of replantation should proceed in an orderly manner with a two-team approach. The first team dissects the avulsed scalp and identifies temporal or occipital vessels for anastomosis, and the second team harvests vein grafts and dissects out the superficial temporal and/or occipital vessels. All anastomoses must be performed outside the zone of injury. Careful inspection of the intima using microscopic magnification will locate a safe area to anastomose. The artery is repaired first, particularly if the ischemia time is greater than 6 to 10 hours. Two arteries and as many veins as possible are anastomosed. It is, however, important to remember that the entire scalp can survive on a single superficial temporal artery via its rich vascular collateral network. Contraindications to scalp replantation include severe avulsion injury with an inability to identify the vascular pedicle, an ischemic time greater than 30 hours,[33] serious concomitant injuries, or a prohibitive medical history precluding a long operative intervention. Patients with scalp avulsions will typically have an extensive amount of blood loss and should be resuscitated prior to and during operation.

Microvascular tissue transfer for scalp reconstruction has also allowed almost the entire skull to be covered with a single microvascular transfer, albeit with non-hair-bearing skin. Indications for microvascular tissue transfer are a wound too large for local flaps, poor vascularity of the surrounding tissues, previous radiation, osteomyelitis of the skull, and/or coverage of a foreign body.[16] The advantages of free tissue transfer are

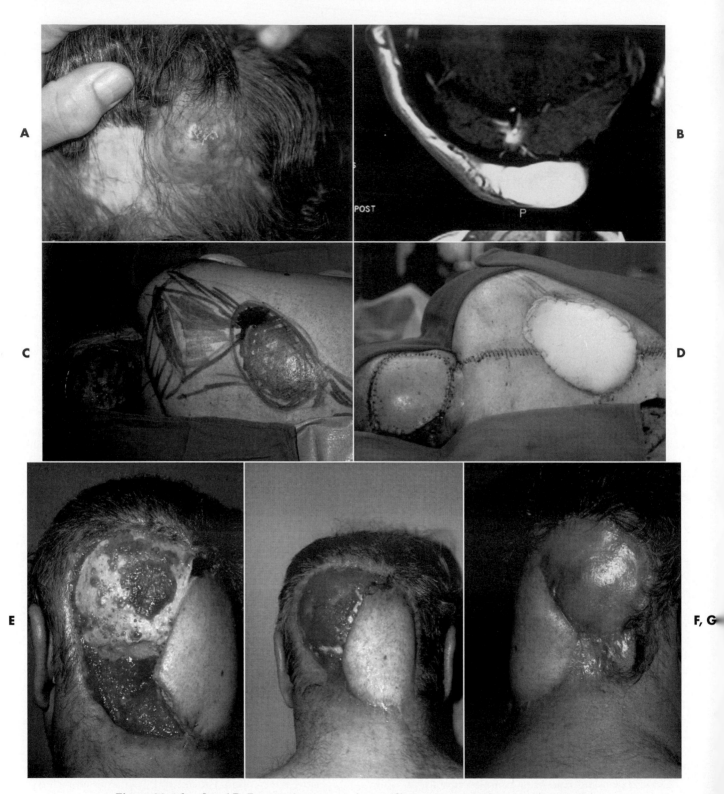

Figure 90-16. **A** and **B,** Extensively recurrent dermatofibrosarcoma protuberans in the occipital scalp of a 48-year-old man. The tumor abutted the periosteum but did not invade the calvarium. **C** and **D,** Resection included a large amount of full-thickness occipital scalp and cervical skin and muscle carried out at the subperiosteal layer. The defect was reconstructed with a large trapezius musculocutaneous flap. The donor site was covered with a split-thickness skin graft. **E** and **F,** A seroma beneath the flap became infected several weeks after discharged and resulted in delayed necrosis of the distal portion of the previously viable flap. Wound care with local debridement and moist dressings of saline allowed granulation tissue to form from the openings of the emissary veins and the arteries, which completely covered the bone over 3- to 4-week period. **G,** Split-thickness skin grafts over the granulation tissue have provided durable stable coverage.

the enhanced vascularity of the transferred tissue, especially muscle, when compared to pedicle flaps; the variety of donor tissues available for transfer (i.e., skin, muscle, bone, and combination thereof); and the ability to cover essentially any size defect and to do a simultaneous cranioplasty. The transfer of large, well-vascularized muscle has been particularly useful in cases where posttraumatic scarring or radiation or infection is present.[6,37] The disadvantages are the need for microsurgical expertise, the non-hair-bearing tissue that is transferred, and the potential donor site deformity. The first free tissue transfer described was the use of the omentum to cover a scalp defect following excision of a neurofibroma.[43] Since then, numerous flaps have been reported.[18] These include the latissimus dorsi with or without serratus anterior flap,[52] subscapular system

free flaps (see Figure 90-19), the rectus abdominis muscle flap,[28] the radial forearm flap,[12] the scapula and parascapula flaps,[13] and also the scalp itself as a free flap donor site with hair-bearing skin[47] (Figure 90-17).

Although several series report successful use of the superficial temporal vessels as recipient vessels, it is our strong preference to use vessels in the neck. For the posterior scalp the occipital vessels can be dissected from beneath the digastric to the external carotid and will reveal the postalveolar area. Similarly, careful dissection of the facial artery out of the submandibular gland and from behind the digastric back to its origin on the external carotid will gain enough length to extend into the midpreauricular area. By following the posterior facial vein into the parotid and preauricular area and the external jugular

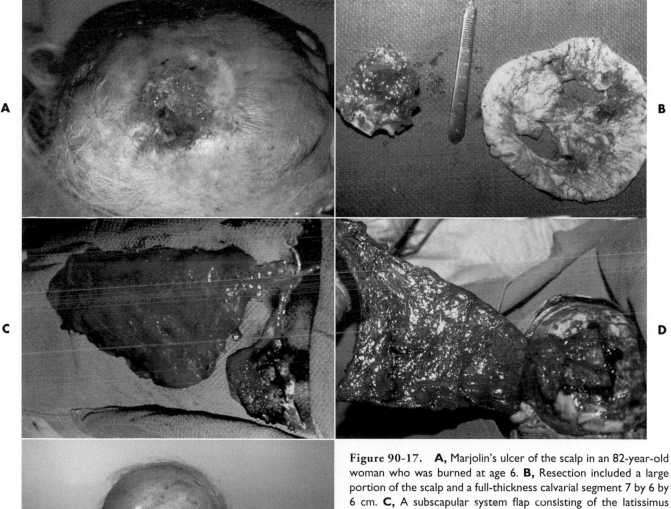

Figure 90-17. **A,** Marjolin's ulcer of the scalp in an 82-year-old woman who was burned at age 6. **B,** Resection included a large portion of the scalp and a full-thickness calvarial segment 7 by 6 by 6 cm. **C,** A subscapular system flap consisting of the latissimus dorsi muscle and a segment of distal scapula 7 by 6 by 6 cm based on the angular artery was designed. **D,** The vascularized scapula was used to fill the calvarial defect and the latissimus provided soft tissue coverage and a vascularized bed for split-thickness skin grafts. Microvascular anastomosis was between occipital artery, posterior facial veins, and thoracodorsal vessels. **E,** Stable scalp and calvarial reconstruction 2 years after surgery.

into the postauricular area, further mobility is obtained. The choice of which flap to use depends on the type of tissue required, the length of the pedicle needed, and an evaluation of the donor site deformity. The serratus muscle flap, designed to use distal muscle slips and harvesting of the vessels to the subscapular level, gives the longest pedicle, usually enough to reach over the anterior scalp. Latissimus and serratus muscles are extremely useful, and muscle bulk usually atrophies with tissue to match the contour of the remaining scalp and skull.

The latissimus dorsi/serratus muscle flap is an excellent choice for scalp reconstruction. It is a large muscle complex capable of covering almost the entire scalp despite postoperative atrophy (Figure 90-18). It is useful in cases of bacterial infection where muscle is required. The donor site deformity

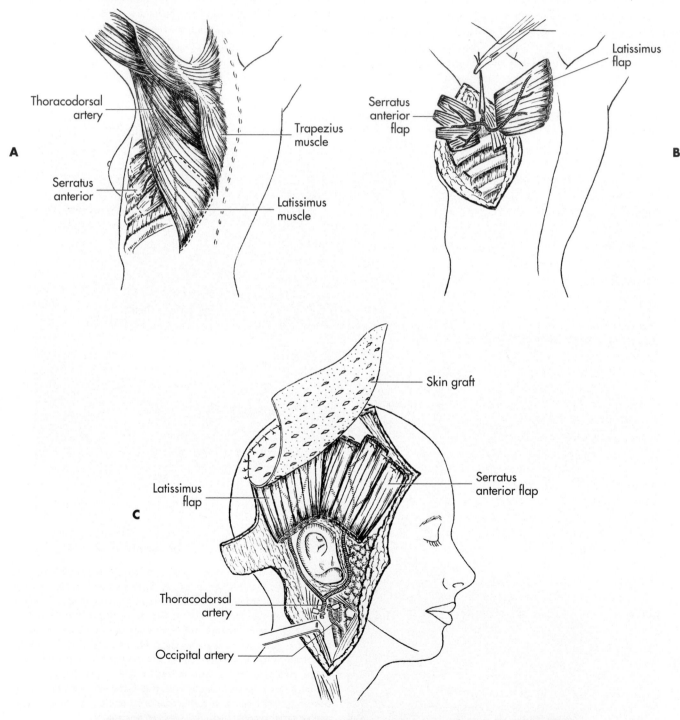

Figure 90-18. **A,** The combined latissimus serratus muscle flap based on the thoracodorsal vessels and the crossing branch that runs on top of the serratus muscle. **B,** Dissection of the vessels off the muscle for a short distance allows a freer arc of rotation for both muscles. **C,** Microvascular anastomosis is usually performed in the neck, and the vessels can be placed in the periauricular and postauricular position for maximum coverage of the scalp.

is minimal, the color match when the muscle is skin grafted is cosmetically acceptable, and the muscle is able to tolerate postoperative radiation well.[52] The omentum provides reasonable coverage of the scalp, is large, has a long pedicle, and can cover almost the entire scalp with well-vascularized tissue, but requires laparotomy with subsequent risk of adhesions, wound dehiscence, and bowel obstruction. The radial forearm flap provides a long pedicle, but it is a fasciocutaneous flap and is limited in size.

The scapula and parascapula flaps offer a long pedicle all the way to the subscapular system, minimal donor site deformity, and a fairly large skin paddle. The disadvantages are that patient positioning may be problematic, especially with combined neurosurgical cases, and that these flaps can be quite bulky and do not atrophy over time.

Although not as large as the latissimus muscle, the rectus abdominis is an easily accessible muscle with minimal donor deformity, has a large pedicle, and is easily contoured to fit the convexity of the skull.[8]

When hair-bearing tissue is critical, the scalp itself can be used as a donor site. These cases are probably best reserved for restoration of the anterior hairline.

OUTCOMES

There are presently no good outcome studies available for scalp reconstruction. There is, however, plenty of literature suggesting good to excellent results with the various techniques outlined. Certainly the indications for the procedure (i.e., trauma versus tumor extirpation) influence the overall long-term result and patient satisfaction, as well as quality of life, and each procedure described has its own set of potential complications. Simple repair of scalp lacerations should, in general, provide very satisfying results; however, careful attention must be paid to the blood supply of the scalp, especially with complex lacerations as seen in the patient in Figure 90-6. This patient subsequently underwent loss of approximately 30% of her scalp and required a free tissue transfer for final coverage (see Figure 90-4). Excessive blood loss and the potential for a depressed scar if the galea is not repaired are the most significant problems seen. Complications associated with the use of scalp flaps include partial or complete flap loss and secondary alopecia, dehiscence secondary to excessive tension, and hematoma formation, which may potentiate the other complications. Recognition of preoperative risk factors such as diabetes and smoking history, careful attention to preoperative planning, elevation of the scalp with three to four flaps, potential incorporation of the delay phenomenon when long narrow pedicle flaps are used to enhance vascularity, and adequate drainage of the wounds all help to obviate some of these complications. In the execution of a rotation scalp flap, the design of the flap is perhaps the most critical parameter to ensure success.[7]

Major complications of tissue expansion include infection, hematoma, implant exposure, and deflation. Minor complications include pain, cellulitis, seromas, and resulting widened scars.[37] The major complication rate in a large series of head and neck expansion was 6%,[6] although it was believed to be lower than other series because of standardization of preoperative and intraoperative planning and removal of the periprosthetic capsule with careful anchoring of the expanded flap to deeper tissues. The overall complication rate of expansion for scalp reconstruction is probably closer to 15% to 25%. Exposure of an implant does not necessarily preclude further expansion. A clinical decision should be made at that point as to whether the implant exposure is secondary to infection. If not, expansion may be continued with extreme caution.

Complications and outcome with the use of free tissue transfer are usually directly related to survival of the transferred tissue. Free flap survival in most series has averaged 90% to 95%.[13,18,47,54] Although the ideal postoperative monitoring method is not clear, we feel that hourly Doppler checks of the pedicle and an assessment of the flap's color can provide a good outcome, particularly in the crucial first 24 to 48 hours postoperatively. As is true for other methods of reconstruction described in the chapter, the underlying bony reconstruction must be stabilized to optimize results. If an infection is present, the bone should be thoroughly debrided and staged bony reconstruction performed. Similarly with irradiated tissue, removal of as much affected tissue as possible and coverage with a muscle flap are preferable.

The future for scalp reconstruction probably will reflect progress in tissue engineering. Currently, tissue-engineered skin is widely used for burn coverage as well as for coverage of large congenital nevi. Tissue-engineered cartilage is undergoing clinical trials for reconstruction of articular defects of the knee. It might be possible in the future to produce tissue-engineered hair-bearing skin for scalp reconstruction. Further advances could be made in techniques providing rapid tissue expansion versus the 6- to 8-week procedure that is routinely carried out today. Experimental work with angiogenic factors to enhance the vascularity of currently available flaps may also improve results obtained with pedicle flaps for scalp reconstruction.

REFERENCES

1. Achauer BM: Scalp reconstruction. In Achauer BM, editor: *Burn reconstruction,* New York, 1991, Thieme Medical Publishers, p 13.

2. Albert BS, Buncke HJ Jr, Mathes SJ: Surgical treatment of the totally avulsed scalp, *Clin Plast Surg* 9:145, 1982.

3. Argenta LC, Dingman RO: Total reconstruction of aplasia cutis congenita involving scalp, skull, dura, *Plast Reconstr Surg* 77:650, 1986.

4. Argenta LC, Watanabe MJ, Grabb WC: The use of tissue expansion in head and neck reconstruction, *Ann Plast Surg* 11:31, 1982.

5. Arnold PG, Rangarathnam CS: Multiple scalp flap reconstruction: Orticochea revisited, *Plast Reconstr Surg* 69(4):605, 1982.

6. Azzoloni A, et al: Skin expansion in head and neck reconstructive surgery, *Plast Reconstr Surg* 90:799, 1992.

7. Bardach J: Scalp reconstruction using local flaps and free skingrafts. In Bardach J, editor: *Local flaps and free skingrafts in head and neck reconstruction,* St Louis, 1992, Mosby, p 193.

8. Borah GC, Hidalgo DA, Wey PD: Reconstruction of extensive scalp defects with rectus free flaps, *Ann Plast Surg* 34:281-287, 1985.

9. Bucholz RW, Carlton A, Holme R: Interporous hydroxyapatite as a bone graft substitute in tibial plateau fractures, *Clin Orthop* 240:53-62, 1985.

10. Burke JF, Banouc CC, Quinby WC: Primary excision and immediate grafting: a method for shortening illness, *J Trauma* 14:389-395, 1974.

11. Cassanova R, Cavalcante D, Grotting JC, et al: Anatomic basis for vascularized outer table calvarial bone grafts, *Plast Reconstr Surg* 78:300, 1986.

12. Chicarelli ZN, Ariyan S, Cuono CB: Reconstruction of extensive tissue defects of the scalp by microsurgical composite tissue transplantation, *Plast Reconstr Surg* 77:577, 1986.

13. Chiu DTW, Sherman JE, Edgerton BW: Coverage of the calvarium with a large parascapular flap, *Ann Plast Surg* 42:60, 1989.

14. Delagénière H, Lewin P: A general method of regaining loss of bony substance and of reconstructing bone by osteoperiosteal grafts taken from the tibia, *SGO* 30:441, 1920.

15. Dingman RO, Argenta LC: The surgical repair of traumatic defects of the scalp, *Clin Plast Surg* 9(2):131, 1982.

16. Elliot LF, Jurkiewicz MJ: Scalp and calvarium. In Jurkiewicz MJ, Krizer TJ, Mathes SJ, et al, editors: *Plastic surgery—principles and practice,* St Louis, 1990, Mosby, pp 419-440.

17. Freund RM: Scalp, calvarium and forehead reconstruction. In Ashton S, Beasley RW, Thorne CUM, editors: *Grabb and Smith's plastic surgery,* Philadelphia, 1997, Lippincott-Raven, p 473.

18. Furnas H, Lineweaver WC, Alpert BS, et al: Scalp reconstruction by microvascular free tissue transfer, *Ann Plast Surg* 24(5):431, 1990.

19. Gillies H: Note on scalp closure, *Lancet* 2:310, 1944.

20. Glasson DW, Duncan GH: Aplasia cutis congenita of the scalp: delayed closure complicated by massive hemorrhage, *Plast Reconstr Surg* 75:423, 1985.

21. Gloster HM, Brodland DG: The epidemiology of skin cancer, *Dermatol Surg* 22:217, 1996.

22. Grossman HJ, Singer O, Greeley PW, et al: Surgical separation in craniopagus, *JAMA* 153:201, 1953.

23. Habal MB: Bone grafting the orbital floor for post-traumatic defects, *J Craniofac Surg* 3:175-180, 1992.

24. Habal MB, Redi HA: Bone graft and bone induction substitutes, *Clin Plast Surg* 2(4):525, 1994.

25. Hallock GG, Trevaski AE: Refinement of the subcutaneous pedicle flap for closure of forehead and scalp defects, *Plast Reconstr Surg* 75:903, 1985.

26. Harrison SH: Exposure of the skull from burns, *Br J Plast Surg* 4:279-292, 1952.

27. Huang TT, Larson DL, Lewis SR: Burn alopecia, *Plast Reconstr Surg* 60:763-767, 1977.

28. Jones NF, Sekhar LN, Schramm VL: Free rectus abdominal muscle flap reconstruction of the middle and posterior cranial base, *Plast Reconstr Surg* 78:471, 1986.

29. Juri J: TPO and TPOP scalp flaps. In Strauch B, Vasconez LO, Hall-Fundley EJ, editors: *Grabb's encyclopedia of flaps,* ed 2, Philadelphia, 1998, Lippincott-Raven, p 19.

30. Juri J: Use of parieto-occipital flaps in the surgical treatment of baldness, *Plast Reconstr Surg* 55:456, 1975.

31. Juri J, Juri C: Aesthetic aspects of reconstructive scalp surgery, *Clin Plast Surg* 8:243, 1981.

32. Kazanjian VH: Repair of partial losses of the scalp, *Plast Reconstr Surg* 12:325, 1953.

33. Kaixiang C, Su Zhai, et al: Microsurgical replantation of the avulsed scalp: report of 20 cases, *Plast Reconstr Surg* 97:1099, 1996.

34. Lai CS, Lui SD, et al: The subgaleal periosteal turnover flap for reconstruction of scalp defects, *Ann Plast Surg* 30:267-271, 1993.

35. Lever WF, Schaunburg-Lever G: *Histopathology of the skin,* ed 6, Philadelphia, 1983, JB Lippincott.

36. Manders ER, et al: Skin expansion to eliminate large scalp defects, *Ann Plast Surg* 12:305, 1984.

37. Manders ER, Schenden MJ, Furrey JA: Soft tissue expansion: concepts and complications, *Plast Reconstr Surg* 74:495, 1984.

38. Manson PN, Crawley WA, Hoopes JE: Frontal cranioplasty: risk factors and choice of cranial vault reconstructive material, *Plast Reconstr Surg* 77:888, 1986.

39. Marchac D: Deformities of the forehead, scalp and cranial vault. In McCarthy JG, editor: *Plastic surgery,* Philadelphia, 1990, WB Saunders, pp 1538-1574.

40. Mathes ST, Nahai F: Reconstructive surgery—principles, anatomy, technique. In Mathes ST, Nahai F, editors: *Trapezius flap,* New York, 1997, Churchill Livingstone, p 651.

41. McCann J, O'Donoghue S, Ghazal SKA, et al: Microvascular replantation of a completely avulsed scalp, *Microsurgery* 15:639, 1994.

42. McCarthy JC, Zide BM: The spectrum of calvarial bone grafting: introduction of the vascularized calvarial bone flap, *Plast Reconstr Surg* 74:10, 1984.

43. McLean DH, Buncke HJ Jr: Autotransplant of omentum to a large scalp defect with microsurgical revascularization, *Plast Reconstr Surg* 49:268, 1972.

44. Miller GD, Anstee EJ, Snell JA: Successful replantation of an avulsed scalp by microvascular anastomoses, *Plast Reconstr Surg* 58:133, 1976.

45. Müller W: Zur frage der temporaren schadelresektion an stelle der trepanation, *Zentralbl Chir* 17:65, 1890.

46. O'Connell JE: Craniophagus twins: surgical anatomy and embryology and their complications, *J Neurol Psych* 39:1, 1976.

47. Ohmori K: Application of microvascular free flaps to scalp defects, *Clin Plast Surg* 9:263, 1982.

48. Orticochea M: Scalp flaps. In Strauch B, Vasconez LD, Hall-Fundley EJ, editors: *Grabb's encyclopedia of flaps,* ed 2, Philadelphia, 1998, Lippincott-Raven, pp 13-18.

49. Orticochea M: Repair of partial losses of the scalp, *Plast Reconstr Surg* 24:184, 1971.

50. Orticochea M: New three flap scalp reconstruction technique, *Br J Plast Surg* 24:184-188, 1971.

51. Orticochea M: Four flap scalp reconstruction technique, *Br J Plast Surg* 20:159, 1967.

52. Pennington DG, Stern HS, Lee KK: Free flap reconstruction of large defects of the scalp and calvarium, *Plast Reconstr Surg* 83:655, 1985.

53. Ranev D, Shindarsky B: Operative treatment of deep burns of the scalp, *Br J Plast Surg* 12:305-312, 1969.

54. Robson MC, Zachary LS, et al: Reconstruction of large cranial defects in the presence of heavy radiation damage and infection utilizing tissue transferred by microvascular anastomoses, *Plast Reconstr Surg* 83(3):438, 1989.

55. Sadove AM, Moore TS, Eppley BL: Total scalp, ear, and eyebrow avulsion: aesthetic adjustment of the replanted tissue, *J Reconstr Microsurg* 6:223, 1990.

56. Sahai S, Soeda S, Terayama I: Subcutaneous pedicle flaps and scalp defects, *Br J Plast Surg* 41:255-261, 1988.

57. Santoni-Rugii P: Repair of skull defects by outer table osteoperiosteal free grafts, *Plast Reconstr Surg* 74:10, 1969.

58. Scotto J, Fears TR, Fraumeni JF: Incidence of non melanoma skin cancer in the United States, *NIH Publication No. 83-2433,* Washington, DC, 1983, Government Printing Offices.

59. Shestak KC, Ramasastry SS: Reconstruction of defects of scalp and skull. In Cohen M, editor: *Mastery of plastic surgery,* Boston, 1994, Little, Brown, pp 830-859.

60. Shively PE, Bermant MA, Bucholz RD: Separation of craniopagus twins utilizing tissue expanders, *Plast Reconstr Surg* 78:765, 1985.

61. Stron SS, Yomamura BA: Epidemiology of non-melanoma skin cancer, *Clin Plast Surg* 24(4):627-636, 1997.

62. Stuzin JM, Wagstrom L, Kawamoto HR, et al: Anatomy of the frontal branch of the facial nerve, *Plast Reconstr Surg* 83:265, 1989.

63. Temurena W: The use of periosteal flaps in scalp and forehead reconstruction, *Ann Plast Surg* 25:450, 1990.

64. Tolhurst DE, et al: Surgical anatomy of the scalp, *Plast Reconstr Surg* 87:603-612, 1991.

65. Vadhure TR: Multiple pinwheel scalp flaps. In Strauch B, Vasconez LD, Hall-Fundley EJ, cditors: *Grabb's encyclopedia of flaps,* ed 2, Philadelphia, 1998, Lippincott-Raven, pp 11-12.

66. Vinocur CD, Wentraub WH, Wilensky RJ, et al: Surgical management of aplasia cutis congenita, *Arch Surg* 14:1160, 1976.

67. White TC: Late complications following cranioplasty with alloplastic plates, *Ann Surg* 128:743, 1948.

68. Worthen EF: Scalp flaps and the rotation forehead flap. In Strauch B, Vasconez LD, Hall-Fundley EJ, editors: *Grabb's encyclopedia of flaps,* ed 2, Philadelphia, 1998, Lippincott-Raven, pp 5-10.

69. Worthen EF: Regeneration of the skull following a deep electrical burn, *Plast Reconstr Surg* 48·1-4, 1971.

70. Zhan S, Chang T, Guan W, et al: Microsurgical replantation of the avulsed scalp: report of six cases, *J Reconstr Microsurg* 9:121, 1993.

CHAPTER

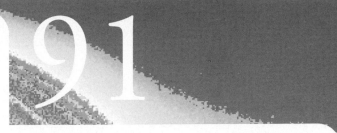

Skull Base: Orbit, Anterior, Lateral

Stephen P. Beals

INTRODUCTION

The development of skull base surgery in the past decade has made possible complete resection of tumors of this region that were previously thought to be incurable. Safe avenues of exposure through complex anatomy, where critical structures were once thought to be insurmountable obstacles for curative resection, have been discovered, allowing single-stage resection of complex tumors with shorter operating times and low patient morbidity. Moreover, major advances in imaging techniques, anesthesia, monitoring of the brain and cranial nerves, reconstructive techniques, postoperative intensive care monitoring, instrumentation technology, and localization devices have complemented these surgical innovations. Despite these developments, skull base surgery remains exceedingly demanding and challenging.

An essential principle in conducting cranial base surgery is the multidisciplinary team approach. No single surgical discipline has the skills and training to manage all aspects of the patient with a skull base tumor. The rarity of skull base tumors demands centralization of care by a skull base team so that an adequate number of patients can be cared for in order to maintain a high skill level, to conduct research that continues to refine surgical techniques, and to understand outcome. Coordinated care by a skull base team improves communication between physicians and results in a superior treatment plan, giving the patient the best chance for a successful outcome. The core specialties include neurosurgery, head and neck surgery, plastic surgery, and neurotology. Additional specialists in the fields of neurology, endovascular radiology, radiation oncology, chemotherapy, ophthalmology, and neurorehabilitation also make contributions to the skull base team. The team functions best with the help of an administrative coordinator and medical director who can organize patient care and facilitate communication between the specialists and the patient. The team should meet on a regular basis to evaluate patients and plan their care. This format also facilitates follow-up and discussion of morbidity and mortality, and fosters development of research protocols.

THE PATHOLOGY OF SELECTED TUMORS

See Table 91-1 for the pathology of selected tumors.[4,64]

PATIENT EVALUATION

Tumors of the skull base often grow silently to an alarming size before symptoms bringing medical attention are noted by the patient. At the time of presentation, the history and physical examination provide a significant amount of information regarding location and extent of the tumor. Presenting signs and symptoms may be vague, depending on the location in the skull base, the type of tumor, and the tumor's size. Benign tumors usually cause symptoms by compressing adjacent tissues in the orbital area, causing proptosis, diplopia, epiphora, and conjunctival exposure. In the paranasal sinus and nasal cavity, obstruction can result in sinusitis, nasal airway obstruction, mucocele, otitis media due to eustachian tube obstruction, and epistaxis in the case of vascular tumors.

Malignant tumors, which are invasive, may present with headache, focal seizures, loss of cranial nerve function (including blindness), anosmia, diplopia, ptosis, altered facial sensation and animation, tinnitus, hearing loss, speech and swallowing dysfunction, and facial mass or swelling.

After initial clinical evaluation, computed tomography (CT) scan with contrast and magnetic resonance imaging (MRI) with T1-and T2-weighted images are indicated. A CT scan provides the greatest information about bony involvement. In general, benign tumors show displacement of bone and malignant lesions show invasion and lysis. MRI provides the most information regarding soft tissue details and anatomic extent of the tumor margins. Angiography may be critical to understand the degree of vascularity of the tumor and involvement of the carotid artery and other critical vascular structures.

Text continued on p. 1550

Table 91-1.
Pathology of Selected Tumors

BENIGN EXTRACRANIAL TYPE	PATHOLOGY	ORIGIN	INCIDENCE	AGE/SEX
Inverted papilloma	Benign growth of epithelium; invades into stroma	Nasal, sinus; ethmoid, middle turbinate	0.5-4% of nasal tumors	White males, age 40-70
Angiofibroma	Benign vascular lesion with spindle or stellate fibrocytes in connective tissue stroma	Lateral margin posterior nares near sphenopalatine foramen	Rare in US & Europe, common in Orient and Far East	Adolescent males
Salivary gland pleomorphic adenoma	Encapsulated, smooth, firm; epithelial, mesenchymal elements	Parotid, minor salivary glands, palate, nasopharynx	65% of parotid tumors	F > M, over 50
Paraganglioma	Encapsulated, densely adherent, well-differentiated epithelial cells, neurosecretory granule	Chemoreceptor system; carotid vagal, jugulo-tympanic bodies	60% carotid body	F:M 3:1, age 30-60
Mucocele	Blocked sinus; expansive mucin collection	Frontal and ethmoidal sinus		Adult
Cholesteatoma	Stratified epithelial lining surrounding desquamated keratin	Temporal bone, CPA		All
Pituitary adenoma	Chromophobe adenoma; 50% can produce growth hormone, prolactin-type factor, thyrotrophic	Pituitary, Rathke's pouch	10% of all intracranial neoplasms	Adult

Data from Barnes L, Kapadia SB: The biology and pathology of selected skull base tumors, *J Neurooncol* 20:213-240, 1994; and Ross DA, Sasaki CT: Pathology of tumors of the cranial base, *Clin Plast Surg* 22:407-416, 1995.
CN, Cervical nerve.
CPA, Cerebellar pontine angle.

CAUSE	CLINICAL PRESENTATION	NATURAL HISTORY	TREATMENT	OUTCOME
Unknown; possible human papillomavirus	Can be associated with squamous cell carcinoma with recurrence (13%)	Pressure erosion of bone	Surgical resection	27-73% recurrence if incompletely excised
Unknown; possible hormonal sensitivity	Epistaxis, nasal obstruction; intracranial = 10-20%	Grows along tissue planes	Surgical resection, preoperative embolization	Local recurrence 5-25%
Unknown	Slow-growing painless mass	Parapharyngeal extension to skull base	Surgical resection, preserve normal structures	Recurrence 5-50%, malignant degeneration 2-5%
Unknown; familial pattern	Pulsatile tinnitus, hearing loss	Progressive CN deficit, painless, hearing loss, Horner's syndrome	Surgical resection, preoperative embolization	2-13% malignant
Inflammatory, trauma or bony or soft tissue growth	Headache	Intracranial extension, meningitis, brain abscess	Surgical resection with reconstruction of defect	Adequate surgery curative
Congenital: epithelial nests, acquired: chronic middle ear disease	Meningitis, brain abscess	Erosion into ossicles and intracranial	Surgical resection	Adequate surgery curative
Unknown; possible genetic alteration	Endocrine abnormalities, visual disturbance	Can be invasive directly to dura, bone, CNs, pharynx, sinuses, can be ectopic	Surgical resection; radiation for recurrence and inoperable tumors	

Continued

Table 91-1.
Pathology of Selected Tumors—cont'd

BENIGN EXTRACRANIAL TYPE	PATHOLOGY	ORIGIN	INCIDENCE	AGE/SEX
Craniopharyngioma	Distinguished from amelo-blastoma of jaw by irregular calcified masses and foci of metaplastic bone or cartilage	Unobliterated portions of the fetal craniopharyngeal duct	Child: 9% of intracranial neoplasms Adult: 2.5-4% of intracranial neoplasms Child: 54% of sella-chiasmal lesions	M = F, peak: 5-10 yrs and 55-65 yrs
Meningioma	Meningothelial arachnoid cells found in arachnoid villi adjacent to dura; four histologic types	Parasagittal, lateral cerebral convexities, sphenoid ridge, at CN foramina	2nd most common brain tumor, 13-18% of all intracranial tumors	Female 65%, peak age 45
Schwannoma	Nerve sheath; encapsulated, adjacent to nerve fibers	Cranial nerves, CPA, foramina	95% are acoustic neuroma	
Ossifying fibroma	Marrow replacement by whorls of spindle cells with osteoblasts rimming the fibroosseous tissue	Contour-altering lesion of facial bones		3rd decade
Fibrous dysplasia	Fibroosseous tissue replaces medullary bone, monostotic, polyostotic, Albright's syndrome	Ribs, femur, tibia, maxilla, mandible, skull, frontal, sphenoid	25% have head and neck involvement	<30 monostotic M = F; polyostotic M:F = 1:3
Osteoma	Smooth, well-encapsulated, extensive with osteoplastic active at margin	Frontal bone perpendicular plate of ethmoid	0.45% of patients getting radiographs, most common fibroosseous lesion of skull	F:M = 3:1, median age 60s

Data from Barnes L, Kapadia SB: The biology and pathology of selected skull base tumors, *J Neurooncol* 20:213-240, 1994; and Ross DA, Sasaki CT: Pathology of tumors of the cranial base, *Clin Plast Surg* 22:407-416, 1995.

CAUSE	CLINICAL PRESENTATION	NATURAL HISTORY	TREATMENT	OUTCOME
Unknown	Endocrine abnormalities and lethargy	Depends on rate of growth	Surgical resection; radiation if only partially resectable	Recurrence common; radiation and/or reoperation
Unknown	Headaches, seizure, visual impairment	Slow growing, noninvasive, some are aggressive	Surgical resection	Curable with complete resection; late recurrence possible
Unknown	Symptoms correlate with CN VIII; sensorineural hearing loss, tinnitus	Growth rate is variable	Early surgical resection	Curable with complete resection
Unknown	Contour change, compression of normal structures	Slow growth, progressive	Total surgical resection	Low recurrence rate
Unknown	Painless, asymptomatic swelling	1 in 200 osteosarcoma; primary growth in adolescence; impingement of foramina	Functional consideration determines debulking vs. resection	20-30% recurrence with debulking
Unknown	Usually asymptomatic		Surgical resection if symptomatic	

Continued

Table 91-1.
Pathology of Selected Tumors—cont'd

BENIGN EXTRACRANIAL TYPE	PATHOLOGY	ORIGIN	INCIDENCE	AGE/SEX
Osteoblastoma	Dark red, gritty tissue; interconnecting osteoid islands rimmed by osteoblasts, vascular stroma	Infrequent in head/neck; 75% in jaw, cervical vertebrae, nasal	3% of benign bone tumors	2nd decade
Chordoma	Dysontogenetic neoplasm; lobulated, partially translucent, mucoid; no absolute histologic findings	Embryonic notochord	1/3 occur in skull base; 1% of intracranial tumors	M > F, 20-40 years
Congenital dermoid	Nasal anomaly; tract or cyst lined by epithelium can run from skin to dura; ectoderm and mesoderm origins, stratified epithelium and adnexal structure	Nose, forehead, anterior fontanels, orbits, periorbital, tongue, neck; lines of embryonic fusion	1 in 20,000-40,000 births	Congenital
Squamous cell carcinoma	Well to poorly differentiated	Paranasal sinuses	80% of malignant tumors of paranasal sinuses	M : F = 2 : 1, >40
Adenoid cystic carcinoma	Epithelial origin, circumscribed, unencapsulated; four histologic patterns	Salivary and lacrimal glands	4% of salivary gland tumors	M = F, 40s
Rhabdomyosarcoma	Malignant myoblasts	Orbit, mouth, pharynx, face, neck, ear, sinus	Most common soft tissue neoplasm in child	Mean age 6

Data from Barnes L, Kapadia SB: The biology and pathology of selected skull base tumors, *J Neurooncol* 20:213-240, 1994; and Ross DA, Sasaki CT: Pathology of tumors of the cranial base, *Clin Plast Surg* 22:407-416, 1995.

CAUSE	CLINICAL PRESENTATION	NATURAL HISTORY	TREATMENT	OUTCOME
Unknown		Known nasal lesions >2.5 cm; one with intracranial extension	Surgical resection	20% recurrence
Unknown	Affects CN's	Extensive bony destruction	Surgical resection, radiation	High recurrence rate
Unknown	Distortion of local tissues, mass, asymptomatic, risk of infection	Growth with patient	Surgical resection	Adequate surgical resection curative
Unknown	Sinus obstruction, inflammation, CN I-VI involvement	Silent growth until large	Surgical resection, radiation	Poor prognosis
	Mass, parotid, orbit, skull base	Neural invasion with skin lesions, enters skull base	Surgical resection, radiation	Poor prognosis, high rate of local recurrence, metastases
	Proptosis	Painless tumor of orbit	Radiation, chemotherapy, surgery for diagnosis or resection of early lesion	

Continued

Table 91-1.
Pathology of Selected Tumors—cont'd

BENIGN EXTRACRANIAL TYPE	PATHOLOGY	ORIGIN	INCIDENCE	AGE/SEX
Hemangiopericytoma	Mesenchymal; highly vascularized, spindle cells	Nasal, sinus, pterygopalatine fossa, infratemporal fossa	Uncommon	
Esthesioneuroblastoma	Neural crest cells of olfactory epithelium; fleshy, pink areas of necrosis; calcification; neurocytes, neuroblasts	Upper nasal cavity	Rare	20-50 years, slight male predominance
Malignant schwannoma	Fusiform or nodular mass, infiltrative, spindle casts in interlacing fasciales	Retromaxillary, pterygomandibular region common	Higher incidence and earlier age in von Recklinghausen's disease	M = F, 40-50
Chondrosarcoma	Blue/white, lobular tissue, mucoid character	Skull base, more lateral than chordoma; also, sinus, facial bones	Rare	M = F, 12-80 (mean 32)
Osteogenic sarcoma	Sarcomatous stroma, production of osteoid and bone		Rare	2nd-3rd decade
Metastatic	Breast, lung, prostate, lytic vs. hyperostotic			

Data from Barnes L, Kapadia SB: The biology and pathology of selected skull base tumors, *J Neurooncol* 20:213-240, 1994; and Ross DA, Sasaki CT: Pathology of tumors of the cranial base, *Clin Plast Surg* 22:407-416, 1995.

CAUSE	CLINICAL PRESENTATION	NATURAL HISTORY	TREATMENT	OUTCOME
Unknown	Biologic behavior related to size and location	Cribriform plate, oropharynx more likely to metastasize	Surgical resection, pre-operative embolization	
Unknown	Nasal obstruction, epistaxis, anosmia, epiphora, proptosis, diplopia	Growth through cribriform plate; neck node metastases	Surgery, radiation, chemotherapy	Younger patients have low rate of recurrence but high metastasis and worse outcome
	Painful, functional nerve deficit		Surgical resection	Recurrence 50-80%, increases with von Recklinghausen's disease
Unknown, associated with radiation therapy	Nasal stuffiness, discharge, epistaxis, diplopia	Clinically like chordoma	Surgical resection	50-60% 5-year survival
Unknown	Swelling, nasal stuffiness, obstruction, epistaxis, pain	Mass	Surgical resection, radiation, chemotherapy	60% 5-year survival
			Depends on tumor type	

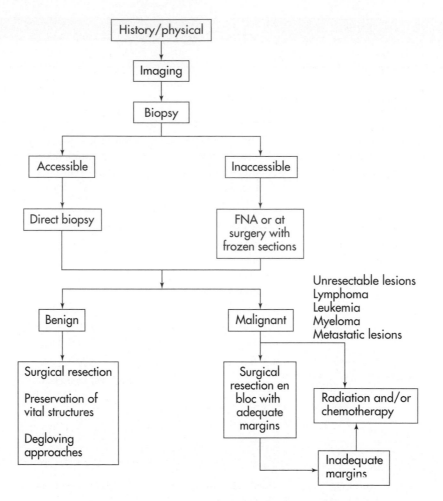

Figure 91-1. Treatment plan for skull base surgery.

For accessible tumors, a direct biopsy is desirable before the final treatment plan is determined. For inaccessible lesions, fine-needle aspiration, which may be CT-guided, is sometimes possible. If not, the surgical plan for resection is undertaken. Prior to full exposure or sacrifice of any critical structures, a biopsy with frozen section is taken. If there is any doubt about the diagnosis or the appropriateness of full surgical resection, the procedure is staged.

Although the vast majority of cranial base tumors require surgical resection as the primary means of treatment, some are inoperable. Certain tissue types lend themselves more to treatment with radiation and/or chemotherapy. Examples of these types of tumors include lymphoma, leukemia, myeloma, rhabdomyosarcoma, and some metastases (Figure 91-1).

INFORMED CONSENT

The patient with a skull base tumor usually comes with significant fear and anxiety. Although great assurance and confidence can be given because of the success of new techniques and technology, the potential for devastating morbidity and mortality remains, including the risk of anesthesia, bleeding, infection, failure of adequate wound healing, and cerebrospinal fluid (CSF) leak. Depending on tumor location and the approach utilized for resection, problems may include neurologic deficits, which can be life-threatening or can result in lifelong functional deficits. Systemic complications may also occur, based on the patient's associated preexisting medical condition.

Other potential complications include those associated with orbital adnexa, such as altered blink dynamics, epiphora due to nasal and lacrimal duct obstruction, and enophthalmos. Midface complications include malocclusion, palatal fistula, nasal airway obstruction, and abnormal speech. Maxillofacial prosthetics, which may play a role in patient reconstruction and rehabilitation, have their own inherent complications. Hardware complications can occur, necessitating removal of plates and screws. Radiation and previous surgery increase the risk of wound-healing problems, and therefore increase the risk of CSF leak and infection. Recurrence of tumor may necessitate the need for secondary surgery or the addition of radiation or chemotherapy.

Tissues of the face that are traversed by transfacial approaches, and thus potentially adversely affected, include the skin; facial muscles and bones; the dentition; paranasal sinuses; the nasal cavity; the soft and hard palates; tongue; eustachian tubes and superior pharyngeal constrictor muscles; nerves that provide sensation and animation of the face; speaking, chewing, and swallowing mechanisms; and the ocular and adnexal tissues that are responsible for tear production and drainage, blink dynamics, and ocular movement. The carotid and vertebral arteries are also potentially at risk.[34]

OPERATIONS

GENERAL PRINCIPLES

Modular disassembly of functional aesthetic units of the face has become an accepted approach for accessing pathways to skull base regions. The principles of disassembly are part of Tessier's contribution to the development of craniofacial surgery. He demonstrated that intracranial and extracranial approaches can be combined without undue risk of infection, that orbits can be osteotomized, that the globes can be moved without causing blindness, and that the facial bones can be stripped of periosteum, osteotomized, repositioned, and still survive.[81] Applications of these principles for exposure to resection of skull base tumors began in the 1970s and have evolved to accepted but complex facial disassembly techniques. The concept of wide exposure, despite its seeming more radical, has been a major advance. It allows better visualization of tumors and critical structures, and diminishes the need for prolonged retraction on the brain. In referring to brain surgery, Nofziger[56] stated, "The surgical treatment of the lesion itself often involved less time and effort than exposure of it and closure of the wound." This quotation accurately depicts the situation of skull base surgery today. Although the tendency may be to displace the minimum amount of tissue possible for access to the tumor, the wider exposure permitted by a more radical approach actually adds safety to the procedure. Complete removal of the tumor and visualization of vital structures are enhanced with a wider exposure, although it may be more time consuming and require more effort than removing the tumor itself.

Noting the advantages of transfacial approaches, Janecka[34] states:

"(1) Facial anatomy is developed through the embryonic fusion of nasal, frontal, maxillary, and mandibular processes. Normally, the fusion takes place in the midline or in the paramedian region, thus, logically presenting optimal lines of separation of facial units for a surgical approach, permitting the least traumatic displacement.

(2) The primary blood supply to the 'facial units' is through the external carotid system, which also has a lateral-to-medial direction of flow, thus ensuring viability of displaced surgical units.

(3) The midface includes multiple 'hollow' anatomic spaces (oronasal cavity, nasopharynx, paranasal sinuses) that facilitate the relative ease of surgical access to the central skull base.

Box 91-1.
Skull Base Approaches

ANTERIOR
Intracranial
Transfrontal (Level I)
Transfrontal nasal (Level II)
Transfrontal nasal-orbital (Level III)

Extracranial
Transnasomaxillary (Level IV)
Transmaxillary (Level V)
Transpalatal (Level VI)

Combined
ANTEROLATERAL
Minifacial Translocation
Medial
Lateral

Standard Facial Translocation
Expanded Facial Translocation
Medial and inferior extended
Posterior extended
Bilateral

Data from Beals SP, Joganic EF, Holcombe TC, Spetzler RF: Secondary craniofacial problems following skull base surgery, *Clin Plast Surg* 24(3):565-581, 1997; and Janeka IP. Facial translocation approach. In Janecka IP, Tiedeman K, editors: *Skull base surgery, anatomy, biology, technology*, Philadelphia, 1997, Lippincott-Raven.

---

(4) The displacement of facial units approach to the central cranial base offers much greater tolerance to postoperative surgical swelling, as opposed to similar displacement of the content of the neurocranium.

(5) The reestablishment of the normal anatomy, following repositioning of the facial units during the reconstructive phase of surgery involves considerable functional as well as aesthetic achievement."

However, transfacial approaches also have certain disadvantages; these include:

"(1) Contamination of the surgical wound with oropharyngeal bacterial flora.

(2) The need for facial incisions and subsequent scar development.

(3) Emotional considerations for the patient related to 'surgical facial disassembly.'

(4) The potential need for supplementary airway management (postoperative endotracheal intubation, temporary tracheostomy)."[34]

Selecting the best approach can seem difficult because of the large number of choices available (Box 91-1). The major factor determining the approach is the anatomic site of the lesion and its extension. A secondary factor is the histologic type of the tumor. Benign tumors, which primarily displace normal tissue, can be removed through a more limited approach and still achieve gross total removal and protection of vital structures.

Malignant tumors require an adequate margin of excision for hope of cure, and thus require a radical approach. Benign tumors are more amenable to degloving types of procedures. Malignant tumors more often require facial incisions to achieve adequate exposure and resection, especially those with an extracranial and a more lateral origin or extension. Complete excision of malignant tumors with a primary intracranial component and/or in the midline position can be selectively and adequately accomplished with degloving procedures.

PREOPERATIVE PREPARATION

Thorough preoperative preparation of the patient for cranial base tumor resection through a transfacial approach is essential to minimize risk and achieve curative resection of the tumor. Presentation of the patient's case to the skull base team ensures a coordinated and comprehensive treatment plan that all responsible surgeons have agreed on. The surgical approach is decided on at that time, directing the remaining preoperative workup, including patient positioning, preparation for reconstruction, and incisions.

All patients should have clinical photographs. Patients requiring interruption of the dental arch for exposure require cephalometric x-rays, dental models, and splint fabrication. Those patients requiring resection of a portion of the dental arch need a temporary prosthesis. Routine labs and type and cross for 4 to 6 units of blood are prepared. Cryoprecipitate is also requested in anticipation of use in fibrin glue. The patient has a CT scan or MRI on the way to the operating room for ISG wand referencing.

In the operating room, hypotensive anesthesia is planned. Monitoring and venous access lines are placed. The patient is orally intubated or a temporary tracheostomy is performed. When oral intubation is used, a reinforced tube is utilized and is secured to the lower dentition with 26-gauge stainless steel wire.

Prophylactic antibiotics are given in meningicidal doses. Somatosensory evoke potential monitoring is utilized. A lumbar drain is sometimes placed preoperatively at the discretion of the neurosurgeon. The patient's head is positioned in pins to maintain stability for use of the ISG localizing wand and the operating microscope. The corneas are protected with temporary tarsorrhaphy sutures. Prepping and draping of the entire head, face, and upper neck are performed to allow the widest possible exposure of the craniofacial skeleton. Additional sites are prepped at this time as anticipated need for reconstructive tissues.[8]

ANTERIOR SURGICAL APPROACHES

The central and paracentral skull base and anterior cranial fossa can be approached through anterior transfacial approaches (Figure 91-2). These approaches have evolved over the past 20

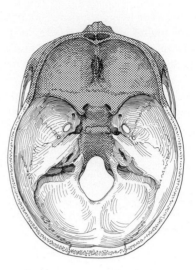

Figure 91-2. Region of tumor sites in the anterior skull base and clivus that can be exposed by direct anterior transfacial routes. (Courtesy Barrow Neurological Institute, Phoenix.)

years, with contributions from many surgeons.* The following represents a compilation of these approaches and a system for their use in approaching this region at different levels (Table 91-2).

Direct anterior approaches to the midline skull base and anterior cranial fossa have advantages over lateral and anterolateral approaches:

(1) Access is through the relatively avascular midline plane.

(2) Vital neurovascular structures, the temporomandibular joint, and muscles of mastication are avoided.

(3) Facial incisions are infrequently needed because of the wide exposure possible by degloving.

The configuration of the skull base, which is approximately perpendicular to the vertical plane of the face, dictates that tumors that have anterior extension be approached from a more superior approach, while posteriorly located tumors with a more superior extension be addressed through an inferior approach.

Anterior transfacial approaches can be divided into six levels to aid the decision-making process (Figure 91-3 and Table 91-3).[5-8] The superior three approaches (transfrontal, transfrontal nasal, transfrontal orbital) are intracranial and build from the supraorbital bar concept (Figure 91-4). Subfrontal access as achieved by removal of the supraorbital bar is extended vertically to include the entire midline skull base inferiorly to the craniocervical junction by removing the nasal complex and medial orbital walls on the supraorbital bar. Horizontal exposure is increased by adding the lateral orbital walls and orbital roofs to the frontonasal segment. Exposure can be increased further in the transnasal and transorbital approaches with a circumferential cribriform plate osteotomy, which allows retraction of the cribriform plate while leaving the dura intact. This approach is possible when the cribriform

---

*References 1, 3, 10, 12-19, 23, 24, 29-31, 33, 36, 39-42, 44, 45, 47-49, 51, 52, 58, 59, 61, 62, 65, 67, 70, 72, 73, 76, 78-80, 83, 85-87.

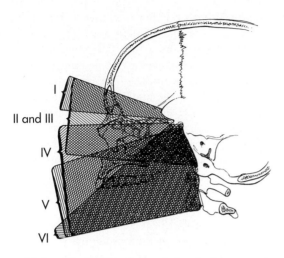

Figure 91-3. Summation of the six levels demonstrating that the anatomic site of the tumor and direction of growth determine the level of transfacial exposure. (Courtesy Barrow Neurological Institute, Phoenix.)

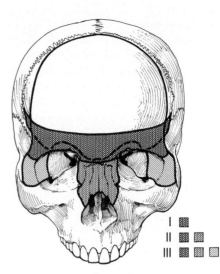

Figure 91-4. The three intracranial approaches are variations of the supraorbital bar. (Courtesy Barrow Neurological Institute, Phoenix.)

Table 91-2.
Facial Translocation Approaches

LEVEL	APPROACH	ANATOMIC SITE OF LESION	FIGURE
I	Transfrontal	Anterior cranial fossa	91-6
II	Transfrontal nasal	Anterior cranial fossa, nasopharynx, clivus tumors with anterior growth	91-7
III	Transfrontal nasal-orbital	Larger anterior cranial fossa or nasopharyngeal lesion, clivus tumors with anterior growth	91-8, 91-17
IV	Transnasomaxillary	Nasopharyngeal lesions, large clivus lesions that extend anteriorly, posteriorly, or inferiorly	91-14
V	Transmaxillary	Clivus lesions with superior and inferior extensions, small nasopharyngeal lesions	91-15, 91-17
VI	Transpalatal	Lower clivus region lesions	91-16

For additional information see Beals SP, Hamilton MG, Joganic EF, et al: Classification of transfacial approaches in the treatment of tumors of the anterior skull base and clivus, *Plast Surg Forum* XVI:211-213, 1993; Beals SP, Joganic EF: Transfacial exposure of anterior cranial fossa and clival tumors, *BNI Quarterly* 8(4):2, 1992; Beals SP, Joganic EF, Hamilton MG, et al: Classification of transfacial approaches in the treatment of tumors of the anterior skull base and clivus. In Monasterio FM, editor: *Craniofacial surgery*, ed 5, Bologna, Italy, 1994, Monduzzi Editors; and Beals SP, Joganic EF, Hamilton MG, et al: Posterior skull base transfacial approaches, *Clin Plast Surg* 22:491-511, 1995.

plate is not invaded by tumor and its resection is not required to achieve adequate margins. Preservation of the dura also has the advantage of diminishing the risk of CSF leak, simplifying skull base reconstruction, and saving olfaction, in most cases.[22,75]

The inferior three approaches (transnasomaxillary, transmaxillary, and transpalatal) are extracranial and provide varying degrees of exposure to the midline skull base when an intracranial approach is not needed (Figure 91-5). The transnasomaxillary approach provides exposure of the entire midline skull base but requires a facial incision. The transmaxillary approach accesses the lower half of the midline skull base, as well as the retromaxillary area, and the transpalatal approach provides access to the lower third of the skull base and the craniovertebral junction region. Overlapping exposure can be provided by these six levels of transfacial exposure, providing flexibility and choice to deal with a variety of anatomic sites of tumors. Each level can be used in isolation or in combination with another level or an intracranial or lateral approach for single- or multiple-stage tumor resection.

Intracranial Approaches

The position of the bicoronal incision in the midaspect of the calvarium or posterior to this is essential to preserve adequate length of pericranial and frontogaleal flaps for potential use for skull base reconstruction following tumor resection.

Reflection of the anterior scalp flap is performed by micro-needle dissection,[21] since it is more hemostatic and preserves the important pericranial and temporalis tissues for possible

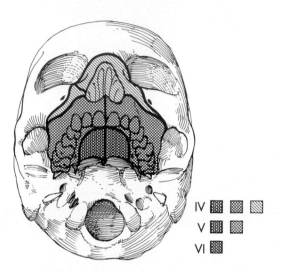

Figure 91-5. The extracranial approaches provide increasing exposure as more of the maxilla is added. (Courtesy Barrow Neurological Institute, Phoenix.)

use as flaps (Figure 91-6). The scalp flap is reflected to the superior orbital rims on either side, then inferiorly into the temporalis region beneath the intermediate temporalis fascia to avoid the frontalis innervation. The pericranial flap can either be raised anteriorly, based on its axial blood supply, or laterally, based on the temporalis muscle. The pericranium is scored against the calvarium at the midline or asymmetrically if it is anticipated that a laterally based pericranial flap of greater length is needed from one side. The entire pericranium can be carried from one temporalis muscle if needed. Even if the pericranial flap is not needed for skull base reconstruction, its attachment to the temporalis muscles is useful in reattaching the temporalis muscles in their anatomic position in the temporal fossa.

For Levels II and III (Figures 91-7 and 91-8), the pericranium and temporalis muscles are reflected, the periorbita and the periosteum in the region of the nasal process of the maxilla are stripped, taking great care to preserve the nasolacrimal ducts. The medial canthal ligaments are detached. The upper lateral cartilages are taken down from their attachment on the inferior side of the caudal margin of the nasal bones. Nasal mucosa is dissected from the underside of the nasal bones.

The bifrontal craniotomy is then performed and dura retracted from the anterior cranial fossa. If preservation of the cribriform plate is anticipated, the posterior margin of the bifrontal craniotomy must be at the level of the coronal suture and must extend laterally and inferiorly to the skull base in the temporal region. This placement is necessary to allow

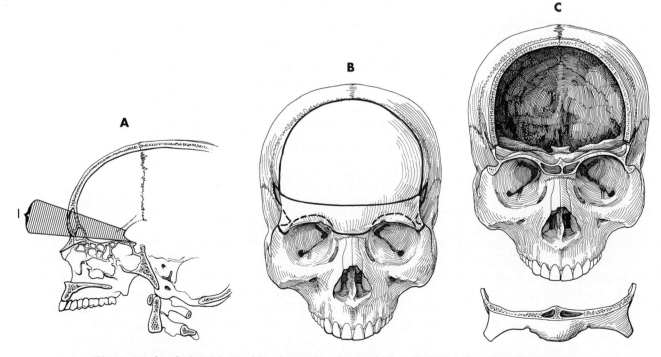

Figure 91-6. **A,** Level I transfrontal exposure for anterior cranial fossa. **B** and **C,** The Level I exposure requires removal of the supraorbital bar. (**A** to **C** courtesy Barrow Neurological Institute, Phoenix.)

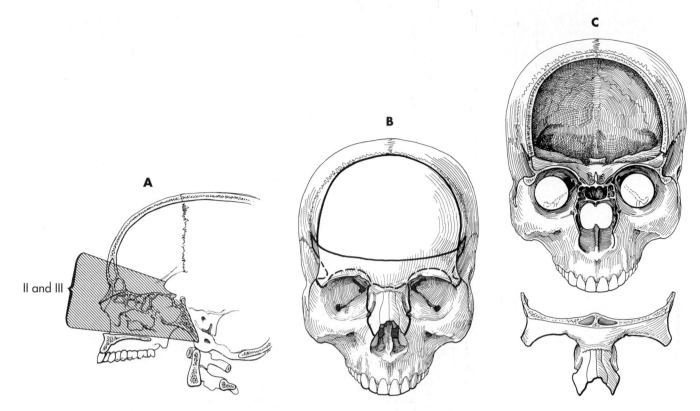

Figure 91-7. **A,** Level II transfrontal nasal exposure for anterior approach to the anterior cranial fossa and clivus. **B** and **C,** The Level II exposure requires removal of the frontonasal fragment. (**A** to **C** courtesy Barrow Neurological Institute, Phoenix.)

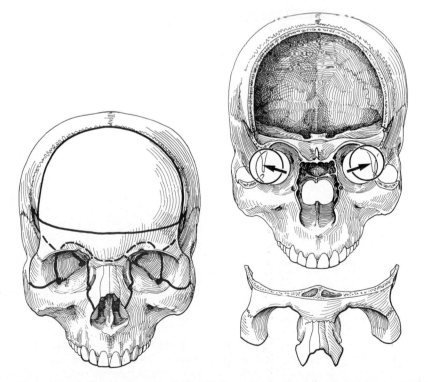

Figure 91-8. Level III transfrontal nasal-orbital exposure for larger anterior cranial fossa, nasopharyngeal, and clival lesions. This approach is similar to Level II (see Figure 91-7, *A* and *B*), except that it provides for a wider exposure by allowing lateral retraction of the globes. The Level III exposure requires inclusion of the lateral orbital walls on the frontonasal fragment (frontonasal-orbital unit). (Courtesy Barrow Neurological Institute, Phoenix.)

perpendicular access of the reciprocating saw to the planum sphenoidale.

When the dissection is complete, the osteotomy lines are marked (see Figures 91-7, *B,* and 91-8, *A*). Inclusion of the majority of superior orbital roof on the fragment facilitates retraction of the globes and increases the ease of performing the cribriform plate osteotomy (Figure 91-9). The osteotomies are then performed in the same order on both sides, with great care taken to preserve the periorbita, optic nerve, and dura, as well as the nasolacrimal duct and nasal mucosa. After the osteotomies are completed with a reciprocating saw, an

osteotome is used, positioned anteriorly and inferiorly through the crista galli osteotomy site to separate the bony septum. The fragment can now be mobilized and then removed and set aside (Figures 91-6, *C,* 91-7, *C,* and 91-8, *B*).

Preservation of the cribriform plate is possible with a circumferential osteotomy (see Figure 91-9). Parasagittal and anterior cuts have already been made in the process of removing the frontonasal-orbital fragment. After the posterior osteotomy is performed, an inferior cut is made, preserving a 1 cm cuff of nasal mucosa and septum. The cribriform plate is thus freed and can be elevated with the dura.[8,75]

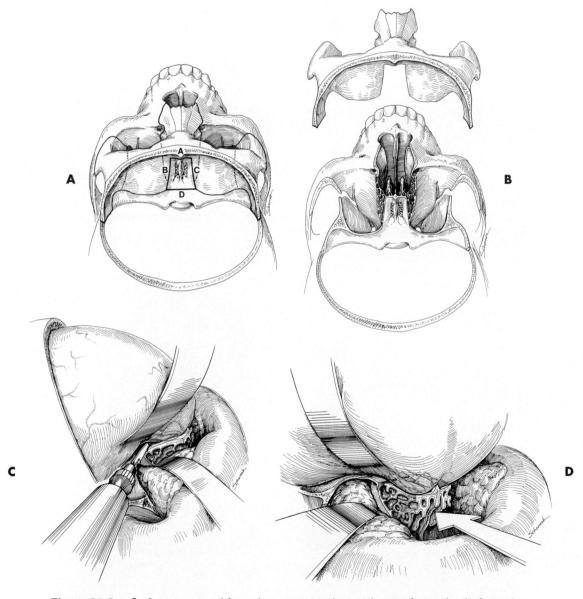

Figure 91-9. A, Anterior cranial fossa demonstrating the initial circumferential cribriform plate osteotomies. *A,* Anterior osteotomy; *B* and *C,* parasagittal osteotomy; *D,* posterior osteotomy through the planum sphenoidale. The additional lines indicate osteotomy cuts for removal of the frontonasal-orbital unit. **B,** All osteotomy cuts except for "D" are performed to allow removal of the frontonasal-orbital unit. **C,** The final osteotomy cut ("D", planum sphenoidale) is performed with appropriate retraction of the frontal lobe dura and paranasal soft tissues. **D,** After dividing the trabeculae and leaving a generous cuff of mucosa intact, the intact cribriform plate unit is released from the skull base. (**A** to **D** courtesy Barrow Neurological Institute, Phoenix.)

Superior ethmoid sinus mucosa, as well as posterior septum, can be resected in order to achieve complete access to the region of the tumor. The advantage of the Level III approach is that, in removing the lateral orbital walls, the globes can be retracted laterally to achieve more central interorbital access to the tumor. If the tumor size does not require this degree of exposure, the lateral orbital walls can be left intact, removing only the nasal-medial orbital wall complex with the supraorbital bar (Level II approach, see Figure 91-7). If the tumor is more localized to the anterior cranial fossa, the supraorbital bar alone can be removed (Level I approach, see Figure 91-6).

If the tumor has invaded the interorbital space, usually a bilateral approach is desired to achieve the ideal exposure for ease of resection. In some situations in which the tumor is smaller or oriented more to the medial orbital region, a unilateral approach may be adequate. Resection of soft tissue and nasal orbital skeletal tissues depends on the involvement

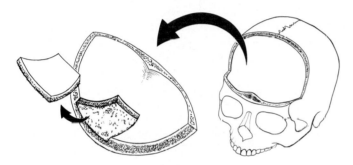

Figure 91-10. Cranial bone grafts are harvested from the frontal bone for orbital and skull base reconstruction. (Courtesy Barrow Neurological Institute, Phoenix.)

of the tumor. This approach is flexible and needs to be individualized according to the anatomic site of the tumor and its extension, as well as to the surgeon's preference.

After tumor resection, reconstruction is addressed. If needed, the skull base and orbital walls are reconstructed with split cranial grafts. Grafts can usually be harvested from the inner table of the bifrontal bone flap (Figure 91-10). Interosseous light gauge wire fixation is appropriate for this region.

Sealing of the extracranial and intracranial interface is important. Depending on the location and size of the defect, regional flaps such as pericranial or temporalis muscle can be used and should be inset and sutured in place after replacement of the frontonasal-orbital unit (Figure 91-11). If the cribriform plate has been sacrificed, it is ideal to place a flap on the nasal and intracranial side of the bone graft, but this is not always possible. If the Level I approach is used, a pericranial flap either laterally or anteriorly based is placed on the skull defect, traversing either above or below the supraorbital bar (Figure 91-12). In the Level II and III approaches, access beneath the fragment is not possible. The flap must access the defect between the bifrontal bone flap and frontonasal-orbital fragment. If the cribriform plate is preserved, a single flap is used to cover the osteotomy defect. Either an anteriorly based or laterally based flap can be used. Either must be split to cover all sides of the cribriform plate osteotomy, or alternatively, a slit can be made for it to drop through (Figures 91-11 and 91-13).[9,53,69,77]

When this fragment is replaced, it is rigidly fixed except at the osteotomy through the nasal process of the maxilla, where interosseous light gauge wire fixation is utilized. Great effort is taken to place small plates in concealed areas so that they will not ever be visible or palpable (Figures 91-11, C, 91-12, C, and 91-13, C).

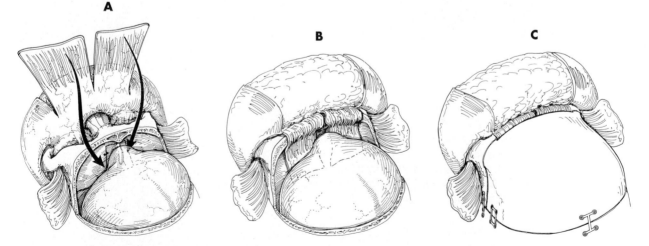

Figure 91-11. The frontogaleal flap can be split (**A**) to cover the cribriform plate osteotomy (**B**). The flap courses over the frontonasal-orbital fragment (**C**). (**A** to **C** courtesy Barrow Neurological Institute, Phoenix.)

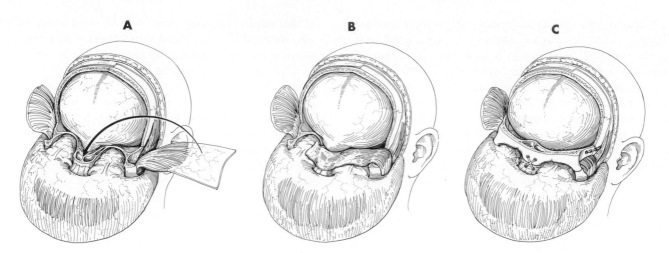

Figure 91-12. **A** and **B,** Laterally-based pericranial flaps can be used to cover either the extracranial or intracranial side of the skull base defect. **C,** It can course over or under the supraorbital fragment. (**A** to **C** courtesy Barrow Neurological Institute, Phoenix.)

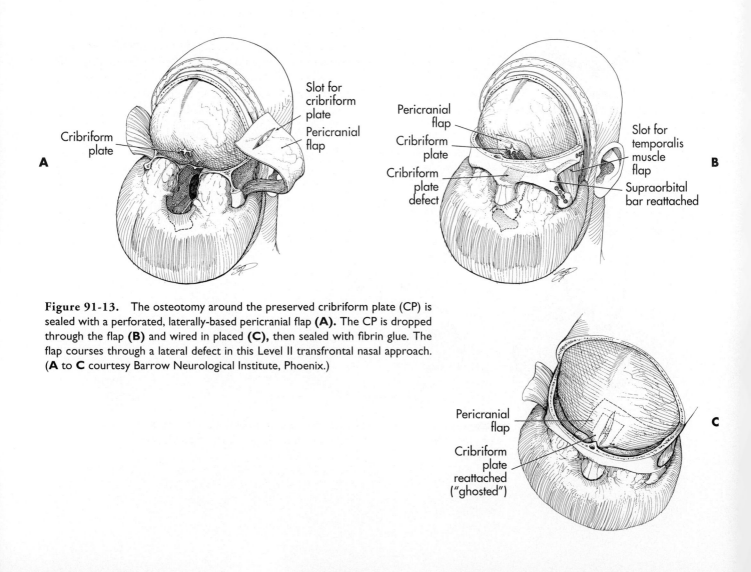

Figure 91-13. The osteotomy around the preserved cribriform plate (CP) is sealed with a perforated, laterally-based pericranial flap **(A).** The CP is dropped through the flap **(B)** and wired in placed **(C),** then sealed with fibrin glue. The flap courses through a lateral defect in this Level II transfrontal nasal approach. (**A** to **C** courtesy Barrow Neurological Institute, Phoenix.)

Fibrin glue can be used to seal the flap margins in an effort to obtain a watertight closure. The upper lateral cartilage must be reattached to the caudal margins of the nasal bones in order to prevent a saddle-nose deformity. This is accomplished by drilling holes in the bony margin and suturing the cartilages to the bone with nonabsorbable suture.

The medial canthal ligament is repaired by transnasal wiring. Prior to replacing the frontal bone in adults, the frontal sinuses are obliterated. The frontal bone can be reattached with plates or wires. The unused temporalis muscle or pericranial flaps are reattached in their anatomic position with direct sutures to drill holes in the bone along the superolateral orbital rim. After generous irrigation of the region with 0.5% peroxide and 0.25% Betadine, followed by bacitracin solution, the scalp is closed with galeal and skin sutures.

Extracranial Approaches

TRANSNASOMAXILLARY APPROACH (Level IV, Figure 91-14). The nasomaxillary region is exposed through a right modified Weber-Fergusson incision with extension across the glabella and opposite subciliary margin (Figure 91-14, *B*). A bilateral buccal sulcus incision is also made. The periosteum

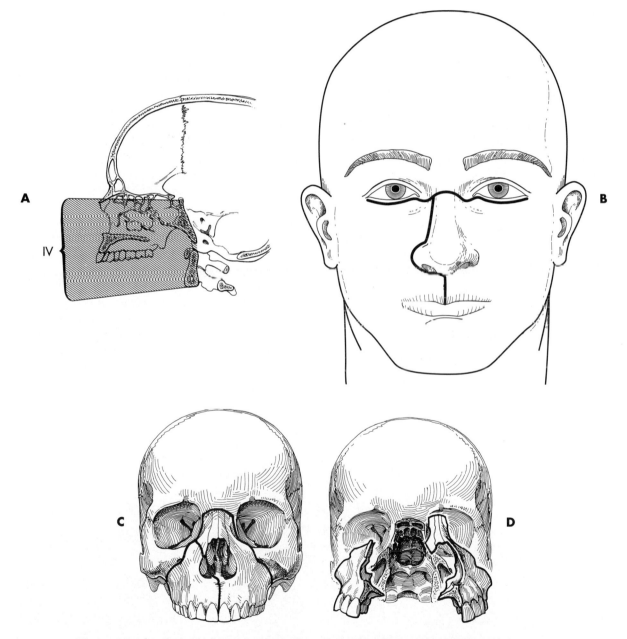

Figure 91-14. **A,** Level IV transnasomaxillary approach yields a wide exposure of the entire central skull base from the radix to the cranial cervical junction. A similar degree of exposure can usually be obtained with a combination of the Level III and Level V exposures. **B,** Incisions for the transnasomaxillary approach. **C** and **D,** The Level V exposure requires a LeFort II osteotomy, then splitting of the maxillary fragment. (**A** to **D** courtesy Barrow Neurological Institute, Phoenix.)

is stripped in preparation for a LeFort II osteotomy. The piriform aperture and orbital and nasal floor are exposed. The nasolacrimal duct and infraorbital nerves are isolated.

Osteotomy lines are marked for a LeFort II osteotomy (Figure 91-14, *C*). Plates are then adapted for a perfect passive fit at the zygomatic buttress, inferior orbital rims, and radix. Also, a plate adapted to the anterior nasal floor adds stability after the palatal split. A screw is placed on each side of the osteotomy, and the remaining holes are drilled. The plates are then removed, labeled, and set aside.

The LeFort II osteotomy is performed and the fragment mobilized (Figure 91-14, *D*). The fragment is split at the nasal process of the maxilla on the right and the midline of the hard and soft palates. The lesser (right) fragment and the greater (left) fragment containing the nose can then be retracted as needed to gain exposure for tumor resection. If the exposure is limited by tethering of the nasolacrimal ducts, one or both can be divided, then repaired over tubes after tumor resection. If more lateral exposure is needed, the pterygoid plates can be outfractured, resected, or retained on the maxillary fragment. The mirror image approach can be chosen if it gives a better angle of approach to the tumor.

After tumor resection, the skull base defect may require reconstruction with a fat graft or bone graft prior to mucosal closure.

The occlusal splint is used to reorient the fragments. The preregistered plates are applied. The soft palate and oral mucosa are repaired. The facial incisions are closed. If desired, the orotracheal tube can be transferred to the nose before reassembly by removing the coupler and passing the tubes retrograde through the nostril on one side. The splint is used for 10 to 14 days. A liquid diet is recommended for 4 weeks.

TRANSMAXILLARY APPROACH (Level V, Figure 91-15). An upper buccal sulcus incision is made, leaving a generous cuff of muscular mucosa on the gingival side, and the anterior maxilla is stripped. This is continued posterior to the pterygomaxillary suture line, anteriorly to the inferior orbital rims, carefully preserving the infraorbital nerve, and along the piriform aperture. The mucosa from the piriform aperture and lateral nasal walls as well as nasal floor is stripped, and the anterior nasal spine region is exposed.

When the dissection of the anterior maxilla is complete, the LeFort I osteotomy level is determined (see Figure 91-15, *B*). In children this should be high, essentially at the level of the inferior margin of the infraorbital foramen, and in adults above the nasal floor and parallel to the occlusal plane. Plates are then adapted for perfect passive fit on each side. A screw is placed on each side of the LeFort I osteotomy site and the remaining holes are drilled. The plates are removed and labeled.

A LeFort I osteotomy is then performed with a reciprocating saw. The lateral nasal wall and septum are osteotomized with guarded osteotomes, and the pterygomaxillary fissure is separated with a curved osteotome. The LeFort I fragment is then down-fractured with finger pressure and mobilized with disimpaction forceps. Depending on the tumor location, the tumor may be visible at this point, and the degree of exposure needed for removal of the tumor is reevaluated. Smaller tumors may not require any further maxillary osteotomy to provide adequate exposure for complete resection.

If more exposure is needed, the palate can be split at the midline and the two fragments retracted laterally (see Figure 91-15, *C*). Depending on tumor location, the vomer and quadrilateral cartilage, as well as inferior turbinates, may require partial resection to yield the desired exposure. If with maximum fragment retraction adequate lateral exposure is not achieved, one or both pterygoid plates can be resected. Some tumors will require maxillectomy to achieve cure.

After tumor resection, the defect is evaluated for reconstruction; in the case of sella turcica, sphenoidal, or clival midline defects, a dermal fat graft or bone graft may be required prior to mucosal closure.

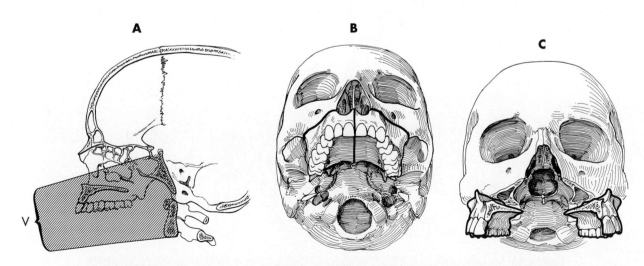

A

B

C

Figure 91-15. A, Level V transmaxillary exposure provides exposure of the clivus and nasopharyngeal area. **B** and **C,** The Level V exposure requires a LeFort I osteotomy and splitting of the palate for further exposure. (**A** to **C** courtesy Barrow Neurological Institute, Phoenix.)

When tumor resection and reconstruction are completed, the palatal fragments are returned to their anatomic position with the help of an occlusal splint. The fragments are snapped into the splint, and the preregistered plates are retrieved and placed, first across the nasal floor. Perfect anatomic reposition of the fragments should have been achieved. Secure muscular mucosal realignment and closure of the soft palate are critical and can be done either before or after the maxillary repositioning, depending on the surgeon's preference. No nasal pack is required.

The splint should be left intact for 10 to 14 days. It can be left out for the first 3 days if there is concern about palatal mucosal swelling against the crosspiece. Routine oral care for LeFort I osteotomy is used, and the patient is kept on a liquid diet for 4 weeks, transitioned to a soft diet for 4 weeks, and then returned to a regular diet 8 weeks postoperatively.

TRANSPALATAL APPROACH (Level VI, Figure 91-16).

An upper buccal sulcus incision is made and the nasal floor is exposed. A midline palatal mucosal incision is made, also splitting the soft palate. The mucosa may be back-cut anteriorly along the junction of the rough and smooth periosteum, allowing wide mobilization of the entire hard palate on the oral side. The levator muscle is taken down from the posterior margins of the hard palate. The osteotomy can skirt just medial to the greater palatine arteries or the arteries can be sacrificed and the osteotomy taken laterally (see Figure 91-16, B).

The hard palate is cut with a reciprocating saw, skirting along the alveolar bone. The remaining attachments to the septum and lateral nasal walls are separated with guarded osteotomes, and the hard palate is removed. Exposure to the clivus is created through the nasal mucosa (see Figure 91-16, C).

After tumor resection, the skull base defect may require reconstruction with a fat or bone graft. The hard palate is

sometimes thick enough to split, yielding a suitable bone graft for clival reconstruction.

Small two- or three-hole plates in three locations are applied to the hard palatal fragment before anatomic repositioning. The palatal mucosa and soft palate are closed and the buccal sulcus incision is closed.

Combined Surgical Approaches

Any of the intracranial approaches can be combined with the transmaxillary or transpalatal approaches if the anatomic site of the tumor dictates. The Level III (transfrontal nasal-orbital) and Level V (transmaxillary) approaches provide wide exposure of the anterior cranial fossa and midline skull base and are usually preferred over the Level IV (transnaso-maxillary) approach because a facial incision is avoided (Figure 91-17).

When combined intracranial and extracranial exposures are used, the intracranial approach is performed first. The tumor is removed from the region of the vital skull base structure and dural integrity is established. The extracranial approach is then performed to remove the remaining portion of the tumor. Skull base and orbital reconstruction and fragment reassembly are then addressed.

Orbital Reconstruction

Orbital reconstruction, and that of adjacent skeletal units, may be required if extensive resection is needed to remove the tumor. Cranial bone grafts are preferred, and can be obtained from the frontalis flap if a craniotomy has been performed. If not, a parietal craniotomy can be performed to harvest bone for orbital reconstruction. Split-rib grafts also have advantages for orbital reconstruction in that they can be bent into the circular configuration of the orbit. When orbital exenteration is required, the temporalis muscle flap must be transposed into the orbit to facilitate socket reconstruction for a prosthesis.

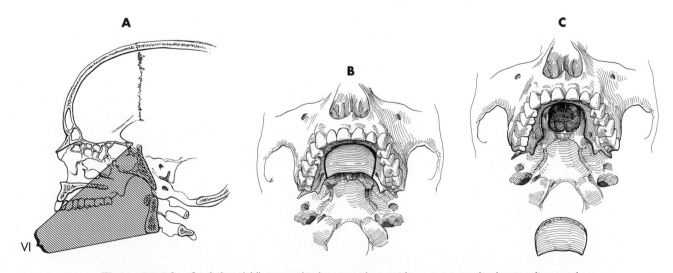

Figure 91-16. A, A Level VI transpalatal approach provides access to the lower clivus and upper cervical region. **B** and **C,** The Level VI exposure requires removal of the hard palate. (**A** to **C** courtesy Barrow Neurological Institute, Phoenix.)

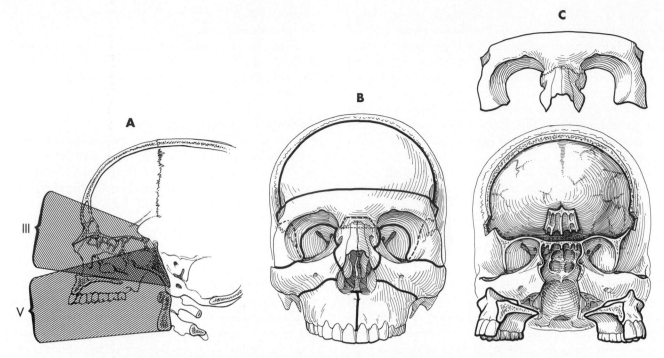

Figure 91-17. **A,** Combination of the Level III and V approaches provides wide exposure of the anterior skull base and clivus. **B** and **C,** The combination of the two approaches is illustrated with preservation of the cribriform plate. (**A** to **C** courtesy Barrow Neurological Institute, Phoenix.)

Patient Examples

(1) A 16-year-old young man presented with nasal obstruction and nosebleeds. A subsequent work-up revealed the presence of a large angiofibroma that filled the midline interorbital space, and coursed posteriorly and inferiorly through the soft palate level in the midline. A transfrontal nasal-orbital approach was utilized and complete tumor resection was accomplished. A circumferential cribriform plate osteotomy was utilized. Five years postoperatively, the patient has had no evidence of recurrence, and has had no complications from the exposure (Figure 91-18). Olfaction was preserved.

(2) A 16-year-old young man presented with nasal obstruction and severe life-threatening hemorrhage from the nose. Work-up revealed the presence of a very large angiofibroma that coursed from the nasopharynx into the midline of the skull base region anteriorly, filling the interorbital region and coursing inferiorly into the retromaxillary region on the right. Symptoms also included loss of olfaction. The patient underwent a combined transfrontal nasal-orbital (Level III) and transmaxillary (Level V) approach (Figure 91-19), and complete resection of the tumor was possible. Reassembly restored facial and occlusal integrity. Additionally, the circumferential cribriform plate osteotomy was utilized and the patient experienced return of olfaction within 2 weeks following surgery. Four years postoperatively, the patient is free of recurrent tumor. Cannulation of the nasolacrimal duct on the right side was required because of persistent epiphora.

ANTEROLATERAL APPROACHES

The anterolateral approaches to the skull base have been developed and championed by Janecka.[32-34,36,37] The facial translocation approach is based on creation of composite facial units, which are designed along key neurovascular anatomy and aesthetic lines. The individual units are additive as greater exposure is required (Table 91-3).[34]

Minifacial Translocation

MEDIAL MINIFACIAL TRANSLOCATION. The medial minifacial translocation approach is indicated for lesions of the medial orbit, sphenoid, ethmoid sinus, and inferior clivus. A skin incision is made along the lateral aspect of the nose with a triangular design as it courses over the medial canthal ligament and then onto the inferior aspect of the eyebrow. Exposure is then accomplished with an osteotomy of the ipsilateral nasal bone and nasal process of the maxilla, leaving the medial canthal ligament, lacrimal duct, and skin attached. A rectangular opening is created, the lateral margin being just medial to the inferior orbital nerve. Repair is accomplished with rigid fixation (Figure 91-20).

LATERAL MINIFACIAL TRANSLOCATION. The lateral minifacial translocation is indicated for lesions of the infratemporal fossa. This is exposed through an excision that courses from the medial canthus horizontally to the preauricular area and then vertically along the preauricular line anterior to the ear. An osteotomy of the zygomatic arch and malar eminence is

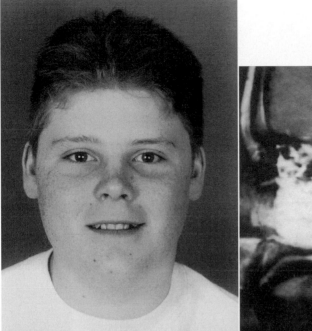

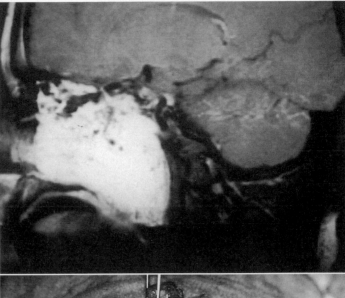

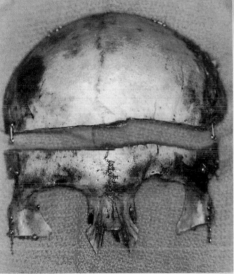

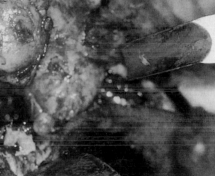

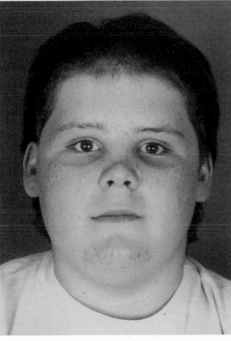

Figure 91-18. A 16-year-old young man **(A)** with angiofibroma **(B)** had Level III exposure for resection **(C** and **D)**. Three months postoperative **(E)**. **(A** to **E** courtesy Barrow Neurological Institute, Phoenix.)

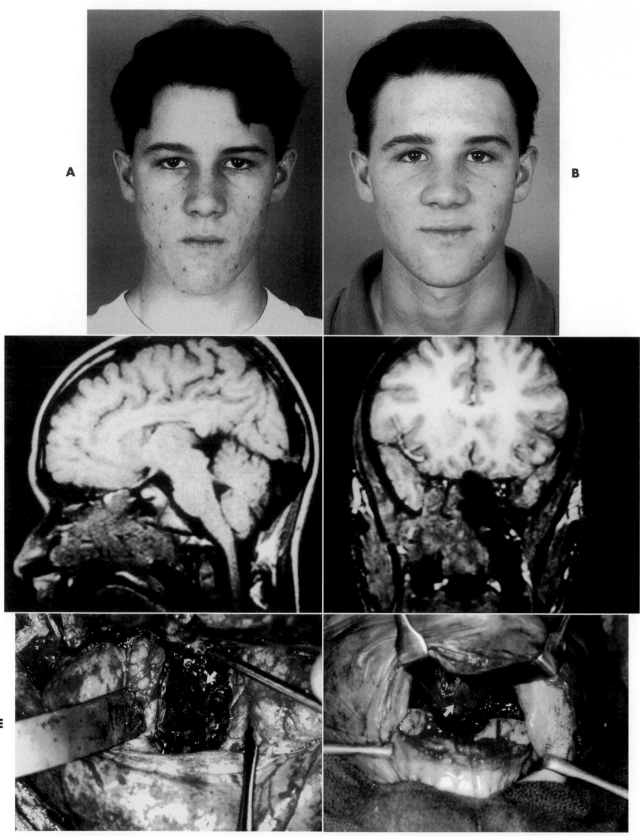

Figure 91-19. **A,** A 16-year-old young man with angiofibroma underwent combined Level III and Level V approaches with preservation of the cribriform plate. **B,** Appearance 1-year after operation. **C,** Sagittal MRI demonstrating large nasopharyngeal mass. **D,** Coronal MRI showing retromaxillary extension. **E,** Exposure of the tumor *(arrow)* obtained with the Level III approach. The frontal lobe dura is at the bottom, and the retractor blade is positioned on the medial aspect of the left globe. **F,** Extended exposure of the tumor obtained with the Level V approach *(arrow)*. (**A** to **F** courtesy Barrow Neurological Institute, Phoenix.)

Table 91-3.
Facial Translocation Approaches[34]

APPROACH	ANATOMIC SITE OF LESION	FIGURE
Medial mini	Medial orbit, sphenoid sinus, ethmoid sinus, inferior clivus	91-20
Lateral mini	Infratemporal fossa	91-21
Standard	Anterolateral skull base, infratemporal fossa, orbit	91-22
Medial extended	Ipsilateral infratemporal fossa, central and paracentral skull base bilaterally, clivus, optic nerves, precavernous carotid arteries, nasopharynx	91-23
Medial and inferior extended	Preceding exposure with inferior extension into upper cervical region	91-24
Posterior extended	Adds exposure of ear, temporal bone, posterior fossa	91-25
Bilateral	Both infratemporal fossae, central skull base, entire paracentral skull base, both distal cervical internal carotid arteries, full clivus, inferior to C2-3 with palatal split, to C3-4 with mandibular split	91-26

For additional information see Janeka IP: Facial translocation approach. In Janecka IP, Tiedeman K, editors: *Skull base surgery, anatomy, biology, technology*, Philadelphia, 1997, Lippincott-Raven.

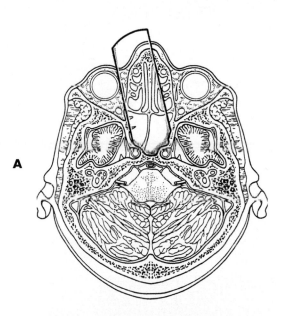

A

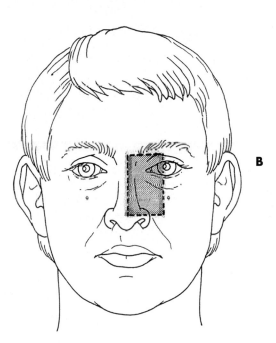

B

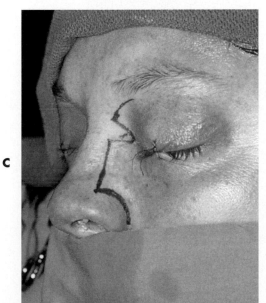

C

Figure 91-20. Medial minifacial translocation. **A,** Surgical field in axial view. **B,** Surgical field in coronal view. **C,** Skin incision. (**A** to **C** from Janeka IP: Facial translocation approach. In Janecka IP, Tiedeman K, editors: *Skull base surgery, anatomy, biology, technology*, Philadelphia, 1997, Lippincott-Raven.)

accomplished, and the mandibular condyle is either displaced or resected (Figure 91-21).

Standard Facial Translocation

The standard facial translocation approach yields access to the entire anterolateral skull base. This approach is based on the concept of a vascularized facial composite, allowing wide exposure of this region and simplified reconstruction through a paranasal skin incision. It can be extended to include the upper lip if the exposure is warranted. The incision courses horizontally from the nose to the inferior fornix of the lower lid and then across the lateral canthus. The incision can end within 1.5 cm of the lateral canthus for more anterior tumors. It can be extended to the preauricular area for wider exposure. If this extension is necessary, the frontal branches of the facial nerve are identified and transected after being placed in silicone tubing. Reconstruction of the facial nerve is accomplished by reconnecting the transected tube ends. Depending on the need for exposure, the osteotomy, correlating to a LeFort I-II, can be utilized, or a midpalatal osteotomy is performed when the entire maxilla is being displaced. The inferior orbital nerve is identified and electively sectioned in the floor of the orbit. It is tagged and repaired during the reconstructive phase of the procedure. Reconstitution of the facial bones is accomplished with rigid fixation (Figure 91-22).

Expanded Facial Translocation

MEDIAL EXTENDED FACIAL TRANSLOCATION. The medial extended facial translocation combines the standard translocation and adds the nose and the medial half of the opposite face (the lateral margins of the infraorbital nerve). As in the standard translocation, it can be rotated at the LeFort I

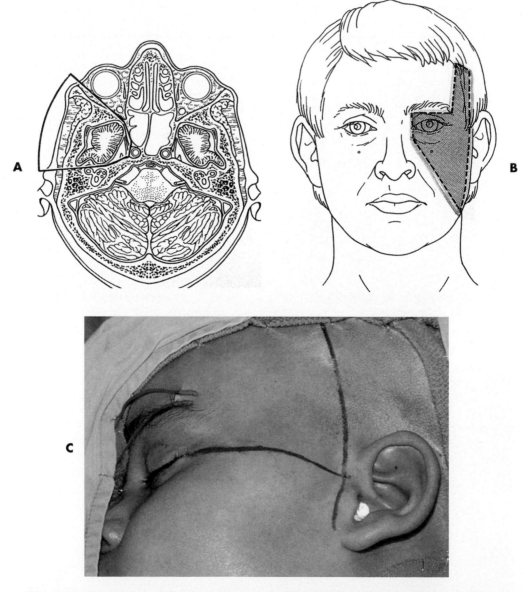

Figure 91-21. Lateral minifacial translocation. **A,** Surgical field in axial view. **B,** Surgical field in coronal view. **C,** Skin incision. (**A to C** from Janeka IP: Facial translocation approach. In Janecka IP, Tiedeman K, editors: *Skull base surgery, anatomy, biology, technology,* Philadelphia, 1997, Lippincott-Raven.)

level, so it can include ipsilateral palate and upper lip incision. The paranasal incision is made on the contralateral side. This approach is useful for lesions of the ipsilateral infratemporal fossa/central and paracentral skull base bilaterally, the entire clivus, optic nerves, precavernous internal carotid arteries bilaterally, and the nasopharynx. This access also allows reconstruction of the skull base with the temporalis muscle flap. Reconstruction is accomplished with rigid fixation with the aid of an occlusal splint. Prophylactically, intranasal silicone stents as well as nasolacrimal stents are utilized (Figure 91-23).

MEDIAL AND INFERIOR EXTENDED FACIAL TRANS-LOCATION. This approach adds exposure inferiorly to the level of the upper cervical region. The skin incision is the same in the midface region, and a lower lip incision is added in a zigzag configuration, conforming to the natural skin tension lines. This incision extends horizontally into the upper neck. A mandibular split is accomplished via mandibular osteotomy performed just medial to the mental foramen in a step configuration. Preregistration of the plate prior to the osteotomy, including the drilling of holes, ensures anatomic reconstruction and preservation of the preoperative occlusion (Figure 91-24).

POSTERIOR EXTENDED FACIAL TRANSLOCATION. This extension provides an approach to the anterior and posterior aspects of the temporal bone and allows control of key neurovascular structures. It incorporates the ear,

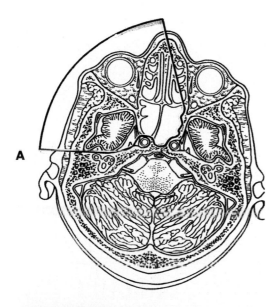

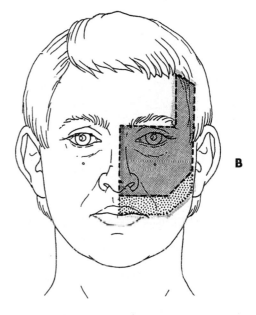

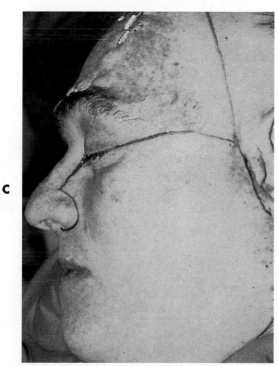

Figure 91-22. Standard facial translocation. **A,** Surgical field in axial view. **B,** Surgical field in coronal view. **C,** Skin incision. (**A** to **C** from Janeka IP: Facial translocation approach. In Janecka IP, Tiedeman K, editors: *Skull base surgery, anatomy, biology, technology,* Philadelphia, 1997, Lippincott-Raven.)

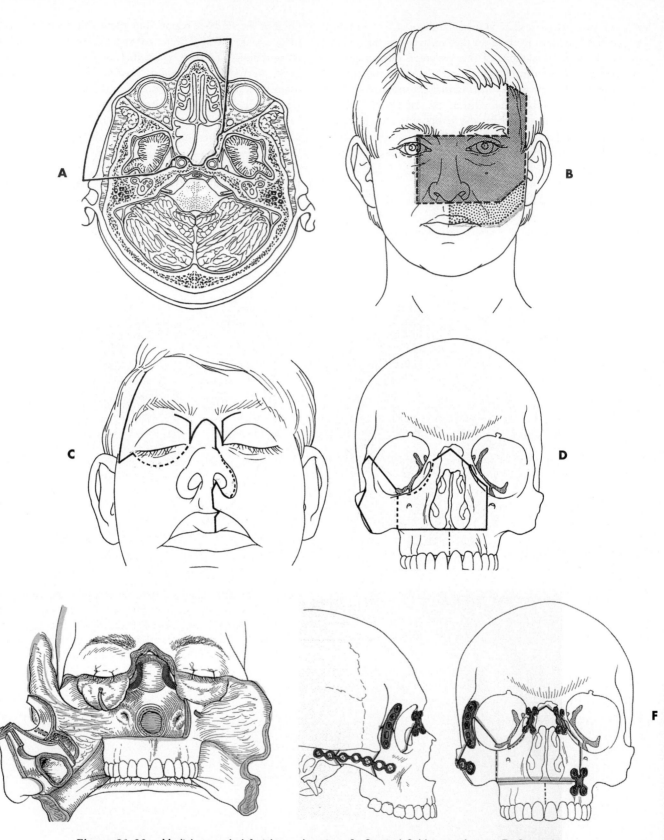

Figure 91-23. Medial extended facial translocation. **A,** Surgical field in axial view. **B,** Surgical field in coronal view. **C,** Skin incision. **D,** Osteotomy of nasomaxillary and orbitozygomatic regions. **E,** Surgical field of exposure showing both cavernous carotids, eustachian tubes, and clival dura. **F** Rigid fixation of osteotomies. (**A** to **F** from Janeka IP: Facial translocation approach. In Janecka IP, Tiedeman K, editors: *Skull base surgery, anatomy, biology, technology,* Philadelphia, 1997, Lippincott-Raven.)

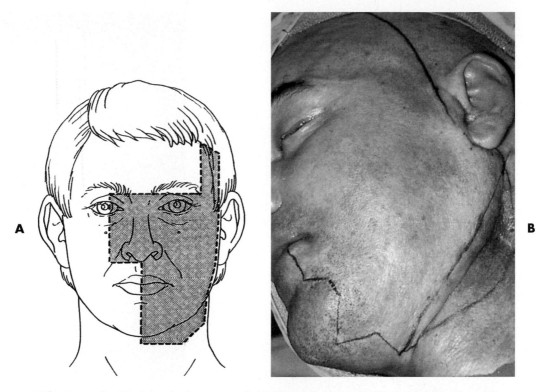

Figure 91-24. Medial and inferior extended facial translocation. **A,** Surgical field in coronal view. **B,** Skin incision. (**A** to **C** from Janeka IP: Facial translocation approach. In Janecka IP, Tiedeman K, editors: *Skull base surgery, anatomy, biology, technology,* Philadelphia, 1997, Lippincott-Raven.)

temporal bone, and posterior fossa. The standard translocation incision is extended posteriorly just above the external ear and curves inferiorly over the occipital bone through the neck (Figure 91-25).

Bilateral Facial Translocation

This approach provides exposure to both infratemporal fossae and the central as well as the paracentral skull. Both distal and cervical internal carotid arteries are exposed. The addition of a palatal split provides an inferior approach to approximately the level of cervical vertebrae 2 and 3. A further inferior extension can be accomplished with the addition of a mandibular split to reach cervical vertebrae 3 and 4. The temporalis muscle flap can be used to cover the skull base. Craniotomies can be added to these approaches as needed to protect or gain additional access to the intracranial component (Figure 91-26).

Reconstruction

After resection of the tumor of the cranial base, repair of the dura is critical to minimize postoperative CSF leak and related complications. If the dura can be repaired primarily, it is also reinforced with fibrin glue. If a defect exists, it is repaired with autogenous fascia lata or pericranium. A second layer, consisting of a vascularized pericranial flap, is also placed, and every effort should be made to try to suture this directly to the dura or adjacent soft tissue or bone utilizing drill holes. If the bony defect of the skull base is small, and if it has adequate soft tissue closure and does not need rigid support for the intracranial structures, it can be left unrepaired. For larger defects, a bone graft is required in addition to soft tissue repair. Other facial and orbital bones sacrificed for exposure or for tumor resection can also be reconstructed with autogenous cranial bone grafts. This is preferable to alloplastic material.

The temporalis muscle flap can be utilized to repair the skull base. Its reach is facilitated by release of the coronoid process. Care must be taken not to devascularize its arterial supply coming from the posterior aspect of the sigmoid notch of the mandible. Use of a temporalis muscle flap will create an aesthetic defect in the temporal fossa that can be reconstructed at a later stage with autogenous bone grafts, dermal fat graft, or an alloplastic implant. Exposure of the temporalis muscle in the nasopharynx is well tolerated, and since coverage with mucosa occurs rapidly, skin graft is not necessary. A watertight closure to the surrounding soft tissue utilizing the durable temporalis fascia is important.

The vascularized facial segments are returned to anatomic position with the aid of a dental occlusal splint and rigid fixation. Sectioned nerves and skin are repaired.

POSTOPERATIVE MANAGEMENT

Following surgery, the patient must be managed in a neurosurgical intensive care unit environment to enable close surveillance and monitoring. Postoperative CT scans or MRIs are obtained to evaluate the brain, thoroughness of resection of the tumor, and the presence of any dead space or intracranial air. In patients in whom a tracheostomy can be avoided, an

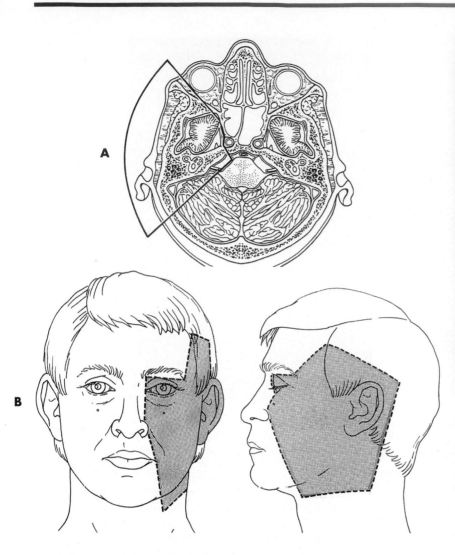

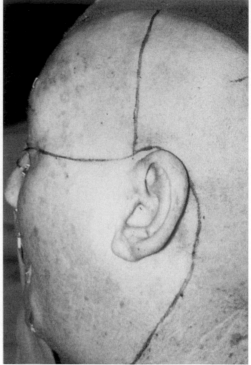

Figure 91-25. Posterior extended facial translocation. **A,** Surgical field in axial view. **B,** Surgical field in coronal and sagittal views. **C,** Skin incision. (**A** to **C** from Janeka IP: Facial translocation approach. In Janecka IP, Tiedeman K, editors: *Skull base surgery, anatomy, biology, technology,* Philadelphia, 1997, Lippincott-Raven.)

endotracheal tube is retained until swelling has decreased to ensure an adequate airway. Prophylactic antibiotics are continued. A lumbar drain is used for CSF management. Postoperative surveillance and early intervention are essential in successful management of a postoperative CSF leak. Because the wound is often concealed, surveillance can be difficult. A CT scan or MRI is not always helpful.[2] Direct observation by endoscopy at the bedside should be performed routinely, and reexploration of the wound may be required to be definitive. Patients with preexisting medical problems must be prepared carefully prior to surgery and carefully managed in the postoperative period to minimize related complications. Enteral or parenteral nutrition is essential in the early postoperative period for best healing and to help reduce the incidence of sepsis.

Patient Example

(1) A 35-year-old woman presented with adenoid cystic carcinoma of the right ethmoid sinus. The tumor extended into the right orbit and into the maxillary and sphenoid sinuses. Intracranially, it involved the cavernous sinus and dura (Figure 91-27). Because the right internal carotid artery was involved, the surgery was staged. The first stage required

bypass of the right internal carotid artery using a saphenous-vein graft placed between the internal carotid artery above the bifurcation and the middle cerebral artery. The graft traversed subcutaneously from the neck, preauricularly, and then through a temporal craniotomy. The plastic surgeon was present at this procedure to place the scalp incision optimally and to dissect the local temporalis and pericranial flaps to be used in the second procedure.

One week later, the second stage was performed. Through a right anterolateral intracranial-extracranial approach, gross total resection of the tumor was accomplished. An orbital exenteration and resection of the cavernous sinus and a 10×10-cm area of frontotemporal dura were required. The large anterior and middle cranial fossa defect extended into the nasopharynx and oropharynx (see Figure 91-27, *B*). Reconstruction utilized local pericranial and temporalis flaps against the pharynx and sinuses and a rectus abdominis free flap against the intracranial compartment (see Figure 91-27, *C*).

The rectus abdominis free flap was a composite of muscle, posterior rectus sheath, and peritoneum that was tailored to the dural defect (Figure 91-28). This vascularized dural replacement was sutured in a watertight closure, and fibrin glue was

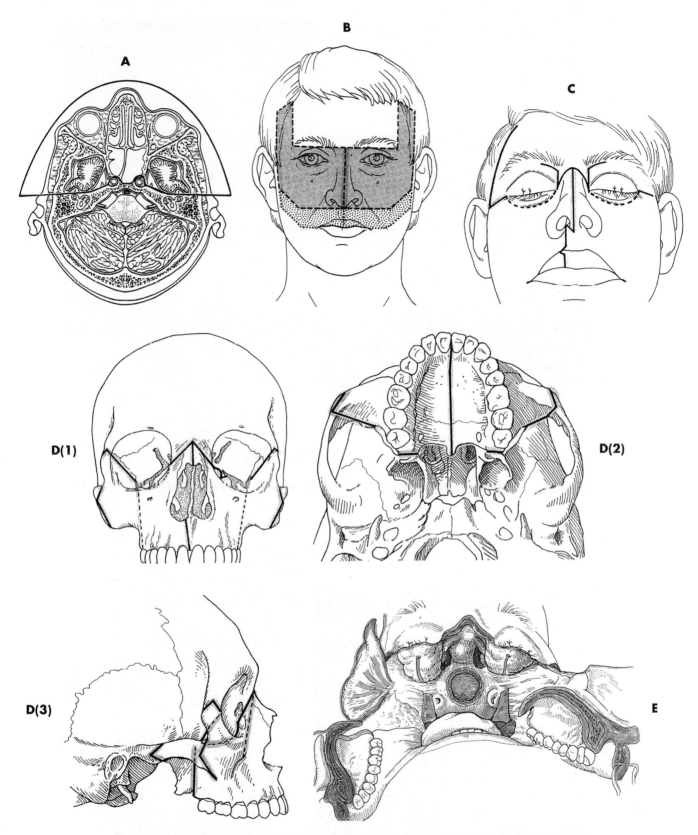

Figure 91-26. Bilateral facial translocation. **A,** Surgical field in axial view. **B,** Surgical field in coronal view. **C,** Skin incisions. **D,** Osteotomies. Anterior, inferior, and lateral views. **E,** Surgical field showing wide central and paracentral views. (**A** to **E** from Janeka IP: Facial translocation approach. In Janecka IP, Tiedeman K, editors: *Skull base surgery, anatomy, biology, technology,* Philadelphia, 1997, Lippincott-Raven.)

Figure 91-27. **A,** MRI shows tumor of ethmoid, orbit, and cavernous sinus. **B,** An anterolateral approach with orbital exenteration is used for tumor resection. **C** and **D,** The large frontotemporal dural defect is closed with a composite free rectus abdominis flap using the peritoneum for the vascularized dural repair. *Continued*

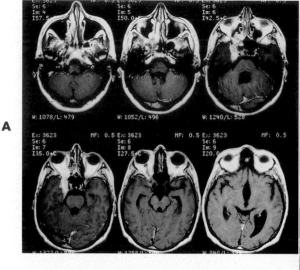

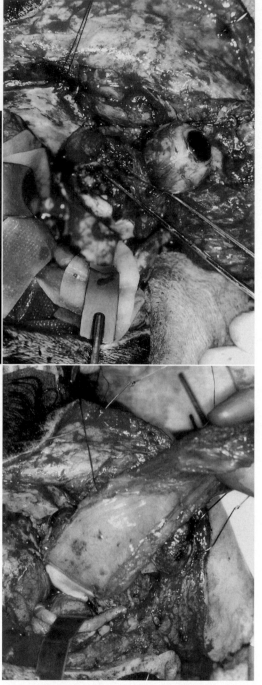

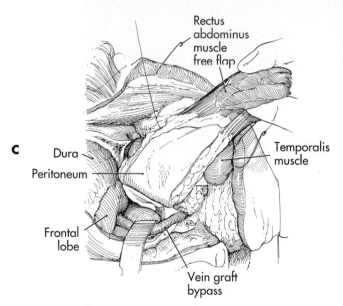

used. The vascular pedicle was anastomosed in the neck utilizing the jugular vein end-to-side and a branch of the external carotid artery (see Figure 91-27, *D*). A portion of the flap was left exposed preauricularly and skin grafted to allow for monitoring. No bone grafts were used (see Figure 91-27, *F*).

The combination of local flaps and free flaps filled the dead space completely. An ocular prosthesis was placed in a conjunctiva-lined socket (see Figure 91-27, *E*). A lumbar drain was placed. To completely isolate the aerodigestive tract, a temporary gastric feed tube and tracheostomy were placed.

The patient had an uncomplicated postoperative course except for acute acalculous cholecystitis that required surgical management. Early in the postoperative course, swelling of the free flap appeared to be causing a significant shift of the brain as evaluated by CT. The patient remained asymptomatic.

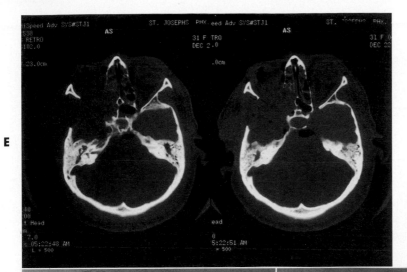

Figure 91-27, cont'd. **D** to **E,** CT scan shows extent of resection. **F** and **G,** Patient 4 months after resection. (**A** to **G** courtesy Barrow Neurological Institute, Phoenix.)

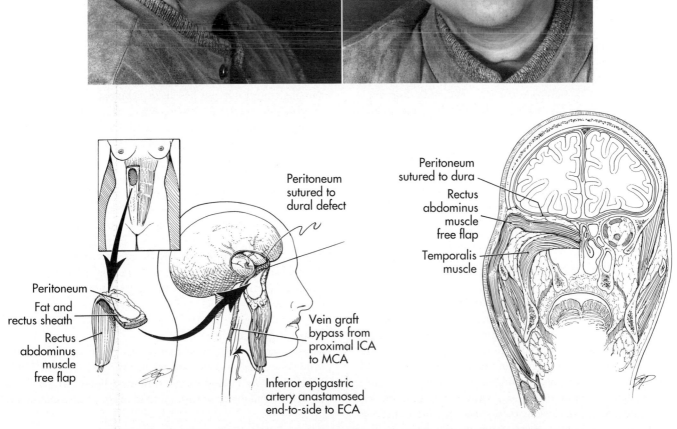

Figure 91-28. The rectus abdominis free flap was a composite of muscle, posterior rectus sheath, and peritoneum. **A,** The peritoneum was used as a dural graft. **B,** The temporalis muscle was folded below the rectus flap to aid in eliminating dead space. (**A** and **B** courtesy Barrow Neurological Institute, Phoenix.)

Box 91-2.
Sources for Technology

Howmedica, Inc.
359 Veterans Blvd.
Rutherford, NJ 07070-2584

Micro 100, by Amsco-Hall Surgical
Santa Barbara, CA 93101

Midas Rex
3001 Ray Street
Ft. Worth, TX 76111

Carl Zeiss
1 Zeiss Drive
Thornwood, NY 10594

KLS-Martin
P.O. Box 50249
Jacksonville, FL 32250-0249

ISG Localizing Wand, by ISG Technologies
Mississauga, Ontario, Canada

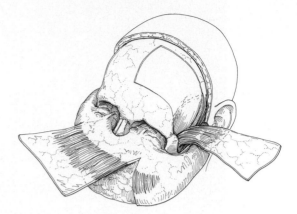

Figure 91-29. Frontogaleal flap can be used for secondary skull base coverage. (Courtesy Barrow Neurological Institute, Phoenix.)

frontogaleal flap (Figure 91-29), which is reserved for last resort, and free flap reconstruction (see Figure 91-28)* are more frequently necessary in secondary resection.

TECHNOLOGY

Somatosensory evoke potential is used for intraoperative monitoring. The ISG wand is utilized for localizing tumor margins and critical structures. The Zimmer micro 100 reciprocating saw is utilized for facial osteotomies, and the drill attachment for placement of plates and screws. KLS-Martin rigid fixation is utilized for maxillary and mandibular osteotomies. Specialized maxillary plates are available that allow fixation with only one plate on each side. Superrigid titanium plates are tailormade for fixation along the anterior border of the mandible using unicortical screws. These are low-profile plates with three holes on each side of the osteotomy. Luhr panfixation plates made by Howmedica are ideal for midface, periorbital, and calvarial fixation. The Midas Rex system is utilized for craniotomy. Microsurgical dissection is ideal with the Zeiss microscope on a Contraves stand (Box 91-2).

SECONDARY PROCEDURES

Secondary Surgery for Tumor Recurrence

Recurrent tumor is sometimes amenable to reoperation, and the patient should undergo the same evaluation and scrutiny by the skull base team. The choice of approach is again determined by the anatomic site of the lesion and its extension, and can be a repeat of the same approach if appropriate. Repeating the same incision and osteotomies is not a problem if indicated. Secondary reconstruction becomes more challenging because local flap options have usually been used. A

Radiation and Previous Surgery

Preoperative and postoperative radiation has a profound effect on wound healing and can add to the incidence of wound complications. Chances for wound healing are improved if the most reliable reconstruction possible is utilized when radiation is anticipated. This usually means free flap reconstruction with anastamosis performed outside the zone of radiation.

OUTCOMES

COMPLICATIONS

Although great success has been achieved in exposure and resection of previously unresectable, deep-seated skull base lesions, the tumor's effect on the skull base and adjacent vital structures may leave the patient with devastating complications, loss of function, and aesthetic appearance, all at an enormous cost.[9,43,55,71] As we continue to redefine resectability, resection of more advanced tumors is attempted, resulting in more complex procedures and larger defects that require multicomponent reconstruction. The intracranial compartment sealed by the cranial base is a privileged space that is violated by skull base tumors and the process of resecting them. Reestablishing this boundary that is impenetrable to bacteria from adjacent sinuses and the digestive tract remains a challenge.

Neurologic Deficits

Most serious complications that are life-threatening and result in lifelong functional deficits are neurologic in origin.[38,46,68] Wide exposure is essential to minimize brain retraction, to ensure meticulous hemostasis, and to allow good visualization

---

*References 11, 27, 53, 66, 77, 82.

and access for complete tumor removal. Wide exposure also gives the space needed to reconstruct the dura with a watertight closure.

Wound Complications

Skull base defects are among the most challenging wounds that a plastic surgeon confronts. To support the brain, to contain CSF, and to create a compartment sealed from contamination are the goals of reconstruction. This unforgiving area is often made worse by radiation, previous surgery, or dead space, and can yield a high rate of wound complication despite maximum efforts. Success requires diligence and attention to detail. Infection and poor vascularity of tissues can contribute to poor healing and result in CSF leak, flap failure, and palatal fistula. A Valsalva's maneuver due to coughing, sneezing, or nose blowing can break the seal of the cranial base closure for some period of time following surgery. Orbital and facial cellulitis, pneumocephalus, and sinoscalp fistulas have all been reported and have required secondary reconstruction. Local flaps and granulation tissue in a poorly vascularized area cannot be expected to seal a defect. An appropriate choice of reconstructive technique and appropriate use of free tissue transfer are required. Wound surveillance can be difficult in the immediate postoperative period because the deep aspects of the wound are concealed. Direct observation with endoscopy at the bedside can be performed routinely. Reexploration of the wound may be required if sepsis is suspected or if CSF leakage persists despite lumbar drainage.

Postoperative swelling in the facial area, although extensive, has not been a long-term problem, and does not contribute to morbidity in and of itself. However, intracranial edema can be devastating. When placing free flaps in the intracranial compartment, there is a potential for intolerable pressure on the brain in this closed space. Close surveillance is critical, and return to surgery for temporary removal of the bone flap may be necessary.

Dead space is the enemy of any skull base reconstruction. An attempt should be made at the time of reconstruction to eliminate this wherever possible.

CSF Leak

A CSF leak is the Achilles heel of any skull base reconstruction, and can occur despite ideal repair.[54] A lumbar drain is used routinely for 3 to 5 days to diminish CSF pressure during the early healing phase.[74] Prophylactic antibiotic coverage is essential. If a CSF leak persists, localization studies are undertaken to assist in planning exploration of the wound. If the leak is not resolved with conservative measures in 3 to 5 days, the skull base defect must be reexplored and the site of the leak repaired. If the defect is small and the adjacent tissues are healthy, direct repair is performed. Reinforcement with a fat and muscle graft and fibrin glue is ideal. If a local flap is still available, it can be used to reinforce the leak repair.

If the defect is large, or is due to fat necrosis or infection, secondary reconstruction is undertaken after wound debridement. Microvascular free tissue transfer is usually needed for secondary reconstruction.

Management of Surgical Approach–Related Complications

Displacement of facial units for exposure of the skull base can result in technique-related complications apart from the skull base tumor itself or its resulting defect.[9]

MALOCCLUSION. Malocclusion following transmaxillary (Level IV, V) approaches is usually related to technique and is avoidable. Transmaxillary approaches to the skull base must be treated with the same respect and precision as an elective orthognathic procedure to preserve the preoperative occlusion. In patients who undergo a two-piece transmaxillary (Level V) approach, a fixation plate or lag screw placed between the two fragments is essential. A plate can be placed on the nasal floor anteriorly or across the anterior nasal spine region. A splint with a palatal crosspiece offers greater postoperative control of the fragments. Postoperative intermaxillary fixation has not been used. If a postoperative malocclusion occurs and is beyond the realm of correction orthodontically, reosteotomy at an appropriate time postoperatively is necessary to correct the malocclusion.

EPIPHORA. Approaches that require an osteotomy near the region of the nasolacrimal duct or require actual transection of the duct may result in epiphora postoperatively. A surgeon should look for disruption during the reconstructive phase and repair and cannulate as indicated. If transection was required, the duct can be repaired over tubes during the reconstructive phase of the procedure. If persistent epiphora occurs postoperatively, workup is indicated, and occasionally a dacryocystorhinostomy is needed.

OCULAR-ORBITAL. Orbital walls and thus orbital volume must be restored to normal at the time of reconstruction to maintain symmetry and globe position. This restoration can be difficult when a large portion of the orbit is removed in the course of tumor resection. Nevertheless, the same principles apply. If enophthalmos results postoperatively, a secondary reconstruction of the orbit with autogenous bone grafts or rib grafts is indicated. Strabismus can occur following orbital surgery and may require surgical correction. Orbital reconstruction and ocular prosthesis are indicated in cases of orbital exenteration.

Motor or sensory nerves that require transection for exposure are repaired directly and have a high success rate for recovery.[34] In cases of facial nerve deficit, secondary nerve grafting, facial reanimation procedures, or static suspension may be indicated.

PALATAL FISTULA. A palatal fistula can occur following a palatal split procedure for transfacial approach and is usually technique-related. Secondary repair may be necessary using palatal flaps to line the nasal and oral sides of the fistula.

SPEECH ABNORMALITIES. Speech abnormalities can occur, not only due to neurologic complications, but also to use of a transpalatal approach. Usually, speech improves spontane-

Table 91-4.
Evolution of Cranial Base Surgery (First Period [1960s-1970s])

	KETCHAM ET AL.[42]*		VAN BUREN ET AL.[84]†		KETCHAM ET AL.[41a]‡	
	PATIENT NO.	%	PATIENT NO.	%	PATIENT NO.	%
Histology						
SCCA	7	37	7	22	17	31
Sarcoma	7	37	10	31	14	26
Adenocarcinoma	0	0	3	9	6	11
Adenoid cystic CA	1	5	0	0	2	4
Surgery						
Primary	6	32	17	53	12	22
Salvage	13	68	15	47	42	78
Margins: positive	9	47	N/A		17	31
Radiation therapy	10	53	N/A		33	61

From O'Malley BWJ, Janecka IP: Evolution of outcomes in cranial base surgery, *Semin Surg Oncol* 11:221-227, 1995.
SCCA, Squamous cell cancer; *CA*, cancer; *CSF*, cerebrospinal fluid; *CNS*, central nervous system; *NED*, no evidence of disease; *f/u*, follow-up; *DOC*, died of other causes; *N/A*, not applicable.
*19 patients studied.
†32 patients studied.
‡54 patients studied.

Continued

ously as the soft palate and nasopharynx heal. Speech evaluation with nasoendoscopy is helpful to elucidate the cause. Irregularities and concavity of the clival and vertebral junction in the region of the nasopharynx can result in velopharyngeal insufficiency.

LONG-TERM RESULTS

Long-term results are now being evaluated by skull base surgery teams.* O'Malley and Janecka have recently reviewed the results of treatment of skull base carcinomas and sarcomas over the past 40 years.[35,57] They have designated three periods of time that reflect the advances of skull base surgery. In the first, pioneer era (1960s to 1970s), 3- and 5-year survivals of 52% and 49% were achieved by attempting to resect tumors without pterygopalatine or intracranial extension (Table 91-4). Improved surgical techniques in the second era (1970s to 1980s) allowed resection of more extensive tumors that

included intracranial invasion, raising the 3-year survival to 57% to 59%, with limited reports of 5-year survivals in the range of 49% (Table 91-5). With further refinement and introduction of the team approach, the third era (1980s to 1990s) had improved results, increasing the 5-year survival to 56% to 70% (Table 91-6).

The definition of unresectability continues to change as techniques continue to evolve, particularly in the management of the carotid system. According to O'Malley and Janecka, tumor involvement of the carotid artery itself is not a contraindication, but invasion into the "dominant" carotid system should preclude surgery in most cases. Additionally, general contraindications include substantial invasion into the dominant temporal lobe and bilateral optic nerve or chiasm involvement. The histology of tumors also impacts the decision on resectability. More aggressive tumors that demand a need for a large surgical margin and therefore involvement of critical intracranial structures render some tumors, such as squamous cell carcinoma, undifferentiated tumor, sarcomas, and melanomas, unresectable. Furthermore, elderly patients and those with significant preexisting medical illness tolerate

*References 20, 25, 26, 28, 50, 57, 60, 63, 84.

Table 91-4.
Evolution of Cranial Base Surgery (First Period [1960s-1970s])—cont'd

	KETCHAM ET AL.[42]*		VAN BUREN ET AL.[84]†		KETCHAM ET AL.[41a]‡	
	PATIENT NO.	%	PATIENT NO.	%	PATIENT NO.	%
Complications						
Infections	4	21	13	41	27	54
Meningitis/abscess	2	11	4	13	8	15
Bone flap	1	5	9	28	10	19
CSF leak	0	0	15	47	17	31
CNS deficit/bleeding	1	5	1	3	6	11
Perioperative mortality	1	5	2	6	2	4
Results						
NED (30 month f/u)	(n = 17) 9	53	(n = 30) 10	33	27	50
Local control at last f/u	13	68	21	66	N/A	
Distant metastases	6	32	11	34	N/A	
DOC	2	11	2	7	8	15
Survival						
3-year		53		56		52
5-year	N/A		N/A			49

these major procedures poorly, and thus, they may not be suitable candidates.

COST

Due to the complexity of these procedures, the length of time in the operating room, and the need for postoperative intensive care monitoring, the cost for these procedures can be enormous. Although no studies have been done comparing costs, it is estimated that a typical procedure could exceed $100,000.

AESTHETIC CONSIDERATIONS

The very basis of transfacial approaches to the skull base is to maintain aesthetic facial units in the process of exposure. For the most part, this has been a resounding success, and patients can expect to have very little, if any, change in their facial features. The exception occurs in patients who have direct tumor involvement of the facial skeleton and skin. Reconstruction of major facial units following resection can be satisfactory, and prosthetic reconstruction is also an option in some cases.

PATIENT SATISFACTION

The question of "Is it worth it?" is a fair one in surveying the extensive surgery and recovery that is necessary to address these tumors. While reported series have shown increased survival rates and decreased complications rates, the answer appears to be "yes." However, the question is best answered by the individual patient who previously had no hope for treatment of his or her deep-seated skull base tumor.

Table 91-5.
Evolution of Cranial Base Surgery (Second Period [1970s-1980s])

	VAN TUYL AND GUSSACK[84a]*		SISSON ET AL.[73b]†		CHEESMAN ET AL.[13a] LUND AND HARRISON[47a]‡	
	PATIENT NO.	%	PATIENT NO.	%	PATIENT NO.	%
Histology						
SCCA	8	38	32	53	7	8
Sarcoma	3	14	4	7	14	15
Adenocarcinoma	2	10	5	8	25	27
Adenoid cystic CA	0	0	10	17	9	10
Surgery						
Primary	18	86	58	97	31	34
Salvage	3	14	0	0	61	66
Margins: positive	N/A		N/A		N/A	
Radiation therapy	21	100	53	85	40	44
Complications						
Infections	10	48			4	4
Meningitis/abscess	4	19			2	?
Bone flap	6	29			2	2
CSF leak	4	19			3	3
CNS deficit/bleeding	0	0			5	5
Perioperative mortality	1	5			4	4
Results						
NED (30 month f/u)	12	57	22	37	46	50
Local control at last f/u	12	57	28	47	58	63
Distant metastases	8	38	3	5	7	8
DOC	0	0	N/A		0	0
Survival						
3-year		57	N/A			59
5-year	N/A			49	N/A	

From O'Malley BWJ, Janecka IP: Evolution of outcomes in cranial base surgery, *Semin Surg Oncol* 11:221-227, 1995.
SCCA, Squamous cell cancer; *CA,* cancer; *CSF,* cerebrospinal fluid; *CNS,* central nervous system; *NED,* no evidence of disease; *f/u,* follow-up; *DOC,* died of other causes; *N/A,* not applicable.
*21 patients studied.
†60 patients studied.
‡92 patients studied.

Table 91-6.
Evolution of Cranial Base Surgery (Third Period [1980s-1990s])[57]

	SHAH ET AL.[73a]*		JANECKA ET AL.[37a]†		JANECKA ET AL.[37b]‡	
	PATIENT NO.	%	PATIENT NO.	%	PATIENT NO.	%
Histology						
SCCA	11	15	36	31	13	26
Sarcoma	15	21	37	31	18	36
Adenocarcinoma	10	14	7	6	4	8
Adenoid cystic CA	3	4	16	14	7	14
Surgery						
Primary	40	56	43	36	23	46
Salvage	31	44	75	63	27	54
Margins: positive	15	21	51	43	11	22
Radiation therapy	47	66	118	100	50	100
Complications						
Infections	20	28	5	4	0	0
Meningitis/abscess	1	1	1	1	0	0
Bone flap	9	13	0	0	0	0
CSF leak	2	3	5	4	1	2
CNS deficit/bleeding	4	6	5	4	3	6
Perioperative mortality	2	3	3	2	0	0
Results						
NED (30 month f/u)	37	52	70	60	30	60
Local control at last f/u	50	70	99	84	41	82
Distant metastases	18	25	29	25	5	10
DOC	1	1	7	6	1	2
Survival						
3-year	N/A			67		74
5-year		56		65		70

From O'Malley BWJ, Janecka IP: Evolution of outcomes in cranial base surgery, *Semin Surg Oncol* 11:221-227, 1995.
SCCA, Squamous cell cancer; *CA*, cancer; *CSF*, cerebrospinal fluid; *CNS*, central nervous system; *NED*, no evidence of disease; *f/u*, follow-up; *DOC*, died of other causes; *N/A*, not applicable.
*71 patients studied.
†118 patients studied.
‡50 patients studied.

REFERENCES

1. Altemir FH: The transfacial access to the retromaxillary area, *J Maxillofac Surg* 14:165, 1986.

2. Anand VK, Arrowdood JPJ, Patel RB, et al: Significance of MRI changes after surgery of the skull base, *Otolaryngol Head Neck Surg* 109:35, 1993.

3. Anand VK, Harkey LH, Al-Mefty O: Open-door maxillotomy approach for lesions of the clivus, *Skull Base Surg* 1(4):217, 1991.

4. Barnes L, Kapadia SB: The biology and pathology of selected skull base tumors, *J Neurooncol* 20:213-240, 1994.

5. Beals SP, Hamilton MG, Joganic EF, et al: Classification of transfacial approaches in the treatment of tumors of the anterior skull base and clivus, *Plast Surg Forum* XVI:211-213, 1993.

6. Beals SP, Joganic EF: Transfacial exposure of anterior cranial fossa and clival tumors, *BNI Quarterly* 8(4):2, 1992.

7. Beals SP, Joganic EF, Hamilton MG, et al: Classification of transfacial approaches in the treatment of tumors of the anterior skull base and clivus. In Monasterio FM, editor: *Craniofacial surgery*, ed 5, Bologna, Italy, 1994, Monduzzi Editors, p 215.

8. Beals SP, Joganic EF, Hamilton MG, et al: Posterior skull base transfacial approaches, *Clin Plast Surg* 22:491-511, 1995.

9. Beals SP, Joganic EF, Holcombe TC, Spetzler RF: Secondary craniofacial problems following skull base surgery, *Clin Plast Surg* 24(3):565-581, 1997.

10. Belmont JR: The LeFort I osteotomy approach for nasopharyngeal and nasal fossa tumors, *Arch Otolaryngol Head Neck Surg* 114:751, 1988.

11. Besteiro JM, Aki FE, Ferreira MC, et al: Free flap reconstruction of tumors involving the cranial base, *Microsurgery* 15:9, 1994.

12. Blacklock JB, Weber RS, Lee Y-Y, et al: Transcranial resection of tumors of the paranasal sinuses and nasal cavity, *J Neurosurg* 71:10, 1989.

13. Brown AM, Lavery KM, Millar BG: The transfacial approach to the postnasal space and retromaxillary structures, *Br J Oral Maxillofacial Surg* 29:230, 1991.

13a. Cheesman AD, Lund VJ, Howard DJ: Craniofacial resection for tumors of the nasal cavity and paranasal sinuses, *Head Neck Surg* July/Aug:429-435, 1986.

14. Cocke EW, Robertson JH, Robertson JT, et al: The extended maxillotomy and subtotal maxillectomy for excision of skull base tumors, *Arch Otolaryngol Head Neck Surg* 116:92, 1990.

15. Crockard HA: Surgical access to the base of skull and upper cervical spine by exterior maxillotomy, *Neurosurgery* 29(3):411, 1991.

16. Crockard HA: The transmaxillary approach to the clivus. In Sekhar LN, Janecka IP, editors: *Surgery of cranial base tumors*, New York, 1993, Raven, pp 235-244.

17. deFries HO, Deeb ZE, Hudkins CP: A transfacial approach to the nasal-paranasal cavities and anterior skull base, *Arch Otolaryngol Head Neck Surg* 114:766, 1988.

18. Derome PJ: The transfacial approach to tumors invading the base of the skull. In Schmidek MH, Sweet WH, editors: *Operative neurosurgical techniques*, ed 2, Orlando, 1988, Grune & Stratton, pp 619-633.

19. Derome PJ, Akerman N, Anquez L, et al: Les tumers spheno-ethmoidales, *Neurochir* [Suppl] 18:1, 1972.

20. Dos Santos LRM, Cernea CR, Brandao LG, et al: Results and prognostic factors in skull base surgery, *Am J Surg* 168:481, 1994.

21. Farnworth TK, Beals SP, Manwaring KH, et al: Comparison of skin necrosis in rats using a new microneedle electrocautery, standard-size needle electrocautery, and the Shaw hemostatic scalpel, *Ann Plast Surg* 31:164, 1993.

22. Fearon J, Bruce D: Preservation of olfaction with a cribriform plate osteotomy, *Plast Surg Forum*, Washington, September 20-24, 1992.

23. Fearon JA, Munro IR, Bruce DA: Transfacial approaches to the cranial base, *Clin Plast Surg* 22:483, 1995.

24. Fujitsu K, Saijoh M, Aoki F, et al: Telecanthal approach for meningiomas in the ethmoid and sphenoid sinuses, *Neurosurgery* 28:714, 1991.

25. Gay E, Sekhar LN, Rubinstein E, et al: Chordomas and chondrosarcomas of the cranial base: results and follow-up of 60 patients, *Neurosurgery* 36:887, 1995.

26. Irish JC, Gullane PJ, Gentilli F, et al: Tumors of the skull base: outcome and survival analysis of 77 cases, *Head Neck* 16:3, 1994.

27. Izquierdo R, Leonetti JP, Origitano TC, et al: Refinements using free-tissue transfer for complex cranial base reconstruction, *Plast Reconstr Surg* 92:567, 1993.

28. Jackson IT, Bailey H, Marsh WR, et al: Results and prognosis following surgery for malignant tumors of the skull base, *Head Neck* 13:89, 1991.

29. Jackson IT, Marsh WR, Bite U, et al: Craniofacial osteotomies to facilitate skull base tumor resection, *Br J Plast Surg* 39:153, 1986.

30. Jackson IT, Marsh WR, Hide TAH: Treatment of tumors involving the anterior cranial fossa, *Head Neck Surg* 6:901, 1984.

31. James D, Crockard HA: Surgical access to the base of skull and upper cervical spine by exterior maxillotomy, *Neurosurgery* 29:411, 1991.

32. Janecka IP: Classification of facial translocation approach to the skull base, *Otolaryngol Head Neck Surg* 112:579, 1995.

33. Janecka IP: A new approach to the cranial base. *Proceedings of the 14th World Congress of Otolaryngology, Head and Neck Surgery, Madrid, Spain, September 10-15, 1989*, Amsterdam, 1990, Kugler & Ghedini.

34. Janecka IP: Facial translocation approach. In Janecka IP, Tiedeman K, editors: *Skull base surgery, anatomy, biology, technology*, Philadelphia, 1997, Lippincott-Raven, pp 183-219.

35. Janecka IP, Sekhar LN: Surgical management of cranial base tumors: a report on 91 patients, *Oncology* 3:69, 1989.

36. Janecka IP, Sen CH, Sekhar LN, et al: Facial translocation: a new approach to the cranial base, *Otolaryngol Head Neck Surg* 103:413-419, 1990.

37. Janecka IP, Sen CH, Sekhar LN, et al: Facial translocation for cranial base surgery, *Keio J Med* 40(4):2115-2220, 1991.

37a. Janeka IP, Sen CH, Sekhar LN, et al: Cranial base surgery: results in 183 patients, *Otolaryngol Head Neck Surg* 110:539-546, 1994.

37b. Janecka IP, Sen CH, Sekhar LN, Curtin HD: Treatment of paranasal sinus cancer with cranial base surgery: results, *Laryngoscope* 104:553-555, 1994.

38. Jennings KS, Siroky D, Jackson CG: Swallowing problems after excision of tumors of the skull base: diagnosis and management in 12 patients, *Dysphagia* 7:40, 1992.

39. Johns ME, Kaplan MJ, Jane JA, et al: Supraorbital rim approach to the anterior skull base, *Laryngoscope* 94:1137, 1984.

40. Kawakami K, Yamanouchi Y, Kubota C, et al: An extensive transbasal approach to frontal skull-base tumors, *J Neurosurg* 74:1011, 1991.

41. Kennedy DW, Papel ID, Halliday M: Transpalatal approach to the skull base, *Ear Nose Throat J* 65:125, 1986.

41a. Ketcham AS, Chretien PB, VanBuren JM, et al: The ethmoid sinuses: a re-evaluation of surgical resection, *Am J Surg* 126:469-476, 1973.

42. Ketcham AS, Wilkinsen RH, Marron JM, et al: A combined intracranial facial approach to the paranasal sinuses, *Am J Surg* 106:698, 1963.

43. Kraus DH, Shah JP, Arbit E, et al: Complications of craniofacial resection for tumors involving the anterior skull base, *Head Neck* 16:307, 1994.

44. Lauritzen C, Vallfors B, Lilja J: Facial disassembly for tumor resection, *Scand J Plast Reconstr Surg* 20:201, 1986.

45. Lee J-P, Tsai M-S, Chen Y-R: Orbitozygomatic infratemporal approach to lateral skull base tumors, *Acta Neurol Scan* 87:403, 1993.

46. Levine TM: Swallowing disorders following skull base surgery, *Otolaryngol Clin North Am* 21:751, 1988.

47. Lewis WJ, Richter HA, Jabourian Z: Craniofacial resection for large tumors of the paranasal sinuses, *Ear Nose Throat J* 8:539, 1989.

47a. Lund VJ, Harrison DFN: Craniofacial resection for tumors of the nasal cavity and paranasal sinuses, *Am J Surg* 156:187-190, 1988.

48. Mann WJ, Gilsbach J, Seeger W, et al: Use of a malar bone graft to augment skull base access, *Arch Otolaryngol* 111:30, 1985.

49. Maran AGD: Surgical approaches to the nasopharynx, *Clin Otolaryngol* 8:417, 1983.

50. McCaffrey TV, Olsen KD, Yohanan JM, et al: Factors affecting survival of patients with tumors of the anterior skull base, *Laryngoscope* 104:940, 1994.

51. Miller HS, Petty PG, Wilson WF, et al: A combined intracranial and facial approach for excision and repair of cancer of the ethmoid sinuses, *Aust [NZ] Surg* 43(2):179, 1973.

52. Munro IR: The transfacial approach for tumors of the midline skull base, *Presented at the American Association of Plastic Surgeons, 69th Annual Meeting,* Hot Springs, Va, May, 1990.

53. Musto TA, Corral CJ: Soft tissue reconstructive choices for craniofacial reconstruction, *Clin Plast Surg* 22:543, 1995.

54. Myers DL, Sataloff RT: Spinal fluid leakage after skull base surgical procedures, *Otolaryngol Clin North Am* 17:601, 1984.

55. Nguyen TT, Delashaw JB Jr: Complications of skull base surgery, *Clin Plast Surg* 22:573, 1995.

56. Nofziger HC: Brain surgery, *Surg Gyn Ob* 46:241-248, 1928.

57. O'Malley BWJ, Janecka IP: Evolution of outcomes in cranial base surgery, *Semin Surg Oncol* 11:221-227, 1995.

58. Panje WR, Dohrmann III GJ, Pitcock JK, et al: The transfacial approach for combined anterior craniofacial tumor ablation, *Arch Otolaryngol Head Neck Surg* 115:301, 1989.

59. Persing JA, Jane JA, Levine PA, et al: The versatile frontal sinus approach to the floor of the anterior cranial fossa, *J Neurosurg* 72:513, 1990.

60. Poe DS, Jackson CG, Glasscock ME, et al: Long-term results after lateral cranial base surgery, *Laryngoscope* 101:372, 1991.

61. Price JC: The midfacial degloving approach to the central skull base, *Ear Nose Throat J* 65:174, 1986.

62. Raveh J, Turk JB, Lädrach K, et al: Extended anterior subcranial approach for skull base tumors: long-term results, *J Neurosurg* 82:1002, 1993.

63. Richtsmeier WJ, Briggs RJS, Koch WM, et al: Complications and early outcome of anterior craniofacial resection, *Arch Otolaryngol Head Neck Surg* 118:913, 1992.

64. Ross DA, Sasaki CT: Pathology of tumors of the cranial base, *Clin Plast Surg* 22:407-416, 1995.

65. Sandor GKB, Charles DA, Lawson VG, et al: Trans oral approach to the nasopharynx and clivus using the LeFort I osteotomy with midpalatal split, *Int J Maxillofac Surg* 19:352, 1990.

66. Sasaki CT: Pectoralis flap reconstruction in resection of anterior skull base tumors, *Auris-Nasus-Larynx (Tokyo)* 12:S143, 1985.

67. Sataloff RT, Bowman C, Baker SR, et al: Transfacial resection of intracranial tumor, *Am J Otol* 9:222, 1988.

68. Sataloff RT, Myers DL, Kremer FB: Management of cranial nerve injury following surgery of the skull base, *Otolaryngol Clin North Am* 17:577, 1984.

69. Scher RL, Cantrell RW: Anterior skull base reconstruction with the pericranial flap after craniofacial resection, *Ear Nose Throat J* 71:210, 1992.

70. Schramm VL Jr, Myers EN, Marron JC: Anterior skull base surgery for benign and malignant disease, *Laryngoscope* 89:1077, 1979.

71. Schwaber MK, Netterville JL, Coniglio JU: Complications of skull base surgery, *Ear Nose Throat J* 70:648, 1991.

72. Sekhar LN, Janecka IP, Jones NF: Subtemporal-infratemporal and basal subfrontal approach to extensive cranial base tumors, *Acta Neurochir (Wien)* 92:83, 1988.

73. Shah JP: Surgical approach to carcinoma of the nasal cavity, paranasal sinus with extension to the base of the skull, *Clin Bull* 82(2):61, 1978.

73a. Shah JP, Kraus DH, Arbit E, et al: Craniofacial resection for tumors involving the anterior skull base, *Otolaryngol Head Neck Surg* 106:387-393, 1992.

73b. Sisson GA, Toriumi DM, Atiyah RA: Paranasal sinus malignancy: a comprehensive update, *Laryngoscope* 99:143-150, 1989.

74. Snow RB, Kuhel W, Martin SB: Prolonged lumbar spinal drainage after resection of tumors of the skull base: a cautionary note, *Neurosurgery* 28:880, 1991.

75. Spetzler RF, Herman JM, Beals S, et al: Preservation of olfaction in anterior craniofacial approaches, *J Neurosurg* 79:48, 1993.

76. Spetzler RF, Pappas CTE: Management of anterior skull base tumors, *Clin Neurosurg* 37:490, 1991.

77. Spinelli HM, Persing JA, Walter B: Reconstruction of the cranial base, *Clin Plast Surg* 22:555, 1995.

78. Stell PM, Wood GD: The LeFort I osteotomy as an approach to the nasopharynx, *Clin Otolaryngol* 9:59, 1983.

79. Sundaresan N: Craniofacial resection for paranasal sinus tumors, *Indian J Cancer* 16(3/4):74, 1979.

80. Sundaresan N, Shah JP: Craniofacial resection for anterior skull base tumors, *Head Neck Surg* 10:219, 1988.

81. Tessier P, Guiot G, Rougerie J, et al: Osteotomies, cranio-naso-orbitofaciales pour hypertelorisme, *Ann Chir Plast* 12:103, 1967.

82. Thomsom JG, Restifo RJ: Microsurgery for cranial base tumors, *Clin Plast Surg* 22:563, 1995.

83. Uttley D, Moore A, Archer DJ: Surgical management of midline skull-base tumors: a new approach, *J Neurosurg* 71:705, 1989.

84. Van Buren JN, Ommaya AK, Ketcham AS: Ten-years experience with radical combined craniofacial resection of malignant tumors of the paranasal sinuses, *J Neurosurg* 28:341, 1968.

84a. Van Tuyl R, Gussack GS: Prognostic factors in craniofacial surgery, *Laryngoscope* 101:240-244, 1991.

85. Wei WI, Lam KH, Sham JST: New approach to the nasopharynx: the maxillary swing approach, *Head Neck* 13:200, 1991.

86. Weissler MC: Transoral approaches to the skull base, *Ear Nose Throat* 70(9):587-592, 1991.

87. Wood GD, Stell PM: The LeFort I osteotomy as an approach to the nasopharynx, *Clin Otolaryngol* 9:49, 1983.

CHAPTER

Prosthetic Reconstruction

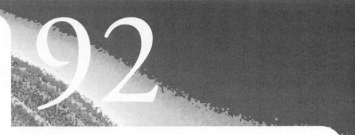

Gordon H. Wilkes
John F. Wolfaardt

INTRODUCTION

Over the past 15 years, the introduction of osseointegrated implants has radically altered the value of facial prosthetics to the surgeons concerned with reconstruction of the head and neck. This chapter will consider this development as it relates to reconstruction of defects of the ears, orbits, and midface. (Although osseointegrated implants are central to any discussion on jaw reconstruction, this subject is not addressed in this chapter.)

The history of facial prosthetics provides a fascinating lesson in the ingenuity of mankind in dealing with facial disfigurement.[7] In the past, technologic limitations frequently made facial prosthetics the method of last resort for both the surgeon and patient. The introduction of osseointegration biotechnology to head and neck reconstruction has forever altered this perspective. Craniofacial osseointegrated implant–supported prostheses now provide previously unavailable treatment options that can enhance the patient's quality of life.

HISTORICAL PROBLEMS WITH FACIAL PROSTHETICS

Historically, the essential problems that have always challenged the success of facial prostheses are the retention of the prosthesis and the inadequacies of facial prosthetic materials. For a facial prosthesis to be successful, it must meet the criteria of predictable retention, functional performance, aesthetic acceptability, and biocompatibility.[49]

In the past many materials have been used to construct facial prostheses, including metals, alloys, ceramics, waxes, resins, and rubbers. Silicone materials were introduced to facial prosthetics in 1960,[6] providing potential to produce a resilient prosthesis with useful durability. Many other materials have been investigated but silicones remain the material of choice for constructing facial prostheses.[21] More recent developments in materials, their manipulation, coloring, and techniques of prosthesis construction have greatly advanced the aesthetic and functional value of facial prostheses.

Facial prostheses have been retained by mechanical means, but in the past the majority of patients have relied on adhesives. Mechanical retention has depended on the engagement of divergent undercuts within the defect or the use of external devices such as spectacle frames or elasticized retention. Despite such ingenuity, these methods have seldom been of real value to patients. The use of adhesives continues to be plagued by concerns for damage to tissue surfaces, difficulty of manipulation, unpredictable performance, damage to the prosthesis, and additional cost to the patient.[9,29] The crudeness of these approaches to facial prosthesis retention remained the primary factor in limiting the success of facial prosthetic reconstructions.

Autogenous reconstruction of facial defects may at times be precluded, undesirable, or delayed. In these circumstances, prosthetic reconstruction becomes the treatment of choice. With the introduction of percutaneous osseointegration biotechnology to facial prosthetics, there was opportunity to provide secure and predictable retention without jeopardizing the integrity of the skin or prosthesis,[9] providing patients with previously unavailable reconstructive opportunities. Autogenous reconstruction and craniofacial osseointegration should not be seen as competing technologies but rather as complementary techniques that are essential to the successful management of patients requiring head and neck reconstruction.

HISTORY OF CRANIOFACIAL OSSEOINTEGRATION

Nephrology, cardiology, neurology, otolaryngology, orthopedic surgery, and plastic and reconstructive surgery have all demonstrated a need for a permanent percutaneous connection. As recently as 1981, according to the literature there were no studies that consistently demonstrated percutaneous devices being maintained in man or animals for longer than 3 months without failure due to infection.[40]

In 1975, based on the principles of osseointegrated dental implants, Albrektsson et al postulated that a skin-penetrating implant may be possible.[2] The principles of osseointegration

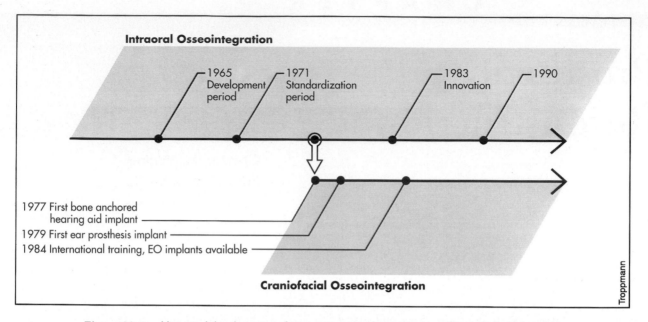

Figure 92-1. Historical development of osseointegration biotechnology. Through the Brånemark experience osseointegrated implants have been subjected to over 30 years of scientific scrutiny. Craniofacial applications were more recently introduced, with the first patient being treated in 1977.

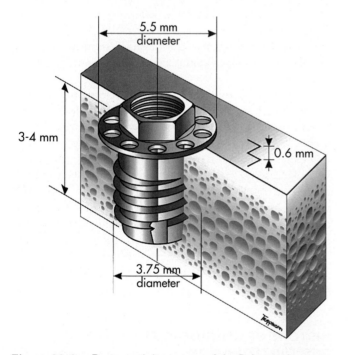

Figure 92-2. Design and dimensions of the Brånemark craniofacial osseointegration implant.

are well documented, and the outcomes of this modality of treatment in the management of edentulousness were already scientifically established in the early 1980s in longitudinal[1] and replication studies[50] (Figure 92-1). Based on the pioneering work by Brånemark and his co-workers, the first clinical trial on skin-penetrating osseointegrated implants was conducted in 1977 at Sahlgrenska Hospital in Göteborg, Sweden, where specifically designed implants (Figure 92-2) were

placed in the mastoid region to support a bone-conduction hearing aid.[2,37] In 1979, the first implants were placed in the mastoid region to retain an auricular prosthesis.[38] In May 1984, the biotechnology was released internationally with the training of interested clinicians in Göteborg.[48] The Swedish health system approved the bone anchored hearing aid in February of 1988. A state-of-the-art conference was held on September 1, 1988 in Göteborg to consider bone anchored implants in the head and neck region.[44] A report on this landmark conference was produced by the Swedish Council on Technology Assessment in Health Care.[19] This report remains as a founding document to the introduction of craniofacial osseointegration in head and neck reconstruction. From 1990 onward, numerous reports have confirmed the efficacy and predictability of craniofacial osseointegration.

ADVANTAGES OF CRANIOFACIAL OSSEOINTEGRATION

Reconstruction with craniofacial osseointegration has several advantages (Box 92-1). The surgical procedures are relatively short, straightforward, and can often be done on an outpatient basis under local anesthesia. There is seldom need to create a donor site. The technique is less demanding of the surgeon, the results are more consistent, and there is less postoperative morbidity. The prosthesis usually has greater similarity of form and color than usually achieved with an autogenous reconstruction. If, for whatever reason, a prosthesis is deemed unsatisfactory, a new prosthesis can be made to correct any shortcomings, usually a much simpler option than repeat autogenous reconstruction.

Box 92-1.
Advantages of Craniofacial Osseointegration

SURGICAL
Surgical procedure predictable
Surgical procedure relatively short and straightforward
Usually outpatient/short stay procedure
Short learning curve to consistent result
Can be performed under local anesthesia
Seldom need to create donor operative site
Less postoperative morbidity
Rescue option for failed autogenous reconstructions
Tumor resection site surveillance

PROSTHETIC
Predictable retention of prosthesis
Design options for retention system
Lower long-term costs than with adhesive retention
Increased prosthesis durability
Enhanced prosthesis aesthetics
Ease of placement
No skin damage
More successful incorporation of prosthesis into body image

Box 92-2.
Indications for Craniofacial Osseointegrated Implant–Retained Facial Prostheses

GENERAL INDICATIONS
No systemic/local factors that could obviously influence bone remodeling capacity
Age alone is not a contraindication
Patient who cannot tolerate a long surgical procedure
Patient who is a poor anesthetic risk
Compliant patient
No psychiatric or substance abuse conditions
Smoking is a relative contraindication
Radiation therapy is a relative contraindication
Tumor surveillance
Cognitive, visual, and dextrous ability to maintain osseointegrated implants
Geographic accessibility

INDICATIONS FOR EAR RECONSTRUCTION
Major cancer resection
Radiotherapy to area of reconstruction
Absence of lower half of ear
Severely compromised local tissue
Microtia
Costal cartilage calcification
Salvage procedure for failed autogenous reconstruction
Patient preference

INDICATIONS FOR ORBIT AND MIDFACE RECONSTRUCTION
Orbital exenteration
Severe enophthalmos with compromised vision
Extension of midface defect to oral cavity
Defects resulting in severe loss of facial contour

INDICATIONS FOR NOSE RECONSTRUCTION
Following removal of adequate autogenous reconstruction due to tumor recurrence
Failed autogenous reconstruction
Significant scarring in autogenous donor sites
Patient preference

INDICATIONS FOR CRANIOFACIAL OSSEOINTEGRATION

Craniofacial osseointegration provides invaluable treatment options for reconstruction of the ear, orbit, and midface. Indications and contraindications of craniofacial osseointegration can be separated into those that are general and those that are specific to the ear, orbit, and midface (Box 92-2).

GENERAL INDICATIONS

Osseointegration involves micromodeling at periosteal and endosteal surfaces, and remodeling at the bone-implant interface. Associated with these processes is a cellular and noncellular mineralization of remodeled bone. Any local or systemic process that influences these phenomena may jeopardize the integration of the implant. The literature cites many local and systemic factors that hold potential to interrupt the integrity of the bone-implant interface, yet few of these appear to be objective contraindications. Age alone is not a contraindication; patients as young as 2 to 3 years of age[15] and as old as 80 years of age are known to have been treated. Patient compliance is an important consideration in treatment selection in osseointegration, since the patient must be able to maintain the implants with a daily hygiene routine and be willing to return for follow-up visits. Certain psychiatric conditions and substance abuse may be contraindications to

treatment. Smoking is associated with a higher osseointegrated implant failure rate, so cessation of tobacco habits is advisable.[3] Dexterity and vision to accomplish hygiene routines or the availability of caregivers to perform these tasks is mandatory. Geographic accessibility is an important issue because follow-up assessment of the patient is important. Combined modality cancer therapy may considerably alter the individual implant success rate. The role of chemotherapy remains uncertain.[47] Radiation therapy can significantly reduce the individual implant success rate, and hyperbaric oxygen therapy may be required prior to implant placement.[13,14] The need for tumor surveillance is facilitated by having a prosthesis that is removable, thereby allowing for examination of the resection site.

INDICATIONS FOR EAR RECONSTRUCTION

Although treatment selection for ear reconstruction remains controversial, appropriate guidelines for when to select an autogenous or craniofacial osseointegrated implant approach are being developed.[42] Total loss of an ear following major cancer resection (Figure 92-3),[43] associated therapeutic radia-

tion, posttraumatic scarring, or severe burns may have compromised local tissues, making autogenous techniques difficult and thus favoring a craniofacial osseointegration approach (Figure 92-4). This may also apply to an absence of the lower half of the ear with poor surrounding tissue. In older adults where the costal cartilage has undergone calcification, autogenous reconstruction is very difficult and

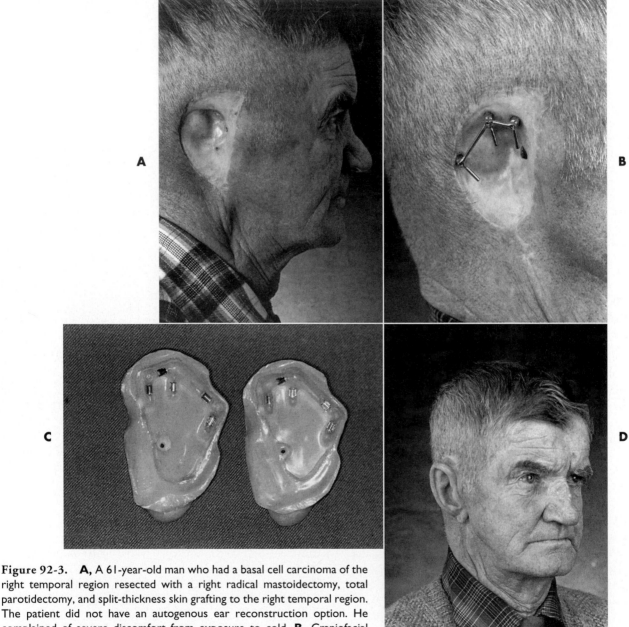

Figure 92-3. **A,** A 61-year-old man who had a basal cell carcinoma of the right temporal region resected with a right radical mastoidectomy, total parotidectomy, and split-thickness skin grafting to the right temporal region. The patient did not have an autogenous ear reconstruction option. He complained of severe discomfort from exposure to cold. **B,** Craniofacial osseointegrated implants were placed into the osseous rim of the defect and connected with a bar superstructure. **C,** The patient is always provided with two prostheses so that a spare prosthesis is always available. The acrylic resin substructure contains the clip retention elements. The only portion of the silicone prosthesis that contacts the skin surface is the anterior aesthetic and conchal bowl margins. **D,** A three-quarter view of the prosthesis connected to the patient. The removable prosthesis allowed for tumor surveillance. The patient no longer experienced discomfort from the cold.

craniofacial osseointegrated implants become the treatment of choice (Figure 92-5). Craniofacial osseointegration also provides an excellent salvage procedure for failed autogenous reconstructions.

Perhaps the most controversial indication surrounds the use of craniofacial implants in the child with microtia. Although it is technically possible to place implants in the young child and although early results are encouraging, the follow-up is relatively short. Autogenous reconstruction does not preclude the later use of craniofacial osseointegrated implants, but the creation of scarring in the area of a microtia associated with implantation precludes many later methods of autogenous approach. Given the medicolegal changes in several international jurisdictions arising from revisions in the statutes of limitations, those involved in auricular reconstruction would be well advised to fully inform patients of all treatment options.

An adhesive-retained auricular prosthesis is almost relegated to historical significance only. It certainly cannot be considered a "test" for an osseointegrated reconstruction. It offers none of the advantages of implant-retained prosthesis (i.e., ease of placement, predictable retention, enhanced aesthetics, increased longevity of the prosthesis, and no ongoing insult to the skin).

INDICATIONS FOR ORBIT, NOSE, AND MIDFACE RECONSTRUCTION

When the contents of the orbit have been radically disrupted or lost, the options for autogenous reconstruction are limited (Figure 92-6). Attempts at reconstruction of severe enophthalmos with a visually compromised eye do not always produce satisfactory results. When orbital contents are lost or when the defect extends beyond the orbit, flaps may be moved into the site but the results are sometimes less than aesthetic. When tumor surveillance is required, covering of the defect with a flap makes clinical examination of the site difficult and precludes self-examination. In all the above instances, craniofacial osseointegration may be useful (Figure 92-7).

In the midface, autogenous options might exist but where the defect extends to the oral cavity or orbit, osseointegrated implants may offer the most appropriate treatment option. In the isolated nasal defect, osseointegrated reconstruction is also a viable treatment option. Many of the same controversies in treatment selection between autogenous and craniofacial osseointegrated auricular reconstruction also exist when choosing the most appropriate technique for nasal reconstruction. Often patients do not want to

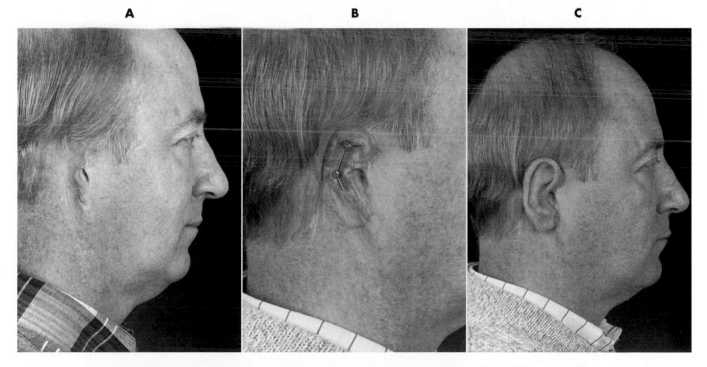

A   **B**   **C**

Figure 92-4. **A,** This 50-year-old man was involved in a motor vehicle accident, which resulted in total avulsion of the right ear. **B,** Two craniofacial osseointegrated implants were installed in the mastoid region and connected with a bar superstructure. The soft tissue surrounding the abutments has been flattened and thinned. There should be no relative motion between the periabutment tissue and the abutment. Note that the tragus has been maintained. **C,** The completed bar and clip-retained auricular prosthesis in position on the patient. Maintaining the tragus reduced the length of the anterior aesthetic margin.

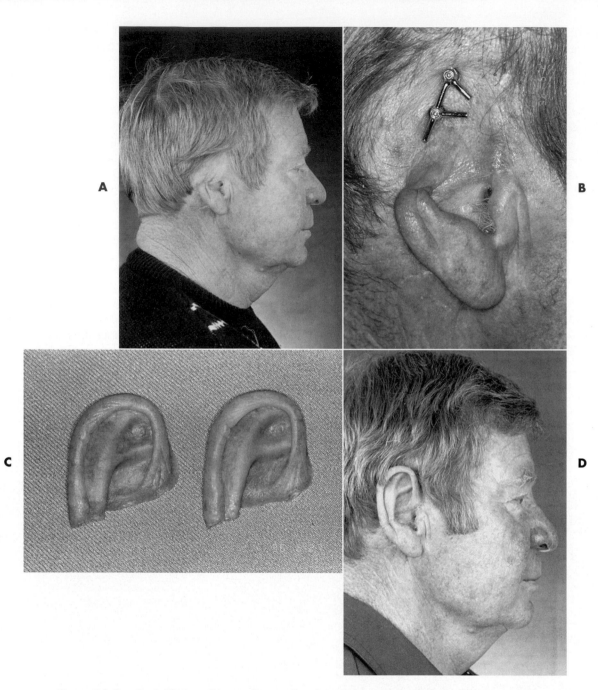

Figure 92-5. **A,** A 68-year-old man diagnosed with melanoma of the right ear. The upper half of the ear was resected, leaving the tragus, conchal bowl, lobule, and inferior helix and antihelix intact. Likely calcification of the costal cartilage made an osseointegrated implant–retained auricular prosthesis the treatment of choice. **B,** Two craniofacial osseointegrated implants were placed and connected with a bar superstructure. **C,** The two sectional auricular prostheses are intrinsically colored to match the skin. The color match was achieved with spectrophotometry and color formulation software. **D,** Profile view of the completed sectional auricular prosthesis.

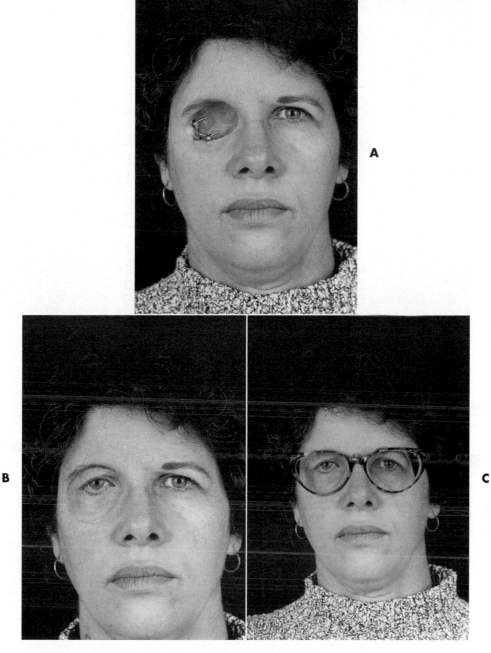

Figure 92-6. **A,** A 43-year-old woman who underwent a right orbital exenteration. The orbit was lined with a split-thickness skin graft, and the superior and inferior orbital rims lined with remnants of the upper and lower eyelids respectively. The upper eyebrow was drawn inferiorly into the orbit, resulting in a brow ptosis. The patient had attempted to wear an orbital prosthesis retained by intrinsic mechanical retention. This prosthesis resulted in repeated breakdown of the split-thickness skin graft, which produced great discomfort that prevented the patient from wearing the prosthesis. The ptosis was corrected with a brow lift. Craniofacial osseointegrated implants installed into the lateral and inferior orbital rims were connected with a bar superstructure. **B,** The completed bar and clip retained orbital prosthesis in position on the patient. The patient was able to wear the prosthesis continuously during waking hours without discomfort. **C,** The completed prosthesis with a spectacle frame used to enhance the aesthetic effect.

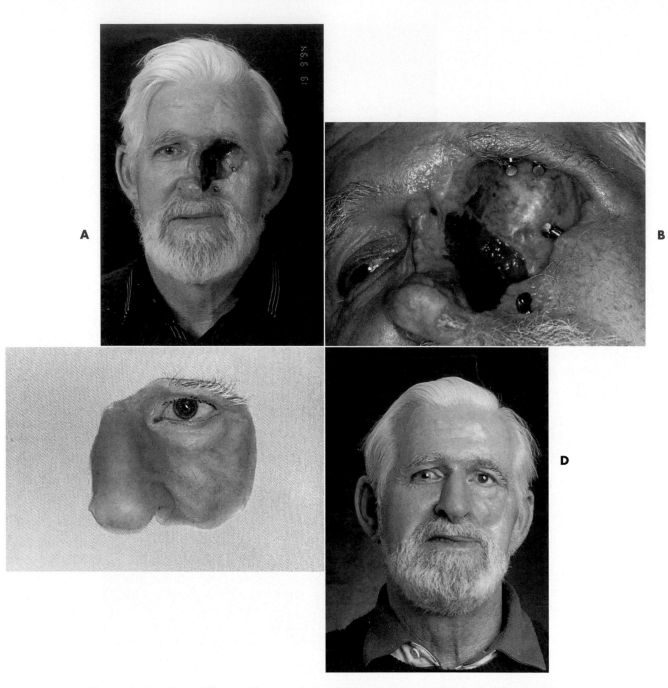

Figure 92-7. A, A 75-year-old man who underwent resection of a basal cell carcinoma resulting in exenteration of the left orbit and resection of the left face and nose. **B,** Craniofacial osseointegrated implants were installed in the supraorbital rim, the malar region, and the anterior maxilla. Special abutments have been connected to allow for magnet retention to be used away from the long axis of the implants. **C,** The silicone prosthesis is lightweight and only has contact with the tissues along the margin of the prosthesis. **D,** The magnet-retained prosthesis in position. This patient developed a recurrent lesion on the posterior wall of the defect. Because the prosthesis was removable, the recurrence was readily identified by the patient during daily self-examination. The lesion was resected, a temporalis flap brought in through the lateral orbital wall for coverage of the site of resection, and within 10 days, the patient could resume wearing his prosthesis.

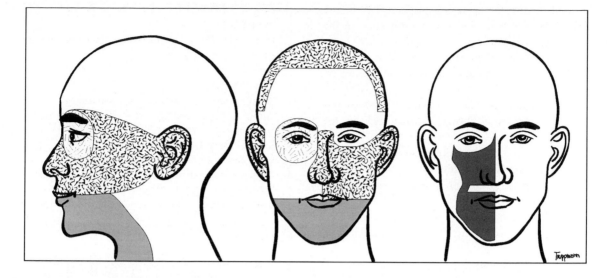

 Osseointegration and/or autogenous reconstruction

 Osseointegration reconstruction

 Autogenous reconstruction (soft tissue defect)

 Autogenous and osseointegration reconstruction

Figure 92-8. A rationale for treatment selection in the head and neck region. (Courtesy BF Conroy, JF Wolfaardt, GH Wilkes.)

undergo a multistaged reconstructive procedure requiring other donor sites with a higher morbidity and a more variable final result. When there has been severe loss of facial contour, reconstruction with an implant-retained facial prosthesis may be the best option. In such instances it may be necessary to use the combination of autogenous vascularized reconstruction of the osseous architecture and subsequent osseointegrated implants to support a facial prosthesis. An anatomic rationale for treatment selection is provided in Figure 92-8.

INFORMED CONSENT

Informed consent is essential to the success of craniofacial osseointegration treatment, not only for medicolegal reasons but also for patient education. In the authors' experience, for informed consent, an ISO 9000 approach to process control of the treatment pathway has been an important development. The intent is to ensure that the patient and family receive proper pretreatment education, are committed to treatment, are compliant, and fully appreciate their commitment to the postsurgery maintenance process. The patient receives formal pretreatment education and is psychologically screened through the work-up phase. The patient is allowed to enter the

treatment phase only when all clinical and patient based parameters are met.

The basic issues that the patient must be advised of are:
- The potential for individual implant success rates in the area of reconstruction.
- That usually two implants are placed to retain an ear prosthesis, three to six for an orbital prosthesis, two to three for a nasal prosthesis, and a variable number for larger defects.
- That surgery is usually conducted in two phases—the first to install the implants and the second 3 to 4 months later to connect the percutaneous abutment.
- That higher individual implant failure rates are associated with radiation therapy.
- That when the patient has been irradiated, additional implants may be installed due to the potential for higher implant failure rate.
- That if radiation therapy was administered, hyperbaric oxygen therapy may be indicated.
- That in irradiated patients, the time between the two phases of surgery is extended to 6 months. The consequence is that the duration of treatment is extended.
- That if osseointegrated implants are installed and the patient learns later in life that he or she is to be irradiated, the percutaneous abutment will need to be disconnected and the implants buried. Once the postradiation soft tissue effects have subsided, the percutaneous implants can be reconnected and the prosthesis returned to service.

- That if an implant fails, it may be possible to replace it. Use of the replacement implant will mean modification of the prosthesis or construction of a new prosthesis.
- That the ideal position for implants as determined during treatment planning may need to be adjusted during surgery. This may affect the ultimate aesthetic result.
- That changes in facial contour and symmetry surrounding the defect site cannot always be corrected by the prosthesis.
- That once the implants are placed, during healing it may not be possible to wear a previous prosthesis.
- That prosthesis construction requires multiple visits of long duration.
- That the prosthesis usually has a life of 2 to 5 years, depending on such factors as how the prosthesis is handled, skin secretions, smoking, and ultraviolet exposure.
- That maintenance visits are initiated after the second phase of surgery (percutaneous abutment connection). These visits are for monitoring the integration of the implant, skin response around the percutaneous abutment, and the condition of the prosthesis. Maintenance visits occur more frequently in the first year; once the skin response is satisfactory the maintenance visits occur annually.
- That in the case of an unscarred microtia, if implants are placed, most likely autogenous reconstruction options are precluded.
- That lifestyle issues may need to be addressed (e.g., head, ear, and eye protection in the work environment; contact sports; recreational activity in fast moving water).
- That smoking can result in a decreased individual implant success rate.

FUNCTIONAL AND PSYCHOSOCIAL CONSEQUENCES OF FACIAL DEFECTS

Absence, mutilation, or loss of a body part from the head and neck region may have a profound and negative impact on an individual, both functionally and psychosocially. The functional deficit associated with a head and neck defect is related to the extent and location of the defect. Because the head and neck area initiates the two main vegetative functions of man, respiration and alimentation (and their corollary functions, speech and swallowing), functional loss can be devastating (Box 92-3). The psychosocial consequences of a facial defect also have significant impact on an individual's quality of life,[30,31] resulting in withdrawal from social contact and destructive reclusive behavior.

Understanding the functional and psychosocial needs of the patient with a head and neck defect is essential to the preparation of the patient for craniofacial osseointegration treatment and will allow the patient to receive realistic expectations. When expectations are not realistic, the treatment should not be initiated.

Box 92-3.
Potential Deficits Associated with Defects of the Head and Neck

FUNCTIONAL
Loss/decreased masticatory function
Secondary occlusal trauma—few natural teeth carrying the load of the full dentition
Loss of taste/smell
Loss/interruption of swallowing reflex
Altered respiration
Loss of hearing/repeated ear infections
Speech defects—articulation problems/altered resonance
Loss/changes in vision
Chronic pain—local/phantom
Altered sensation—anesthesia/paresthesia
Loss/altered secretion control

PSYCHOSOCIAL
Depression
Denial
Interpersonal problems
Alienation
Persecutory ideas
Anxiety
Self-deprecation
Hypochondriasis
Thinking disorders
Social introversion

OPERATIONS

THE MULTIDISCIPLINARY TEAM

Providing craniofacial osseointegration care requires a patient-centered multidisciplinary team. The structure of the multidisciplinary team is considered essential if craniofacial osseointegration care is to be delivered appropriately. The multidisciplinary team can be divided into two levels, the core team and the full team. The core team should consist of a reconstructive surgeon, a prosthodontist, a dental technologist, an anaplastologist, and a nurse/dental assistant (Table 92-1). To optimize the potential of craniofacial osseointegration care, the full multidisciplinary team involves a wide range of clinical skills. The team assembled by the authors is shown in Box 92-4. Many of the issues in relation to craniofacial osseointegration require clinical personnel who possess psychomotor skills and a knowledge base specific to osseointegration biotechnology and more specifically to craniofacial applications. The individuals in the full team are not involved with every patient but are called on when required. These team members must have a distinct and identifiable relationship with and commitment to craniofacial osseointegration care.

Craniofacial osseointegration is protocol driven, and consequently a structured patient management system becomes essential. To meet this challenge, an ISO 9000 patient

Table 92-1.
The Core Team for Providing Craniofacial Osseointegration Care

DISCIPLINE	PRIMARY RESPONSIBILITIES
Reconstructive surgeon	Treatment planning Surgery Maintenance phase of care—surgical procedures
Prosthodontist	Treatment planning Assisting at surgery/involvement in intraoperative decisions Biologic phases of prosthetic treatment Supervision of maintenance phase of care
Dental technologist	Technical phases of prosthetic care
Anaplastologist	Aesthetic phases of prosthetic care
Nurse/dental assistant	Administer structured patient education Maintenance phase of care

Box 92-4.
The Full Multidisciplinary Craniofacial Osseointegration Team

CLINICAL DISCIPLINES
Surgeons
    Plastic and reconstructive surgeon
    Otolaryngologist
    Maxillofacial and oral surgeon
Prosthodontist
Dermatologist
Radiologist
Oral and maxillofacial radiologist
Hyperbaric medicine physician
Audiologist
Speech Pathologist
Dental Technologist
Anaplastologist
Psychologist
Social worker
OR Nurses
Dental assistants

SUPPORTING DISCIPLINES
Biomechanical engineer
Electrolysis technologist

ADMINISTRATIVE STAFF
Quality leader
Quality coordinator
Patient scheduler

management system has been developed for osseointegration. This system defines roles within the multidisciplinary team and provides the framework for treatment planning, active treatment, and maintenance of the patient group.

Internationally, several structures have emerged in teams providing craniofacial osseointegration care. Many of these structures are not patient centered and have become limited by historical professional politics, lack of knowledge of the appropriate role of disciplines, and misguided professional objectives. Clinicians wishing to become involved in providing craniofacial osseointegration care would be well advised to plan the structure of the team with foresight.

PREOPERATIVE TREATMENT PLANNING

An initial consultation is held between the surgeon, prosthodontist, patient, and supporting caregivers. At this consultation, general treatment options are discussed and appropriate written and visual material is supplied to the patient. When the patient decides to proceed with osseointegration treatment, an appointment is made with the prosthodontist for recording of preoperative records. At this visit:

- Charting for the specific osseointegration procedure is planned.
- Standardized preoperative photographic images are recorded.
- Preoperative psychologic profiling is undertaken.
- Desirable implant positions are marked on the skin surface and an impression of the area is recorded.

- In ear reconstruction, if indicated, an audiological assessment is scheduled.
- Imaging of the defect site is undertaken.

From the impression recorded, a diagnostic cast is constructed, which is used to construct templates to guide the surgeon for optimal implant placement.[8] The templates are also used for radiologic studies to determine bone availability. The templates are fashioned in clear resin sheet, have radiopaque markers installed to identify underlying osseous sites on the images, and have holes to locate the desired implant sites. Standard posteroanterior views are used for the orbit to determine the presence and extent of the frontal sinus. Panoramic views may be of assistance in the midface regions. With increasing frequency the primary planning tool is the computed tomography (CT) scanner in conjunction with an implant treatment planning software application. This planning tool allows simulation of the surgery so that the clinically determined implant positions can be related to the availability of underlying bone. The application preferred by the authors is the SIM/Plant System (Columbia Scientific Inc., Columbia, MD). A CT image is recorded according to a specific protocol, and this image is reformatted through the ImageMaster-101 Application (Columbia Scientific Inc., Columbia, MD). The reformatted image is then loaded into the SIM/Plant System where the implant surgery can be simulated. Among other things, this technique identifies desired sites of implant placement; locates vital structures; verifies implant sizes, positions, and angulations; and assesses available bone volumes, general bone densities, and bone densities around the implant. The use of this technology in treatment planning has proved invaluable (Figure 92-9).

Once it is determined that the patient can be accepted into the craniofacial implant program, a pretreatment education visit is scheduled. At this visit a structured approach is used to educate the patient on the full extent of the nature of the proposed treatment. If the patient decides to proceed with treatment, he or she signs a consent form that is specific to craniofacial osseointegration.

SURGICAL TECHNIQUE

The successful integration of osseointegrated implants requires that a stepwise protocol be followed during implant installation, with the operating room staff well educated and trained in the protocol. The instruments should be prepared according to the protocol, and the instrument and implant handling protocol should not be violated during the surgical procedure.[32] Osseointegration biotechnology is very specific in terms of material preparation, surgical protocol, and tissue preparation techniques.

The description of the surgery will provide information specific to the surgical technique and will not address the operating room protocol. The surgical technique is attributed to Tjellström and Bergström[32] unless indicated otherwise.

Surgery is conducted in two phases. The first phase is the installation of the implant and then after 3 or 4 months the second phase is the connection of the percutaneous abutment. In the mastoid region a "one-stage" approach has been used where both phases of surgery are conducted as one procedure. In the orbit and midface regions, and in therapeutically radiated patients, children, and compromised patients, a two-stage approach is used.

Fundamental Principles of Osseointegration Surgery

There are several fundamental principles to be observed with osseointegration surgery:

- The surface of the implant must not be contaminated during the surgical procedure. All powder is removed from gloves with careful glove washing.
- All gauze sponges are dampened with saline solution to bind loose fibers.
- All surgical drills are run for several minutes in a vertical position to dispose of excess oil. The handpieces are then dried with damp gauze sponges.
- Electrocoagulation is used very sparingly or avoided, particularly in the midface and orbit to reduce tissue trauma. This is especially important in the irradiated patient.
- Titanium instruments must not be contaminated. Titanium instruments are always used to manipulate titanium components and should not be allowed to come into contact with other materials.

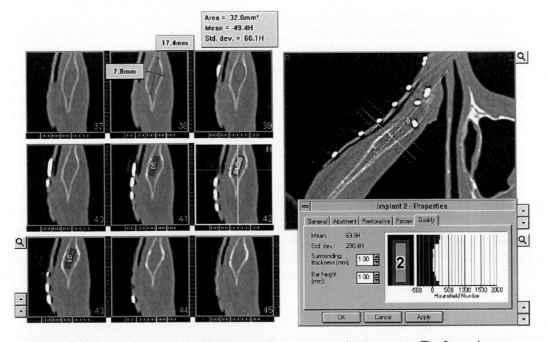

Figure 92-9. CT study with the SIM/Plant implant treatment planning system. The figure shows a study of vascularized scapula flap transferred to the infraorbital rim in a patient who underwent maxillectomy and orbital exenteration. The template with radiopaque markings can be seen along the skin surface of the infraorbital margin. The presence of a bone screw is also evident. Installation of an implant has been simulated and the figure shows the plot of bone density in Hounsfield units around the implant.

PHASE I SURGERY

Patient Preparation

The authors prefer to undertake the two phases of surgery under general anesthesia. When general anesthesia is contraindicated the procedure can be done with sedation and local anesthesia. With children general anesthesia is preferred.

The surgical field is prepared by washing with 10% povidone-iodine topical solution (Purdue Frederick Inc., Pickering, Ontario, Canada). The site is then draped in the usual way. Xylocaine with 1/100,000 adrenaline is infiltrated for hemostasis. If the site of implant installation communicates with the oral cavity, nasal cavity, or a paranasal sinus, it is advisable to apply a plastic adhesive-backed draping to the area.

Technique

The treatment planning template is placed in position and a needle coated with methylene blue is used to mark the position of the implants at the periosteal level. Once the incision line has been designed, sharp dissection is performed down to the level of the periosteum. The periosteum is exposed, and at each planned implant site, a hole 6 mm in diameter is made in the periosteum (Figure 92-10). Implant installation should be completed for one site before moving on to the next site. The first step is to confirm the availability of bone for implant installation by using a guide drill. A guide drill 3 mm in length is first used to drill a guide hole into the bone (Figure 92-11, *A*). Because this guide hole will influence the final angulation of the implant, correct angulation of the guide drill is important. The preparation of the implant sites using the guide drill is carried out at a speed of 2000 rpm. All bone drilling is carried out under abundant irrigation with saline at room temperature. Bone chips should be removed frequently from the flutes of the guide drill. As the guide holes are prepared, they are slightly widened with the drill to improve saline irrigation during the procedure. Once the guide hole

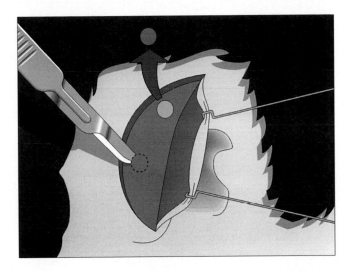

Figure 92-10. Reflected flap for ear reconstruction with osseointegrated implants. Once the sites of implant placement have been determined, a hole approximately 6 mm is made in the periosteum. The incision line should be placed a minimum of 1 cm away from the implant sites. (Courtesy Nobel Biocare.)

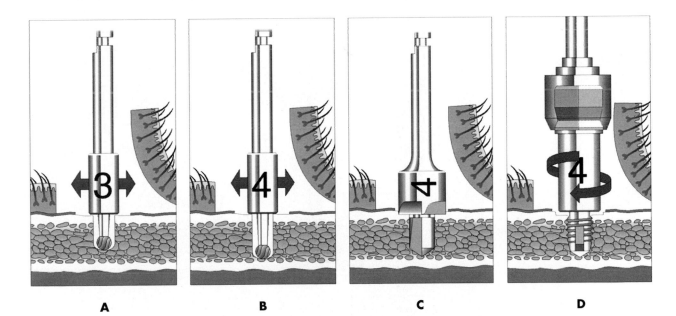

A   **B**   **C**   **D**

Figure 92-11. Preparation of the bone hole to receive the implant. **A,** A 3-mm guide drill is used at 2000 rpm to drill a pilot hole. **B,** If the base of the pilot hole is bony, a 4-mm guide drill is used to lengthen the pilot hole. The shoulder on the guide drills governs pilot hole depth. **C,** The countersink drill widens the bone hole and countersinks the bone for accommodating the flange of the implant. The countersink drill is used at 2000 rpm. The tip of the countersink drill is blunt to prevent tearing of the dura mater. **D,** The tap is used at 15-20 rpm with 30-40 Ncm of torque to create threads in the walls of the bone hole. All bone drilling is done under copious saline irrigation. (Courtesy Nobel Biocare.)

preparation is complete, the quantity and quality of bone in the walls of the guide hole are assessed. The base of the guide hole is repeatedly checked with a blunt instrument to determine that penetration of vital structures has not occurred. When adequate bone is found at the base of the guide hole, drilling is continued with a 4-mm guide drill. Again, the walls and base of the guide hole are assessed continuously.

The next step is to widen the guide hole for threading of the walls of the bone hole with a countersink drill 3 and then 4 mm in length, respectively (Figure 92-11, C), which not only widens the bone hole for threading but also prepares a flat countersunk area on the bone surface that allows the flange of the implant to have maximum contact with the bone surface. The tip of the countersink drill is blunt to limit the risk of damaging any soft tissue at the base of the bone hole.

Threading of the bone hole, the next step, is carried out at 15 to 20 rpm (Figure 92-11, D). The drilling unit controls the drill speed, and the drill torque should be adjusted on the drill unit to suit the quality of bone encountered. In compact cortical bone, a setting of 30 to 40 Ncm is recommended. In softer bone, the torque should be reduced accordingly. The titanium tap is connected to the drill handpiece, and it is of great importance that the tap is not touched with anything but a titanium-coated instrument. Abundant saline irrigation is essential during the tapping process. The tap is started with slight pressure against the prepared hole and its direction carefully oriented. If tapped in an unacceptable direction, the

bone hole probably cannot be retapped, and consequently the site will have to be abandoned. Once the tap is removed from the bone hole, if it is to be reused, the threads are cleaned with a titanium-cleaning needle and rinsed with saline.

The osseointegrated implant is supplied in a titanium cylinder that is housed in a sterile glass container. This container is opened over a titanium bowl. Again, there should be no contact between the titanium cylinder or implant and any surface that is not titanium. The implant is placed into a titanium organizer and picked up with a titanium implant mount (Figure 92-12, A). The implant mount is then connected to an adapter on the drilling handpiece (Figure 92-12, B), and the implant is threaded into the bone hole at 15 to 20 rpm and with appropriate torque without cooling for the first thread or two to prevent saline entering the space beneath the implant. If saline accumulates in the space as the implant is seated, it would be compressed into the marrow space in the bone. Once the first few threads have passed into the bone, saline irrigation is used until implant installation is complete. If great resistance is encountered during implant installation, the implant is removed and the source of resistance determined. Once the implant is fully seated with the drilling unit, a manually applied cylinder wrench is sometimes used for the final seating of the implant (Figure 92-12, C), taking care to prevent excessive torque, which could result in stripping of the bone threads. The implant mount is removed with caution so as not to loosen the implant in the bone threads, leaving the implant in place.

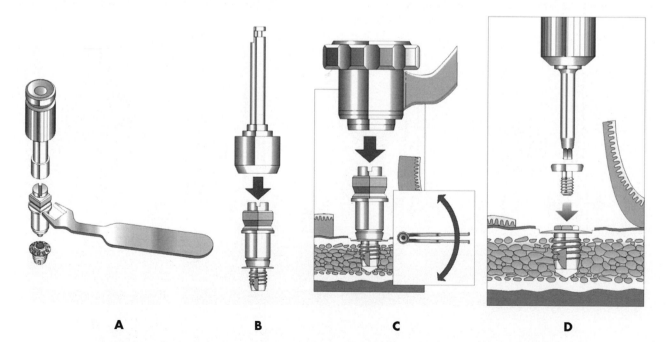

A **B** **C** **D**

Figure 92-12. Implant Installation. **A,** The craniofacial osseointegrated implant is connected to an implant mount. **B,** The implant mount is loaded into an adapter on the drilling unit handpiece. **C,** The implant is fed into the threads of the bone hole. A cylinder wrench is used to seat the implant fully. Again, this procedure is carried out under copious saline irrigation, but irrigation is only initiated after a few threads have entered the bone hole so as to prevent saline being compressed ahead of the implant during implant seating. **D,** The hexagonal head of the implant is covered with a cover screw and the soft tissues are closed. (Courtesy Nobel Biocare.)

The final step is to place a cover screw into the internal threads in the implant (Figure 92-12, *D*) to prevent bone ingrowth into the internal threads. The standard cover screw covers the hexagonal head of the implant, protecting it from bone overgrowth. If the tissues to be closed over the implant are thin or friable, a smaller space screw can be inserted. This screw only closes the internal threads of the implant and does not protect the hexagonal head of the implant.

The periosteum over the implant site is repositioned and sutured with resorbable sutures. When implant installation has been completed, the incision line is closed.

Postoperative Management

A standard dressing is placed over the surgical site for 1 to 2 days. The patient can usually return to normal activity 1 to 2 days after surgery.

In the mastoid and orbit region, the implants are left to heal for a period of 3 to 4 months to allow for the osseointegration process to occur. In the midface or in a therapeutically radiated patient, this period will be extended to 6 to 9 months.

PHASE II SURGERY

Objectives

There are a number of objectives to be achieved at Phase II surgery:

- The implants installed at Phase I surgery should be located and the percutaneous abutment should be connected.
- There should be no relative motion between the skin and the percutaneous abutment. To achieve this, the subcutaneous tissue should be removed so that the overlying skin is firmly attached to the periosteum.
- The skin surrounding the percutaneous abutment should be hairless. The absence of relative motion of the skin to the abutment and a hairless zone extending at least 1 cm around each abutment are two important prerequisites for establishing and maintaining a reaction-free skin penetration.
- Where the implant sites approach the hairline, thought should also be given to soft tissue preparation to account for slumping of the scalp due to the effect of gravity. This may require undermining the scalp under the hairline and removing subcutaneous tissue. The overlying hair-bearing tissue should be firmly attached to the underlying periosteum to prevent migration of hair-bearing scalp tissue into the site of the implant.
- Prior to Phase I surgery and particularly at Phase II surgery, careful consideration must be given to the position of the margins of the prosthesis. The surgeon should review this matter with the prosthodontist, since preparation of the soft tissue bed surrounding the abutments may have a profound effect on the design of the prosthesis, function, and aesthetic result. There are a number of issues to be considered:
  - In the case of an ear prosthesis, the ideal situation is to have a flat tissue bed surrounding the percutaneous abutments. Where possible, the only cartilaginous remnant to be maintained is the tragus. If this is possible, the anterior aesthetic margin of the prosthesis consists only of the area of the root of the helix and the lobule area.
- In ear reconstruction, it is best to leave any remaining cartilaginous remnants in place. Then at Phase II surgery, once the implants have been located and it is confirmed that they have integrated, the cartilaginous remnants can be removed.
- In the case of an orbit, the walls of the orbit have usually been grafted with a split-thickness skin graft. The implants are best positioned on the inner surface of the orbital rim so that the percutaneous abutment does not procline and, in doing so, interfere with the construction of the orbital prosthesis. This position of the orbital implants will frequently mean that the flange of the implants is covered in part by the split-thickness skin graft lining the walls of the orbit, which is unlikely to survive over the implant flange, creating a hygiene hazard that the patient cannot maintain. To overcome this, adequate soft tissue coverage should be brought into the area to fully cover the flanged implant. In doing this, however, it is important not to produce ptosis of the eyebrow.
- In defects of the orbit and midface, it is difficult to conceal the aesthetic margin of the prosthesis. Careful thought must therefore be given to the soft tissue contours surrounding the defect.
- In preparing the soft tissue surrounding the abutments, it is not desirable to create a step deformity between the surrounding tissue and the tissue adjacent to the abutment.

Patient Preparation

The choice of anesthesia discussed in the section on Phase I surgery applies to Phase II surgery. Prior to preparing and draping the patient, the surgical site is carefully assessed to locate the sites at which implants were placed. Photographic images recorded at the time of implant placement are extremely helpful in designing the position of the skin incision. The skin incision should be positioned at least 10 mm away from the site of the implant (Figure 92-13). Consequently, a different incision line from that used for Phase I surgery may be needed.

Technique

Once the flap is raised, the subcutaneous tissue is reduced to leave a very thin skin layer. Any hair follicles present in the skin flap should be removed. To avoid creating steps in the soft tissue around the implant site, a subcutaneous tissue reduction is performed along the periphery of the surrounding tissue (Figure 92-14, *A*). The objective is to develop a gradual sloping edge toward the implants. If the periosteal layer is thick, it should also be thinned. The skin edges are sutured down to the periosteum. At this point, the skin should be less than 1 mm thick so that the head of the implant should be visible through the overlying skin. If not, further subcutaneous tissue reduction should be undertaken.

If the skin overlying the site of the implant is deemed unsuitable or carries excessive hair follicles that cannot be removed, a non–hair-bearing skin graft may be required.

A skin punch or 4-mm-diameter disposable biopsy punch is used to punch holes over the site of the implants (Figure

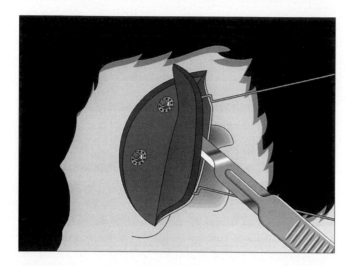

Figure 92-13. Abutment connection. The site at which the implants were installed is determined. The incision line is placed to pass a minimum of 10 mm away from the sites of abutment connection. (Courtesy Nobel Biocare.)

92-14, *B*). The cover screws are then removed, and the head of the implant is checked and cleaned to ensure that all soft tissue debris is removed. The abutments are available in lengths of 3, 4, and 5.5 mm. The abutment is placed over the head of the implant and rotated until it is fully seated onto the hexagonal head of the implant (Figure 92-14, *C*). The internal screw of the abutment is then tightened into the implant.

Plastic healing caps are then screwed into the internal screw of the abutment. The plastic healing caps are 6.5 or 14 mm in diameter, depending on the space between the abutments. Once the healing caps are screwed down into place, antibiotic ointment–soaked gauze dressing is wound underneath the healing caps to prevent hematoma during the initial healing period (Figure 92-14, *D*).

Postoperative Management

At the completion of surgery, a dressing is applied over the healing caps. This dressing is removed and replaced by a smaller dressing on the day after surgery. Antibiotics are not usually required at Phase II surgery.

Five to seven days after surgery, the healing caps and gauze pressure dressing are removed. The area is cleaned with great care and the wound is aerated for an hour. The healing caps are then replaced, and a new antibiotic ointment–soaked gauze is put in place to maintain slight pressure on the periabutment

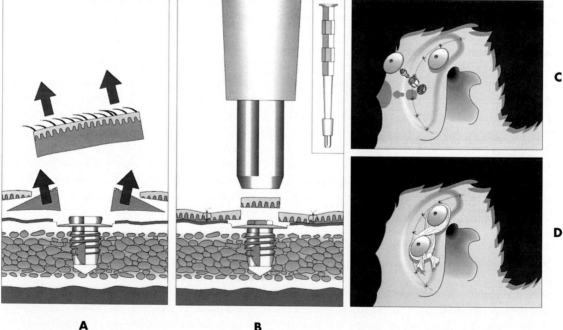

A   **B**

Figure 92-14. Soft tissue reduction and abutment connection. **A,** Hair-bearing tissue should not surround the abutment, and a hairless zone 10 mm from the abutment should be created. The periabutment tissues should be thinned to eliminate relative motion between the periabutment soft tissue and the abutment. Additionally, a step in the soft tissues surrounding the abutment should not be created. **B,** The soft tissue flap is sutured in place, and a tissue punch is used to expose the head of the implant. **C,** An abutment of the correct length is selected and connected to the implant with the abutment screw. A plastic healing cap is screwed onto the abutment. **D,** An antibiotic-soaked gauze is wound around the plastic healing caps to produce pressure on the periabutment tissues. (Courtesy Nobel Biocare.)

tissue. This dressing is left in place for another 5 to 7 days when the healing caps and gauze are removed and the area is left open. The patient is then placed on a maintenance schedule to be discussed below.

ONE-STAGE SURGERY

The two-stage procedure described is considered the clinical routine; however, more recently, one-stage surgery has been conducted under certain circumstances.[33,34] It is suggested that the one-stage procedure only be used in the mastoid region in selected cases that meet the following criteria[32]:

- The patient is an adult.
- The patient has not been therapeutically irradiated.
- The cortical layer of bone is >3 mm in thickness (a 4-mm implant is used)
- Surgery is uneventful and has no contact with the dura mater or the wall of the sigmoid sinus.

The surgical technique is essentially the same, except that Phase I surgery and Phase II surgery are conducted in the same operation, requiring that both the skin and periosteum be lifted at the same surgery. Cover screws are not required, since the abutments are connected and healing caps placed.

Postoperative Management

Postoperative care is essentially the same as that described following routine Phase II surgery. It is very important that the gauze dressing placed under the healing cap not produce excessive pressure on the flap because with the one-stage procedure both the periosteal and skin layers are vulnerable and there is a higher incidence of periabutment soft tissue necrosis.[33]

Following one-stage surgery, the implant-abutment assembly must be protected from any mechanical insult for at least 3 to 4 months to allow the osseointegration process to occur. Initial mechanical stability of the implant-abutment assembly is thus very important. The patient should be advised to sleep on the opposite side of the head and to avoid any mechanical insult to the abutment. Three to four months of healing is allowed before the initiation of prosthesis construction.

MAINTENANCE PROTOCOL

Following removal of the gauze dressing from beneath the healing caps, the area is left open. The patient is advised to apply antibiotic ointment (mupirocin) once a day to the periabutment tissue and not to wash the area. The maintenance protocol is initiated 2 weeks following Phase II surgery. By this stage the large diameter healing caps have been replaced with healing caps the same diameter as the abutment. At the 2-week visit, the area is very gently cleaned.

The patient returns for maintenance visits 1 month, 3 months, 6 months, 12 months, 18 months, and 24 months after Phase II surgery, and annually thereafter. At these visits, several parameters are monitored (i.e., level of hygiene control around the percutaneous abutment; response of skin; the mechanical stability of the abutment-implant assembly; the duration that the prosthesis is worn on a daily basis). The patient's hygiene routine is reviewed and any appropriate alteration in strategy made.

The maintenance visits form an essential part of craniofacial osseointegration care and are extremely valuable from a preventative point of view, ensuring that contact is never lost with the patient and that the patient understands the need for a lifetime commitment to maintenance of the implants.

PROSTHETIC MANAGEMENT

Four to six weeks after Phase II surgery, the tissues have healed sufficiently well to initiate prosthetic treatment. There are a variety of approaches to prosthetic care that again vary with different anatomic sites. The following section outlines some of the general stages in auricular prosthesis construction. For a more detailed description of prosthetic techniques, the reader is referred elsewhere.[36,45,46]

Impression copings are connected to the abutments with guide pins (Figure 92-15, A). Impression material is then used to record the skin surface and the abutments. Material that will set to a rigid form, such as impression plaster, is applied around the impression copings and guide pins (Figure 92-15, B).

Once the impression has set, the guide pins are unscrewed and the impression is removed. Abutment replicas are then connected to the impression copings. A cast of the impression is then poured in white die stone (Figure 92-15, C).

The cast is recovered from the impression, and this forms the working cast (Figure 92-15, D). The surface of the working cast is a replica of the patient's tissues, with the abutment replicas providing a precise representation of the abutments on the skin surface. From the planning templates, the relationship of the abutments to the overlying prosthesis can be determined. The bar superstructure is designed to lie under the antihelix. Gold cylinders are connected to the abutment replicas with gold screws, with a gold bar to connect the gold cylinders. An acrylic resin substructure is then constructed to house the retention clips that connect to the gold bar (Figure 92-16, A). The design of the retention elements of the prosthesis addresses the biomechanics of bone loading.[9,10]

The prosthesis is sculpted in wax and related to the acrylic resin substructure. When anatomically acceptable, with the skin-contacting margins of the prosthesis correct, a mold is constructed using a lost wax technique (Figure 92-16, B).

Silicone elastomer is colored to match the patient's skin color (Figure 92-16, C). The surface of the acrylic resin substructure is chemically primed so that the silicone elastomer bonds to the acrylic resin. The various colored elements of silicone elastomer are introduced into the mold, and the mold is closed for processing.

The prosthesis is recovered from the mold, trimmed, and fitted to the patient (Figure 92-16, D). Minor adjustments to the color of the prosthesis can be made with extrinsic colorants.

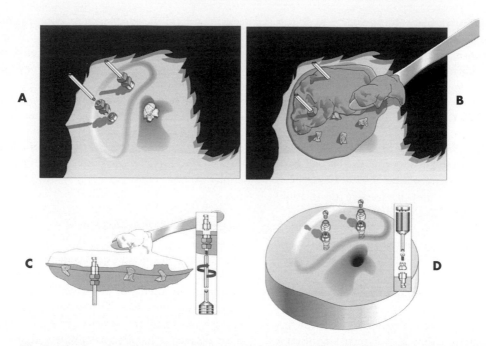

Figure 92-15. Impression recording and cast construction. **A,** Impression copings are connected to the abutment with long guide pins. **B,** An impression is recorded first in a resilient impression material, and this is backed with a rigid supporting material. **C,** The guide pins are unscrewed and the impression recovered. Abutment replicas are connected to the impression copings in the impression. The cast is then poured in a die stone. **D,** The cast is recovered from the impression and gold cylinders are connected to the abutment replicas with gold screws. (Courtesy Nobel Biocare.)

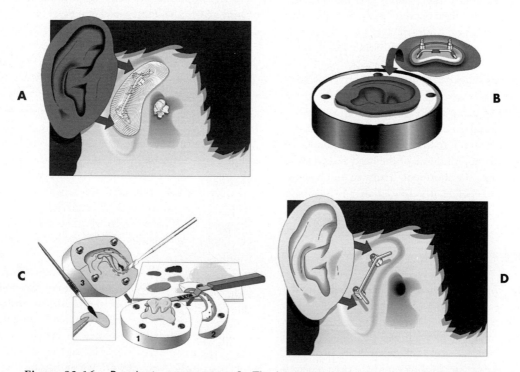

Figure 92-16. Prosthesis construction. **A,** The bar superstructure is constructed. An acrylic resin substructure, which houses the clip retention elements, is constructed. The prosthesis is sculpted in wax to locate on the acrylic resin substructure. **B,** A mold is constructed and this is usually done in gypsum products as a two-part or multipart mold. **C,** Using a lost wax technique, the wax pattern of the prosthesis is eliminated from the mold. Silicone is then colored to match the patient's skin and this is layered into the mold. **D,** The prosthesis is recovered from the mold, trimmed, finished, and fitted on the patient. (Courtesy Nobel Biocare.)

ANCILLARY AUTOGENOUS PROCEDURES

Although craniofacial osseointegration is well documented in the literature, in most cases the reports view osseointegrated reconstruction in isolation from autogenous reconstruction. Many patients present with complex deformities that can best be managed by a combination of both autogenous and osseointegration techniques. Often in these situations, patients have both bony and soft tissue defects that must be addressed in conjunction with the osseointegration procedure. In a series of 27 patients treated with craniofacial osseointegration, 14 required ancillary procedures.[20] The many procedures that have been employed are listed in Box 92-5. Examples of ancillary autogenous procedures are provided in Figures 92-17 and 92-18. An important discussion currently is the reconstruction of maxillary defects as an ancillary autogenous procedure for osseointegration. The goals of the ancillary procedures in combined orbital-maxillary defects are to decrease the size of the facial prosthesis, place the prosthesis margins at the junction of a facial aesthetic unit, decrease the size of the maxillary obturator, improve facial contour, and bring viable bone into the region for implant placement. Many

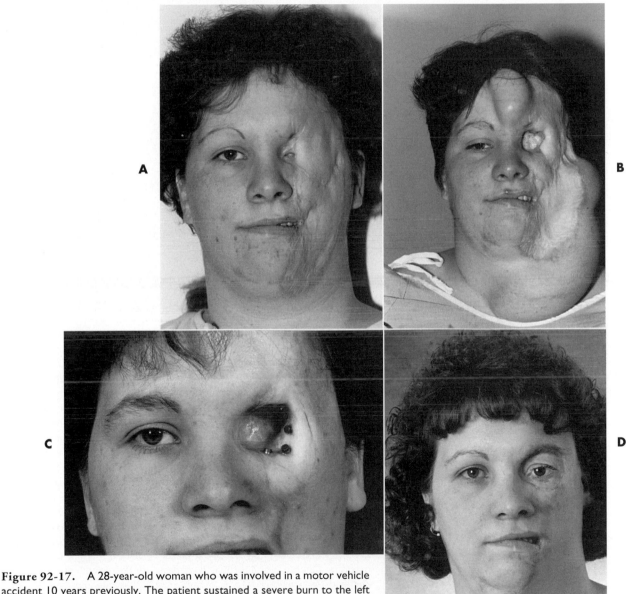

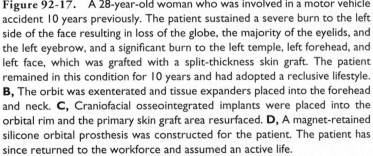

Figure 92-17. A 28-year-old woman who was involved in a motor vehicle accident 10 years previously. The patient sustained a severe burn to the left side of the face resulting in loss of the globe, the majority of the eyelids, and the left eyebrow, and a significant burn to the left temple, left forehead, and left face, which was grafted with a split-thickness skin graft. The patient remained in this condition for 10 years and had adopted a reclusive lifestyle. **B,** The orbit was exenterated and tissue expanders placed into the forehead and neck. **C,** Craniofacial osseointegrated implants were placed into the orbital rim and the primary skin graft area resurfaced. **D,** A magnet-retained silicone orbital prosthesis was constructed for the patient. The patient has since returned to the workforce and assumed an active life.

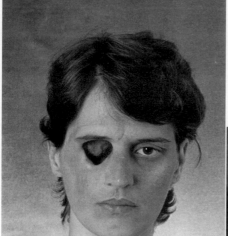

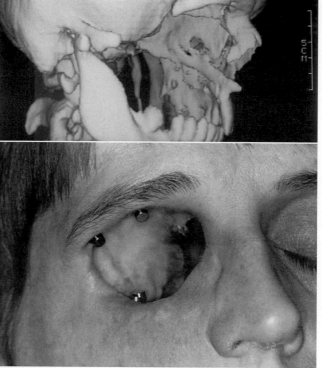

Figure 92-18. **A,** A 34-year-old woman who had an osteosarcoma of the right maxilla resected with a maxillectomy and right orbital exenteration. **B,** Three-dimensional CT scan reconstruction shows the extent of the defect. The defect involved the loss of the maxilla on the right side, and loss of the contents, floor, and lateral wall of the right orbit, with extension along the zygomatic arch to just anterior to the articulatory eminence of the temporomandibular joint. **C,** The three-quarter view demonstrates the serious loss of facial contour associated with the defect. It is not possible to construct a prosthesis for this patient without surgical reconstruction of the facial contours, since the prosthesis would not be able to compensate for the lost contours of the face. **D,** A vascularized scapula flap has been used to reconstruct the right facial contour. Craniofacial osseointegrated implants have been placed into the superior orbital rim and longer intraoral implants have been placed into the vascularized scapula flap. This approach has the added advantage of reducing the size of the maxillary obturator and allowing the maxillary obturator and orbital prosthesis to be treated as separate elements that may be linked. **E,** Profile view to illustrate improvement in facial contour. The vascularized scapula bone flap has produced a manageable facial contour for the prosthetic reconstruction.

approaches have been advocated for immediate or delayed reconstruction of the maxilla. In a comparative study of bone thickness in four vascularized bone flaps it was found that in males the iliac crest, scapula, fibula, and radius all had adequate bone volume for implant placement.[11] In elderly females, the scapula and radius did not have adequate bone volume to place osseointegrated implants. More recently, Brown[4] has distinguished between low level and high level defects of the maxilla and advocates the use of the deep circumflex iliac artery (DCIA) free flap where osseointegrated implants are to be considered. When a high level defect extends laterally, as in Figure 92-18, *B*, a greater length of bone is required to span the defect. In this type of defect the authors advocate the use of a vascularized scapula bone flap.

OUTCOMES

In the assessment of outcomes with craniofacial osseointegration care, the focus has been on individual implant success rates and skin response. More recently, other parameters have been reported, including patient response to craniofacial osseointegration care.

INDIVIDUAL IMPLANT SUCCESS RATES

In a study evaluating treatment outcomes on 389 percutaneous abutments in 174 patients,[2] 49 patients were treated with auricular prostheses, 18 with orbital prostheses, two with nasal prostheses, and the remainder with bone anchored hearing aids. Six of the 389 implants inserted were not integrated at Phase II surgery; five of the six failures were determined to be in irradiated bone. It was concluded that the individual implant success rate in nonirradiated bone was 99.7%, and in therapeutically radiated bone 85.3%; the overall success rate was 98%.

Ten-year follow-up results on 94 patients treated for auricular replacement with craniofacial implants were reported

by Tjellström.[38] Thirty patients had been followed for longer than 5 years and 52 for more than 3 years. A total of 303 implants had been placed for ear replacement, and 244 percutaneous abutments had been connected with no patient being lost to follow-up. The lower number of abutments connected as opposed to implants placed was attributed to the early experience of additional implants being placed in case of implant failure. Initially, three or four implants were placed in the mastoid, and this study confirmed the current practice of only two implants being needed to retain an auricular prosthesis.

Parel and Tjellström[28] reviewed the craniofacial osseointegration work of one Swedish and 13 U.S. centers. They considered implants inserted into patients who had received radiation therapy versus those who had not been treated with radiotherapy. The study confirmed that implant placement in the mastoid region provided high success, with a combined-center success rate of 98.3% in nonradiated patients. The combined-center success rate with orbital implants in nonradiated patients was reported as 93.9%. Success rates in the midface and in therapeutically radiated patients proved more variable. The combined-center individual implant success rate was 61.1% for irradiated patients. In some anatomic locations the number of patients treated was too small to draw firm conclusions. It was concluded that the therapeutically radiated patient should be approached with caution and in an environment that fully appreciates the risks associated with external beam therapy.

A study undertaken in 1992 assessed craniofacial osseointegrated implants used for retaining facial prostheses over a 5-year period.[27] In this study, which included 70 auricular and 17 orbital prosthesis patients, the prosthesis was worn for at least 6 months. The study found that integration in the orbit was not as successful as in the mastoid region, which had a more predictable 95% success rate for implants that had been inserted and then exposed, loaded, and connected. Osseointegrated implants in the orbit that were connected through the skin achieved an individual implant success rate of 72%. An important observation was that failures in the mastoid occurred within 6 months after insertion, whereas orbit failures tended to occur later, sometimes as late as 6 years after insertion. Of the 19 implants in the orbit that failed, 16 were in therapeutically radiated bone. The success rate in therapeutically radiated orbits was 62.7% and in nonradiated orbits 92.1%. This study was significant because it attempted to prescribe criteria for evaluating individual implant success in craniofacial osseointegration (Box 92-6) and it identified that installation of implants in therapeutically radiated bone was a challenge.

A 1993 study considered the early Canadian results and combined them with the Swedish and U.S. results.[48] In all three countries, similar rates of individual implant success in nonradiated patients were noted with a combined success rate of 97.5%. In the irradiated group, the success rate was 69.4%. The success rate in irradiated patients was highest in Canada, declining respectively in the United States and then Sweden; the differences were primarily attributed to duration of follow-up, with the longest follow-up period being in Sweden and the shortest in Canada. As the follow-up time increased, the success rate was expected to decline for irradiated patients. It must be kept in mind that at the time of publication of this study, hyperbaric oxygen therapy was not routinely considered in the management of the therapeutically radiated patient treated with osseointegrated implants.

In 1995 the U.S. Food and Drug Administration (FDA) approved the Brånemark craniofacial implant system. Tolman and Taylor[39] reported on the results of a prospective trial initiated in 1988 in the United States for the FDA. This involved 24 centers and 145 patients provided with craniofacial osseointegrated implant–retained facial prostheses. Throughout the life of the study 115 patients were evaluated and reviewed for at least 30 months. Of the 452 implants, 318 were inserted in the auricular, 98 in the orbital, and 36 in the nasal regions. Of these, 77 implants were not evaluated because they were not uncovered. The success rates reported for the nonradiated group followed throughout the study were very similar to those reported in previously cited studies: auricular 99% (85 patients); nasal 94% (6 patients); and orbital 100% (14 patients). The results in the irradiated patients differed from previously discussed studies in that fewer losses in the orbit were noted. The success rates reported in irradiated patients followed throughout the study were: auricular 100% (2 patients); nasal 100% (1 patient); and orbital 90% (7 patients).

Tjellström and Granström[33] reported their results, which compared patients treated with one- and two-stage procedures for bone anchored hearing aids and auricular prostheses. In the one-stage surgery approach a 16% skin graft failure was found and thought due to compromised vascularity of the graft, a result of the graft and underlying periosteum being elevated at the same time. The two-stage procedure group showed no graft failure. The two groups were found to differ only in terms of graft necrosis and not implant success. This work recommends the use of a 4-mm-long implant for one-stage procedures and that the one-stage procedure be used only for the mastoid. One-stage procedures should not be undertaken in children or in irradiated bone.

Hyperbaric oxygen therapy has been shown to significantly mitigate the loss of craniofacial osseointegrated implants in irradiated bone. In 1994, Granström and co-workers[14,16,18] found that with the use of hyperbaric oxygen therapy, no implant losses had occurred during a 5-year follow-up period involving 48 implants placed in irradiated orbital, nasal, and temporal regions. Furthermore, they noted that when radiotherapy or chemotherapy was administered to areas where osseointegrated implants had already been installed, skin dehiscence sometimes occurred and two of 32 implants were lost with induction of chemotherapy.[17] They concluded that implants should be disconnected and buried if they are to be irradiated.

SKIN RESPONSE

Skin response to percutaneous craniofacial abutments has been considered an important parameter of success and is evaluated by a five-point scale that emanated from the work of Holgers et al[23] in 1987 and has been adopted widely (Box 92-7). Holgers et al[24] studied 136 implants for auricular prostheses over a 3- to 66-month period. A total of 708 observations of skin response were made, of which 647 observations (91.4%) were negative and 27 (3.8%) demonstrated slight redness. In a further study, Holgers et al[23] evaluated 313 observations on 67 bone anchored hearing aid abutments, of which 292

Box 92-6.
Criteria for Success for Craniofacial Osseointegrated Implants as Proposed by Jacobsson et al[27]

- Individual unattached implants should be immobile when tested clinically.

- Soft tissue reactions around skin-penetrating abutments should be of types 0 (reaction free) or 1 (slight redness, not demanding treatment) in more than 95% of all observations.

- Individual implant performance should be characterized by the absence of persistent and/or irreversible signs and symptoms such as pain, infections, neuropathies, or paresthesia.

- In the context of the above, a success rate of 95% in the mastoid process and 90% in the orbital region, in nonirradiated bone tissue, at the end of a 5-year observation period should be a minimum criterion for success.

Box 92-7.
Classification of Skin Response to Percutaneous Craniofacial Osseointegrated Abutments

0 = No irritation: Epithelial debris removed if present

1 = Slight redness: Temporary local treatment

2 = Red and slightly moist tissue; no granuloma formation: Local treatment; extra controls

3 = Reddish and moist; sometimes granulation tissue: Revision surgery is indicated

4 = Removal of skin-penetrating implant necessary due to infection

From Holgers K-M, Paulsson M, Tjellström A, et al: Selected microbial findings in association with percutaneous titanium implants, *Int J Oral Maxillofac Implants* 9:565-570, 1994.

(93.3%) showed no reaction and 13 (4.2%) showed slight redness.[22,25] In 1994, Holgers[26] published a monograph based on doctoral work that examined skin response to skin-penetrating titanium implants, grading skin response, as well as morphologic, microbiologic, and immunologic changes.

Tjellström[38] reported on 244 percutaneous abutments used to retain auricular prostheses. The skin response was assessed at three periods separated by 2-year intervals. The three periods sequentially reported grading of no reaction as 92.9%, 88.8%, and 89.3% over the 4 years. Of great interest was the finding that 15% of patients accounted for 70% of skin reactions, suggesting that a small group of patients account for the majority of observed adverse skin reactions.

Tjellström et al[35] considered the skin response in eight pediatric patients ranging from 6 to 11 years of age. Assessment of 113 observations of skin response on 26 percutaneous abutments revealed 95 (84.1%) observations of no skin response. It was noted that behavioral problems and lack of compliance with hygiene measures were encountered with two of the subjects on reaching adolescence.

Skin response was assessed in seven patients treated with BUD implants (BUD Industries, East Aurora, NY): five patients with auricular prostheses; one with an orbital prosthesis; and one with a hair replacement prosthesis. The parameters assessed were sebaceous crusting, presence of a peri-implant exudate, skin cultures, implant mobility, and tissue response characterized by type, thickness, contour and attachment, mobility, and reaction. Interestingly, these researchers proposed a four-point grading of skin response based more on a typical inflammatory response. The study reported that two patients had an adverse skin response, one patient having a mild response and the other moderate to severe. Cultures grew normal skin flora except for the two patients with adverse skin reactions who grew *Staphylococcus aureus.* This finding was in agreement with that of Holgers.[26]

Based on the Holgers grading system, Tolman and Taylor[39] discussed the findings of 1872 observations of skin response during a 30-month period of assessment of patients with orbital, nasal, and auricular prostheses. It was found that 4% of observations recorded an adverse tissue response.

QUALITY OF LIFE

Outcome assessments of craniofacial osseointegrated implants have been preoccupied with the integrity of the bone-implant interface and the skin-abutment interface, since these are critical to tolerance of the implant.

More recently, there has been growing interest in documenting patient perceptions of treatment. Those involved in providing craniofacial osseointegration care share the common subjective experience that the vast majority of patients, if properly educated to have appropriate levels of expectation, seem delighted with their implant-retained facial prosthetic reconstructions. Although there is a developing surge of interest in measuring patient responses to craniofacial osseointegration treatment, little scientific data on the subject exist.

Of 94 patients assessed in one study on ear reconstruction with craniofacial implants, only two patients were found to not wear their prostheses.[38] The study did not indicate why they chose not to wear them.

Tolman and Taylor[39] attempted to evaluate patient-perceived changes after undergoing craniofacial osseointegration treatment. A questionnaire was administered at enrollment into the study and at 6 and 18 months after prosthesis connection. A telephone survey was also conducted on 30 patients. According to the questionnaire, at the time of enrollment, only 50% of patients with a nonimplant-retained prosthesis considered the prosthesis stable. Eighteen months after craniofacial implant prosthesis connection, 93% of patients rated the implant prosthesis stable. A summary of the results of the questionnaire is provided in Table 92-2. Of the 30 patients who

Table 92-2.
Patient-Perceived Changes After Craniofacial Osseointegration Treatment[39]

PARAMETER EVALUATED	BEFORE CRANIOFACIAL OSSEOINTEGRATION TREATMENT (%)	18 MONTHS AFTER CRANIOFACIAL OSSEOINTEGRATED IMPLANT PROSTHESIS CONNECTED (%)
Prosthesis stability	50	93
Acceptable appearance of prosthesis	31	72
Self-conscious about prosthesis	36	77
Insertion of prosthesis	39	91
Removal of prosthesis	58	91
Ability to clean area	55	65
Activities not limited by prosthesis	38	83
Removal of prosthesis no more than once a day	68	89

Table 92-3.

Swedish Comparison of Costs for Nonimplant- Versus Craniofacial Osseointegrated Implant–Retained Prosthesis Treatment Over a 10-, 25-, and 70-Year Period[19]

PROSTHESIS TYPE	SAVINGS ACHIEVED WITH CRANIOFACIAL OSSEOINTEGRATION		
	10-YEAR SAVINGS (%)	25-YEAR SAVINGS (%)	70-YEAR SAVINGS (%)
Auricular/nasal	36	46	49
Orbital	34	46	50

Table 92-4.

Initial Cost of Nonimplant- Versus Craniofacial Osseointegrated Implant–Retained Prostheses

PROSTHESIS TYPE	NONIMPLANT RETAINED ($CANADIAN)	CRANIOFACIAL OSSEOINTEGRATED IMPLANT RETAINED ($CANADIAN)
Auricular	2800	8823
Nasal	2800	10,424
Orbital (including ocular prosthesis)	4600	12,830
Expected life of prosthesis	1 year	+2-3 years

participated in a telephone poll, 19 wore the prosthesis more than 12 hours per day; 3, 8 to 12 hours; 3, 4 to 8 hours; and 5, less than 4 hours. Remarkably, 24 of the 30 patients viewed the prosthesis as an extension of themselves. The authors concluded that craniofacial osseointegration demonstrated a significant improvement in quality of life when compared to previous retention systems for facial prostheses.

The authors have developed a questionnaire that considers issues related to the prosthesis and quality of life. The patient is asked to respond on a five-point scale so that 60% represents an equivocal response. The results of the responses of 24 patients who had worn a craniofacial implant–retained prosthesis for not less than a year found an average response to treatment of 84%.

COSTS OF CARE

Because implantable biotechnologies carry significant cost, financial impact is an important consideration in introducing craniofacial osseointegration care. In this regard, it is of value to consider the relative costs of autogenous recon-

struction, craniofacial osseointegration, and adhesive-retained prostheses.

A 1989 Swedish report compared the cost of providing nonimplant- versus implant-retained prostheses over a 10-, 25-, and 70-year period (Table 92-3).[19] Over time, there were substantial savings found with the craniofacial implant–retained prostheses. The Swedish report also concluded that the costs of autogenous and craniofacial implant ear reconstructions with 10-year follow-ups were comparable.

At first glance, the adhesive-retained prosthesis appears far less costly an approach. This prosthesis will usually require replacement at least annually, a result of its degradation from the adhesive and the solvent used to remove the adhesive. The craniofacial osseointegrated implant–retained prosthesis has, in the authors' experience, a life expectancy in excess of 2 to 3 years. The costs of providing an adhesive-retained prosthesis and a craniofacial osseointegrated implant–retained prosthesis are provided in Table 92-4. The costs of an auricular reconstruction over a 20-year period are calculated in Table 92-5. In Table 92-5, it is noted that a break-even point for adhesive- and craniofacial osseointegrated implant–retained prostheses is 5 years; thereafter

Table 92-5.
Long-Term Costs of Treatment for an Auricular Reconstruction

TIME INTERVAL (YEARS)	ADHESIVE RETAINED ($CANADIAN)	CRANIOFACIAL OSSEOINTEGRATED IMPLANT RETAINED ($CANADIAN)	AUTOGENOUS RECONSTRUCTION ($CANADIAN)
1	4200	8823	12,673
5	11,200	10,923	
10	21,000	17,523	
20	39,200	26,223	
Maintenance Costs*	4000	3525	
Total Costs	43,200	29,748	
Potential Savings (%)†	31%		

*Maintenance costs over 20 years.
†Potential savings when comparing a craniofacial osseointegrated– with an adhesive-retained auricular prosthesis over 20 years.
Note: 1. Costs are calculated on present value and are not inflation adjusted.
  2. Adhesive-retained prostheses costs are based on annual replacement with a new mold being constructed every third year.
  3. Craniofacial osseointegrated–retained prostheses costs include all hospitalization and surgery costs (at the rate for Alberta residents). The costs are based on a new mold being constructed at every third prosthesis remake.
  4. Autogenous reconstruction includes all hospitalization (at the rate for Alberta residents) and surgery costs.

the osseointegration approach provides savings in the cost of care.

THE FUTURE

Craniofacial osseointegration provides patients with options for care that were not believed possible even a relatively short time ago. The individual implant success rate and the skin response to the percutaneous abutment have been documented for over 15 years. Internationally, percutaneous craniofacial osseointegration biotechnology is now in routine use for bone anchored hearing aids and for facial reconstruction. There is a great deal of innovation surrounding the use of this biotechnology, and it provides fertile ground for future research and development that will spill over into many other disciplines. In common with all osseointegration applications, work is needed to further understand, enhance, and control the process of osseointegration. Chemical and biomechanical modulation of the bone-implant interface will continue to be a focus for future research. The biomechanics of craniofacial osseointegration is in its infancy but is an area considered of great significance for the future. Defining the risks associated with local and systemic factors that may affect the bone-implant interface will be important. The modulation of the skin-abutment interface is relatively unexplored and needs much research. In the craniofacial applications, better definition of treatment options will provide an important challenge. A more complementary relationship between osseointegrated implant and autogenous options needs to be fostered through clinical and research endeavors. Objective methods of assessment of the potential of an individual's bone to integrate an osseointegrated implant must be made clinically usable. Imaging tools for implant planning are emerging and proving to be extremely helpful in treatment planning, but need further development and interfacing with engineering applications for designing prosthesis superstructures. Interfacing imaging with computer numerically controlled (CNC) tools for cast and prosthesis construction, improvement of facial prosthetic materials, and the development of active facial prostheses are fertile areas for future research and development. Assessment of the clinical parameters and the patient response to treatment is an area requiring immediate investigation, as are the effects on growth and the potential for complications arising from a lifetime presence of a skin-penetrating abutment on pediatric patients.

There are many other areas of research related to craniofacial osseointegration biotechnology that provide important opportunities for developments. These developments will have broad impact on reconstructive and rehabilitative care throughout medicine in the future. Combined with innovations in key areas such as tissue engineering, surface control, numerical process control, materials, and implantable devices, prosthetic reconstruction will in the future provide patients with remarkable functional and aesthetic opportunities.

ACKNOWLEDGMENTS

We would like to thank Dr. Anders Tjellström, Dr. Gösta Granström, and Dr. Kerstin Bergström for their assistance with the description of the craniofacial osseointegration technique. Additionally, we wish to recognize them for the collegial manner in which they teach, research, and collaborate. We wish also to thank Nobel Biocare AB, Göteborg, Sweden, for allowing us to use illustrations from their *Operating Theatre Manual*. These illustrations (Figures 92-10 to 92-16) were from those produced by Fredrik and used with Nobel Biocare's permission.

REFERENCES

1. Adell R, Lekholm U, Rockler B, et al: A 15-year study of osseointegrated implants in the treatment of the edentulous jaw, *Int J Oral Surg* 10:387-416, 1981.

2. Albrektsson T, Brånemark P-I, Jacobsson MD, et al: Present clinical applications of osseointegrated percutaneous implants, *J Plast Reconstr Surg* 79:721-730, 1987.

3. Bain CA, Moy P: The association between the failure of dental implants and cigarette smoking, *Int J Oral Maxillofac Implants* 8:609-615, 1993.

4. Brown JS: Deep circumflex iliac artery free flap with internal oblique muscle as a new method of immediate reconstruction of maxillectomy defect, *Head Neck* 18:412-421, 1996.

5. Casselman JW, Vrielinck LGJ, Rathé J: Preoperative computed tomography (CT) evaluation of the temporal bone in patients with external and internal ear deformation within the perspective of endosseous implant surgery. In Ars B, editor: *Congenital external and middle ear malformations: management,* Amsterdam, 1992, Kugler, pp 12-26.

6. Conroy BF: The history of facial prostheses, *Clin Plast Surg* 10:689-707, 1983.

7. Conroy BF: A brief sortie into the history of cranio-oculofacial prosthetics, *Facial Plast Surg* 9:89-115, 1993.

8. Coss P, Wolfaardt JF, Wilkes GH: Surgical templates for auricular reconstruction, *J Facial Somato Prosthet* 2:131-136, 1996.

9. Del Valle V, Faulkner MG, Wolfardt JF, et al: Mechanical evaluation of craniofacial osseointegration retention systems, *Int J Oral Maxillofac Implants* 10:491-498, 1995.

10. Del Valle V, Faulkner MG, Wolfaardt JF: Craniofacial osseointegrated implant-induced strain distribution: a numerical study, *Int J Oral Maxillofac Implants* 12:200-212, 1995.

11. Froedel JL, Funk GH, Capper DT, et al: Osseointegrated implants: a comparative study of bone thickness in four vascularized bone flaps, *J Plast Reconstr Surg* 92:449-455, 1993.

12. Gitto CA, Plata WG, Schaaf NG: Evaluation of the peri-implant epithelial tissue of percutaneous implant abutments supporting maxillofacial prostheses, *Int J Oral Maxillofac Implants* 9:197-206, 1994.

13. Granström G: The use of hyperbaric oxygen to prevent implant loss in the irradiated patient. In Worthington P, Brånemark P-I, editors: *Advanced osseointegration surgery: applications in the maxillofacial region,* Chicago, 1992, Quintessence, pp 336-345.

14. Granström G, Bergström K, Tjellström A, et al: A detailed analysis of titanium implants lost in irradiated tissues, *Int J Oral Maxillofac Implants* 9:1-10, 1994.

15. Granström G, Bergström K, Tjellström A: The bone-anchored hearing aid and bone-anchored epithesis for congenital ear malformations, *Otolaryngol Head Neck Surg* 109:46-53, 1993.

16. Granström G, Jacobsson M, Tjellström A: Titanium implants in irradiated tissue: benefits from hyperbaric oxygen, *Int J Oral Maxillofac Implants* 7:15-25, 1992.

17. Granström G, Tjellström A, Albrektsson T: Postimplantation irradiation for head and neck cancer treatment, *Int J Oral Maxillofac Implants* 8:495-501, 1993.

18. Granström G, Tjellström A, Brånemark P-I, et al: Bone-anchored reconstruction in the head and neck cancer patient, *Otolaryngol Head Neck Surg* 108:334-343, 1993.

19. Hallèn O, Magnusson S, Jacobsson M, et al: *Bone-anchored implants in the head and neck region,* Report from a conference, 1988, The Swedish Council on Technology Assessment in Health Care.

20. Harris L, Wilkes GH, Wolfaardt JF: Autogenous soft-tissue procedures and osseointegrated alloplastic reconstruction: their role in the treatment of complex craniofacial defects, *Plast Reconstr Surg* 98:387-392, 1996.

21. Heller HL, McKinstry RE: Facial materials. In McKinstry RE, editor: *Fundamentals of facial prosthetics,* Arlington, 1985, ABI, pp 79-97.

22. Holgers K-M, Paulsson M, Tjellström A, et al: Selected microbial findings in association with percutaneous titanium implants, *Int J Oral Maxillofac Implants* 9:565-570, 1994.

23. Holgers K-M, Tjellström A, Bjursten L-M, et al: Soft tissue reactions around percutaneous implants: a clinical study of soft tissue conditions around skin-penetrating titanium implants for bone-anchored hearing aids, *Am J Otol* 9:56-59, 1988.

24. Holgers K-M, Tjellström A, Bjursten L-M, et al: Soft tissue reactions around percutaneous implants: a clinical study of soft tissue conditions around skin-penetrating titanium implants for bone-anchored auricular prostheses, *Int J Oral Maxillofac Implants* 2:35-39, 1987.

25. Holgers K-M, Tjellström A, Thomsen P, et al: Morphologic evaluation of clinical long-term percutaneous titanium implants, *Int J Oral Maxillofac Implants* 9:689-697, 1994.

26. Holgers K-M: *Soft tissue reactions around clinical skin-penetrating titanium implants,* Göteborg, Sweden, 1994, University of Göteborg, Thesis Monograph.

27. Jacobsson M, Tjellström A, Fine L, et al: A retrospective study of osseointegrated skin-penetrating titanium fixtures used for retaining facial prostheses, *Int J Oral Maxillofac Implants* 7:523-528, 1992.

28. Parel SM, Tjellström A: The United States and Swedish experience with osseointegration and facial prostheses, *Int J Oral Maxillofac Implants* 6:75-79, 1991.

29. Parel SM: Diminishing dependence on adhesives for retention of facial prostheses, *J Prosthet Dent* 43:552-560, 1980.

30. Pruzinsky T: The psychology of plastic surgery: advances in evaluating body image, quality of life, and psychopathology, *Adv Plast Reconstr Surg* 12:153-172, 1996.

31. Stephanson S: Psychological dimensions in rehabilitative treatment of craniofacial deformities (thesis), 1994, University of Alberta, p 7.

32. Tjellström A, Bergström K: Operating theatre manual: craniofacial rehabilitation, Göteborg, Sweden, 1995, Nobel Biocare.

33. Tjellström A, Granström G: One-stage procedure to establish osseointegration: a zero to five years follow-up report, *J Laryngol Otol* 109:593-598, 1995.

34. Tjellström A, Granström G: The one-stage procedure for implants in the mastoid. In Albrektsson T, Jacobsson M, Tjellström A, editors: *Third international winter seminar: implants in craniofacial rehabilitation and audiology,* Göteborg, Sweden, 1993, Department of Handicap Research, University of Göteborg, p 46.

35. Tjellström A, Jacobsson M, Albrektsson T, et al: Use of tissue integrated implants in congenital aural malformations, *Adv Otorhinolaryngol* 40:24-32, 1988.

36. Tjellström A, Jansson K, Brånemark P-I: Craniofacial defects. In Worthington P, Brånemark P-I, editors: *Advanced osseointegration surgery: applications in the maxillofacial region,* Chicago, 1992, Quintessence, p 293-312.

37. Tjellström A, Linström J, Hallén O, et al: Osseointegrated titanium implants in the temporal bone, *Am J Otol* 2:304-310, 1981.

38. Tjellström A: Osseointegrated implants for replacement of absent or defective ears, *Clin Plast Surg* 17:355-366, 1990.

39. Tolman DE, Taylor PF: Bone-anchored craniofacial prosthesis study, *Int J Oral Maxillofac Implants* 11:159-168, 1996.

40. von Recum AF, Park JB: Permanent percutaneous devices, *CRC Crit Rev Bioeng* 5:37-77, 1981.

41. Watson RM, Coward T, Forman GH, et al: Considerations in treatment planning for implant-supported auricular prostheses, *Int J Oral Maxillofac Implants* 8:688-694, 1993.

42. Wilkes GH, Wolfaardt JF: The auricular defect—treatment selection. In Brånemark P-I, Tolman DE, editors: *Osseointegration in craniofacial reconstruction,* Chicago, 1998, Quintessence.

43. Wilkes GH, Wolfaardt JF: Osseointegrated alloplastic versus autogenous ear reconstruction: criteria for treatment selection, *Plast Reconstr Surg* 93:967-979, 1994.

44. Williams E: *A matter of balance,* ed 1, Novum Grafiska AB, Goteborg, Sweden, 1992, Akademiförlaget, p 145.

45. Wolfaardt JF, Coss P, Levesque R: Craniofacial osseointegration: technique of bar and acrylic resin substructure construction for auricular prostheses, *J Prosthet Dent* 76:603-607, 1996.

46. Wolfaardt JF, Coss P: An impression and cast construction technique for implant-retained auricular prostheses, *J Prosthet Dent* 75:45-49, 1996.

47. Wolfaardt JF, Granström G, Friberg B, et al: A retrospective study on the effects of chemotherapy on osseointegration, *J Facial Somato Prosthet* 2:99-107, 1996.

48. Wolfaardt JF, Wilkes GH, Parel SM, et al: Craniofacial osseointegration: the Canadian experience, *Int J Oral Maxillofac Implants* 8:197-204, 1993.

49. Wolfaardt JF, Wilkes GH: Craniofacial osseointegration, *J Can Dent Assoc* 60:805-809, 1994.

50. Zarb GA, Symington JM: Osseointegrated dental implants: preliminary report on a replication study, *J Prosthet Dent* 50:271-276, 1983.

CHAPTER

Facial Reanimation

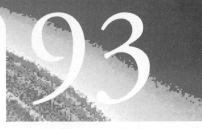

Ronald M. Zuker
Barry L. Eppley

INTRODUCTION

Facial paralysis causes a very visible deformity with widespread consequences from both a functional and psychosocial standpoint. The absence or reduction in function of the facial muscles can lead to an inability to control the facial orifices, the eye and mouth, leading to corneal exposure or chronic irritation of the eye, as well as an oral droop with resultant incompetence manifested by drooling and pocketing of food within the mouth. This deformity may be further accentuated by hyperactivity of the remaining muscles of the ipsilateral (incomplete unilateral facial paralysis) or opposite (complete unilateral facial paralysis) face. From a psychosocial viewpoint, the lack of facial muscular movement can affect self-confidence, professional advancement, social interaction, and the enjoyment of life (Figure 93-1).

The origin of facial paralysis may be congenital or acquired. In the congenital or developmental form, the facial musculature does not develop. This may not be complete and, in fact, usually there is some facial activity. These are mostly unilateral facial palsies and, more rarely, bilateral (e.g., Möbius' syndrome). The most common of the acquired deformities is Bell's palsy, which usually results in spontaneous and complete recovery without the need for surgical intervention. This leaves posttraumatic injuries, neoplastic involvement and resection, and other postinfective conditions (e.g., Ramsay Hunt syndrome) of the facial nerve as postnatal causes of dysfunction.

The anatomy of the facial nerve and the muscles that it innervates has been well described in many articles and surgical textbooks. From a functional and reconstructive standpoint, the facial muscles (17 in number) are essentially a series of three sphincteral mechanisms that operate the eye, nose, and mouth and provide both contraction and expansion of these orifices. This complex three-dimensional muscular arrangement can make restoration of any orifice function difficult, and often unsatisfactory, with any one operation (Figure 93-2).

INDICATIONS

In acute facial nerve transections or resections, primary nerve repair and nerve graft provide for the most complete recovery of muscle function and are superior to any method of secondary reconstruction. Injuries to the facial nerve distal to a line dropped perpendicular from the lateral canthus may not need to be repaired or reconstructed because of the numerous anastomotic branches at that level (see Figure 93-2). Although complete return of motion of the affected muscles is possible, the intricate kinetic harmony of the facial motions is sometimes marred by synkinesis or mass muscle movement, especially when main trunk injuries are repaired. When, however, lack of facial nerve innervation to the muscles is long-standing (greater than 18 to 24 months), the neuromuscular end plates undergo fibrosis and the possibility of reinnervating the affected musculature is lost. In this group of patients, secondary reconstructive procedures to provide either static suspension or muscle transfer/transplants for more dynamic activity must be done.

The operative indications and techniques utilized for facial reanimation are different, depending on the orifice involved. In the periorbital region, most procedures are of a static or minimally dynamic nature, are relatively easy to perform in terms of operative time and invasiveness, and can be carried out almost regardless of patient age or medical condition. Reanimation of the mouth, however, has a wide variety of options that need to be carefully selected for each individual patient; among the deciding factors are the patient's degree of lip droop, functional impairment, age, health, and desire for repositioning versus dynamic activity.

A wide array of operations for facial orifice reconstruction have been described.[18] These procedures can be categorized into those designed to correct ocular and oral deformities, those that provide for static suspension to improve facial asymmetry at rest, and those that result in either eyelid or oral commissure motion with facial animation. In general, static procedures are indicated in older patients with chronic facial palsies in whom more complex methods of facial reanimation would not be well tolerated or would have a low rate of success

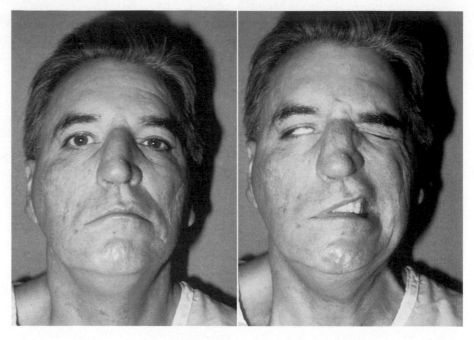

Figure 93-1. Complete right-sided unilateral facial nerve palsy of 4 months' duration caused by neoplastic infiltration by adenoid cystic carcinoma of the parotid gland. **A,** At rest, note flattening of frontalis wrinkles, elevation of upper lid secondary to unopposed levator action, slight lower lid ectropion, flattening of the nasolabial crease, shift of the right nasal ala toward the unaffected left side, and mild drooping of the commissure. **B,** On activation of the contralateral normal side, these changes are accentuated, causing a grotesque asymmetry.

A, B

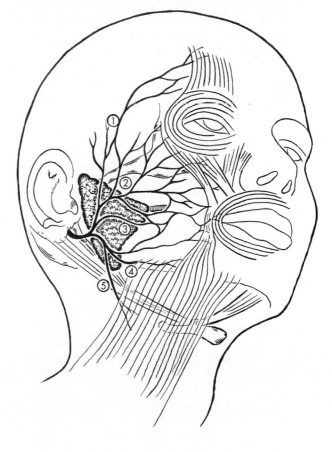

Figure 93-2. Anatomy of the facial nerve. The main trunk branches at the pes anserinus into various patterns of the five main branches. In the midface, there are numerous distal anastomoses between the buccal and zygomatic branches; however, the temporal and marginal mandibular branches have few interconnections with adjacent branches. *1,* Temporal branch; *2,* zygomatic branches; *3,* buccal branches; *4,* marginal mandibular branch; *5,* cervical branch.

(Figure 93-3), or in partial nerve palsies that may be mitigated by lesser procedures (Figure 93-4).

Facial reanimation implies that the facial musculature can be restored to dynamic activity or that motion can be created around the involved facial orifice. To be accurate therefore, most facial paralysis operations do not result in muscle reani-

mation. Short of metal insertions (weights, magnets, or springs) in the upper eyelid, only muscle transfers or transplants can produce dynamic motion. The transplantation of a single skeletal muscle cannot be expected to reproduce the intricate and coordinated movements of the facial musculature. Muscle transplantation can, however, be directed toward oral commis-

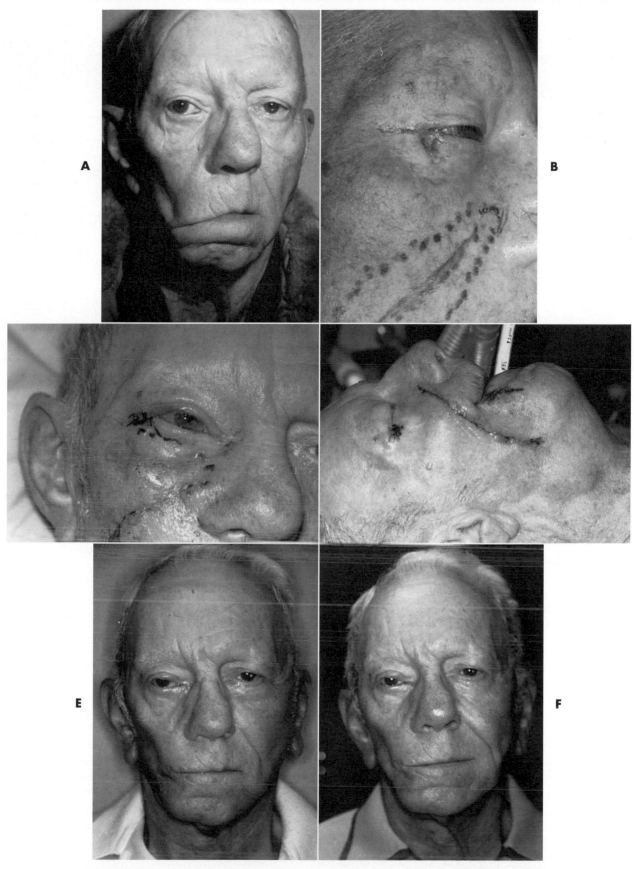

Figure 93-3. **A,** Chronic complete right facial palsy of 20 years' duration secondary to acoustic neuroma. Note more pronounced commissure drooping than in Figure 93-1, where there was still some muscle tone. The ectropion had been addressed by previous canthoplasty but still resulted in chronic intermittent corneal exposure and irritation. **B** to **D,** Z-plasty lateral canthoplasty and resuspension of eyelid combined with resection of the nasolabial skin and elevation of the commissure. **E,** Results at 3 months. **F,** Result at 1 year.

A   **B**   **C**

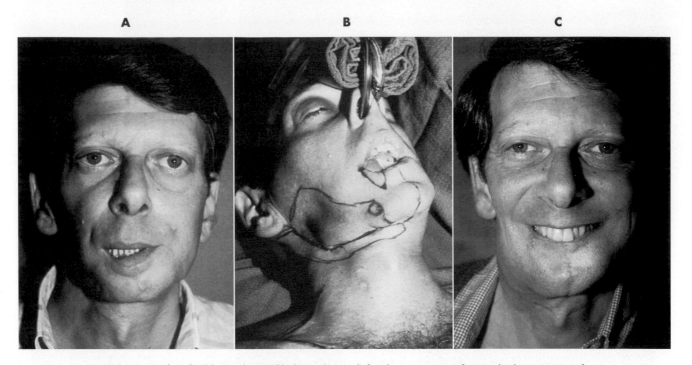

Figure 93-4. **A,** Marginal mandibular palsy and facial asymmetry after radical resection of osteogenic sarcoma of the mandible and reconstruction with fibula osteocutaneous free flap. **B,** Operative plan included deepithelialized lateral thigh free flap to restore facial contour and resection of denervated orbicularis oris and advancement of the functioning muscle to the commissure to improve appearance, speech, and oral continence. **C,** Postoperative result.

sure and upper lip activation. It is this lack of commissure and upper lip activation that is the most obvious deformity in facial paralysis. It is precisely this problem that muscle transplantation addresses most effectively.

OPERATIONS

Dynamic oral procedures have traditionally consisted of transferring segments of the muscles of mastication by the trigeminal nerve to replace lost activity of the levator, zygomaticus, and risorius muscles (lip elevators). The masseter and temporalis muscles have been the most commonly used and they can provide some motion and improve facial and oral commissure symmetry. A strip of temporalis muscle and fascia may be used if the contralateral pattern of lip elevation is more superiorly oblique (Figure 93-5) or the masseter may be used if the motion is more horizontal. Rubin advocates the use of both muscles to better control the vector of commissure movement as well as its length of excursion.[12] Similarly, the anterior belly of the digastric muscle has been used to augment lip depression and eversion of the lower lip (Figure 93-6). This type of reconstruction produces immediate results because it does not depend on a nerve graft or reinnervation; however, the transfer of regional muscles of mastication does not produce a natural spontaneous smile, and abnormal movements of the lip and cheek can occur

during chewing. Postoperative training techniques to maximize muscle control may be difficult and tedious. These operations therefore are best suited to the older patient who can better tolerate the lack of spontaneous facial movement and who desires more immediate postoperative facial effect.

Currently, the development and refinement of microsurgical techniques have made it possible to transfer distant muscle segments for facial reanimation. Although the success in recreating eyelid motion has been limited, several procedures have been developed that reliably reproduce both dynamic and spontaneous elevation of the upper lip and commissure (smile reconstruction). Tamai et al[15] initially described the procedure in a dog model and later Harii et al[4,5] adapted it to facial paralysis. Since then the procedure has evolved to include modification of the size of the muscle, the technique of insertion, and its method of innervation.[3,10] Although Harii initially used the gracilis muscle, numerous other muscles (e.g., serratus, pectoralis minor, latissimus dorsi, extensor hallucis brevis, extensor carpi radialis brevis) have been tried for smile reanimation.[6,7,9,16,17] The fundamental concept, however, remains the same. A muscle from a distant location is transplanted to the face where it is positioned, revascularized to regional vessels, and reinnervated.

The reinnervation process of a free muscle transplant differentiates the types of operations within this technique. The use of the facial nerve is central to the success of the procedure. If a viable ipsilateral facial nerve segment is available, this nerve segment can be directly anastomosed to a new muscle transplant. If no ipsilateral nerve segment is available, a cross-facial

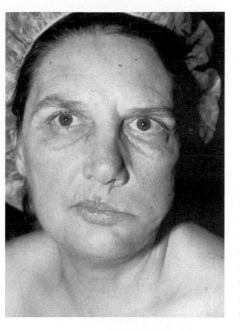

A

Figure 93-5. **A,** Patient with unilateral facial palsy after acoustic neuroma. **B,** Diagram of temporalis muscle fascia transfer. The temporalis muscle is dissected free of the temporal bone and transposed over the zygoma. Strips of the fascia are dissected off from proximal to distal but left attached to the muscle at its distal end. These strips are inset into the atrophic muscles of upper and lower lips. Clenching the teeth, the normal action of the temporalis muscle, pulls on these inset fascial strips, raising the commissure. Significant training is necessary for the patient to create a reasonable smile. **C** and **D,** Preoperative and postoperative (animated) view of patient treated by temporalis transfer to orbicularis oris and orbicularis oculi.

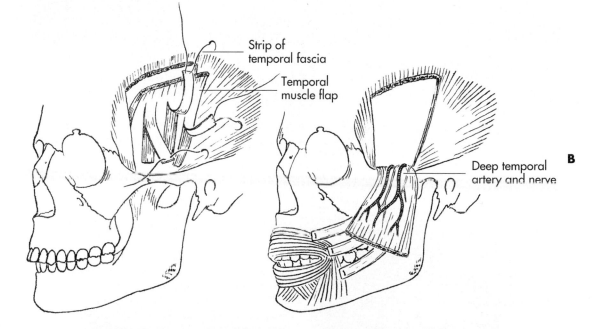

Strip of
temporal fascia

Temporal
muscle flap

Deep temporal
artery and nerve

B

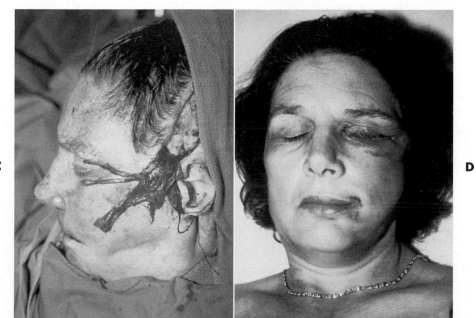

C

D

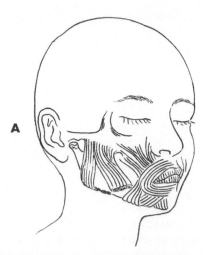
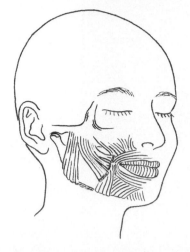

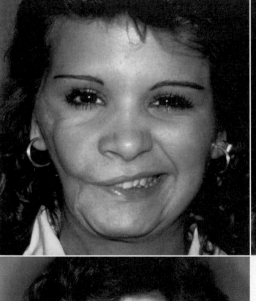

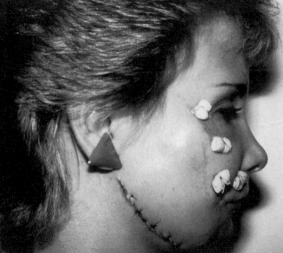

Figure 93-6. A, Diagram of masseter transfer. A portion of, or all of, the masseter muscle is detached from its insertion on the angle of the mandible reflected medially and inset into the orbicularis and adjacent tissues above and below the commissure. **B,** Patient with lower facial palsy secondary to penetrating facial wound in animated expression. **C,** Masseter reflected after exposure through cervical incision. **D,** Animated expression after transfer.

nerve graft can be initially done by sacrificing selective segments of the contralateral normal facial nerve to bring in spontaneous activity to remaining distal nerve trunks or to a muscle transplant that is placed at a second stage. Terzis[16a] has recently introduced the baby-sitter principle wherein muscle tone in the denervated facial muscles is preserved by anastomosis to a branch of the hypoglossal or accessory nerve until axonal regeneration in a cross-nerve graft allows facial-to-facial nerve anastomosis. The idea of bringing across facial nerve function from the normal side, where none is available on the paralyzed side, was initially described in 1971 by Scaramella[13] and Smith.[14] This concept was then expanded and initially used for direct

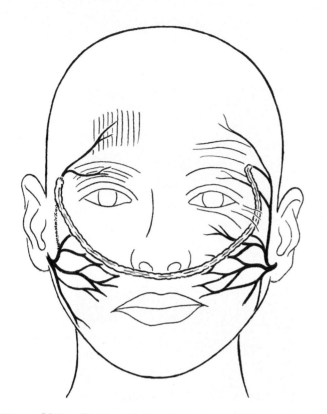

Figure 93-7. Diagram of cross-facial nerve graft from temporal branch to temporal branch for elevation of brow after injury to the temporal branch. Spontaneous symmetrical movement is best achieved when corresponding nerve branches are connected.

neural coaptation[1] (Figure 93-7). Later the concept of cross-facial nerve grafting was combined with free muscle transplantation, and the now commonly used two-stage facial reanimation was described.[11,19,21] In rare cases where no facial nerve is available bilaterally, a different regional motor nerve (segments of the 5th, 11th, or 12th cranial nerves) must be used. Free muscle activation can be successfully achieved, but spontaneity with emotional expression is impossible without facial nerve input.

SURGICAL TECHNIQUE

Our preferred method for facial reanimation involves a functioning muscle transplant using a segment of the gracilis muscle.[8] The innervation will vary according to the situation.[20] If the ipsilateral nerve is not available, the contralateral facial nerve should be used and a cross-facial nerve graft performed as a first stage. With the patient under general anesthesia without neuromuscular relaxation, the contralateral facial nerve is approached through a preauricular incision. In the subcutaneous plane, the buccal branches of the facial nerve are identified at the anterior edge of the parotid fascia. Under nerve stimulation, an accurate mapping of the function of these nerve branches is obtained and those that innervate the zygomaticus major and minor are selected (see Figure 93-2).

Branches with duplicate function are divided and thus distal muscle function is unaffected. After the nerve branches

have been identified, a subcutaneous tunnel is made to the contralateral face with the aid of incisions in the nasal vestibule (passing across the upper lip). On the paralyzed side, the dissection is carried high onto the zygoma, so the nerve graft will ultimately be out of the way of the second-stage muscle transplant. After the tunnel has been made, a red rubber catheter is placed to assist the passage of the nerve graft. The nerve graft is harvested from the leg (sural nerve) through either a longitudinal incision, small horizontal step ladder incisions, or endoscopically, dependent on surgeon preference and experience. Regardless of technique, the key is to avoid traction on the nerve to maximize its capability of functional regeneration. Typically, 25 to 30 cm of sural nerve length is needed for a tensionfree cross-facial graft. The deficit in sural nerve harvest consists only of a small area of numbness on the lateral foot, which is well tolerated by the patient. The graft is then passed through the red rubber catheter with the aid of a wire and the catheter removed, leaving the nerve in place. It is usually preferable to reverse the nerve graft in order to speed axonal crossing as much as possible. The nerve is then tacked with a colored permanent suture in the preauricular area on the paralyzed side (to find it during the second stage), and a microneural fascicular repair to the previously identified branches of the facial nerve is done under high magnification (Figure 93-8, *A*). It will take approximately 1 year for a sufficient number of axons to cross to the end of the nerve graft on the paralyzed side. This can be followed clinically by tapping the skin over the nerve anastomoses on the normal side and locating the distal response (Tinel's sign).

The second-stage muscle transplant is more complex. Immediate preoperative markings of the vector are made, and magnitude of commissure movement with smiling on the normal side is marked out. In addition, the position of the nasolabial crease on the normal side is transferred to the paralyzed side and will serve to aid in the placement of the anchoring sutures during muscle placement. Only through careful preoperative evaluation with these markings can the best position of the muscle transplant be determined.

On the paralyzed side, a preauricular incision with a submandibular extension is made. The cheek flap is elevated to the oral commissure. The pocket is dissected sufficiently high up to the zygoma and into the temporal region so that appropriate positioning of the muscle is possible. In the lower portion of the dissection, the recipient facial vessels for the muscle transplant are located. The vessels are distally ligated and prepared for microvascular repair. The distal end of the sural nerve graft is found and protected during this dissection. In order to provide additional space for the muscle and avoid excessive fullness to the face, the buccal fat pad is also removed.

Accurate anchorage of the muscle to the lower lip, commissure, and upper lip is extremely important. These anchoring sutures must not be placed too deep to avoid lip inversion nor too superficial to avoid dimpling and lip eversion. Proper placement is on the deep surface of the residual orbicularis muscle if present. Generally, one suture is placed in the lower lip, one suture in the modiolus, and two or

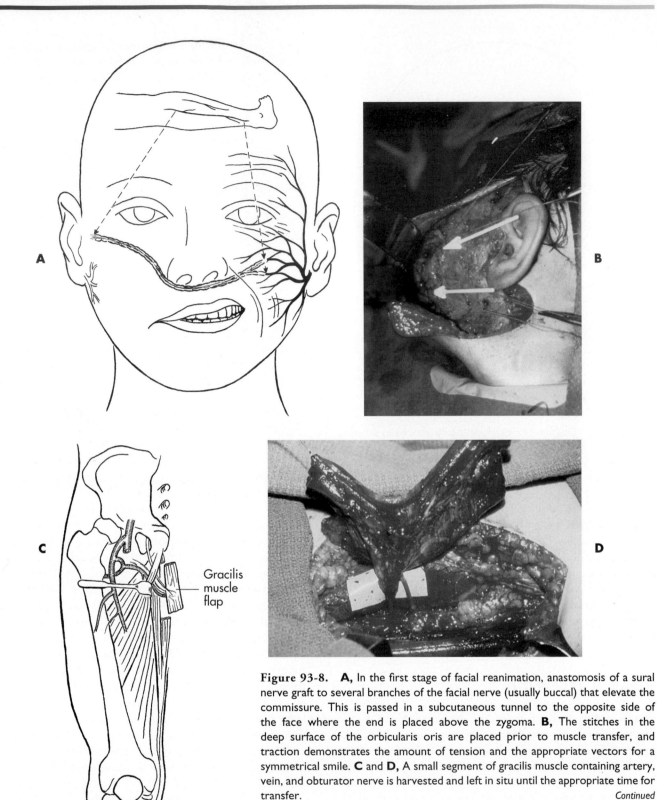

Gracilis
muscle
flap

Figure 93-8. A, In the first stage of facial reanimation, anastomosis of a sural nerve graft to several branches of the facial nerve (usually buccal) that elevate the commissure. This is passed in a subcutaneous tunnel to the opposite side of the face where the end is placed above the zygoma. **B,** The stitches in the deep surface of the orbicularis oris are placed prior to muscle transfer, and traction demonstrates the amount of tension and the appropriate vectors for a symmetrical smile. **C** and **D,** A small segment of gracilis muscle containing artery, vein, and obturator nerve is harvested and left in situ until the appropriate time for transfer. *Continued*

more sutures in the upper lip. After the sutures are placed, the face is ready to receive the muscle (Figure 93-8, *B*).

Dissection of the donor muscle is usually done by a second team concurrently with the facial dissection. Currently, we prefer the use of the gracilis muscle due to its relative constant anatomy, ease of dissection, the lack of functional or contour

deficits from its sacrifice, and the less obvious scar in the medial upper thigh. One disadvantage is the lack of fascial elements for anchorage, which many other muscles have. The gracilis muscle is located superficially just posterior to the adductor longus and is easy to locate with the knee extended and hip flexed with palpation of the origin of the adductor tendon in

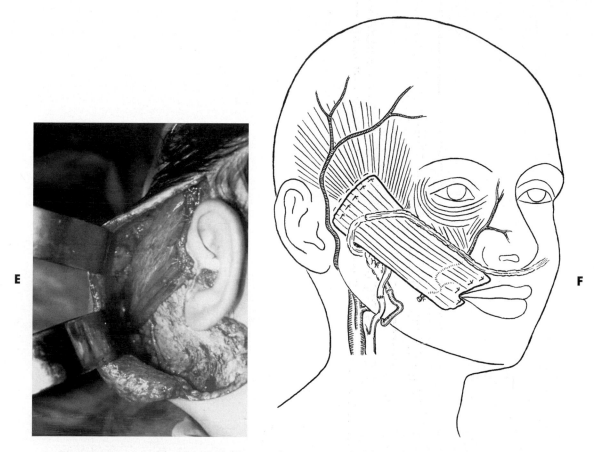

Figure 93-8, cont'd. E and **F,** The muscle is sewn under the appropriate tension to the lip and temporozygomatic fascia, and microvascular anastomosis to the facial vessels in the upper neck reestablishes blood flow. Coaptation of the sural nerve graft and the obturator nerve is performed by microscopic control. Prior to initiating the harvest of the muscle, the presence of viable axons at the distal end of the sural nerve graft is confirmed by frozen section analysis of a small biopsy.

the groin. The gracilis pedicle is located about 10 cm distal to the groin and enters the muscle perpendicularly from the profunda vessels with one artery, two venae comitantes, and a pedicle length of 6 to 8 cm. The motor nerve to the gracilis is a branch of the obturator nerve and enters the muscle at a 45-degree angle from the pedicle and is easily traced proximally with a length of 12 to 14 cm. The length of muscle needed is measured on the face from the modiolus to the tragus and is transferred to the leg with the gracilis muscle on stretch with the knee extended and centered around the pedicle. Typically, the muscle length needed is 9 to 10 cm; however, additional muscle is required for suturing at each end, and an additional 1 cm length of muscle at each end is added to the previous measurement before harvesting. The entire width of the muscle is often not needed and the anterior half may be taken, leaving the posterior portion intact. Prior to harvesting this muscle, however, the obturator nerve is stimulated electrically to ensure that the chosen area is appropriately innervated (Figure 93-8, *C* and *D*). The gracilis muscle is then divided, remaining attached only by its neurovascular pedicle. To aid suturing into the face, mattress sutures are placed in the muscle ends in which the facial anchoring sutures will be passed. The pedicle is then

sectioned as close to the profunda as possible and the muscle transplanted to the face (Figure 93-8, *E*). The oral commissure anchoring sutures are placed through one end of the muscle (with the pedicle exiting inferiorly) and the proximal portion sutured into the zygomatic arch, temporal and preauricular regions simulating the direction of the zygomatic major muscle pull on the normal side. With the muscle fixed into position, it is revascularized with end-to-end anastomoses to the facial artery and vein. Lastly, the motor nerve is repaired under high magnification, with the anastomosis carried out on the superficial portion of the muscle at its proximal end (Figure 93-8, *F*).

This operation differs significantly if the facial paralysis is bilateral. In either congenital bilateral facial paralysis (e.g., Möbius' syndrome) or acquired bilateral facial paralysis (e.g., bilateral acoustic neuromas), no facial nerve input is available and spontaneous movement with facial expression is not possible. However, a significant degree of facial animation can still be achieved with muscle transplantation. The muscle is innervated by another regional motor nerve such as a segment of the nerve to the masseter muscle (V), a fascicle of the hypoglossal nerve (XII), or a fascicle of the accessory nerve (XI). Our preference is one to two fascicles of

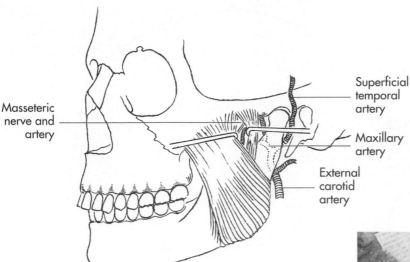

A

Masseteric nerve and artery

Superficial temporal artery

Maxillary artery

External carotid artery

Figure 93-9. **A,** Several terminal branches of the trigeminal nerve enter the masseter muscle from the deep surface at the upper aspect of the muscle. **B,** When the nerve is used to power a gracilis transfer it is isolated by splitting the muscle and carefully dissecting it from the deep surface.

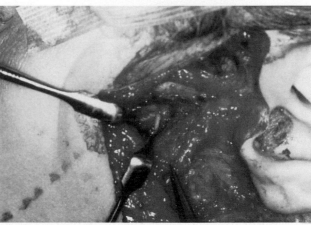

B

the masseteric nerve, which can be found by dissecting through the sigmoid notch of the mandible and locating them on the under surface of the muscle (Figure 93-9). This is in very close proximity to the muscle transplant and within easy reach of its obturator nerve branches. As no cross-facial nerve is needed in bilateral facial paralysis, only a single-stage muscle transfer reconstruction is needed per side. We prefer to only do one side at a time, and thus it still takes two stages to complete bilateral facial paralysis repair. However, the two stages can be fairly close together, and it is often possible to complete both stages in less than 1 year.

Postoperative management after this procedure is similar to that of any other free tissue transfer. Emphasis is placed on avoiding any external pressure at the sites of nerve and vessel repairs. A commissure stabilization device,[2] either preoperatively fabricated from dental models and stabilized intraorally (Figure 93-10, *A*) or fashioned intraoperatively as a hook sutured to the temporal scalp (Figure 93-10, *B*), is used to protect the muscle insertion at the commissure from postoperative pull from the opposite normal commissure. This should be used for up to 3 weeks after surgery. After the muscle begins activation, which generally starts 10 to 12 weeks postoperatively as axonal crossing from the graft completes ingrowth into the muscle, an exercise program is initiated. This is directed toward increasing the range of motion and improving symmetry during smiling. In some cases, the use of

Figure 93-10. **A,** Intraoral prosthesis with flange designed to prevent excessive traction on the commissure after reconstruction. **B,** Prosthesis for commissure maintenance suspended from head gear.

A   **B**   **C**

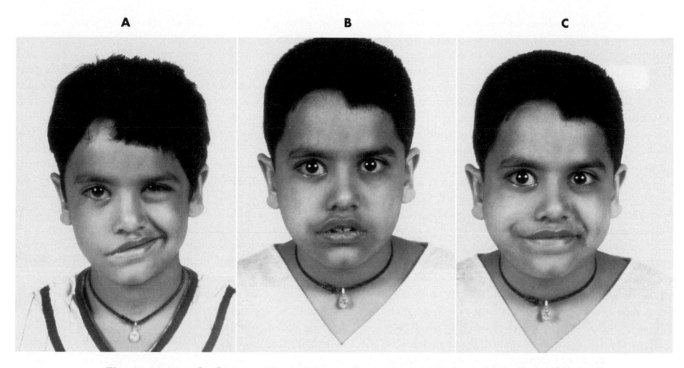

Figure 93-11. A, Patient with complete unilateral congenital facial palsy demonstrating characteristic features. (See Figure 93-1 legend.) **B** and **C,** One year after completion of facial reanimation with cross-face nerve graft and gracilis muscle transfer. At rest **(B)** and with animated smile **(C)**.

biofeedback techniques with the aid of an occupational therapist may be helpful.

SECONDARY PROCEDURES

Secondary procedures needed with free muscle transplantation for facial reanimation are very few. If the direction of muscle pull is improper, or the amount of excursion inadequate, it is extremely difficult to reposition the muscle secondarily. Similarly, excess facial fullness cannot be effectively reduced secondarily without significant risk of muscle injury. Therefore it is far better to properly position the muscle and remove excess fatty tissue during the initial procedure.

If the muscle does not function after an interval appropriate for reinnervation (6 months or less), a major vascular or neural problem has occurred. It is difficult to determine if the problem was devascularization of the muscle or an ineffective cross-facial nerve graft. Biopsy of the cross-facial nerve graft may help to determine if any activity is present and if the potential for reinnervating a muscle exists. If viable regenerating nerve tissue is present, a repeat muscle transplant can be done. If the nerve graft is not viable, a repeat nerve graft would be very difficult because the facial nerve on the normal side has already been dissected. In situations where nothing further can be done from microsurgical techniques, static slings or regional muscle transfers may be considered.

OUTCOMES

The success rate for free muscle transfer to the face exceeds 95% in healthy patients with normal vessels. Success in free muscle facial reanimation, however, only partly depends on survival of the transplant. It also requires reinnervation and a level of postoperative function (muscle excursion) that approximates the smile on the normal side. Excellence in commissure symmetry at rest is usually achieved. With the use of a cross-facial nerve graft from the normal facial nerve, the spontaneity of muscle activation is potentially perfect (Figure 93-11). Function can be expected to appear between 6 to 12 weeks after surgery with flickers of motion of the transplant with contralateral smiling. Optimal muscle function with maximal excursion is usually achieved by the sixth postoperative month. The overwhelming majority of patients are satisfied with the outcome, even though perfect symmetry during motion is rarely achieved. The shortness of the muscle segment involved limits the ability to fully recreate the upper portion of the nasolabial crease. However, the lower portion of the nasolabial crease, as well as the direction and force of pull of the modiolus, should be fairly symmetrical in most cases. With muscle activation, control of lower lip continence and elevation to the point of being capable of bilabial sound production may also occur. Thus improvement in speech will be realized in some patients.

When a nerve other than the facial nerve is used, there is no spontaneity of smile and significant relearning is needed. In bilateral facial paralysis where the motor nerve to the masseter is used in a one-stage facial reanimation with a free muscle transplant per side, the amount of motion obtained is quite impressive. Initially, there was concern that the patient would have to bite down to activate his or her muscle and simulate a smile. However, actual jaw movement is not required and only a thought is enough to lead to contraction of the muscle simulating a smile (Figure 93-12). Young children who are well motivated adapt rapidly and are able to integrate this simulated smile into everyday activities.

The outcome of microneurovascular facial reanimation is also partly affected by the age of the patient. Children and adolescents are ideal for this procedure due to their consistent ability to generate good axonal crossing through nerve grafts and their cerebral capability for reeducation of nerve and muscle function. In addition, the value of a two-stage procedure (unilateral or bilateral facial paralysis) with up to 18 months to achieve the desired result is easily understandable due to their extended lifetimes and the fragile stage of their self-image and personality development. In the young and middle-aged adult, equal functional results can be achieved, but sufficient preoperative education is necessary to realize and accept the time necessary for recovery and attainment of functional results. In the elderly patient, regeneration across a graft and into a muscle segment may be delayed or not occur at all. Although a small number of older patients have had this form of facial reanimation successfully performed, very careful patient selection should be done; most of this population is better served by other regional muscle transfers or static suspension procedures.

The economic issues associated with functioning muscle transplantation may be significant. The surgical procedures are lengthy and most patients spend 4 to 5 days in the hospital with the microneurovascular transfer. In a two-stage facial reanimation procedure for unilateral paralysis, for example, the total billable costs (hospital and physician charges) typically fall between $35,000 and $40,000. Although most third-party payors eventually provide coverage for these procedures, the low number of annual procedures performed and their very low frequency of performance by most surgeons usually require extensive explanation for preoperative approval. However, the gains are enormous in terms of social interaction, self-confidence, and improved quality of life. From an employment standpoint, individuals with a newly acquired facial paralysis may experience difficulties in working with the public or in interpersonal communication fields. With improvement in their facial appearance and function, these problems may be mitigated or completely resolved. This procedure has particularly far-reaching implications to the lifelong economic viability of the child born with facial paralysis.

In conclusion, the results of functioning muscle transplantation in patients who have been treated for facial paralysis have been quite effective, although perfect symmetry with smiling is not always achieved. It is particularly rewarding in severe cases of unilateral facial paralysis and in bilateral paralysis where social interaction is so dramatically affected.

A   **B**   **C**

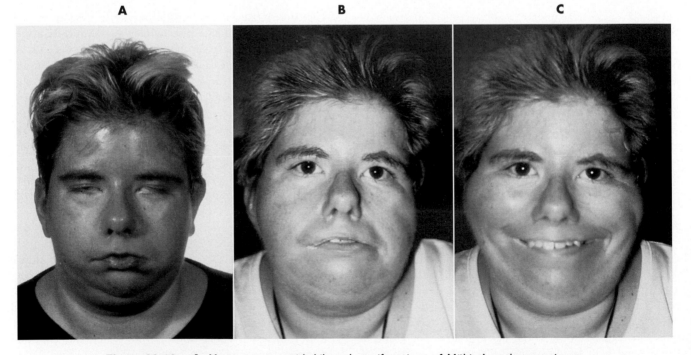

Figure 93-12. **A,** Young woman with bilateral manifestations of Möbius' syndrome prior to bilateral facial reanimation with gracilis muscle transfer powered by masseter branch of trigeminal nerve (at rest). **B** and **C,** One year after completion of facial reanimation. At rest **(B)** and with animated smile **(C).**

The technical demands of the operation and the chance for error at so many dependent parts of the procedures mandate that there be a thorough knowledge of the surgery by an experienced team prior to its undertaking.

REFERENCES

1. Anderl H: Reconstruction of the face through cross-face nerve transplantation in facial paralyses, *Chirurgie Plastica (Berlin)* 2:17-46, 1943.

2. Eppley BL, Hennon D, Sadove AM, et al: A commissure stabilization device for facial reanimation surgery, *Plast Reconstr Surg* 89:1152-1154, 1992.

3. Harii K: Refined microneurovascular free muscle transplantation for reanimation of the paralyzed face, *Microsurgery* 9:169-176, 1988.

4. Harii K: Microneurovascular free muscle transplantation for reanimation of facial paralysis, *Clin Plast Surg* 6:361-375, 1979.

5. Harii K, Ohmori K, Torii S: Free gracilis muscle transplantation with microneurovascular anastomosis for the treatment of facial paralysis, *Plast Reconstr Surg* 57:133-143, 1976.

6. Hata Y, Yano K, Matsuba K, et al: Treatment of chronic facial palsy by transplantation of the neurovascularized free rectus abdominis muscle, *Plast Reconstr Surg* 86:1178-1187, 1990.

7. Mackinnon SE, Dellon L: Technical considerations of the latissimus dorsi flap: a segmentally innervated muscle for facial reanimation, *Microsurgery* 9:36-45, 1988.

8. Manktelow RT, Zuker RM: Muscle transplantation by fascicular territory, *Plast Reconstr Surg* 73:751-755, 1984.

9. Mayou BJ, Watson JS, Harrison DH, et al: Free microvascular and microneural transfer of the extensor digitorum brevis muscle for the treatment of unilateral facial palsy, *Br J Plast Surg* 71:510-518, 1983.

10. O'Brien B, Franklin JD, Morrison WA: Cross-facial nerve grafts and microneurovascular free muscle transfer for long established facial palsy, *Br J Plast Surg* 33:202-215, 1980.

11. O'Brien B, Pederson WC, Khazanchi RK, et al: Results of management of facial palsy with microneurovascular free muscle transfer, *Plast Reconstr Surg* 86:12-24, 1990.

12. Rubin LR: The anatomy of a smile—its importance in facial paralysis, *Plast Reconstr Surg* 53:384-392, 1974.

13. Scaramella L: L'anastomiosi tra I due nerve faciali, *Arch Otolaryngol* 82:209-215, 1971.

14. Smith JW: A technique of facial animation. In Hueston JH, editor: *Transactions of the Fifth International Congress of Plastic and Reconstructive Surgery,* Chatswood, New South Wales, Australia, 1971, Londong, Butterworth, p 83.

15. Tamai S, Komatsu S, Sakamoto H, et al: Free muscle transplants in dogs with microsurgical neurovascular anastomosis, *Plast Reconstr Surg* 46:219-225, 1970.

16. Terzis JK: Pectoralis minor: a unique muscle for correction of facial palsy, *Plast Reconstr Surg* 83:767-776, 1989.

16a. Terzis JK: Babysitters: an exciting new concept in facial animation. In *Proceedings of the VIth International Symposium on the Facial Nerve,* Amsterdam, 1990, Kuslen and Ghedindi, p 525.

17. Terzis JK, Manktelow RT: Pectoralis minor: a new concept in facial reanimation, *Plast Surg Forum* 5:106-110, 1982.

18. Wells MD, Manktelow RT: Surgical management of facial palsy, *Clin Plast Surg* 17:645-653, 1990.

19. Zuker RM: Microvascular management of facial palsy. In Marsh JL, editor: *Current therapy in plastic and reconstructive surgery,* Toronto, 1989, Decker, pp 157-162.

20. Zuker RM, Manktelow RT: Functional and aesthetic muscle transplants, *Adv Plast Reconstr Surg* 9:37-66, 1993.

21. Zuker RM, Manktelow RT: Facial paralysis in children, *Clin Plast Surg* 17:95-103, 1990.

Index

A

S